Volume 1

Pediatric

Orthopedics

SECOND EDITION

Volume 1

Pediatric Orthopedics

SECOND EDITION

MIHRAN O. TACHDJIAN, M.S., M.D.

Professor of Orthopedic Surgery,
Northwestern University Medical School
Attending Orthopedic Surgeon and Former Head
Division of Orthopedics
Children's Memorial Hospital
Chicago, Illinois

1990
W.B. SAUNDERS COMPANY
Harcourt Brace Jovanovich, Inc.
Philadelphia ■ London ■ Toronto ■ Montreal ■ Sydney ■ Tokyo

W. B. SAUNDERS COMPANY
Harcourt Brace Jovanovich, Inc.

Independence Square West
Philadelphia, PA 19106

Library of Congress Cataloging-in-Publication Data

Tachdjian, Mihran O.

Pediatric orthopedics.

Includes bibliographies and index.

1. Pediatric orthopedia.   I. Title. [DNLM: 1. Orthopedics—in
  infancy & childhood. WS 270 T117p]

RD732.3.C48T33 1990   617'.3   87–13006

ISBN 0–7216–8726–1 (set)

Listed here is the latest translated edition of this book together with the language of the translation and the publisher.

Spanish (*1st Edition*)–Nueva Editorial Interamericana S.A. de C.V., Mexico 4 D.F., Mexico

Editor: Edward H. Wickland, Jr.
Developmental Editor: Kathleen McCullough
Designer: Bill Donnelly
Production Manager: Bill Preston
Manuscript Editors: Ruth Barker, Constance Burton, Tina Rebane
Mechanical Artist: Karen Giacomucci
Illustration Coordinator: Peg Shaw
Indexer: Julie Schwager

Pediatric Orthopedics

Volume 1 ISBN   0–7216–8722–9
Volume 2 ISBN   0–7216–8723–7
Volume 3 ISBN   0–7216–8724–5
Volume 4 ISBN   0–7216–8727–X
Complete Set ISBN   0–7216–8726–1

Last digit is the print number: 9   8   7   6   5   4   3   2

Dedicated With Love to
My Wife
Vivian B. Tachdjian

Preface

During the past 18 years, great strides have been made in pediatric orthopedics. A new edition of this book is long overdue. The gestation period of such an *Arbeit* has been prolonged because of the tremendous amount of labor involved in writing a single-author book. The objectives and format of the textbook have not changed from the first edition. I have attempted to present a thorough and comprehensive treatise on the affections of the neuromusculoskeletal system in children.

I have expressed my preferred methods of treatment and surgical procedure based upon my personal experience and the privilege of association with the leaders in pediatric orthopedics throughout the world who have participated in the faculty of the Pediatric Orthopedic International Seminars, which I have directed annually since 1972. The names of the faculty appear in the acknowledgments in the following pages.

The illustrations and operative plates are all original; the majority represent the superb artistry of Mr. Ernest Beck, to whom I am greatly indebted. I also wish to acknowledge Miss Patricia Piescinski for her beautiful drawings.

I wish to thank the entire staff of the W.B. Saunders Company, particularly Miss Ruth Barker, Mr. Albert Meier, Mrs. Kathleen McCullough, and Mr. Edward H. Wickland, Jr.

I would also like to express my gratitude to Mrs. Mikie Boroughf, who assisted in the preparation of this book.

A question frequently posed to me over the years has been, "How do you write such an extensive book?" Every word has been handwritten in my illegible handwriting, readable only by Mrs. Lynn Ridings, without whose assistance and editorial support this work would not have been possible.

MIHRAN O. TACHDJIAN, M.D.

Acknowledgments

I would like to give special thanks to the following people for their help in writing certain sections of this book: Ellen Chadwick, M.D., and Stanford Shulman, M.D.—infectious diseases; Ramiro Hernandez, M.D.—CT scan of the hip; James Donaldson, M.D.—ultrasonography in congenital dislocation of the hip; Andrew Poznanski, M.D.—assistance in imaging findings in various skeletal disorders, especially bone dysplasias; Steven Hall, M.D.—orthopedic aspects of pediatric anesthesia; David McLone, M.D., and Thomas Naidich, M.D.—neurosurgical aspects of myelomeningocele and spinal dysraphism; Dror Paley, M.D.—Ilizarov limb lengthening; George Simons, M.D.—complications of talipes equinovarus; David H. Sutherland, M.D.—gait; and Mary Weck, R.P.T.—physical therapy for cerebral palsy.

I also wish to express my gratitude to the members of the faculty of the Pediatric Orthopedic International Seminars over the past 18 years.

Robert Abrams, M.D.
James Aronson, M.D.
Marc Asher, M.D.
R. Kirklin Ashley, M.D.
Henry H. Banks, M.D.
Riad Barmada, M.D.
Melvin H. Becker, M.D.
Henri Bensahel, M.D.
Anthony Bianco, M.D.
Eugene E. Bleck, M.D.
Prof. Alexander Bliskunov
Walter P. Blount, M.D.
J. Richard Bowen, M.D.
David W. Boyer, M.D.
Robert Bright, M.D.
Prof. Dieter Buck-Gramcko
Wilton H. Bunch, M.D.
Aloysio Campos da Paz, Jr., M.D.
S. Terry Canale, M.D.
Henri Carlioz, M.D.
Nils Carstam, M.D.
Prof. Robert Cattaneo

Mr. Anthony Catterall, F.R.C.S.
Prof. Paul L. Chigot
Eldon G. Chuinard, M.D.
Robert G. Chuinard, M.D.
Stanley M.K. Chung, M.D.
Sherman S. Coleman, M.D.
Mr. Christopher L. Colton, F.R.C.S.
Clinton L. Compere, M.D.
James J. Conway, M.D.
Henry R. Cowell, M.D.
Alvin H. Crawford, M.D.
Burr H. Curtis, M.D.
Prof. George Dall, F.R.C.S.
Prof. G. DeBastiani
Prof. Julio dePablos
Luciano Dias, M.D.
Harold M. Dick, M.D.
Alain Dimeglio, M.D.
James Donaldson, M.D.
John Dorst, M.D.
James Drennan, M.D.
Denis S. Drummond, M.D.

Prof. Jean Dubousset
Mr. Denis M. Dunn, F.R.C.S.
Peter M. Dunn, M.D.
Robert E. Eilert, M.D.
Richard E. Eppright, M.D.
John J. Fahey, M.D.
Albert B. Ferguson, Jr., M.D.
J. William Fielding, M.D.
Mr. John Fixsen, F.R.C.S.
Victor Frankel, M.D.
Nicholas Giannestras, M.D.
Prof. Alain Gilbert
J. Leonard Goldner, M.D.
Neil E. Green, M.D.
William T. Green, M.D.
Paul P. Griffin, M.D.
Donald Gunn, M.D.
John E. Hall, M.D.
Judith G. Hall, M.D.
John E. Handelsman, M.D.
Robert Hensinger, M.D.
Ramiro Hernandez, M.D.
Charles Herndon, M.D.
John A. Herring, M.D.
M. Mark Hoffer, M.D.
Walter A. Hoyt, Jr., M.D.
Mr. J. Rowland Hughes, F.R.C.S.
Prof. Sean P. F. Hughes
Prof. Gabriel Abramovich Ilizarov
Roshen Irani, M.D.
Francois Iselin, M.D.
Preston James, M.D.
Prof. Lutz F.H. Jani
Ali Kalamchi, M.D.
William J. Kane, M.D.
Buni'chiro Kawamura, M.D.
Theodore E. Keats, M.D.
Armen S. Kelikian, M.D.
Hampar Kelikian, M.D.
Mr. J.A. Kenwright, F.R.C.S.
Ara Y. Ketenjian, M.D.
Eugene Kilgore, M.D.
Richard E. King, M.D.
Prof. Predrag Klisiç
Steven Kopits, M.D.
Warren G. Kramer, M.D.
Mr. Douglas Lamb, F.R.C.S.
Prof. Anders F. Langenskiöld
Loren Larsen, M.D.
Franco Lavini, M.D.
Richard E. Lindseth, M.D.
Mr. George Lloyd-Roberts, F.R.C.S.
John E. Lonstein, M.D.
Wood Lovell, M.D.
G. Dean MacEwen, M.D.
John B. McGinty, M.D.
Douglas W. McKay, M.D.
Mr. Brian McKibbin, F.R.C.S.
David McLone, M.D.
John E. Madewell, M.D.
Roger A. Mann, M.D.
Prof. P.G. Marchetti
Prof. S. Matsuno

Peter L. Meehan, M.D.
Malcolm B. Menelaus, M.D.
Michael Michelson, M.D.
Lee W. Milford, M.D.
Edward A. Millar, M.D.
Mr. George P. Mitchell, F.R.C.S.
Prof. Giorgio Monticelli
Raymond T. Morrissy, M.D.
Colin F. Moseley, M.D.
Alf S. Nachemson, M.D.
Ann Nachemson, M.D.
John J. Niebauer, M.D.
John A. Ogden, M.D.
Michael B. Ozonoff, M.D.
Lauren M. Pachman, M.D.
Dror Paley, M.D.
Arsen Pankovich, M.D.
Arthur M. Pappas, M.D.
Klausdieter Parsch, M.D.
Sir Dennis Paterson
Hamlet A. Peterson, M.D.
Guillermo de Velasco Polo, M.D.
Ignacio V. Ponseti, M.D.
Melvin Post, M.D.
Jean-Gabriel Pous, M.D.
Andrew K. Poznanski, M.D.
Charles T. Price, M.D.
Mercer Rang, M.D.
Mr. A.H.C. Ratliff, F.R.C.S.
Inge Reimann, M.D.
L. Renzi-Brivio, M.D.
B. Lawrence Riggs, M.D.
Veijo A. Ritsila, M.D.
John M. Roberts, M.D.
Charles Rockwood, M.D.
Robert B. Salter, M.D.
Robert L. Samilson, M.D.
Shahan K. Sarrafian, M.D.
Michael F. Schafer, M.D.
William L. Schey, M.D.
Keith Schroeder, M.D.
Mr. W.J.W. Sharrard, F.R.C.S.
Stanford T. Shulman, M.D.
Robert S. Siffert, M.D.
Michael A. Simon, M.D.
George W. Simons, M.D.
Clement B. Sledge, M.D.
Wayne O. Southwick, M.D.
Donald P. Speer, M.D.
Prof. Renato Spinelli
Jurgen Spranger, M.D.
Lynn T. Staheli, M.D.
Stanko Stanisavljevic, M.D.
Herbert H. Stark, M.D.
Howard Steel, M.D.
David H. Stulberg, M.D.
Y. Sugioka, M.D.
David H. Sutherland, M.D.
Alfred B. Swanson, M.D.
Prof. W. Taillard
David J. Thompson, M.D.
Georges R. Thuilleux, M.D.
Dietrich Tonnis, M.D.

Levon K. Topouzian, M.D.
Miguel Ferrer Torrelles, M.D.
Prof. Naoichi Tsuyama
Prof. Raoul Tubiana
Vincent J. Turco, M.D.
Prof. M.V. Volkov
Prof. Heinz Wagner
Prof. Isidor Wasserstein
R.S. Watanabe, M.D
Hugh G. Watts, M.D.
Prof. B.G. Weber
Stuart L. Weinstein, M.D

Prof. S. L. Weissman
Dennis R. Wenger, M.D.
G. Wilbur Westin, M.D.
Harvey White, M.D.
Mr. Peter Williams, F.R.C.S.
John C. Wilson, M.D.
Robert Winter, M.D.
Miss Ruth Wynne-Davies, F.R.C.S.
Yasuo Yamauchi, M.D.
Prof. Eduardo Zancolli
Seymour Zimbler, M.D.

Preface to the First Edition

This work was undertaken upon the invitation of its publisher and begun with interest and great personal involvement that have never faltered. Now that its manuscript is complete, I must seize the occasion of this prefatory statement to answer the reader's natural question: Why was it done?

I began with the perhaps-simplistic idea of providing a detailed technical presentation of surgical treatment of disorders of the neuromuscular and skeletal systems in children. I intended to write primarily for the orthopedic surgeon but I hoped also to interest physicians and surgeons of other specialties involved in the care of children.

I had no sooner set out on what proved a long and tortuous path than I began to appreciate that one cannot describe the techniques of surgery without considering also the biological principles of surgery, the dynamics of trauma, and the rationale for surgical intervention. That rationale is itself dependent upon knowledge of neuromuscular physiology and of the biomechanics of motion. One cannot speak of the management of disorder or of the amelioration of congenital defect without understanding disease process and the genesis of musculoskeletal anomaly. The surgeon who operates well performs not only with skill but also with reason; and that reason rests upon a diagnostic acumen fortified by physical examination, pathology, radiology and accurate classification. Similarly, the evaluation of surgery cannot be set out without attention to its possible complications and its aftercare.

On reflection, I realize the project I have undertaken is more ambitious than I had originally envisioned. And so I have written a long and complex book. Its very length and complexity must mean occasional omission and even error. I have tried to guard against them by citing for each important statement significant findings from the vast literature of pediatric orthopedics; but the opinions I have expressed concerning preferred methods of treatment and surgical procedure arise from personal experience and from the privilege of having learned and worked at fine teaching centers.

In another and perhaps more important way I have departed from original intent. I decided to omit chapters on the hand and on orthotics and prosthetics in the conviction that these highly individual subjects should be treated intensively and thoroughly in separate monographs.

I wish to express gratitude to John Dusseau, Editor of the W. B. Saunders Company, for the confidence he invested in me. Without his support, advice, and encouragement, this work would have been impossible.

I wish to express thanks also to the Trust Under Will of Helen Fay Hunter–Crippled Children's Fund, and to Mr. Carl A. Pfau and the Harris Trust and Savings Bank Trustees for their generous support.

The kind indulgence of the Board of Directors of Children's Memorial Hospital in allowing me the necessary time to complete this work is greatly appreciated. I also wish to thank certain of my professional colleagues and members of the orthopedic staff for their sincere cooperation during preparation of this manuscript.

With the exception of a few that have been reproduced from other works, the illustrations and operative plates are all original. The majority represent the superb artistry of Mr. Ernest Beck, to whom I am greatly indebted. I also wish to thank medical artists Wesley Bloom, Jean McConnell, Diane Nelson, and Laurel Schaubert. The diligent work of Miss Helen Silver and Mr. John Kelley of the Photography Department, Children's Memorial Hospital, must be particularly acknowledged.

The entire staff of W. B. Saunders Company, particularly Miss Ruth Barker and Mr. Raymond Kersey, are to be commended for their meticulous work during the preparation and production of the printed book.

Finally, I wish to thank Miss Eleanor Lynn Schreiner, who, in her role as my personal editor, has prepared and finalized the entire manuscript as it has been written during the past four years. Without her assistance and meticulous attention to clarity, this task would have been difficult, if not impossible, to achieve. For her unselfish dedication I shall always be grateful.

I shall conclude in the hope that if the reader learns as much from reading as the writer has from writing this monograph, its attendant trouble and trial will have been amply repaid in the better care of children.

MIHRAN O. TACHDJIAN

Contents

VOLUME 1

1

2

Congenital Deformities 104

VOLUME 2

3

4

VOLUME 3

5

8

Volume 1

1. Introduction

Definition and Scope of Orthopedics

Orthopedics is a branch of medicine and surgery that deals with the preservation and restoration of function of the skeletal and neuromuscular systems. Although the skeleton per se is primarily concerned with the form of the body and its motion, it may be affected by many metabolic and other systemic diseases.

The components of the neuromusculoskeletal system are closely interwoven in their function. Action in one causes a response in the other. For example, many deformities of the skeletal system arise from muscular paralysis in diseases in which the nervous system is the primary area of pathologic change, such as poliomyelitis. During the years of growth, the normal function of muscles is essential to the development of skeletal contours. Abnormalities of muscle function can disturb growth and cause deformities of the bones. Muscles, in turn, respond to diseases of the skeleton. In the instance of an inflamed joint, for example, the muscles that motivate the area respond by a reflex mechanism, a so-called involuntary muscle spasm, to prevent motion in the painful joint. The muscles antagonistic to those in muscle spasm rapidly develop atrophy. If the muscles in spasm are left in their shortened position for a long time, they develop myostatic contracture—permanent shortening of the muscle length. This is seen particularly when there is associated imbalance of muscle strength or when factors that increase fibrosis are present.

The term "orthopaedy" is derived from two Greek works, *orthos*, meaning "straight, upright, or free from deformity," and *paidos*, "a child." It was originally used by Nicholas André, in 1741, as the title of a treatise— *L'Orthopédie, ou l'art de prévenir et de corriger dans les enfants les déformités du corps.*[2] André taught orthopedics as a branch of preventive medicine rather than of surgery. In modern surgical days, one constantly needs to be reminded that "prevention is always better than cure."

Although the name *orthopedics* is barely 250 years old, the diseases of the neuromusculoskeletal system have always been among the major concerns of mankind. The early background of orthopedics is that of surgery and of medicine. All varieties of bone disease existed in prehistoric times, as evidenced by findings in thousands of skeletons unearthed from the caves of Dawn Men of Europe, Asia, and North Africa. Osteomyelitis, bone tumors, arthritis, and others are easily recognized. Fractures were common, and some of them were healed in good alignment. On a portal of Hirkouf's tomb, there is a carving, executed in 2830 B.C., showing the earliest known record of the use of a crutch. A textbook picture of what may well be the residuals of poliomyelitic paralysis is that of an Egyptian prince of the Eighteenth Dynasty with his right lower extremity atrophied and shortened, and the foot in the equinus

1

posture. Surgical operations on bones in prehistoric times are well documented, as skeletons are often well preserved.[3]

Hippocrates gave great attention to the musculoskeletal system; over 40 per cent of the *Corpus Hippocrates* is concerned with it.[7] The diagnosis and treatment of fractures and dislocations were quite well discussed. Traction, splints, and bandages were used. Clubfoot and congenital dislocation of the hip were well known.

The first hospital to specialize in musculoskeletal diseases was founded by Venel, in 1790, at Orbe, Switzerland. It was devoted primarily to the care of tuberculosis and congenital deformities. This was rapidly followed by construction of a number of such hospitals in Europe. In the United States, the first orthopedic hospital was the Good Samaritan, founded in Boston by Buckminster Brown in 1861. In the same year, Lewis Sayre became the first professor of orthopedics in the United States. Appointed to Bellevue Medical College, he organized an orthopedic dispensary at Bellevue Hospital in New York.

Initially, orthopedic surgeons were concerned with disorders of the musculoskeletal system that were of nontraumatic origin, particularly those of the child. During World War I, however, it became evident that the new techniques that they had developed were equally important for the management of disabilities and deformities resulting from trauma, and since then it has become customary to consider all affections of the skeletal and neuromuscular systems as being one field of medicine. Orthopedics has become a broad surgical and medical specialty, interlocking with general surgery, neurosurgery, plastic surgery, vascular surgery, and many aspects of general medicine and pediatrics. Pediatric orthopedics is now established as a subspecialty in orthopedics. The Pediatric Orthopedic Society was founded in 1974 and The Pediatric Orthopedic Study Group in 1975. The two were amalgamated as the Pediatric Orthopedic Society of North America (POSNA) in 1980. The European Pediatric Orthopedic Society was founded in 1981. The *Journal of Pediatric Orthopedics* has been in publication since 1980.

References

1. American Orthopedic Association: Manual of Surgery. 5th Ed., 1979.
2. André, N.: L'orthopédie ou l'art de prévenir et de corriger dans les enfants les déformités du corps. Paris, 1741; London, 1743; Philadelphia, reproduced by Lippincott, 1961.
3. Bick, E. M.: Source Book of Orthopedics. 2nd Ed. Baltimore, Williams & Wilkins, 1948.
4. Blawvel, C. F., and Nelson, F. R. T.: A Manual of Orthopedic Terminology. St. Louis, Mosby, 1977.
5. D'Ambrosia, R. D. (ed.): Musculoskeletal Disorders: Regional Examination and Differential Diagnosis. Philadelphia, Lippincott, 1977.
6. Eddy, D. M., and Clanton, C. H.: The art of diagnosis: Solving the clinicopathological exercise. N. Engl. J. Med., 306:1263, 1982.
7. Hippocrates: The Genuine Works of Hippocrates. Trans. from the Greek (with a preliminary discourse and annotations) by F. Adams. London, Sydenham Soc., 1849.

Diagnosis in Neuromusculoskeletal Disorders

THE ORTHOPEDIC HISTORY

A clinical history skillfully obtained and properly analyzed often holds the key to diagnosis. Many misdiagnoses are due to incomplete or inaccurate histories.

There are certain special problems, however, in taking the history of an infant or a child. First, the child is unable to describe precisely his own subjective symptoms and their temporal relationship. A child's recollection of past events is poor; he tends to live in the present and the future. Though one is compelled to turn to the parents for narration of a sequential history, one should not, however, neglect the child's observations entirely, as a child can often describe his symptoms in a delightfully refreshing and naïve manner, which may be of some historical value relative to his own illness. Second, cooperation is often poor. Patience, kindness, time, and a smile on the examiner's face are essential to ensure a relaxed atmosphere. The physician should conduct the examination in such a manner that it is pleasant for the child and for the anxious parents. Both father and mother should be interrogated whenever possible. One should encourage the parents to relate the problems in their own language. It is essential to convey interest, understanding, and sympathy. An impression of haste should be avoided.

While taking the history, the physician should evaluate the patient as a whole, the reactions of both the child and the parents to his disease and his handicaps, and his relationship to his parents and siblings. A friendly and courteous attitude, the centering of all attention on the patient, accurate and tactful wording of questions—all are important in developing a proper patient-parent-physician relationship.

The orthopedic history, like all clinical histories, usually begins with certain statistical data, which include the child's name, sex, date and place of birth, both father's and mother's names, and the name of the referring physician, his address, and phone number. These data are usually obtained by the nurse or secretary.

Next, the *presenting complaint* is recorded. Common complaints pertaining to the musculoskeletal system are deformity, limp, localized or generalized weakness, swelling, pain, and stiffness of joints. Since the musculoskeletal system is concerned with support and locomotion, many of the symptoms arising from it are brought about by physical stress and motion; interrogation should establish this relation of symptoms to physical activity. The chronological occurrence of the presenting complaint with its exact date and mode of onset should be determined. Questions concerning severity, disability, factors aggravating or alleviating symptoms, and previous treatment should be noted. If there is any history of injury, details of the alleged trauma should be investigated to determine its etiologic significance. Once the foregoing information has been obtained, the physician should determine the time of onset, in terms of the life history of the patient, by taking what may be called *developmental history.*

Prenatal History

During the first trimester of pregnancy, embryogenesis and organogenesis proceed at a maximal rate. Any unusual incident during this period may be of clinical significance. Was there any history of vaginal bleeding to indicate threatened abortion? Were there any infections? The deleterious effects of maternal rubella during the first months of pregnancy with consequent cataract, deafness, heart disease, mental retardation, and seizures are well established. Syphilis, toxemia, and diabetes mellitus in the mother are also associated with a high incidence of abnormalities in the newborn. Was there any herpes—simplex or genital? Is there any history of excessive radiation to the fetus or ingestion of toxic substances and medicines such as the tranquilizer thalidomide? Was there an accident in which the abdominal wall was struck, or in which there was excessive blood loss with critical lowering of the blood pressure?

Fetal movements are usually felt by the mother between the fourth and fifth months of pregnancy. A history of feebleness or absence of fetal movements may be of importance in arthrogryposis multiplex congenita or Werdnig-Hoffmann disease.

Birth History

Information should be obtained as to length of pregnancy, duration of labor, birth weight, and birth length. What was the presentation? Certain conditions, such as congenital dislocation of the hip and congenital muscular torticollis are more frequent in breech deliveries. Was onset of labor spontaneous or induced? Did the mother receive an analgesic or other medications during labor and how long before delivery? Was obstetric anesthesia general, block, or none?

The condition of the infant during the neonatal period should be determined. This is particularly important in children with brain damage and birth defects. What was the Apgar rating? What was the appearance and color of the newborn when first seen by the parents? How many minutes did it take for the infant's first breath and first cry? Was there any cyanosis? Were there any respiratory problems? Was the infant resuscitated? Was there any jaundice, and if present, when was it first noted and when did it disappear? Was any exchange transfusion given? Were there any neonatal convulsions? Was the muscle tone normal, flaccid, or rigid? Was there any opisthotonus? Was the child in an incubator? Did he receive oxygen? Was sucking or feeding normal, feeble, or absent? Did he have to be tube-fed? What was the nature of the cry? Was there any asymmetry of the face or the limbs? When was the infant discharged from the hospital? Did he go home with his mother? Were there any injuries or evidence of trauma? Were there any obvious deformities of the limbs?

Next, milestones of development for posture, locomotion, manipulation, activities of daily living, social development, and speech are determined. When did the infant lift his head, roll, crawl, sit, stand, pull himself to standing position, walk, run, ascend or descend stairs, and hop on one foot without support?

The examiner should habitually inquire about details of development of function of the upper limb. When did the infant hold a bottle, reach for and grasp a toy, transfer objects from hand to hand? When did he offer his arm for coat or foot for socks, feed himself with spoon or fork, pull off or put on clothes? Ambidexterity, i.e., lack of hand preference, is normal during the first two years of life. When an infant demonstrates an unequivocal hand preference before this time some defect in the use of the other hand should be suspected; this may be the first sign of spastic hemiplegia. Exploration of environment by touch and the development of manual skills emerge in an orderly and sequential manner.

Equally important as evidence of the functional adequacy of the neuromusculoskeletal system is the general responsiveness of the infant to parents and objects in the environment. At two months of age an infant smiles when spoken to and vocalizes; at four months he turns his head to sound and recognizes his mother; at eight months he responds to "no"; at ten months he waves bye-bye, plays pat-a-cake, and says da-da and ma-ma. The sounds *a*, *ba*, *da-da*, and *ma-ma* represent the earliest phase of development of the articulatory process and of communication; they are, however, without specific word meaning at this stage.

An interest in picture books and recognition of familiar objects begin at the age of 12 months; the child achieves a vocabulary of four to five words at 15 months, and three-word sentences at 24 months. Inquiry should be made as to age of toilet training (stool and urine). Levels of motor development are presented in Table 1–9 in the appendix to this chapter. Information should be obtained as to whether the child attends school (regular or special) and about his scholastic performance.

A systemic review is carried out next. Is there any unusual bruising or easy bleeding? Is the child subject to hives or eczema; has he any allergies? Past or present medications? Drug reactions? Adverse reaction to anesthesia? Malignant hyperthermia? Previous illnesses and hospitalizations? A family history completes the orthopedic anamnesis.

THE ORTHOPEDIC EXAMINATION

Orthopedic diagnosis requires not only an evaluation of the neuromusculoskeletal system, but also a complete general physical examination.

The orthopedic examination usually follows a definite order unless the symptoms or status of the patient indicate deviation from it. It is imperative to pay scrupulous attention to minute details. The patient is stripped of all clothing and draped to expose the body in use. Standing and sitting heights are measured, and in appropriate cases, e.g., hydrocephalus, the head circumference is measured. In bone dysplasias the upper limb span and the upper and lower limbs

are measured. Normal body measurements are shown in Tables 1–1 and 1–2 in the Appendix to Chapter 1.

Next, if the child has any appliances such as night splints or orthoses, they are examined. Is there any abnormal shoe wear?

Stance and Posture

The first step is inspection of the body as a whole and as a mechanical unit in action. If the child is ambulatory, he is asked to stand, and his natural standing posture and body outlines are observed from the back, front, and side. Are there any obvious defects of the spine or deformities of the limbs? Is there exaggeration or diminution of the normal physiologic anteroposterior curves of the dorsal and lumbar spine? What is the pelvic inclination? Are the shoulders carried behind the pelvis in the lateral view? What is the position of the head, scapulae, shoulders, gluteal and popliteal creases? Are the shoulders balanced over the pelvis? Is there deviation of the trunk to one side? (A plumb line held over the center of the occiput or over the spinous process of the seventh cervical vertebra should pass through the intergluteal cleft.) Are the iliac crests level? Is a lift under one foot required to level the iliac crests and balance the head and shoulders over the pelvis? Is there any scoliosis? Is one hip more prominent than the other? How is the symmetry of the flank creases? If scoliosis is present, the degree and direction of rotation of the involved vertebrae can best be demonstrated by asking the child to bend forward for inspection of his spine from the back. In a structural curve, rotation of the vertebral body is to the convexity of lateral angulation; in a functional curve, it is to the concave side. Is there muscle spasm of the paravertebral muscles? Is there limitation of motion of the vertebral column on forward flexion, extension, lateral bending, and rotation? A Trendelenburg test is performed by asking the patient to stand first on one leg with both hips in extension and the non-weight-bearing knee bent and then to stand on the other leg. Normally, when a person stands on one leg, the contralateral side of the pelvis is elevated with the contraction of the strong ipsilateral hip abductor muscles. When the opposite side of the pelvis drops (a positive Trendelenburg sign) it indicates weakness of the hip abductor muscles (Fig. 1–1).

The general alignment of the lower limbs is also evaluated. Is the child bow-legged or knock-kneed? Is there any pes varus or pes

Opposite side of pelvis stays elevated:

same level as that of tested side

Normal hip abductors

Opposite side of pelvis drops

Weak hip abductors

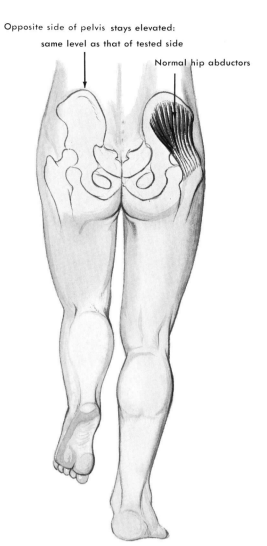 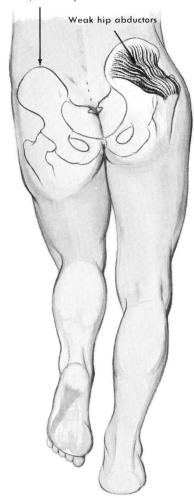

Trendelenburg sign negative

Trendelenburg sign positive

FIGURE 1–1. Trendelenburg test.

(Adapted from von Lanz, T., and Wachsmuth, W.: Praktische Anatomie. Berlin, Julius Springer, 1938, p. 167.)

valgus? Are the longitudinal arches normal, high, or flattened? What is the line of weight-bearing in the lower limbs? Normally, the center of gravity of the body passes from the anterior superior iliac spine to the middle of the patella and the proximal tibial tubercle and falls on the center of the foot, which is between the first and second metatarsals.

If general and local conditions permit, the child is asked to do a deep knee bend, return, and then, standing on one leg, rise to his tiptoes. Next he is asked to walk to demonstrate his gait.

Gait

The primary objective of human locomotion is translation of the body from one place to another by means of bipedal gait. The act of walking is a dynamic and repetitive performance; it occurs with a definite rhythmic sequence of events that take place during a gait cycle. Normal walking is relatively effortless, performed with minimum expenditure of energy.[9, 16, 25]

Gait is an intricate process affected by a number of bodily mechanisms such as trunk sway, arm swing, and head motion. It is dependent on various reflexes—for example, the postural, labyrinthine, and righting reflexes.

GAIT CYCLE

A complete walk cycle is the period between the time when the heel strikes the ground and the next heel-strike of the same limb. The phasic events that take place progressively during a single forward step are expressed as a percentage of the walk cycle, the heel-strikes marking 0 and 100 per cent. The gait cycle consists of two phases—stance and swing (Fig. 1–2 A to D).

Stance Phase. In the stance phase the foot is in contact with the floor and the lower limb is bearing all or part of the body weight (Fig. 1–2 B and E). This phase begins when the heel strikes the floor and ends when the toes rise off the floor. Constituting 60 per cent of the gait cycle, it is further subdivided into four *periods* by five events known as *critical incidents*. The periods in the stance phase are heel-strike, midstance, push-off, and acceleration; the critical incidents are heel-strike, foot-flat, heel-off, knee-bend, and toe-off.

The first period, *heel-strike*, constitutes 15 per cent of the gait cycle; it begins with the first critical incident, *heel-strike*, and terminates with the second critical incident, *foot-flat*.

The second period, known as *midstance* begins with *foot-flat* and ends with the third critical incident, *heel-off*. During this period, the person is balanced on his weight-bearing leg; it lasts for the second 15 per cent of the walk cycle.

The third period, *push-off*, is initiated by *heel-off* (the third critical incident) and terminates with *knee-bend* (the fourth critical incident)—during which the hip and knee are bent, preparing the limb for the swing phase. The *push-off* period constitutes the next 25 per cent of the gait cycle.

The fourth and final period of the stance phase is acceleration; it begins at *knee-bend* and ends at *toe-off*, the final critical incident, marking the termination of the stance phase. The duration of the acceleration phase is 5 per cent of the gait cycle, and its termination marks the completion of 60 per cent of the cycle.

Soon after knee-bend, the contralateral leg has completed its swing phase; its foot is touching the floor, preparing for transfer of the body weight to the new stance limb. It is obvious that the swing foot hits the ground before the opposite stance foot is lifted. During this period the weight borne on the original stance limb

decreases rapidly. The time in which both limbs are on the floor *simultaneously* is known as the *double-support* (or *double-stance*) *phase* (Fig. 1–2 D). In normal walking this period diminishes with increased walking velocity and disappears during running.

Swing Phase. In the swing phase, the foot is not touching the floor, and the body weight is borne by the opposite limb (Fig. 1–2 C and E). Beginning at toe-off and ending at heel-strike, this phase occupies 40 per cent of the walk cycle. It is subdivided into three periods— initial swing, midswing, and deceleration.

The *initial swing* commences with the critical incident of *toe-off* and continues as the foot is elevated from the floor in an arc by hip and knee flexion and the limb moves forward. The initial swing occupies the first 10 per cent of the swing phase.

Midswing begins when the swing limb passes the opposite limb in stance; the knee extends, and the path of the foot is a forward-swinging arc. This period occupies 80 per cent of the swing phase.

The *deceleration* period occurs during the final 10 per cent of the swing phase; the force of gravity and the musculature of the limb smoothly brake the forward-moving swing limb; the heel strikes the ground, and the full sequence of the gait cycle is completed at 100 per cent. This sequence of motions is continually repeated, with the limbs alternating, during normal walking on level ground.

Gait may be described as an interplay between loss and recovery of balance in which the center of gravity of the body shifts constantly. As one pushes forward on his weight-bearing limb, the center of gravity of his body shifts forward, and he tends to fall forward, only to be stopped by the swinging leg, which arrives in its new position just in time.

Other terms are used in analysis of gait. *Stride length* is the distance traveled in the same time span as the gait cycle; *step length* is the distance from the heel of one foot to the heel of the opposite foot during the double-support phase (Fig. 1–2 A). *Cadence* is the number of steps per minute. *Walking velocity* is the speed of movement in a single direction in centimeters per second. *Angular rotation* is rotation of the joint in degrees plotted against percentage of the walk cycle.

A number of forces act upon and modify the human body in forward motion—gravity, counteraction of the floor, muscle forces, and kinetic energy developed with the movement of the body mass.

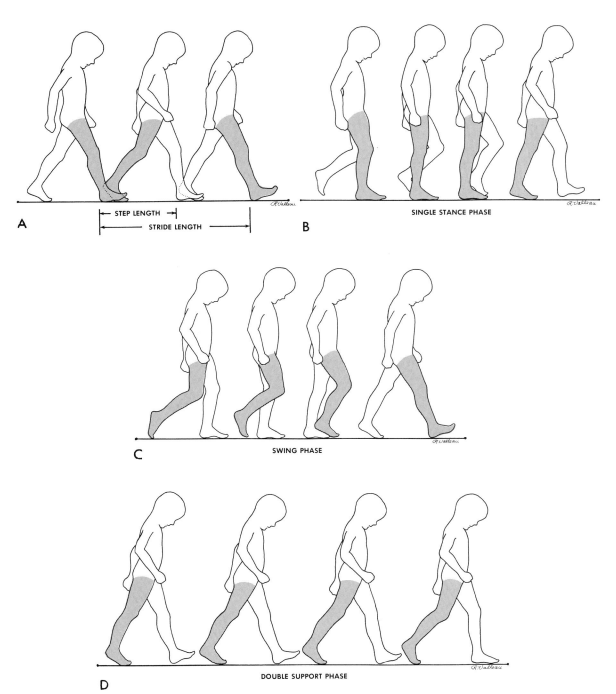

FIGURE 1–2. The gait cycle.

A. *Step length* is measured from the heel of one foot to the heel of the opposite foot during double support. *Stride length* is the distance from foot-strike to foot-strike of the same limb. **B.** Single-stance phase is the period of support by a single limb. **C.** Swing phase is the period in which the foot is off the floor. **D.** Double-support phase is the period in which both feet are on the floor.

Illustration continued on following page

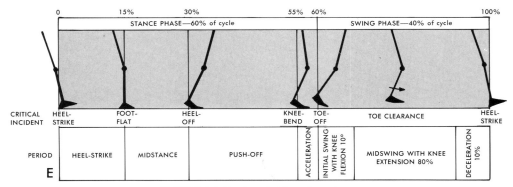

| 0 | 15% | 30% | 55% 60% | 100% |

FIGURE 1–2 Continued. *The gait cycle.*

E. Analysis of a single stride, as explained in the text.

GRAVITY

The location of the center of gravity of the adult body has been estimated to be just anterior to the second sacral vertebra within the true pelvis at a level that is about 55 per cent of the total height of the individual.[19] In normal human gait, the pathway followed by the center of gravity of the body is a smooth, regular curve moving up and down in the vertical plane with an average rise and fall of about 2 inches. The low point is reached at the double-support phase when both feet are on the ground, and the high point at midstance. The center of gravity of the body is also displaced laterally in the horizontal plane during locomotion; the

total side-to-side distance traveled is about 2 inches. The motion is toward the weight-bearing limb and reaches its lateral limit in midstance. When the vertical and horizontal motions of the center of gravity of the body are combined, they are found to describe a double sinusoidal curve.

Reactions Between Foot and Floor. Friction between the floor and the foot affects gait. The force of gravity stabilizes the contact of the foot with the ground, modifying acceleration and deceleration.

The *force plate*, a complex device upon which the patient stands, measures the magnitude and direction of the forces of vertical loading, fore-and-aft shear, medial and lateral shear, and the

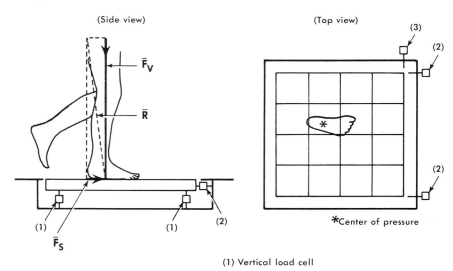

(1) Vertical load cell
(2) Fore-aft shear cell
(3) Medial-lateral shear cell

FIGURE 1–3. *Force plate.*

Side view shows subject in single-limb support phase. Vertical force vector F_v, fore-aft shear vector F_s, and line of application of the floor reaction force, R are shown. The center of pressure (calculated) is illustrated in the top view.

medial and lateral torque.[14, 17, 24, 26] The center of pressure is the instantaneous location of the center of the vertical force on the force plate. The line of application of the floor reaction force (vector $\overline{R}$) is the result of the vertical force (vector $\overline{Fv}$) and fore-aft shear (vector $\overline{Fs}$) (Fig. 1–3 side view). The termination of the floor reaction force vector $\overline{R}$ is at the center of pressure (Fig. 1–3 top view).

In equinus gait, such as occurs in spastic cerebral palsy, the heel may not touch the floor at any time during the gait cycle. It has been proposed that the term "heel-strike" not be used in such a case and the period of contact between the foot and the floor be subdivided into initial contact, contact response, and terminal stance.

Immediately after heel-strike there is a forward peak in the fore-and-aft shear that quickly

reverses as the foot pushes backward on the floor.

Lateral and medial shear recordings demonstrate the lateral shift of the center of gravity in gait.

DETERMINANTS OF GAIT

The six basic determinants of gait as defined by Saunders, Inman, and Eberhart in 1953 are as follows:[21]

Pelvic Rotation—the First Determinant. In normal level locomotion, the pelvis rotates in the horizontal plane 4 degrees forward on the swing limb and 4 degrees backward on the stance limb with a total magnitude of rotation of approximately 8 degrees (Fig. 1–4). Since the pelvis is rigid, the rotation actually occurs at the hip joint, which passes from medial to lateral rotation during the stance phase. The

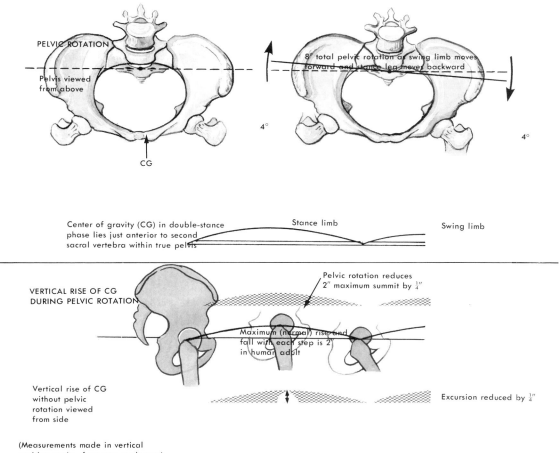

FIGURE 1–4. *Pelvic rotation—the first determinant of gait.*

pelvis and two lower limbs during double-stance phase (swing limb at heel-strike and stance limb at heel-off) form an isosceles triangle. The apex of this triangle determines the height of the center of gravity from the ground. The sides of the bipod intersect the plane of the floor at an angle. Rotating the pelvis in the horizontal plane decreases this angle between the limbs and the floor, thereby relatively "lengthening" the limbs and propping up the bipod. This has the effect of flattening the arc of the pathway of the center of gravity by elevating the extremities of the arc. The stride is lengthened without increasing the drop of the center of gravity at the instant of heel-strike. In this way, the expenditure of energy in locomotion is greatly reduced.

Pelvic Tilt—the Second Determinant. The pelvis also tilts during normal locomotion, listing downward in relation to the horizontal plane on the side opposite to that of the weight-bearing limb (positive Trendelenburg sign) (Fig. 1–5). The angular displacement occurs at the hip joint and is, on the average, 5 degrees. To permit pelvic tilt, the knee joint of the non-weight-bearing limb must flex to allow toe clearance for the swing-through of that limb. Pelvic tilt causes the center of gravity to lower by approximately half. By cutting the vertical displacement of the center of gravity in half and by shortening the pendulum of the limb by knee flexion in the swing phase, energy is saved.

Knee Flexion After Heel-Strike in Stance Phase—the Third Determinant. The supporting lower limb enters the stance phase at heel-

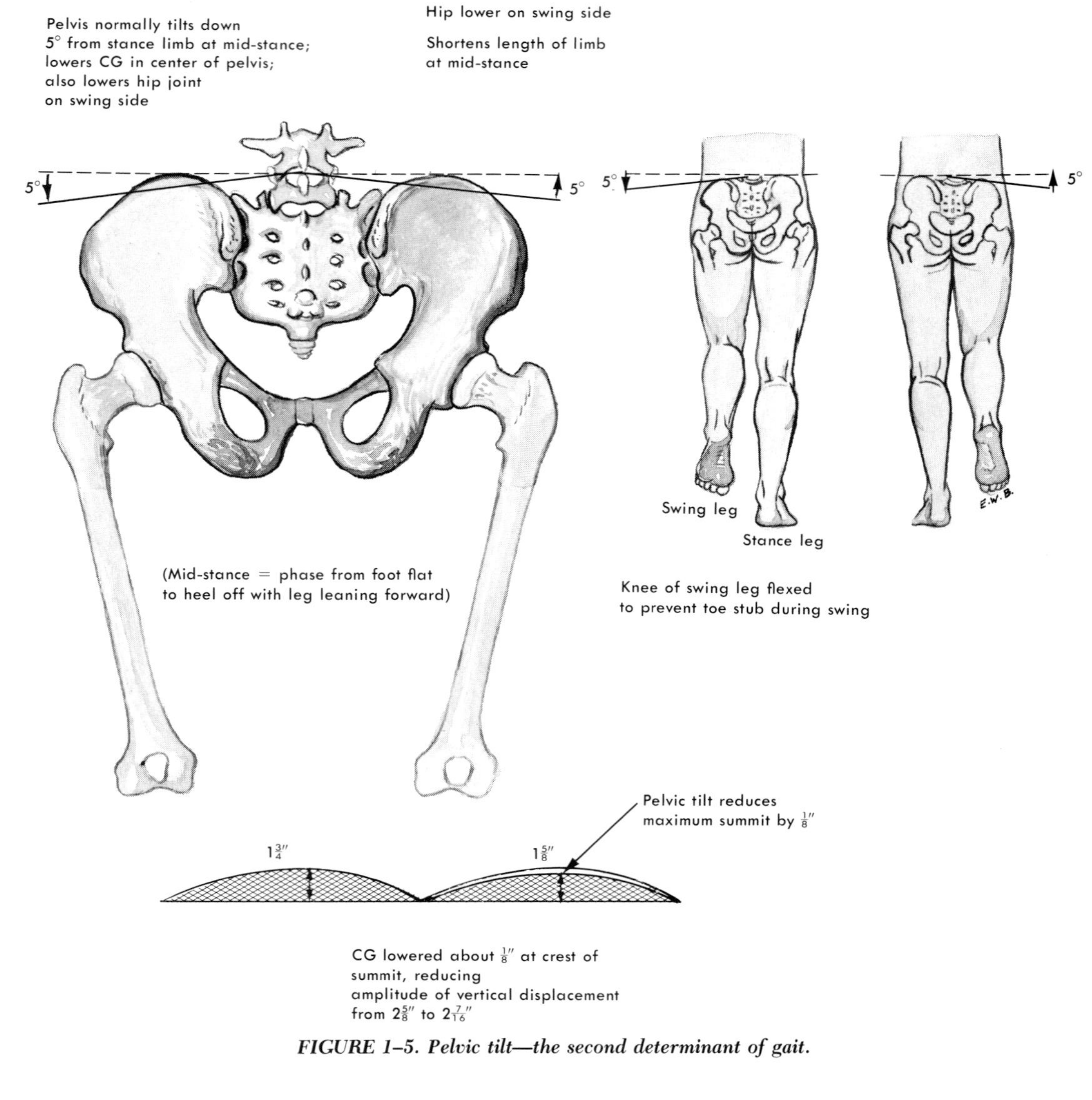

Pelvis normally tilts down
5° from stance limb at mid-stance;
lowers CG in center of pelvis;
also lowers hip joint
on swing side

Hip lower on swing side

Shortens length of limb
at mid-stance

5°   5°   5°   5°

(Mid-stance = phase from foot flat
to heel off with leg leaning forward)

Swing leg

Stance leg

Knee of swing leg flexed
to prevent toe stub during swing

Pelvic tilt reduces
maximum summit by $\frac{1}{8}''$

$1\frac{3}{4}''$ $1\frac{5}{8}''$

CG lowered about $\frac{1}{8}''$ at crest of
summit, reducing
amplitude of vertical displacement
from $2\frac{5}{8}''$ to $2\frac{7}{16}''$

FIGURE 1–5. Pelvic tilt—the second determinant of gait.

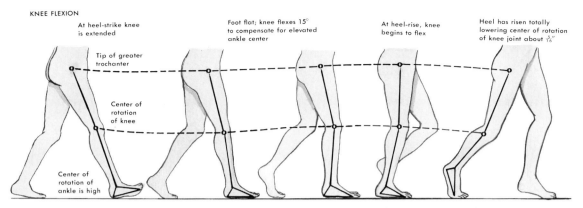

KNEE FLEXION

At heel-strike knee is extended

Foot flat; knee flexes 15° to compensate for elevated ankle center

At heel-rise, knee begins to flex

Heel has risen totally lowering center of rotation of knee joint about $\frac{5}{16}''$

Tip of greater trochanter

Center of rotation of knee

Center of rotation of ankle is high

FIGURE 1–6. *Knee flexion after heel strike in stance phase—the third determinant of gait.*

strike with the knee in full extension, after which the knee joint immediately begins to flex until the foot is flat on the ground (Fig. 1–6). The average degree of knee flexion at this time is 15 degrees. Shortly after midstance, the knee joint passes into extension once more, and this is immediately followed by the second flexion of the knee, beginning simultaneously with heel-rise as the limb is carried into the swing phase. This period of the stance phase in which the knee is first locked in extension, unlocked by flexion, and again locked in extension prior to its final flexion is referred to as the period of *double knee-lock*. This pattern of repeated knee flexion results in reduction of vertical displacement of the center of gravity as the body weight is carried forward over the stance leg, again conserving energy.

It is apparent from the foregoing discussion that pelvic rotation, pelvic tilt, and knee flexion in stance (all three determinants) flatten the arc through which the center of gravity of the body is translated. Pelvic tilt and knee flexion act to depress the summit of the arc, whereas pelvic rotation elevates the extremities of the arc.

Foot and Ankle Motion—the Fourth Determinant. The motions of the foot, ankle, and knee are intimately related in smoothing out the pathway of the center of gravity in the plane of progression (Fig. 1–7). The center of rotation of the ankle joint is located approximately at a point connecting the tips of the medial and lateral malleoli; it traverses an arc formed by the lever arm of the calcaneus. At heel-strike, the foot is dorsiflexed, the center of rotation of the ankle is elevated, and the knee is in full extension. Next, rapid plantar flexion of the foot takes place, and when the foot is flat on the ground through midstance, the center of rotation of the ankle is lowered. The knee is flexed 15 degrees at foot-flat. Then the heel rises from the ground, elevating the center of rotation of the ankle again. These motions of the foot and ankle smooth out the path of the center of gravity when coupled with knee motion, which thus acts as the fifth determinant of gait.

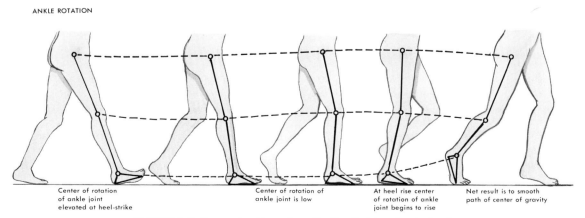

ANKLE ROTATION

Center of rotation of ankle joint elevated at heel-strike

Center of rotation of ankle joint is low

At heel rise center of rotation of ankle joint begins to rise

Net result is to smooth path of center of gravity

FIGURE 1–7. *Foot and ankle motion—the fourth determinant of gait.*

KNEE EXTENSION

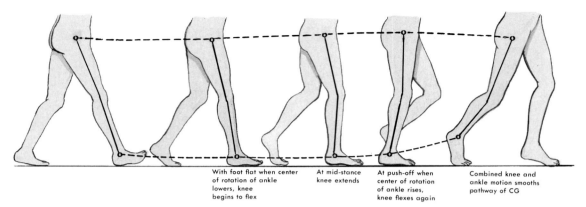

With foot flat when center
of rotation of ankle
lowers, knee
begins to flex

At mid-stance
knee extends

At push-off when
center of rotation
of ankle rises,
knee flexes again

Combined knee and
ankle motion smooths
pathway of CG

FIGURE 1–8. Knee motion—the fifth determinant of gait.

Knee Motion—the Fifth Determinant. The center of rotation of the knee is considered to be a point on the axis connecting the greatest prominences of the medial and lateral femoral condyles. The knee flexes just after heel-strike when the center of rotation of the ankle is elevated, and thereby the center of rotation of the knee is lowered. During midstance the knee is fully extended and its center of rotation raised when that of the ankle is lowered. At push-off the knee flexes again when the center of rotation of the ankle is rising the second time. The foot-ankle and knee motions are combined in such a manner that the ankle rise is largely cancelled out by the knee flexion (Fig. 1–8).

Lateral Displacement of Pelvis—the Sixth Determinant. In bipedal gait the center of gravity of the body must shift from the second sacral vertebra over the supporting foot while the contralateral limb swings forward. As the weight of the body is being shifted from one limb to the other, the pelvis moves laterally in the horizontal plane (Fig. 1–9). If the two limbs were parallel to one another, the necessary shift would be half the interval between the axis of the hip joints, approximately 4 inches. The femoral and tibial axes do not drop vertically from the hip joints, however; the femora are inclined medially at the hip, and the tibiae are aligned vertically at the knee joint. This tibiofemoral relationship narrows the support base and provides sufficient balance. Therefore, the lateral movement of the center of gravity toward the stance foot is reduced to only 1 inch, or a total of about 2 inches displacement per gait cycle.

The final result of the combination of the six determinants of gait is containment of the rise and fall of the center of gravity (vertical displacement), and of side-to-side motion of the pelvis (horizontal displacement) within a 2-inch square box. Exaggerations in the range of any one of these six basic determinants of locomotion are compensated for by reductions in another. The interaction of the six determinants of gait creates a smooth pathway for the forward displacement of the center of gravity of the body.

AXIAL ROTATIONS

During walking the various segments of the lower limb rotate around their long axes.[12, 13, 18] In general, from the swing phase to foot-flat the rotation is medial, and when the foot prepares to leave the floor the rotation is reversed laterally. In gait analysis, a stick attached to the anterior aspect of the pelvic belt is used to measure pelvic rotation. Viewed from the front, the tip and base of the stick are lined up when pelvic rotation is zero degrees. When the tip of the stick is to the right of center, the right side of the pelvis is rotated medially and the left side laterally. As stated previously, the pelvis rotates anteriorly 4 degrees during swing and posteriorly 4 degrees during stance. During the swing phase, the femur rotates laterally about 5 degrees at the hip joint; in the stance phase it rotates medially 3 to 4 degrees. Its total rotation is 8 to 9 degrees during a full gait cycle. Femoral torsion is measured from the front; it is zero when the hip, patella, and ankle are in a straight line; when the patella is facing the body midline from the hip to ankle line, the femur is rotated medially.

At heel-strike with the foot in neutral position the tibia rotates medially to align the ankle with

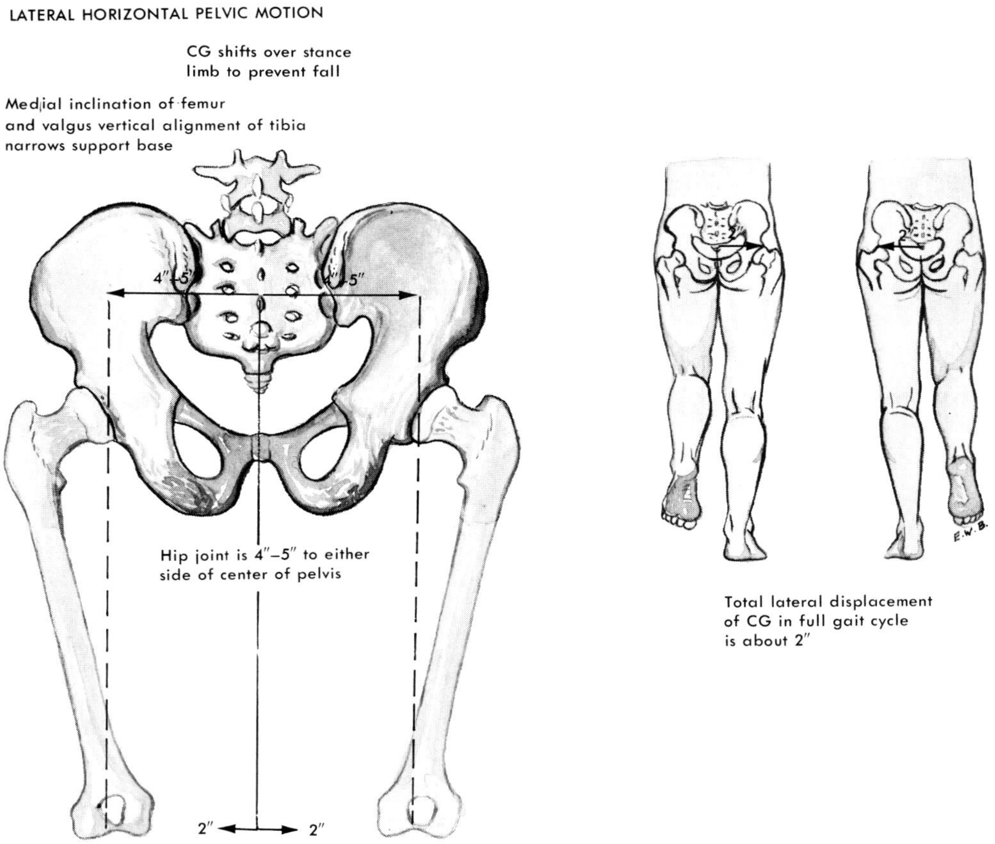

LATERAL HORIZONTAL PELVIC MOTION

CG shifts over stance
limb to prevent fall

Medial inclination of femur
and valgus vertical alignment of tibia
narrows support base

4"–5" 4"–5"

Hip joint is 4"–5" to either
side of center of pelvis

2" 2"

Total lateral displacement
of CG in full gait cycle
is about 2"

FIGURE 1–9. Lateral displacement of pelvis—the sixth determinant of gait.

the foot. At completion of foot-flat it begins to rotate laterally against the fixed foot, and it is at its maximum lateral rotation when the foot leaves the ground. It then begins to rotate medially in preparation for heel-strike. The total rotation of the tibia on the femur is 9 degrees.

In summary, during the act of walking, the weight of the body is supported by one lower limb (stance phase—the foot is on the ground), while the other limb executes the movement of progression (swing phase—the limb is carried into its new position). Normal locomotion represents a heel-toe sequence of support and progression, i.e., the weight of the body is first supported by the heel of the advancing lower limb, next by the foot, until the heel is lifted, and then by the ball of the forefoot. In addition to associated motions of the pelvis, hip, and knee, there are normal swinging movements of the upper limbs—as one lower limb is advanced, the upper limb of the opposite side advances.

MUSCLE ACTION IN GAIT

A source of energy is required for locomotion. The initial energy to start, accelerate, and decelerate the leg segments is supplied by muscle action. Other factors that enter into the cycle are momentum and gravity.

Muscles are grouped about joints as primary extensors, flexors, abductors, adductors, and medial and lateral rotators. Some muscles cross only one joint; others span two or three articulations. Their function changes according to positions of the limb.

In general, the muscles of the lower limb are used to stabilize, accelerate, or decelerate the leg. These muscles function while contracting, lengthening, or maintaining the same length. Electromyographic studies of muscle action during gait have shown that muscles act over very short periods and that during long intervals of the gait cycle they are relaxed, the limb being propelled forward by the pendulum-like action of its own momentum. Concentric contraction of a muscle shortens the distance between its origin and insertion and generates *motor power* to move or lift a part. The force exerted and the work performed can be readily calculated. Another major function of muscles in the lower limb during walking is to act as *shock absorbers* by decelerating a moving limb. Progressive elongation of a muscle by eccentric contraction serves to resist the passive forces that act to move a limb segment in the opposite direction. Muscles also function as stabilizers by isometric contraction and by maintaining a limb in a given position by locking the joints. Therefore, in gait, the muscles of a limb may contract concentrically (shorten the distance between origin and insertion) to provide motor power, contract eccentrically (lengthen the distance between origin and insertion) to perform as shock absorbers, or contract isometrically (no change in the distance between origin and insertion) to act as stabilizers.

Muscle activity is measured by wire electromyography of the lower limb during walking; the electromyograph does not, however, distinguish between the various forms of the muscle's activity of lengthening, shortening, or isometric contraction.

The quadriceps femoris shows activity potential during the deceleration period (the last 10 per cent) of the swing phase and at heel-strike (the initial 15 per cent) of the stance phase (Fig. 1–10). It contracts eccentrically, lengthening and acting as a shock absorber. It permits flexion of the knee until the foot reaches a foot-flat position. It should be noted that the duration of quadriceps activity is short. When the ankle rises at push-off, the knee is again flexed to counterbalance further heel-rise and make the path of the center of gravity smooth. During this very brief period of acceleration in the stance phase and the beginning of swing phase after toe-off, the rectus femoris and vastus intermedius portions of the quadriceps femoris fire again, contracting eccentrically to act as shock absorbers.

At heel-strike the pelvic balancer and trunk supporter groups of muscles (gluteus medius, gluteus minimus, gluteus maximus, erector spinae, and tensor fascia latae) are active. They contract eccentrically, allowing the pelvis to drop 5 degrees. They complete their function by heel-off. During the first 10 per cent of swing phase (initial swing) the tensor fasciae latae contracts concentrically, abducts the hip minimally, and places it in a better position to

initiate hip flexion. The next group of muscles to become active are those that assist in push-off—the triceps surae, posterior tibial, long toe flexors, and peroneus longus. The soleus and gastrocnemius, the most powerful and vital, provide the greatest force. They begin firing immediately after foot-flat, contracting eccentrically and lengthening to stabilize the tibia and allow extension of the knee. Toward the end of midstance they contract concentrically and plantar flex the ankle from 10 degrees of dorsiflexion to neutral position.

Next, the hip accelerators, consisting of iliopsoas, sartorius, tensor fasciae latae, adductor longus, and adductor magnus, contract concentrically. The iliopsoas acts during the period of acceleration in the stance phase, and the other accelerator muscles act during the swing phase.

The foot dorsiflexors (anterior tibial, long toe extensors, and extensor hallucis longus) contract concentrically during swing phase to provide enough force for the foot to clear the floor. They also contract eccentrically after heel-strike to make the descent of the forefoot to the ground smooth.

The decelerator group of the muscles consists of the gracilis, semimembranosus, semitendinosus, and biceps femoris. They contract eccentrically during the last 10 to 20 per cent of the swing phase just prior to heel-strike to decelerate the swinging limb. The brief period of contraction during the initial stance phase provides limb stability.

DEVELOPMENT OF MATURE GAIT

The average milestones of development of locomotion are as follows: the infant sits at 6 months of age, crawls at 9 months, cruises and walks with assistance at 12 months, walks independently at 15 months, and runs at 18 months.[10, 11, 22, 23] On gross inspection the independent gait of the infant has a wide base, the hips and knees are hyperflexed, the arms are held in extension and abduction, and the movements are abrupt. With maturation of the neuromuscular system, gradually the width of the base diminishes, the movements become smoother, reciprocal swing of the upper limbs begins, and step length and walking velocity increase. The adult pattern of gait develops between three and five years of age.[28]

The development of mature gait depends upon maturation of the central nervous system, which progresses cephalocaudally.

Sutherland and associates performed gait studies in 186 normal children between one

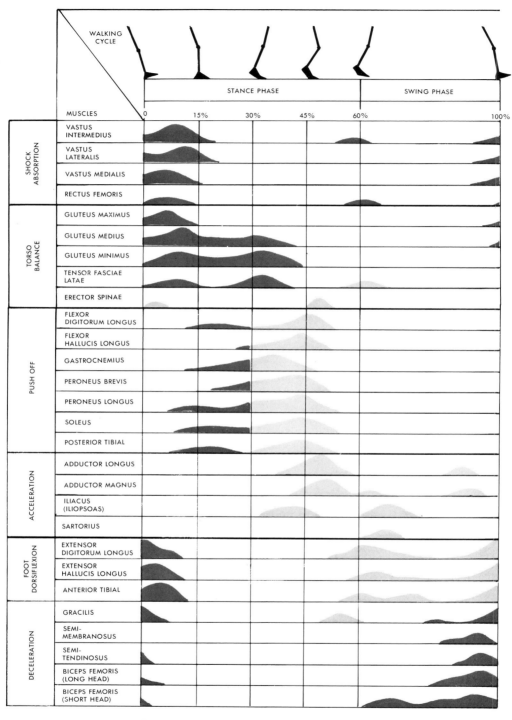

FIGURE 1–10. Muscle action during gait.

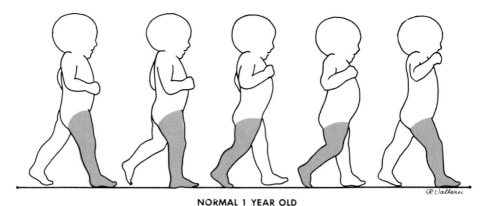

NORMAL 1 YEAR OLD

FIGURE 1–11. Normal gait in one-year-old.

Note the flexed elbows, absence of arm swing, plantar flexion at foot-strike, and increased shoulder sway in this one-year-old girl.

and seven years of age. Electromyograms were obtained by surface electrodes; 12 joint angle and 9 linear measurements were recorded in each lower limb throughout a gait cycle. The data were gathered and processed by high-speed movies, Graf-pen sonic digitizer, and computer and plotter. These investigators found that from two years and on, sagittal plane angular rotations in gait are very similar to and more closely related to those of the adult. Children under two years of age exhibited greater knee flexion and ankle dorsiflexion in stance phase, smaller knee flexion waves, and pronounced lateral rotation of the hips. By 18 months of age reciprocal arm-swing and heel-strike were present. Major determinants indicating maturity of gait are single-stance percentage (an index of limb stability), walking velocity, cadence, and step length. As the child gets older and acquires an adult gait pattern the cadence decreases and walking velocity and step length increase. According to these criteria gait maturity is established by three years of age.[27, 28]

The following examples of normal gait pattern in one-year-old, three-year-old, and six-year-old children are presented by courtesy of Dr. David H. Sutherland of San Diego, California.

A normal one-year-old child walks in a staccato manner (Fig. 1–11). The walking cadence is rapid, but the steps are very short. Walking velocity is approximately half that of an average adult. The elbows are kept flexed, and reciprocal arm movements are not yet present. In the frontal plane a wide base of support can be observed. Foot-strike occurs without initial heel-strike.

GENERAL MEASUREMENTS

	Right	Left
Opp. toe-off (per cent cycle)	12	16
Opp. foot-strike (per cent cycle)	50	48
Single stance (per cent cycle)	38	32
Toe-off (per cent cycle)	66	61
Step length (cm.)	21	21
Stride length (cm.)	42	42
Cycle time (sec.)	.7	.7
Cadence (steps/min.)	171	171
Walking velocity (cm./sec.)	60	60
(m./min.)	36	36

In comparison with a composite of normal adult control subjects, the child has greater hip and knee flexion in the swing phase (Fig. 1–12). Plantar flexion is present at foot-strike, but dorsiflexion is impaired in the early swing phase. There is excessive external rotation of pelvis, femur, tibia, and foot in both stance and swing phases.

All these variations from mature gait are normal initial adaptations to the demands of independent walking.

The gait of a normal three-year-old boy resembles mature gait (Fig. 1–13). Reciprocal arm movements are present. The dynamic base of support is normal. Cadence is slower than that of the normal one-year-old girl, and walking velocity is greater. Limitation of step length still prevents achievement of mature walking velocity.

GENERAL MEASUREMENTS

	Right	Left
Opp. toe-off (per cent cycle)	18	17
Opp. foot-strike (per cent cycle)	52	49
Single stance (per cent cycle)	34	32
Toe-off (per cent cycle)	68	67

NORMAL 1 YEAR OLD

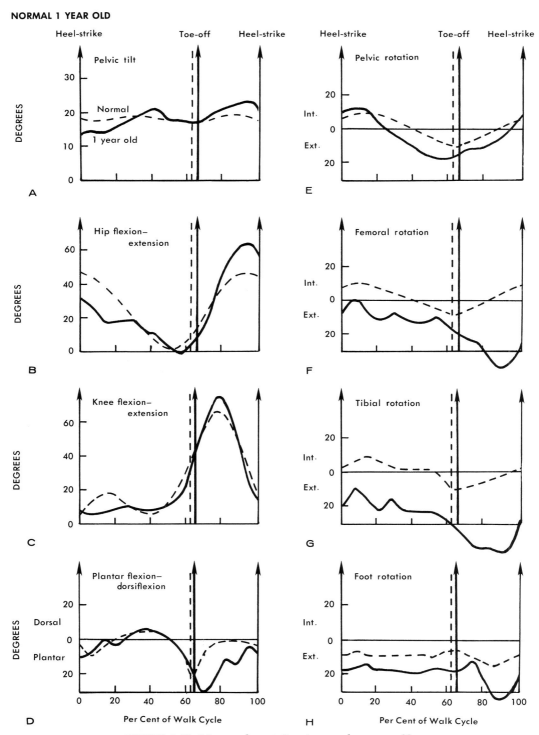

FIGURE 1–12. Joint angular rotations in normal one-year-old.

A. Slight increased sagittal plane pelvic oscillation. **B.** Increased swing phase hip flexion. **C.** Extended knee throughout stance. **D.** Plantar flexion at foot-strike and drop foot in swing. **E** to **H.** Exaggerated lateral rotation of pelvis, femur, tibia, and foot.

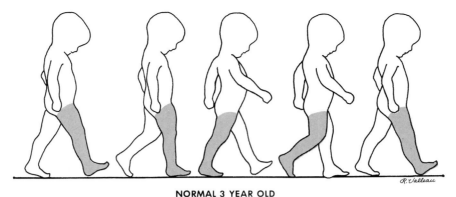

NORMAL 3 YEAR OLD

FIGURE 1–13. Normal gait in a three-year-old boy.

Synchronous arm swing and heel-strike, and apparent trunk stability are indicators of considerable gait maturity.

Step length (cm.)	29	32
Stride length (cm.)	64	61
Cycle time (sec.)	.76	.76
Cadence (steps/min.)	158	158
Walking velocity (cm./sec.)	80	80
(m./min.)	48	48

Although angular rotations of hip and knee are very similar to a composite of those of normal adults, ankle dorsiflexion in stance phase is greater (Fig. 1–14). Fully mature gait will be gained when better control of ankle musculature brings about the normal plantar flexor activity necessary to increase step length.

A normal six-year-old girl walks with a mature gait pattern (Fig. 1–15). Walking velocity, step length, and cadence are appropriately related.

GENERAL MEASUREMENTS

	Right	Left
Opp. toe-off (per cent cycle)	10	11
Opp. foot-strike (per cent cycle)	49	52
Single stance (per cent cycle)	39	40
Toe-off (per cent cycle)	60	63
Step length (cm.)	49	49
Stride length (cm.)	98	98
Cycle time (sec.)	.7	.7
Cadence (steps/min.)	171	171
Walking velocity (cm./sec.)	140	140
(m./min.)	84	84

The increase in pelvic rotation is attributable to rapid free cadence. The first peak vertical force and midstance valley are also increased for the same reason. The rapid cadence is also responsible for increases in fore-aft and lateral shear (Fig. 1–16). Electromyography reveals normal phasic activity of the vastus medialis, vastus lateralis, gluteus maximus, gastrocnemius-soleus, medial and lateral hamstrings, and anterior compartment muscle groups.

The gait of this child differs in no significant qualitative manner from that of a young adult.

PATHOLOGIC GAIT

Clinical appraisal of the gait is important. Abnormalities of gait are often specifically diagnostic. The child is usually asked to walk normally, then to walk on his toes and on his heels, then to run. He may be asked to climb stairs. When disorders of the neuromuscular system are suspected, he may be asked to walk "tandem," i.e., to place one heel directly in front of the toes of the other foot; to follow a line on the floor; to walk forward and backward six steps with eyes open and then with eyes closed; to walk sideward and around a chair. He may be asked to walk rapidly and stop suddenly.

In neurologic diseases one may gain some information by listening to the patient walk. The flopping sound of the gait of a person who has a foot drop, the dragging or scraping characteristic of spasticity, and the stamping in ataxia are well known. Inspection of the patient's shoes, noting the worn places, is of great value. When a patient has appliances, such as crutches or braces, he should be observed walking with their aid.

Abnormalities of gait may be caused by muscle weakness (source of motion), structural deformity of bones and joints (the articulated levers), neurologic disorders (which disturb awareness of need for, action of, and control of motion), and cardiopulmonary diseases (which will affect oxygen supply and energy).

Muscle Weakness. A common cause of pathologic gait is muscle weakness. The type of limp depends upon the location of the weakness and its degree.

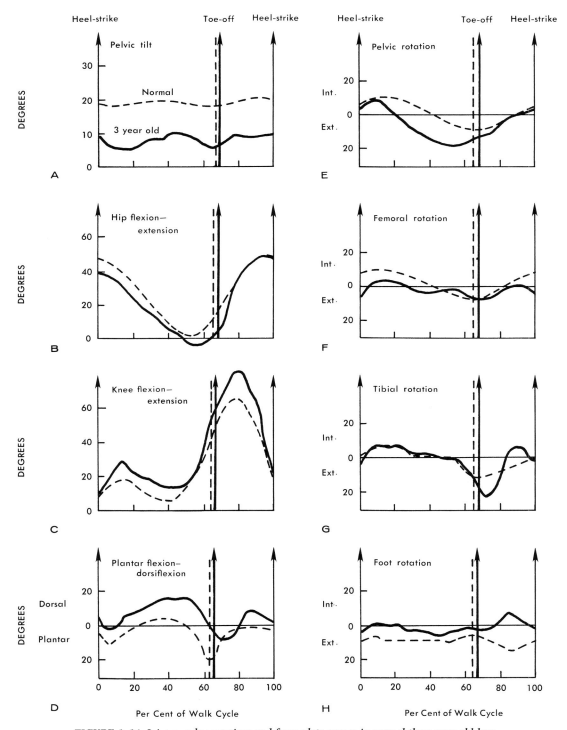

FIGURE 1–14. *Joint angular rotations and force plate curves in normal three-year-old boy.*

A to **D**. The sagittal plane joint angular rotations of this three-year-old boy are comparable to those of normal young adult controls. **E**. Pelvic rotation shows mild exaggeration of stance phase external rotation. **F** to **H**. With the exception of some irregularities of foot and tibial rotations in swing phase, femoral tibial foot rotations are similar to those young adult controls.

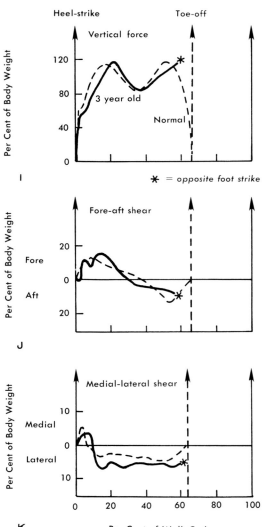

I

* = opposite foot strike

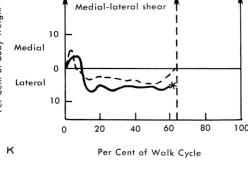

J

K

Per Cent of Walk Cycle

FIGURE 1–14. Continued. Joint angular rotations and force plate curves in normal three-year-old boy.

I, J, and **K.** Force plate curves show that vertical force, fore-aft shear, and medial-lateral shear duplicate adult control values. The curves are terminated at the asterisk because of opposite foot-strike on the plate.

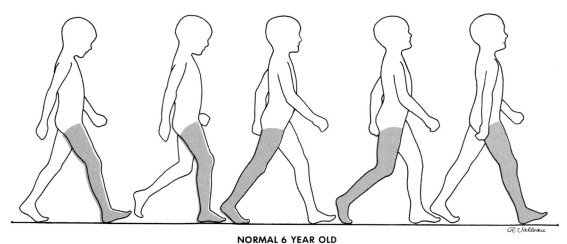

NORMAL 6 YEAR OLD

FIGURE 1–15. The gait pattern of a normal six-year-old girl.

This gait pattern resembles very closely that of a young adult.

NORMAL 6 YEAR OLD

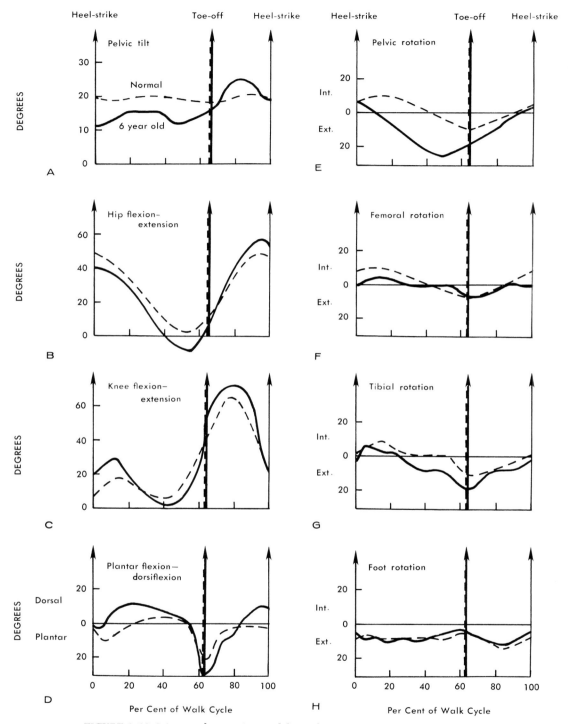

FIGURE 1–16. *Joint angular rotations and force plate curves in normal six-year-old girl.*

A to **D.** The sagittal plane joint angular rotations of this six-year-old girl differ in no significant manner from a composite of curves for young adult controls. **E.** Pelvic rotation is increased by rapid cadence and increased walking velocity. **F** to **H.** Femoral, tibial, and foot rotations are normal.

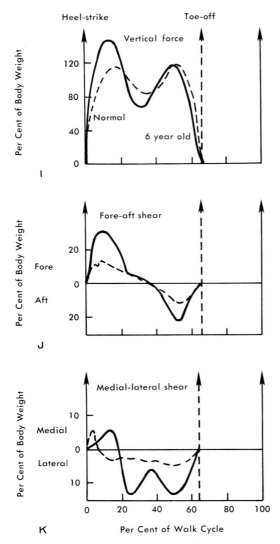

FIGURE 1–16. Continued. *Joint angular rotations and force plate curves in normal six-year-old girl.*

I. Vertical force first peak and midstance valley are increased because of rapid cadence and walking velocity. **J.** Fore-aft shear is increased for the same reason. **K.** Lateral shear is increased because of rapid cadence and walking velocity.

The *gluteus medius* is the principal hip abductor. Normally, when one stands on one leg, the gluteus medius of the same side elevates the pelvis on the opposite side, balancing the trunk over the weight-bearing hip. If the gluteus medius is paralyzed and the patient stands on the paralyzed lower limb, the opposite side of the pelvis drops (positive Trendelenburg test; see Fig. 1–1). As he walks and bears weight on the weak limb, because the paralyzed gluteus medius cannot stabilize the pelvis over the weight-bearing leg, the patient, at each stance phase of gait, lurches his trunk over toward the side of the weak gluteus medius (Fig. 1–17). By lurching his trunk toward and over the hip with gluteus medius paralysis, he brings the center of gravity of the body weight over and beyond the femoral head in order to compensate for the abductor weakness. In gaits in which muscle weakness exists, as a rule, the center of gravity of the body is shifted toward the paralyzed muscle in the stance phase.

The *gluteus maximus* is the principal hip extensor. The patient with paralysis of the gluteus maximus hyperextends his trunk at the hip joint when bearing weight on the affected limb, bringing the center of gravity posterior to the axis of the hip joint. This compensatory mechanism prevents the hip from giving way on flexion.

The *quadriceps femoris muscle* is the principal knee extensor. Strength of the quadriceps muscle is essential for climbing stairs and establishing stability of the knee. A patient with a poor quadriceps can, however, walk almost normally on level ground, provided he does not have flexion deformity of the knee. This can be done because, when weight is borne on the knee, the line of the center of gravity is normally anterior to the center of the joint, enabling the patient to lock the knee in extension in the stance phase. If there is flexion deformity of the knee, it will give way unless he lurches his trunk forward. In this way, the line of weight-bearing through the knee joint is displaced anteriorly so as to lock the knee in the stance phase of gait. This is another example of shifting the center of gravity and of balance to counteract the effect of weak muscles. With zero strength of the quadriceps in the presence of flexion deformity of the knee and a poor gluteus maximus, often the only way the patient can bear weight is by supporting the front of the affected thigh with his hand (Fig. 1–18). This represents an awkward and poor substitute for the paralyzed muscle.

The *gastrocnemius-soleus (triceps surae) muscles* are responsible for the final forward propulsion in the push-off portion of the stance phase. When the gastrocnemius-soleus muscles are paralyzed, the patient has a *calcaneus gait.* There is lack of push-off, and the tibia shifts posteriorly over the talus in the final portion of the stance phase when the limb is trying to take off (Fig. 1–19). To be functionally effective, the gastrocnemius-soleus muscle must be able to lift the body weight. A normal triceps surae muscle is one that enables the patient to rise

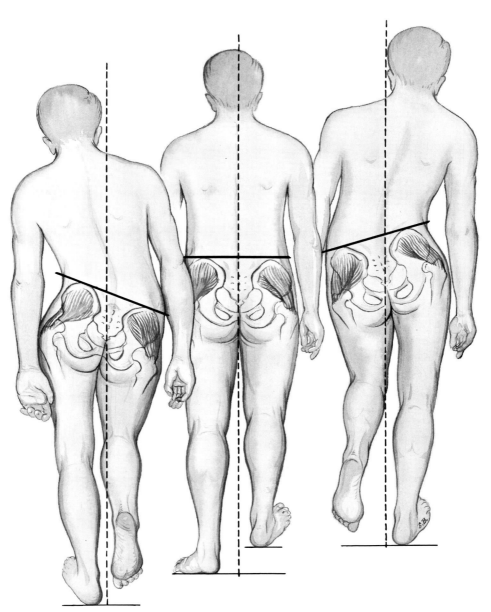

FIGURE 1–17. *Gluteus medius lurch.*

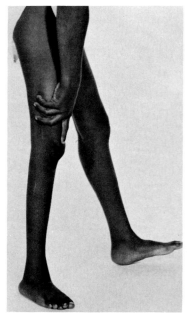 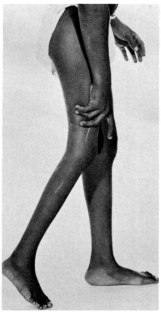 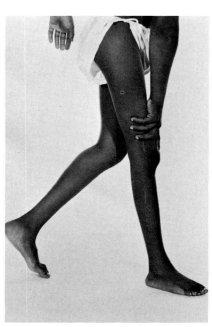

FIGURE 1–18. Quadriceps paralysis.

In quadriceps paralysis associated with flexion deformity of the knee and a poor gluteus maximus, the only way the patient can walk is by supporting the front of his thigh with his hand.

up on his toes through the full range of motion of the ankle at least ten times without either flexing his knees or leaning his trunk forward.

In *drop-foot* or *steppage gait* there is paralysis of the muscles that dorsiflex the foot. In the swing phase, as the patient brings his leg forward, he cannot hold his foot against gravity in dorsiflexion. The pull of gravity and the unopposed action of the antagonist muscles of the calf cause the foot to go into plantar flexion—it drops. In order to clear his toes, the patient externally rotates and raises the whole lower limb to a higher level than normal by flexing the knee and hip. A drop-foot gait is an illustration of abnormality in which the disturbed muscular action is in the swing phase.

Structural Deformities of the Bones and Joints. A *short leg*, depending on its degree, may produce a limp. A leg length discrepancy of one half inch or more may be well hidden by the tilt of the pelvis, as demonstrated by the low shoulder, low iliac crest, and low anterior superior iliac spine on the short side. Other means of compensation for leg length discrepancy are to hold the foot and ankle of the short limb in equinus posture, and the knee and hip of the longer leg in flexion. In *short-leg limp*, the patient's head, shoulder, and pelvis *dip down* as the body weight is borne on the short lower limb.

Ankylosis of the joints of the lower limb will cause a pathologic gait. The type of limp depends upon the joint involved and the position of fusion. When the hip is ankylosed, there is greater motion of the pelvis on the lumbar spine during the swing phase; and when the knee is stiff, the pelvis is elevated (hiked) to clear the foot, again during the swing phase. These are easy to diagnose. The gait resulting from an ankylosed ankle, however, lacks spring and may be difficult to distinguish from the normal.

In an *antalgic limp*, because of the painful affection of the bones or joints of the limb, the stance phase of gait is shortened. On weight-bearing the patient will take quick, soft steps with the painful limb.

In *congenital dislocation of the hip*, the head of the femur does not have a fixed position in the acetabulum and rides high on the side of the pelvis; thus, the action of the gluteus medius is impaired, and its motor strength weakened. The child walks with a gluteus medius limp and Trendelenburg gait.

Neurologic Disorders. Neurologic disorders may cause various abnormalities of gait, some of which may be pathognomonic of certain disease processes. Only the more important and more characteristic of these as seen in pediatric orthopedics are described here.

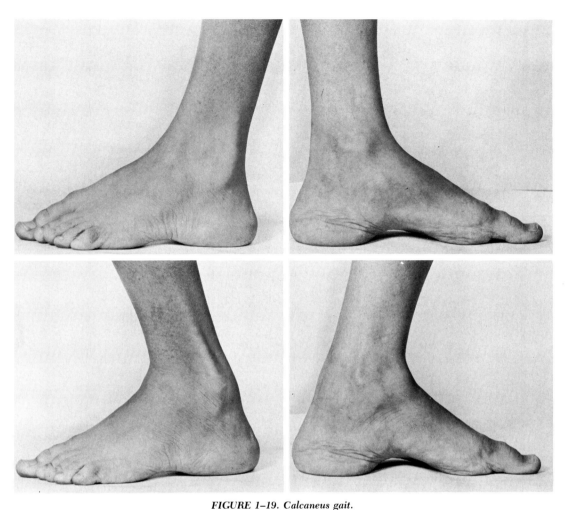

FIGURE 1–19. Calcaneus gait.

Note the posterior shift of the tibia over the talus.

Spastic Gait. In spasticity there are hypertonicity, hyperreflexia, exaggerated muscle stretch reflex, an imbalance of muscle action of certain predisposed muscle groups, and deformity. The distribution of spastic paralysis may be unilateral or bilateral. The resulting abnormalities of gait are typical. The child may have a toe-toe, toe-heel, or plantigrade gait. The anterior tibial muscle may be cerebral zero in motor strength and not contract. When there is associated spasticity of the posterior tibial muscle, the foot may be bent inward (pes varus); when the peroneals are spastic, the foot will be bent outward (pes valgus). The extensor hallucis longus may be hyperactive in an attempt to substitute for the weak anterior tibial muscle. The knee and hip may be held in flexion, or the knee may hyperextend when the heel touches the ground in toe-heel gait.

In spastic paraplegia the child walks with a scissorlike gait—because of exaggerated adduction and internal rotation of the hips due to spasticity of the hip adductors and medial hamstrings, the knees may cross one in front of the other, rubbing together and rolling around each other. There may be a Trendelenburg gait with a drop of the opposite side of the pelvis in stance phase. When walking, the patient does not swing his arms normally. The posture of the upper limb is typical—the elbow is flexed, the shoulder is adducted and internally rotated, the forearm pronated, the wrist flexed, the thumb adducted, and the fingers flexed in the palm. In acquired spastic paralysis the shoulder may be held in abduction, and the anterior tibial muscle in the leg may be hyperactive. Balance and coordination may be impaired. In mild cases, this is demonstrated by the inability of the patient to walk tandem; in severe involvement, the child may be able to walk only on parallel bars or with the assistance of crutches. Presence or absence of a reciprocal pattern of locomotion should be noted. One may have to observe the way in which a child crawls. The worn areas of the shoes may suggest toe walking. A shuffling, scraping sound may be characteristic.

Ataxic Gait. Ataxic gait may be of two types. The gait of *spinal ataxia* is caused by interruption of the proprioceptive pathways in the spinal cord or brain stem. In children, this is encountered in peripheral neuritis and in lesions of the brain stem; in adults, it is commonly seen in tabes dorsalis and in posterolateral and multiple sclerosis. The ataxia results from loss of appreciation of the senses of position and motion of the parts of the body and from lack of spatial orientation. The gait may not be too abnormal when the child walks with his eyes open, as he correlates his visual impulses with proprioceptive ones; however, if there is severe involvement, the child walks with a broad base, throwing out his feet, which come down first on the heel and then on the toes with a slapping sound or "double tap." The sound of the double tap produced by the noisy stamping of the hypotonic feet in two phases is so characteristic that one may diagnose the gait of spinal ataxia merely by hearing the patient walk. Upon close inspection, it is evident that the child is keeping his eyes on the floor and watching his feet while walking. When asked to walk with his eyes closed, he staggers, becomes unsteady, his feet shoot out, and he is unable to walk.

In the gait of *cerebellar ataxia*, ataxia is present with the eyes open or closed. It is caused by disease processes that involve the coordinating mechanisms in both the cerebellum and its connecting systems. The gait is wide-based, unsteady, and irregular. The child staggers and is unable to walk tandem or to follow a straight line on the floor. There may be tremors or oscillatory movements of the entire body. This form of ataxia is encountered in cerebellar lesions. If the disease process is localized in one cerebellar hemisphere, there is persistent deviation or swaying toward the affected side.

In *Friedreich's ataxia*, the ataxia is both spinal and cerebellar in type, as there is involvement of the posterior columns, spinocerebellar tracts, lateral columns, and cerebellum. The absence of the patellar reflex, the presence of a Babinski response, marked nystagmus, and other associated musculoskeletal findings will help to establish the diagnosis.

Dystrophic Gait. The dystrophic gait is encountered in various myopathies. It is most typical of muscular dystrophy. The child is usually brought to the physician with the presenting complaints of difficulty in running and trouble in ascending steps. He stands and walks with marked exaggeration of his lumbar lordosis. There is a pronounced "waddling" element in his gait; he has difficulty in fixing his pelvis. The child throws or rolls his hips from side to side with the stance phase of every forward step to shift the weight of the body. The exaggerated lateral tilting and rotation of the pelvis are largely to compensate for the weakness of the gluteal muscles. Overuse of the trunk and upper limbs in dystrophic gait has led to its being called a "penguin gait." The child has difficulty in getting up from a supine position on the floor; he has to roll to a prone position and "climb up on himself" by placing his hands first on his knees, then on his thighs, and finally on his hips to brace himself. He has marked difficulty in going up steps except with the help of hand pressure on his knees. This is caused by the weakness of the quadriceps and gluteus maximus in particular. In climbing stairs, he often needs a hand rail to pull himself up with his hands.

GAIT ANALYSIS

Gait analysis is performed in special centers in the United States and in Europe as a research tool and, also, to assist in planning an effective therapy program. The following studies are carried out in the analysis. Muscular activity is measured by electromyography. Indwelling electrodes identify the activity of specific muscles; their use is indicated when muscle transfers or releases are contemplated. Surface electrodes measure activity of groups of muscles during a movement. Inspection and traditional testing of muscles by slow stretching is not as reliable as electromyography; this is especially true in cerebral palsy.[15] Perry and Hoffer have clearly demonstrated the value of electromyography in planning surgery in cerebral palsy.[20] Their preoperative and postoperative dynamic electromyographic studies showed that when deforming muscles act exclusively in one portion of a gait cycle or movement of an upper limb, appropriate tendon transfer should be performed; whereas if there is continuous muscle activity, tendon lengthening is indicated. This evaluation is discussed in detail in the section on cerebral palsy.

Other data obtained in the gait laboratory include measurments of movements of the lower limbs in three planes, foot-floor reaction (force plate), joint torque, foot switch, and energy consumption. Gait analysis findings in various affections of the neuromuscular skeletal system are presented in the appropriate sections.

Deformities

The type and actual site of a deformity is now determined. Is it in the soft tissues, the bones, or the joints? How severe is it? Is it fixed, or can it be passively or actively corrected? What are the factors producing it? Is there muscle spasm with the deformity? Is there local tenderness or pain on motion?

Special tests are useful to demonstrate a deformity, particularly in the detection of fixed deformities of the hip, in which limitation of movement may be obscured by motion of the pelvis. It is imperative to observe the pelvis carefully while examining passive motion of the hip joint. A flexion deformity of many degrees may be masked by a forward tilt of the pelvis and excessive lumbar lordosis. In the *Thomas test* the patient is supine and both hips are completely flexed until the lumbar spine is flattened. The hip to be tested is then extended until the pelvis rotates; the angle taken by the tested hip is the degree of flexion deformity (Fig. 1–20). Another method for determining hip flexion deformity is to have the patient lie prone with both hips flexed over the end of the table to flatten the lumbar spine. The surgeon stabilizes the pelvis by placing his forearm over the ilium and lumbosacral spine and, with the opposite hand, extends the tested hip by elevating the thigh toward the ceiling. Motion of the lower spine should be prevented. Normally a hip should extend 30 degrees. If it cannot be brought to neutral position, there is a flexion deformity, which is then measured (Fig. 1–21). If the spine is stiff, or the flexion deformity of the hip is considerable in the standing posture, or both, the knee of the same side is held in flexion, and only the toes touch the ground, causing apparent shortening.

Ober's test is performed to determine the degree of abduction contracture of the hip (Fig. 1–22).[30] The child lies on the side opposite to the one being tested, and the underneath hip and knee are maximally flexed to flatten the lumbar spine. The hip to be tested (with the knee flexed to a right angle) is first flexed to 90 degrees, then fully abducted, and next brought into full hyperextension and allowed to adduct maximally. The knee of the tested limb should always be kept at 90 degrees of flexion. The angle that the thigh makes with a horizontal line parallel to the table represents the degree of abduction contracture. Normally, the limb drops well below the horizontal.

INEQUALITY OF LIMB LENGTH

On inspection, disparity in the length of the lower limbs can be detected by the difference in the level of the popliteal and gluteal creases, the pelvis, and the shoulders as the child stands with both feet together, heels on the ground, and knees fully extended. Next, the examiner places the radial border of his index fingers on the uppermost portion of each iliac crest and the thumb of each hand on the anterior superior iliac spines, and compares the height of the pelvis on the two sides. Blocks of wood of various thickness are placed under the foot of the short limb to make iliac crests and anterior superior iliac spines horizontal. Possible sources of error are bony abnormalities of the pelvis, such as atrophy of the ipsilateral ilium in poliomyelitis.

Then difference in the length of the limbs is measured with a tape with the patient in the supine position. To ensure accurate measurements, it is essential to place the extremities in comparable positions. The *actual leg length* is measured from the under side of the anterior superior iliac spine to the lowest point of the medial malleolus or the plantar surface of the heel—for this, both ankles must be in neutral and identical positions. This is an index of the *real* length of the lower limbs. When the anterior superior iliac spine is not easily palpable or is distorted because of a previous innominate osteotomy, the ischial tuberosity may be chosen as the proximal landmark; the distal point of reference may be either the tip of the medial malleolus or the sole of the heel with the ankle in neutral position. The *apparent length*, an index of the functional length of the lower limbs, is measured from the umbilicus to the lowest point of the medial malleolus, thus taking into consideration the tilt of the pelvis. An adduction deformity of the hip causes an apparent shortening on the side of the contracture; whereas, an abduction deformity of the hip produces an apparent lengthening on the same side (Fig. 1–23).

Whenever there is disproportion between the thigh and leg lengths, they should be measured separately. The medial knee joint line is the intermediate landmark; this is easily located by flexing the knee 45 degrees. Another way to assess disparity between thigh lengths is to determine the level of the knees with the

A.

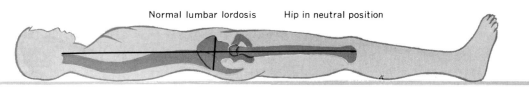

Normal lumbar lordosis   Hip in neutral position

Normal pelvic inclination

B.

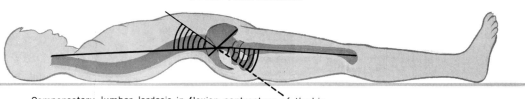

Note increased pelvic inclination

Compensatory lumbar lordosis in flexion contracture of the hip

C.

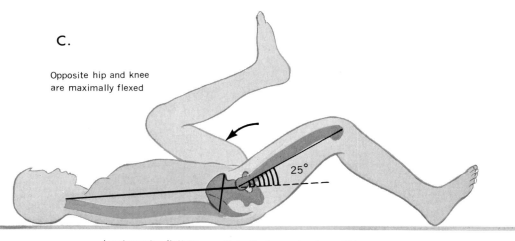

Opposite hip and knee
are maximally flexed

25°

Lumbar spine flattens   Note flexion contracture of hip

FIGURE 1–20. Thomas test.

(Adapted from von Lanz, T., and Wachsmuth, W.: Praktische anatomie. Berlin, Julius Springer, 1938, p. 157.)

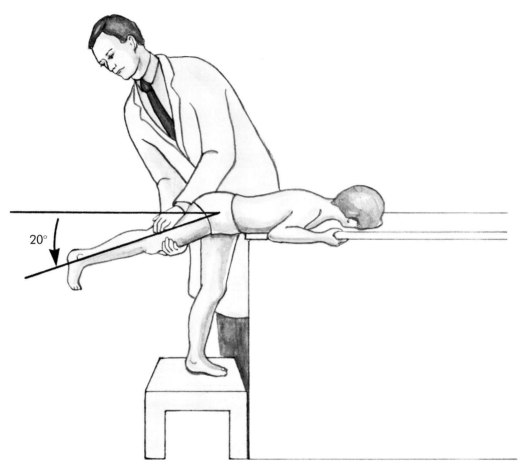

FIGURE 1–21. *Alternate method of determining hip flexion deformity.*

Note the patient lies prone with both hips flexed over the end of the table to flatten the lumbar spine. The tested hip is extended. The degree by which it fails to reach neutral position is the degree of flexion deformity of the hip.

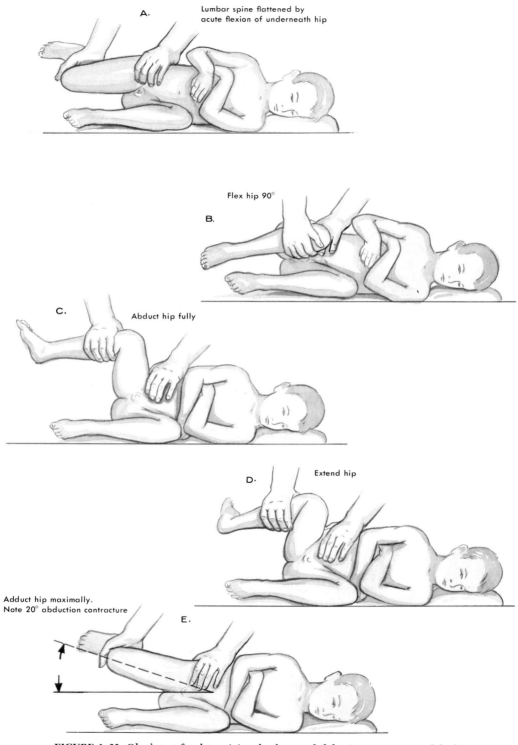

A. Lumbar spine flattened by acute flexion of underneath hip

B. Flex hip 90°

C. Abduct hip fully

D. Extend hip

E. Adduct hip maximally. Note 20° abduction contracture

FIGURE 1–22. *Ober's test for determining the degree of abduction contracture of the hip.*

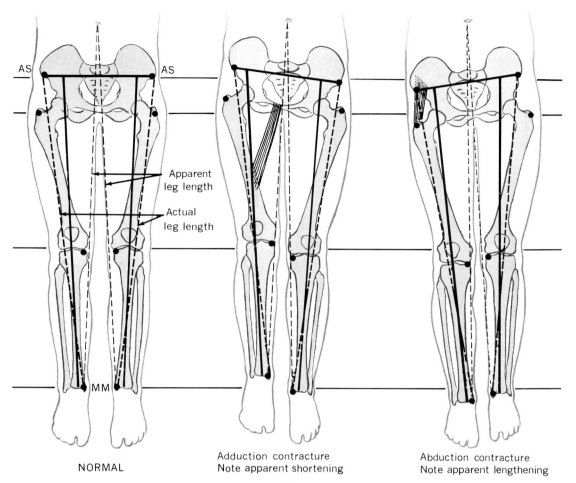

FIGURE 1–23. Measurement of actual and apparent leg lengths.

AS, anterior iliac spine; MM, medial malleolus. (Adapted from von Lanz, T., and Wachsmuth, W.: Praktische Anatomie. Berlin, Julius Springer, 1938, pp. 24–25.)

patient supine and both hips and knees flexed at right angles (Galleazi test). For assessing disparity of leg lengths, turn the patient to prone position with the hips in full extension, knees flexed 90 degrees, and ankles in neutral position to determine the level of the sole of the heels (Ellis test).

The total length of the upper limbs is measured from the posterior tip of the acromion process to the end of the long finger with the elbow, wrist, and fingers in neutral zero degrees extended position. The upper arm is measured from the posterior tip of the acromion to the point of the olecranon; the forearm is measured from the point of the olecranon to the tip of the radial or ulnar styloid process.

The circumference of the calf is measured at its greatest diameter. The thighs are measured at specifically marked identical levels, several inches above the patella or below the anterior superior iliac spine. In the upper limb, the greatest circumference of the forearm and midarm are conventional levels of measurement.

ANGULATION OF BOWING

Terms used in describing angular deformities denote the position of the distal segment of the deformity relative to the proximal unit. *Varus* describes an angulation toward the midline of the body distal to the anatomic part named; whereas, *valgus* describes angulation away from the midline distal to the part named. For example, in cubitus valgus, the forearm is directed away from the midline, distal to the elbow joint; whereas, in cubitus varus, it is bent inward toward the midline of the body. In coxa valga, the angle of the neck and the shaft of the femur is greater than normal, i.e., the distal segment is angulated away from the midline. In coxa vara, it is the reverse.

The angular deformities are measured in degrees and expressed in the same manner as that used for recording joint motions. Other objective measurements are used when indicated. In genu valgum, for example, the amount of knock-knee may be measured by the distance between the medial malleoli, with the knees in full extension, the patellae facing exactly upward, and the medial condyles of the femur brought together with moderate firm pressure to compress excessive subcutaneous fat (Fig. 1–24). Another method used to measure the degree of knock-knee is to determine the angle between the lateral surface of the thigh and leg. Atrophy of the calf, especially of the medial head of the gastrocnemius, and excessive subcutaneous fat on the thigh exaggerate the clinical appearance of knock-knees.

The degree of genu varum is determined in a similar way as that of knock-knees; the distance between the medial femoral condyles is measured with the medial malleoli brought together and firmly compressed. It is imperative for the patellae to face exactly forward, as

medial rotation of the lower limbs at the hips will cause apparent bowlegs.

It is often best to make a tracing or photograph of the deformity for subsequent comparison.

Range of Motion of Joints

The method of measuring and recording joint motion is standardized by the Committee for the Study of Joint Motion of the American Academy of Orthopedic Surgeons and approved by the appointed committees of the Orthopedic Associations of the English Speaking World.[34] It is based on the principles of the Neutral Zero Method, as described by Cave and Roberts.[37] Motion is measured in degrees of a circle with the joint as its center. The anatomic Zero Starting Position of each joint is defined, and the degrees of motion of a joint are added in the direction in which the joint moves from the Zero Starting Position. In the past, much confusion arose because joint motions were measured from various starting positions. This method eliminates the confusion by accepting the extended "anatomic position" of a limb as

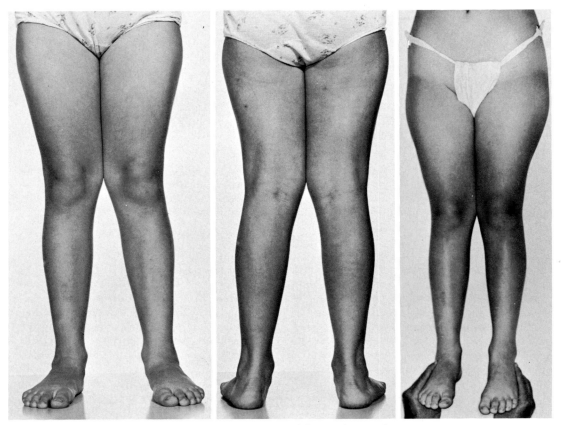

FIGURE 1–24. Measurement of degree of genu valgum.

zero degrees, rather than 180 degrees. For example, when a fully extended elbow joint is bent from the anatomic zero position to a right angle, the range of motion is 90 degrees of flexion.

The range of motion of a joint is determined in both its active and passive ranges. During examination it is important to be gentle, as the motion of a joint may be painful. The limb should be placed in the position that is most comfortable for the child. It is best for the beginner to use a goniometer until he learns to gauge angles accurately by vision. One should remember, however, that the goniometer may give inaccurate information when the bony landmarks are not definite, owing to excess soft-tissue coverage or other causes.

Flexion is the movement of bending a joint, a motion away from the Zero Starting Position. *Extension* is the act of straightening a joint, the return motion to the Zero Starting Position. A distinction is made between the terms *extension* and *hyperextension*. When the motion opposite to flexion is an unnatural one, as it may be at the knee or elbow, the term used is *hyperextension*. *Adduction* is the drawing of the part toward the axis of the body; whereas, *abduction* is motion of the part away from the axis of the body. At the wrist joint, ulnar and radial deviation are used. *Supination* is the act of turning the palm of the hand toward the anterior surface of the body or facing upward. *Pronation* is the turning of the palm of the hand toward the posterior surface of the body or facing downward. *Inversion* is a term applied to an inward turning motion seen primarily in the subtalar joint of the foot. *Eversion* is the opposite motion. *Internal* and *external rotation* are self-explanatory.

A typical hinge joint in which there is "one plane freedom" of motion is the elbow. The Zero Starting Position is the extended straight elbow (zero degrees). The normal range of motions of the elbow are (Fig. 1–25 A): (1) *flexion*—zero to 150 degrees; (2) *extension*—150 degrees to zero (from the angle of greatest flexion to Zero Starting Position); and (3) *hyperextension*—measured in degrees beyond the Zero Starting Position and varying from 5 to 15 degrees. Hyperextension is not present in all persons. Limited motion in the elbow joint is expressed as follows: (1) the elbow flexes 30 degrees to 90 degrees, or (2) the elbow has a flexion deformity of 30 degrees with further flexion to 90 degrees (Fig. 1–25 B).

Examinations of the motions of the hip are more complicated, as it is a ball-and-socket joint capable of three dimensional, compound, or rotatory motion. A common pitfall in determining hip motion is the failure to observe that the pelvis does not rotate or tilt during examination. The examiner should always place one hand on the iliac crest to note the point at which the pelvis begins to move. First the patient lies supine on a firm flat surface with the opposite hip held in full flexion to flatten the lumbar spine and bring out flexion contracture of the hip, if present (the Thomas test). The normal range of flexion is from zero to 110 or 120 degrees. Limited motion in the hip is expressed in the same manner as in the elbow or knee, i.e., (1) the hip flexes from 30 to 90 degrees, or (2) the hip has a flexion deformity of 30 degrees with further flexion to 90 degrees.

Next, rotation of the hip in flexion is determined with the patient still lying supine. The hip and knee of the limb to be examined are each flexed 90 degrees; the thigh is perpendicular to the transverse line across the anterior superior iliac spines of the pelvis. *Medial rotation* is measured by rotating the leg away from the midline of the trunk with the thigh as the axis of rotation, thus producing medial rotation of the hip (normal 35 degrees) (Fig. 1–26 A). *Lateral rotation* of the hip is produced by rotating the leg toward the midline of the trunk with the thigh as the axis of rotation. The terms *internal* (or *inward*) and *external* (or *outward*) should not be used.

In testing *abduction* of the hip, it is imperative that the anterior superior iliac spines be level. The pelvis is held fixed by abduction of the opposite hip and steadied by the examiner's hand, which will detect pelvic motion (Fig. 1–26 C). Abduction is measured in degrees as the outward motion of the limb from the Zero Starting Position. In measuring *adduction*, the examiner should elevate the opposite limb so that the tested leg can pass under it. Rotation of the hip in extension can be measured with the patient supine, but it is best for him to turn over into prone position. His knee is flexed to 90 degrees; the leg is perpendicular to the transverse line across the anterior superior iliac spines. The leg is rotated outward to measure medial rotation (normal range 45 degrees), and inward for lateral rotation (Fig. 1–26 B). Extension of the hip is determined with the patient lying face down with the opposite hip flexed over the end of the table to flatten the lumbar spine. The examiner stabilizes the pelvis by placing his elbow and forearm over the ilium and lumbosacral spine; with his other hand he holds the lower thigh with the knee flexed to

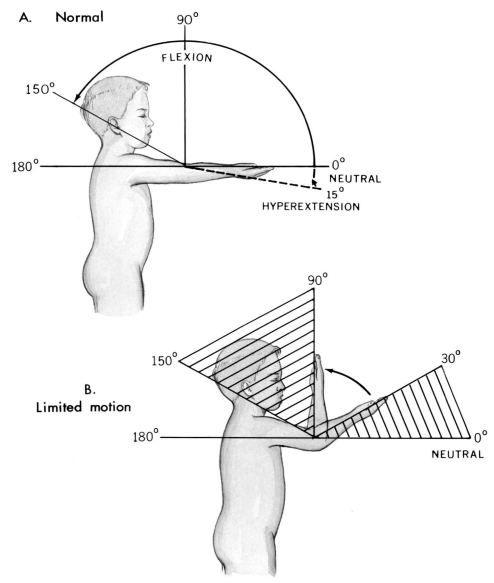

FIGURE 1–25. *Measurement of range of motion of the elbow joint.*

A. Normal. **B.** Limited motion.

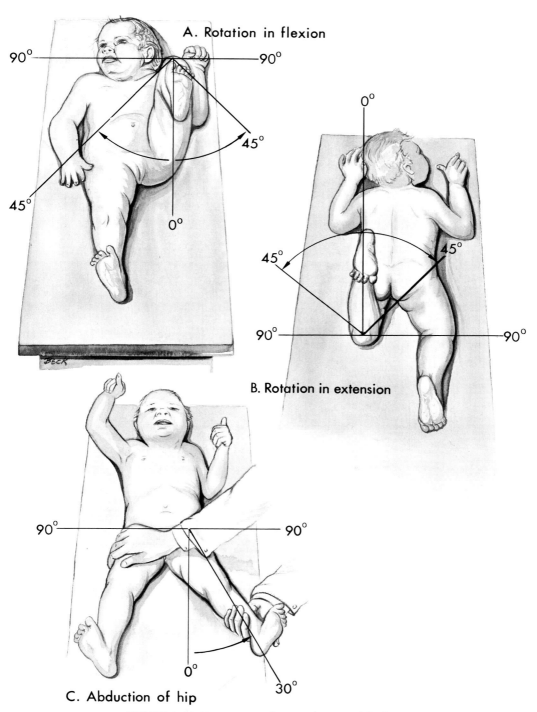

A. Rotation in flexion

B. Rotation in extension

C. Abduction of hip

FIGURE 1–26. *Measurement of range of motion of the hip.*

relax the hamstrings. The tested hip is extended by lifting the thigh toward the ceiling. Motion of the lower spine should be prevented (Fig. 1–27). The normal range of hip extension is about 30 degrees. In the presence of flexion contracture the hip cannot be extended. The Thomas test can also be performed with the patient prone. When a patient is in pain and irritable he may resist flexion of one hip over the end of the table. In such an instance, he may lie prone, a small pillow is placed under the abdomen, and the tested lower limb is extended with the knee slightly flexed.

A gross but rapid way to detect limitation of hip abduction is to ask a patient (either standing or lying supine) to spread his legs apart as far as he can. Normally each hip should abduct about 45 degrees, which is assessed by measuring intramalleolar separation. The standards for amplitude of joint motion as provided by the American Academy of Orthopedic Surgeons manual are for adults. In children, range of joint motion is greater because of joint laxity. Boone and Azen have studied changing patterns of joint motion with increasing age in boys from 18 months to 19 years. Connective tissue becomes progressively more rigid, particularly in and around muscles and tendons, as age increases. Therefore, range of joint motion decreases.

All normal newborns have flexion deformity of the hip and knee because of the intrauterine flexed posture. Usually by four to six months of age, the hip and the knee can be extended to neutral position. Hip abduction decreases with increasing age—on the average, 10 to 15 degrees per decade for the first 20 years. Hip rotation decreases by about 15 to 20 degrees per decade during the first 20 years and by about 5 degrees per decade thereafter.

Children have greater inversion and dorsiflexion of the feet than adults. Because the amplitude of joint motion in the right and left sides is normally similar, it is possible to compare the "healthy" limb with the affected limb.[35]

Motion of the shoulder is subdivided into true glenohumeral motion, pure scapulothoracic motion, and combined glenohumeral and scapulothoracic motion. The term *elevation* defines all upward motions of the humerus in any plane, i.e., vertical raising of the arm in any position of the horizontal plane of abduction or adduction.

In testing range of elevation of the glenohu-

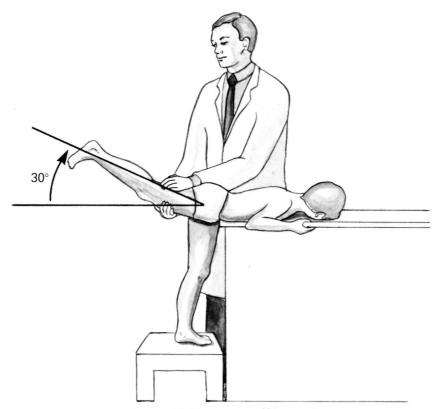

FIGURE 1–27. Measurement of hip extension.

meral joint, it is essential for the examiner to stand behind the patient and fix the scapula by holding its inferior angle (Fig. 1–28 A and B). Motion of the scapulothoracic joint may be further restrained by placing a hand firmly over the acromion of the upper limb being tested. In combined glenohumeral and scapulothoracic

motion, the scapula rotates upward and forward over the chest wall, allowing the shoulder to elevate to 180 degrees (Fig. 1–28 C).

In shoulder elevation the first 20 degrees are pure glenohumeral motion (Fig. 1–29 A). From this point, when the arm is elevated the glenohumeral and scapulothoracic articulations

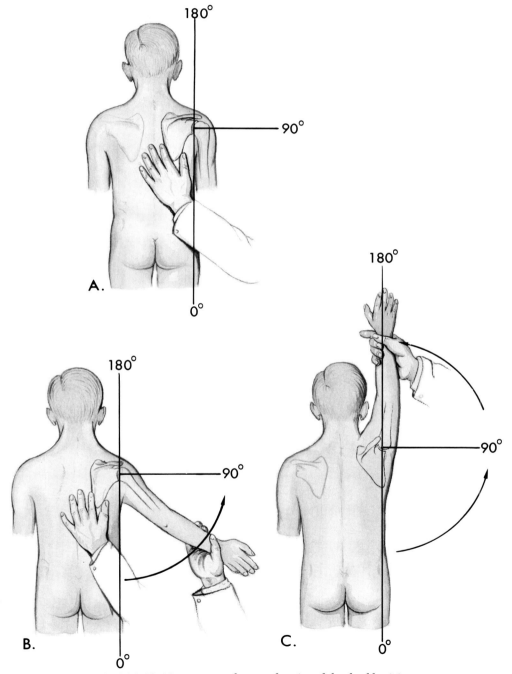

FIGURE 1–28. Measurement of range of motion of the shoulder joint.

(Adapted from Joint Motion–Method of Measuring and Recording. Publication of American Academy of Orthopedic Surgeons, 1965.)

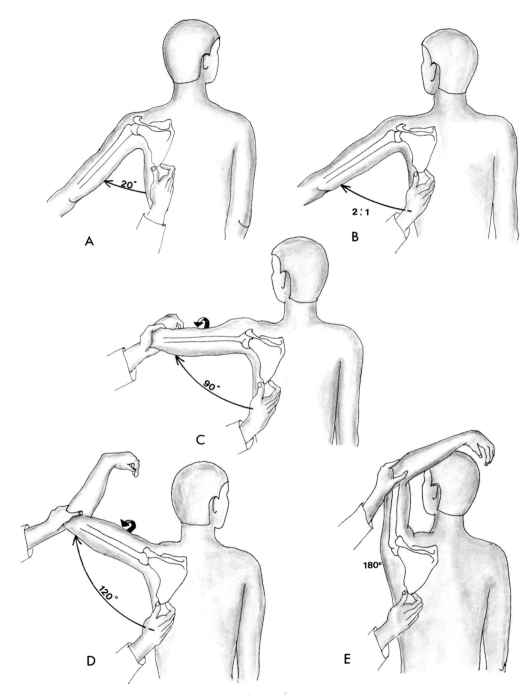

FIGURE 1-29. Elevation of shoulder joint.

    A. The scapula does not move until the arm is elevated to about 20 degrees, i.e., the motion takes place at the glenohumeral joint. **B,** At about 20 degrees of abduction the glenohumeral and scapulothoracic articulations move together in a 2:1 ratio. **C.** True glenohumeral elevation is about 90 degrees. **D.** At about 120 degrees of continued shoulder elevation the surgical neck of the humerus abuts the tip of the acromion process. The humerus rotates laterally to turn its surgical neck away from the acromion, thus allowing full elevation of the shoulder. **E.** Complete elevation of the shoulder joint (combined glenohumeral and scapulothoracic) is 180 degrees. This is made possible by lateral rotation of the humerus.

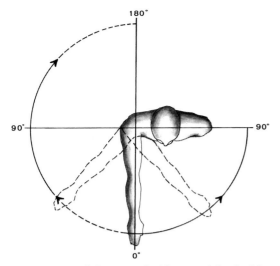

FIGURE 1–30. *Abduction and adduction of the shoulder.*

The terms are limited to describing motions in the horizontal plane from the midsagittal zero position.

move together in a ratio of 2 to 1, i.e., for every 3 degrees of shoulder elevation, 2 degrees occur at the glenohumeral joint and 1 degree at the scapulothoracic joint (Fig. 1–29 B). When the scapula is fixed, pure glenohumeral elevation is about 90 degrees (Fig. 1–29 C). At about 120 degrees of combined shoulder elevation the surgical neck of the humerus abuts the acromion, and full elevation of the shoulder is

allowed by lateral rotation of the shoulder; this turns the surgical neck of the humerus away from the tip of the acromion and increases the articular surface of the humeral head (Fig. 1–29 D and E).

The terms *abduction* and *adduction* of the shoulder describe motion in only the horizontal plane from the midsagittal zero position of the body (Fig. 1–30). Abduction is motion of the arm *away* from the axis, whereas adduction is moving of the arm toward the midsagittal axis of the body. The motions of the shoulder in the sagittal plane are flexion (forward) and extension (backward) (Fig. 1–31). Normally the shoulder will extend to 45 to 55 degrees.

Rotation of the shoulder is measured in the neutral position with the examiner standing in front of the patient. The patient's elbow must be at the side of the body to prevent substitution of adduction for lateral rotation and abduction for medial rotation and is bent 90 degrees. The forearm is rotated medially toward the sagittal axis of the body and laterally away from the body. The shoulder is the axis and the forearm the indicator of motion (Fig. 1–32 A). The normal range of medial rotation is 50 to 60 degrees (the chest wall blocks its motion), and the normal range of lateral rotation is 40 to 45 degrees. Rotation of the shoulder may also be tested with the neutral "zero" position of the shoulder at 90 degrees of elevation and 90 degrees of abduction; in medial rotation the

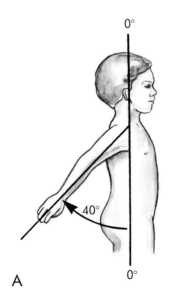

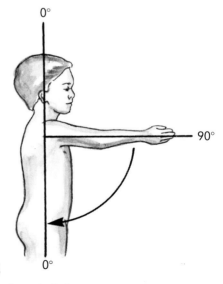

FIGURE 1–31. *Motions of the shoulder in the sagittal plane.*

A. Extension (backward). **B.** Flexion (forward).

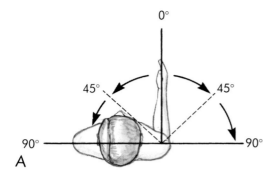

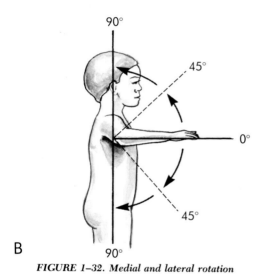

A. With the arm at the side of the body. **B.** With the shoulder at 90 degrees of elevation and 90 degrees of abduction.

FIGURE 1–32. *Medial and lateral rotation of the shoulder.*

arm is moved inferiorly, whereas in lateral rotation it is moved superiorly (Fig. 1–32 B).

A rapid way to assess active range of shoulder motion is to ask the patient to do the following: With his elbows straight and forearms in full supination, to raise both arms vertically and touch his fingers over his head—this tests range of shoulder elevation (Fig. 1–33 A). To place both hands behind his neck and push his elbows posteriorly—this tests range of active horizontal abduction and lateral rotation (Fig. 1–33 B). To reach across his chest and touch the opposite shoulder—this determines the active range of medial rotation and adduction (Fig. 1–33 C). To reach behind his back and touch the lower angle of the opposite scapula—this tests active

range of extension, medial rotation, and adduction (Fig. 1–33 D). To reach behind his head-neck and touch the upper angle of the opposite scapula—this tests the range of elevation, medial rotation, and adduction of the shoulder (Fig. 1–33 E). To reach behind his back and touch his opposite buttock with his hand—this tests extension, adduction, and medial rotation (Fig. 1–33 F).

Motor Power—Muscle Testing

Muscle strength and power may be classified as *kinetic* or *static*, kinetic being the force exerted in changing position, and static being the force exerted in resisting movement. Kinetic power is tested by having the patient carry out movements against the resistance of the examiner or of the force of gravity. Static power is tested by having him resist active attempts by the examiner to move specific parts. *Paresis* or *weakness* is the term used when there is impairment of strength, while the term *paralysis* denotes total loss of strength.

Muscle weakness is manifested not only by loss of kinetic and static power, but also by fatigability, decreased rate and irregularity and clumsiness of motion, tremulousness, incoordination, and diminished ability to perform skilled acts.

If muscle weakness is found, one should determine whether it is *diffuse* or *localized*. Diffuse (or generalized) muscle weakness is encountered in myopathies such as the dystrophies, electrolyte disturbances, toxic and deficiency states, and various types of myositis and myasthenia gravis. If localized (or focal) loss of muscle strength is found, one must determine whether it is due to involvement of a specific *muscle*, of various muscles supplied by one *nerve*, of a group of muscles supplied by a certain *segment of the spinal cord*, of a specific *movement* involving more than one muscle, or of an *entire limb*. Paralysis of one limb is termed *monoplegia*. More than one limb may be involved, in which case the terms used are: *hemiplegia*—one half of the body; *paraplegia*—the lower limbs; *quadriplegia* or *tetraplegia*—all four limbs.

If muscle weakness is present one must determine its degree, character, and cause. Is the paralysis flaccid or spastic? Are there associated sensory changes? What are the reflex changes? What is the degree of muscular atrophy? Is there pseudohypertrophy? Is there fibrillation or fasciculation? When a muscle is maintained in a shortened contracted position for a period

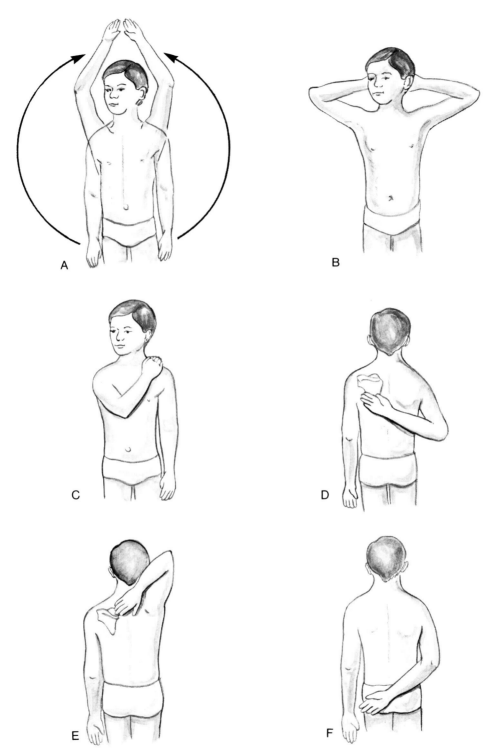

FIGURE 1–33. Rapid way of assessing active range of shoulder motions.

A. Elevation of both shoulders. **B.** Horizontal abduction and lateral rotation. **C.** Medial rotation and adduction. **D.** Extension, medial rotation, and adduction. **E.** Elevation, medial rotation, and adduction. **F.** Extension, adduction, and medial rotation.

of time, a *myostatic contracture* may develop; the muscle cannot be stretched to its original normal length. Myostatic contractures may develop from the overaction of one group of muscles when unopposed by weakened antagonists or following prolonged spasm of muscles, as seen in acute poliomyelitis or in association with spastic paralysis. Contractures may cause deformities of the bones and joints. One should determine whether the deformity itself is increasing the muscle weakness. Is there any pain associated with active or passive motion? Every effort should be made to determine whether limitation or absence of motion is the result of paralysis, involuntary or voluntary muscle spasm, swelling of the joint, or fibrous or bony ankylosis. Finally, one should decide whether the muscle weakness is a reversible process or a fixed state, and whether tendon transfers or transplants can be performed to improve function.

The degree of muscle weakness is objectively graded and recorded on a muscle chart so that the progress of the motor strength can be followed by comparative tests. The original muscle test was developed by Lovett and Martin.[59] The muscle's ability to move the part against gravity or added resistance is used to grade its function. An acceptable classification and the chart used by the author for recording muscle strength are shown in Tables 1–3 to 1–5 in the Appendix to Chapter 1. Innervation of the muscles responsible for movements of the shoulder and upper limb is shown in Table 1–6, and of the muscles responsible for movements of the lower limbs, in Table 1–7.

Examination for muscle weakness in infants and small children is difficult. One can readily detect gross defects in movement by observing the spontaneous activity of the infant and watching the small child play. Methods that stimulate reflexes such as the Moro can also be used.[55, 101]

Neurologic Assessment

A thorough neurologic examination is important in the diagnosis of the disorders of the musculoskeletal system. This is especially true whenever there is evidence of muscle weakness, incoordination, or other disturbances in neuromuscular function. The deep and superficial reflexes, sensory function, cranial nerves, and mental and emotional status should be appraised. For details of neurologic examination, the reader is referred to the works of DeJong, of Thomas, Chesni, and Saint-Anne,

of Paine and Oppé, of Denny-Brown, and of Farmer.*

In the neonatal period and in infancy, a number of primitive reflexes are present and should be examined routinely. For proper appraisal and interpretation of the reactions in the newborn, McGraw presented the following propositions:

1. Two major divisions of the central nervous system controlling neuromuscular functions are (a) the cerebral cortex, and (b) the subcortical nuclei. The subcortical nuclei constitute a more primitive part of the brain than the cortex. The cells of the subcortical nuclei begin to mature and are ready for action much earlier than are the cells in the cortex.

2. At the time of birth the cerebral cortex of the human infant is not functioning to any appreciable degree as a mechanism for controlling behavior. Therefore, the behavior patterns characteristic of the newborn infant are mediated by the subcortical nuclei.

3. Some functions remain essentially under the dominance of subcortical centers throughout life.

4. Some striking behavior patterns of the newborn infant appear to be only residuals of phylogenetic functions which have lost their usefulness to the human species.

5. As the cerebral cortex develops, it exercises a controlling influence over neuromuscular functions and also an inhibitory influence upon activities of the subcortical nuclei.

6. Developmental changes in overt behavior are associated with advancement in cortical maturation. Cortical maturation is reflected in behavior by the suppression or diminution of certain activities and by the emergence and integration of other neuromuscular performances.

7. Development tends to proceed in a cephalocaudal direction.[85]

The important reflexes and reactions are briefly described next and are summarized in Figure 1–34 and Table 1–8 in the appendix. The orthopedic surgeon should be familiar with these, as there is a correlation between functional motor achievement and the underlying reflex structure. The reflexes should not appear to be stereotyped or obligatory in nature.

Hand Grasp Reflex. If the examiner's finger or an object (such as a pencil, rod, or the empty case of a thermometer) is introduced into the palm from the ulnar side, flexor tonus is enhanced and the fingers will flex and grip the object (Fig. 1–35 A). The thumb will not oppose the fingers, but will flex with them if it was in extended position before. If one pulls on the object that the newborn is grasping, the flexor

---

*See references 64, 66, 68, 90, 94.

NEUROPHYSIOLOGIC MATURATION CHART

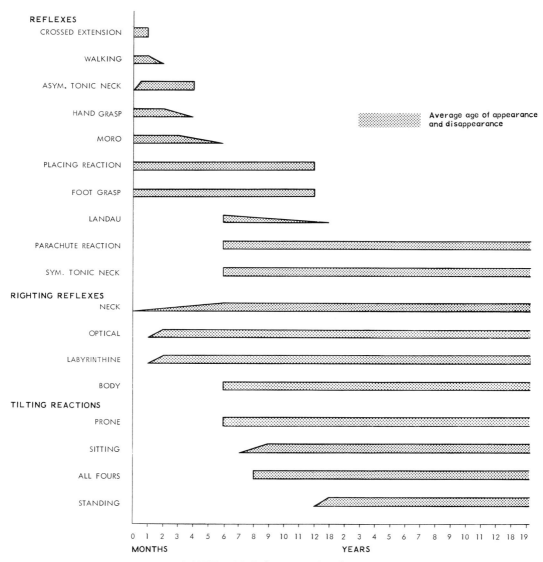

FIGURE 1–34. *Reflex maturation chart.*

tone is increased synergistically in other flexor muscles of the upper extremity and is facilitated by stretch, making his grip so strong that he can be suspended by the object he is holding (Fig. 1–35 B). During the test the head should be in the midline; if it is not, the grasp reflex is more pronounced on the side to which the occiput is directed. The hand will open on tactile stimulation over the dorsum; hence, it should not be touched during the test. This is an example of conflict between reflexes.

The hand grasp reflex is present in the newborn and in very young infants, and it disappears at the age of from two to four months. It is assessed as to its intensity, symmetry, and persistence after it should have disappeared. In older persons, the hand grasp reflex is inhibited by the action of pyramidal and premotor cortices and occurs only as a release phenomenon. In infants, its persistence after four months of age may indicate spastic cerebral palsy. It may be asymmetrical in spastic hemiplegia. The

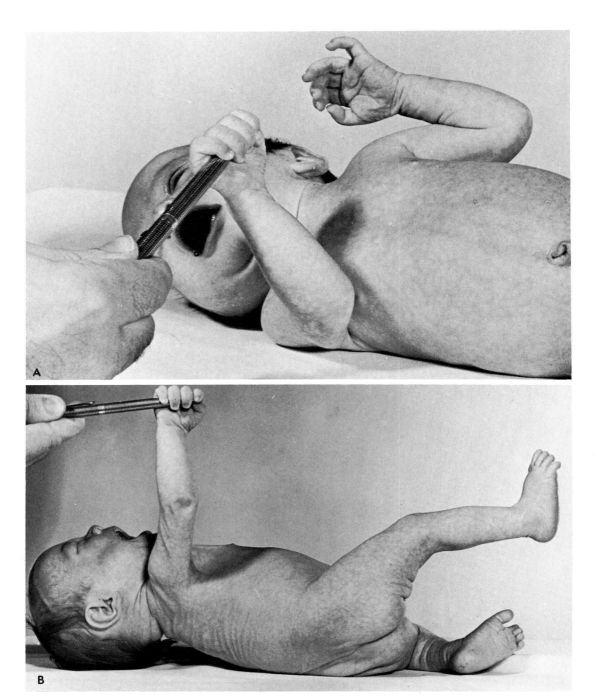

FIGURE 1–35. Hand grasp reflex.

When the reflex is strong, the infant can be suspended by the object he is holding.

hand grasp reflex is strongest at birth, and its absence on one side may indicate flaccid paralysis, such as that seen in obstetrical brachial plexus paralysis.

Plantar Grasp Reflex. There is a very similar grasp reflex in the foot. Tonic flexion and adduction of the toes will occur upon light digital pressure on the plantar surface of the foot, especially in its distal portion just proximal to the toes (Fig. 1–36). The plantar grasp reflex is present in the newborn infant and disappears by the end of the first year, but it may persist in children with birth injuries and retarded development.

Moro Reflex. Since its original description by Moro, in 1918, much has been written about this important reflex.[89] Mitchell presented an excellent review of the literature.[88]

The patient is placed supine with both upper and lower extremities fully extended. The response can be elicited by a variety of stimuli that have in common sudden extension of the neck. One may support the back of the head on the palm of the hand several inches above the table and then suddenly drop the hand (Fig. 1–37 A); or the baby may be gently raised slightly off the table by holding his hands and then rapidly releasing them, causing sudden extension of the cervical spine (Fig. 1–37 B). Other methods are a sharp bang on the table (Fig. 1–37 C) or a sudden tap on the abdomen.

The reflex consists of abduction and extension of all four extremities and extension of the spine, with extension and fanning of the digits except for flexion of the distal phalanges of the index finger and thumb (Fig. 1–37 D). This phase is followed in turn by flexion and adduction of the extremities as if in an embrace. The reflex may also be accompanied by crying.

The Moro reflex is present during the first three months of life; then the response gradually disappears by four to six months of age, probably with the development of myelinization.

Abnormalities of the Moro response may be found in various conditions. It may be asymmetrical in peripheral nerve injury, such as obstetrical brachial plexus paralysis, in fracture of the clavicle or humerus, and in spastic hemiplegia. A positive response after the age of six months indicates delayed maturation of the central nervous system, such as that seen in cerebral palsy. It may be decreased in severe hypertonicity, the increased muscle tone preventing full motion of the extremities. Depending upon the grade of hypertonicity, the hands may fail to open at the height of the reflex, the limbs may move partially, or one may be unable to elicit the reflex because the extremities are so tightly flexed. The Moro reflex may be decreased or absent in conditions of generalized muscle weakness or marked hypotonicity, such as amyotonia congenita. In premature infants, because of the weakness of the antigravity muscles, the extremities tend to fall backward to the bed during the adduction phase.

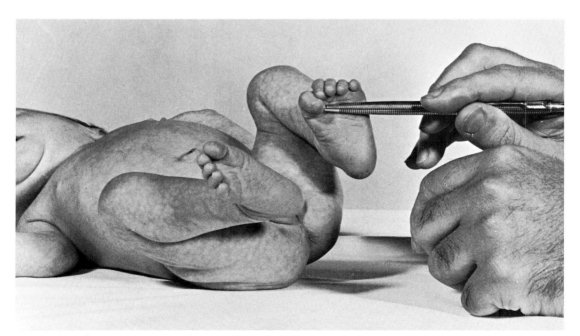

FIGURE 1–36. Plantar grasp reflex.

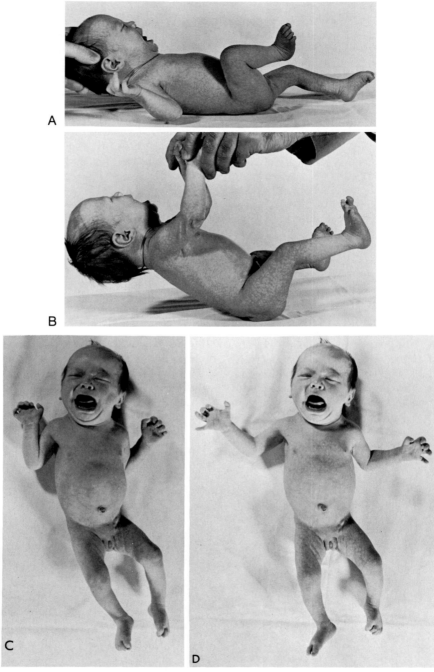

FIGURE 1–37. *Moro reflex.*

Methods of eliciting the reflex by suddenly dropping the head, **A,** sudden extension of the neck, **B,** or a sharp bang on the table, **C** and **D.** The response—note the abduction and extension of the extremities and extension of the spine.

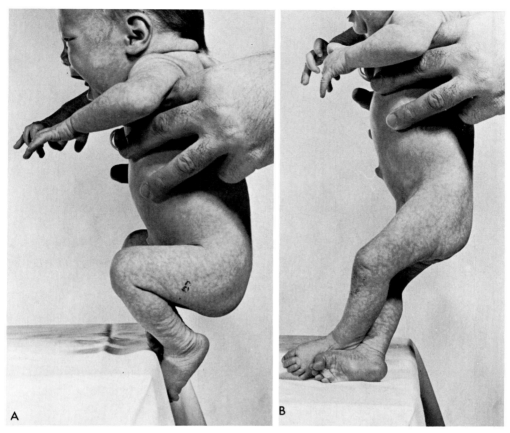

FIGURE 1–38. Placing reaction with lower limbs.

When the anterior aspect of the distal tibia or dorsum of the foot is brought against the edge of the table, **A,** the infant will flex the hip and knee spontaneously, dorsiflex the ankle, and place the foot on the table, extending the lower extremity on contact of the sole with the table, **B.**

Startle Reflex. This should not be confused with the Moro reflex. In the startle reflex, elicited by a sudden loud noise or by tapping the sternum, the elbows are flexed (not extended, as in the Moro response), and the hands remain closed.

Placing Reaction and Walking or Stepping Reflex. To elicit the placing reaction, the infant is supported upright from the waist and the anterior aspect of the distal tibia or dorsum of the foot is brought against the edge of a table. The infant will flex the hip and knee spontaneously, dorsiflex the ankle, and place the foot on the table, extending the lower limb on active or passive contact of the sole with the table (Fig. 1–38). In the upper limb, the placing reaction can be obtained by bringing the dorsum of the ulna against the edge of a table (Fig. 1–39). One should distinguish this from voluntary placing in older children. Normally the placing reaction is consistently present at birth

in full-term infants. Its absence suggests brain damage.

To obtain the walking or stepping reflex, the infant is held upright with the soles of his feet pressing on the table or ground and he is gently moved forward. This initiates reciprocal flexion and extension of the lower limbs, simulating walking (Fig. 1–40). This automatic walking reflex should not be confused with mature, independent walking, as there is neither balancing nor associated movement of the upper limbs. Automatic reflex walking can be elicited only in forward motion; it does not take place to movement backward. The walking reflex disappears in normal children by the age of one to two months.

Crossed Extension Reflex. When one lower limb is held extended at the knee and the firm pressure is applied to its sole by rubbing or stroking, the opposite free leg flexes, adducts, and then extends. There may be fanning of the

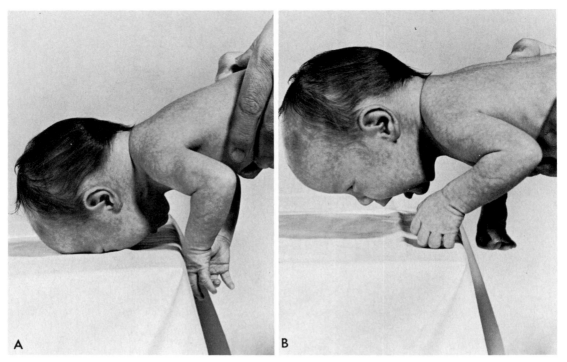

FIGURE 1–39. Placing reaction with upper limbs.

The dorsum of the ulna is brought against the edge of a table, **A,** to elicit the placing reaction, **B.**

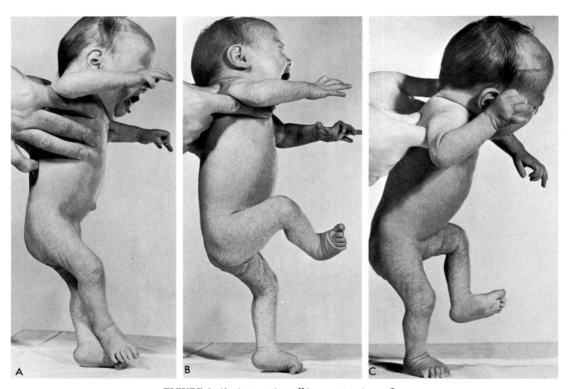

FIGURE 1–40. Automatic walking or stepping reflex.

Holding the infant upright with his feet pressing on the table, **A,** initiates automatic "walking," **B** and **C.**

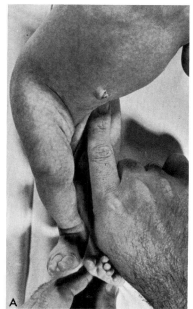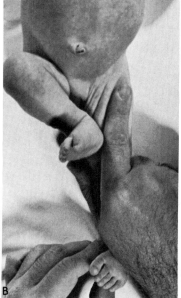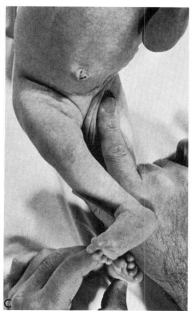

FIGURE 1–41. Crossed extension reflex.

A. Method of stimulation. **B.** Note the flexion and abduction of opposite hip and then, **C,** adduction and extension as if the infant were trying to push away the noxious stimulus.

toes (Fig. 1–41). One gets the impression that the infant is trying to push away the stimulating agent. The stimulation of the sole of the foot causes flexion of the ipsilateral limb, moving it away from the stimulus, and extension of the contralateral limb, moving it toward the stimulus. In newborn infants, one may elicit a similar response by applying strong pressure in the inguinal region, inducing flexion of the ipsilateral limb and extension of the contralateral hip and knee. The crossed extension reflex, or *phénomène d'allongement croisé,* sometimes known as *Philippson's reflex,* is not normally obtained after the first month. Its persistence is indicative of partial, or incomplete, spinal lesion.

Withdrawal Reflex. In the withdrawal reflex, a pinprick applied to the sole of the foot causes dorsiflexion of the ankle, and flexion of the knee and hip, which draws the limb away from the noxious stimulus. The withdrawal reflex is absent or weak in infants born with meningomyelocele and in children with paralysis due to other intraspinal lesions.

Positive Support Response or Leg Straightening Reflex. The patient is held in standing position, and the soles of the feet are pressed to the ground or table several times. When the support response is positive, upon contact of the feet with the ground, the lower limbs and

trunk will go into extension. The legs thereby serve as strong supporting pillars for weight-bearing. The positive support response is normal up to four months of age. For further motor development this reflex should disappear. If it does persist, reciprocal leg movements cannot appear and the infant is neither able to stand nor to walk.

Extensor Thrust. When pressure is applied to the sole of the foot with the lower limb in a flexed position, the infant will suddenly extend the entire leg. This extension is sometimes followed by flexion. The extensor thrust response is normal up to two months of age. Its persistence indicates brain damage and delayed maturation of the central nervous system.

Galant's Reflex or Trunk Incurvation. With the infant in a prone position, the lateral aspect of the back in the lumbar region is stimulated with the index finger (Fig. 1–42). When the reflex is present, the trunk will flex toward the side of the stimulus. A similar response of trunk flexion to the side stimulated is obtained by pricking the outer side of the gluteal area.

Tonic Neck Reflexes. In the decorticate animal, changes in the position of the head relative to position of the body result in reflex modifications of the tonus and position of the limbs.[81] These reflex manifestations are responses to afferent stimuli arising in neck muscles and also

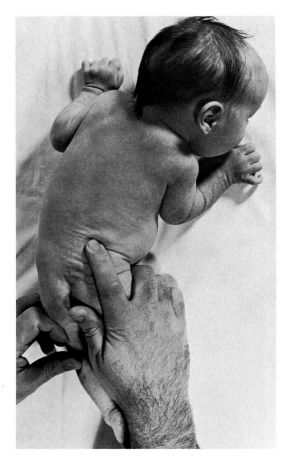

FIGURE 1–42. *Galant's reflex or trunk incurvation.*

to labyrinthine stimuli. Similar reflexes are elicited by carrying out similar maneuvers after section of the cervical nerve roots.

There are both asymmetrical and symmetrical tonic neck reflexes. To elicit the *asymmetrical tonic neck reflex*, the infant is placed in the supine position, and the head is rotated without flexion to one side, kept rotated for five to ten seconds, and then rotated to the other side. In the presence of a positive response, the arm on the side toward which the chin is rotated becomes rigid and goes into extension and the leg may go into extension as well, whereas on the "occiput" side, the arm goes into flexion and the leg may also flex (Fig. 1–43). The grasp reflex may be more readily elicited on the side of flexion. The asymmetrical tonic neck reflex normally disappears by the age of four to six months. In pathologic states, such as severe cerebral palsy, it persists and may even increase. Increased extensor tonus on the "chin" side and increased flexor tonus on the "occiput" side may be the only finding when the positive response is weak.

In the *symmetrical tonic neck reflex*, when the head and neck are extended, the arms extend and the legs go into flexion, whereas when the neck is flexed, the arms flex and the legs go into extension. The symmetrical tonic neck reflex is tested by having the patient rest in prone position over the examiner's knee. On flexion of the neck-head, the arms flex or flexor tone increases, and the legs extend or extensor tone increases. On extension of the head-neck, the arms extend or extensor tone increases, and the legs flex or flexor tone increases (Fig. 1–44). The symmetrical tonic neck reflex is normally present by six months of age. There is no absolute time for its disappearance.

Landau Reflex. To elicit the Landau reflex, the child is held in the air in the prone position with the examiner's hand supporting him under his abdomen and thorax. The child's body should be parallel with the floor. One should note whether the neck, spine, and hips assume a hyperextended position or whether the child hangs them lifelessly. The head is first flexed and then extended and the respective positions

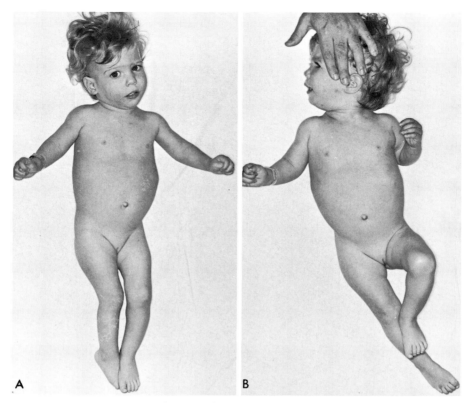

FIGURE 1–43. *Asymmetrical tonic neck reflex persisting in a child with cerebral palsy.*

A. The arm on the side toward which the chin is rotated goes into extension, whereas, **B,** the arm on the opposite side goes into flexion.

of the limbs and trunk are noted. The Landau reflex is positive when, on passive flexion of the head with the body in extended position, the trunk, arms, and legs go into flexion; and, when the head is extended, the limbs and body are brought into the extended position.

The presence of a Landau reflex is normal from six months to two and one half years of age. If elicited beyond two and a half years of age, delayed reflex maturation is suggested.

Parachute Reaction or Protective Extension of Arms Reflex. The patient is suspended in the air by the waist in the prone position, and his head is moved suddenly toward the floor. When a positive response is present, the child will immediately extend his arms and wrists to protect his head, as if to break the force of the fall (Fig. 1–45). The parachute reaction appears at about six months of age and remains throughout life. It can be obtained in blindfolded children, as it does not depend on vision. Absence of response indicates severe brain damage.

Righting Reflexes. These are complex reflexes, of which there are several distinct types.

Neck Righting Reflex. To obtain this reflex, the child is placed supine with the head in mid-position and all four limbs fully extended. The head is rotated to one side, and this position is maintained to the count of 10. When the reflex is present the body will rotate *as a whole* in the same direction as the head; when it is absent the body will not rotate. The afferent impulses in this reflex originate in the musculotendinous and other deep structures in the neck; they are mediated through the upper three cervical nerves and segments, acting principally on the head and neck, and secondarily on the body as a whole. The neck righting reflex is normally present between birth and six months of age. If it is absent after the first month, delayed reflex maturation is again indicated.

Body Righting Reflex. To elicit this reflex, the same test position and stimulus are used, but on rotation of the head, the body, instead of rotating as a whole, rotates cephalocaudally in segments, i.e., the head turns, then shoulders and trunk, and finally the pelvis. This reflex appears at six months of age.

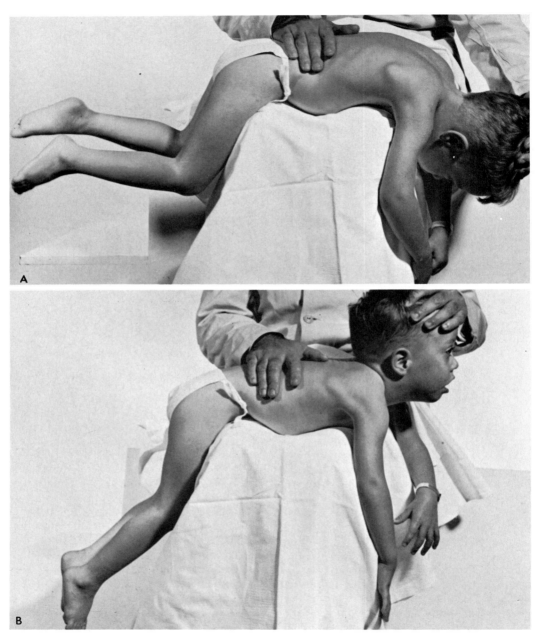

FIGURE 1–44. *Symmetrical tonic reflex in a child with cerebral palsy.*

A. Position of child to test reflex. **B.** On extension of the head and neck the arms extend and the legs flex; on flexion of the head and neck the arms flex and the legs extend.

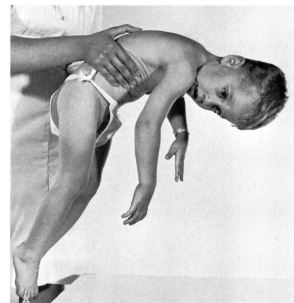

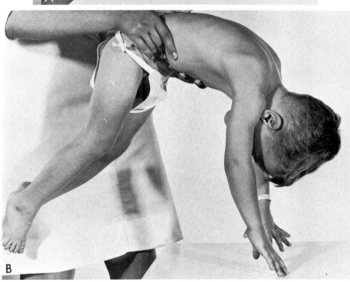

FIGURE 1–45. Protective extension of arms reflex.

When the patient is suspended prone, **A,** and his head is suddenly moved toward the floor, his arms and wrists extend to break his fall, **B.**

Labyrinthine Righting Reflexes. In testing labyrinthine righting reflexes, the patient is blindfolded to rule out optical righting reflexes. First, the child is held in *prone* position in space; when the reflex is present, the head will extend, bringing the face perpendicular to the floor. The labyrinthine righting reflex in prone position appears at one to two months of age and persists throughout life. When it is absent after two months of age, delayed neurophysiologic maturation is suggested. Next, the blindfolded child is placed in *supine* position in space. The presence of the reflex is indicated by extension of the neck and head, bringing the

face perpendicular to the floor. This reflex appears at six months of age and continues throughout life. Then, the child, again blindfolded, is held vertically in space by supporting him at his pelvis. When the patient is tilted to the right or to the left, the head will automatically right itself to the vertical position with the mouth horizontal if the reflex is present. This reflex appears at about six to eight months of age and persists throughout life.

Optical Righting Reflexes. Tests are performed with the child's eyes open (Fig. 1–46). The test positions and stimuli are similar to those for labyrinthine righting reflexes; namely,

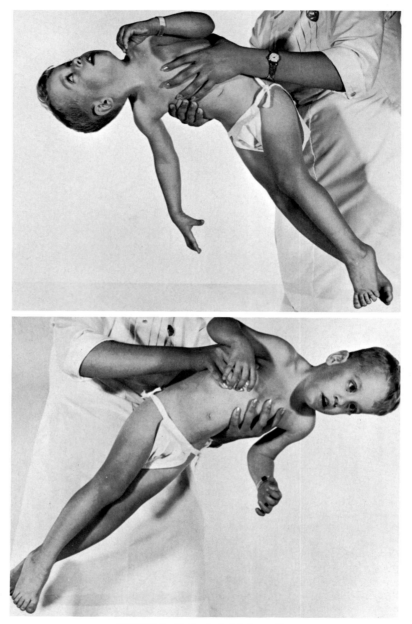

FIGURE 1–46. Optical righting reflex.

The reflex is absent in this six-year-old child with spastic cerebral palsy. It should normally appear at six to eight months of age and persist thereafter.

prone and supine, and tilting of the head to the right and left. The optical righting reflexes appear at the same age as labyrinthine righting reflexes.

Oral Reflexes. The following two reflexes are present in all full-term newborns. Their absence is indicative of a severe developmental defect or marked prematurity. The *sucking reflex* is elicited by introducing a nipple or a finger into the mouth.

The *"rooting"* or *"search" reflexes* are the same as the "cardinal points reflexes" of the French writers. When the infant's cheek touches the breast, he "roots" for milk, enabling him to find the nipple without being directed to it. When the corner of the mouth is lightly stimulated by a finger, the lower lip is lowered on the same side, and the tongue moves toward it. When the examiner's finger slides away from that point, the head rotates to follow it. If the center of the upper lip is lightly touched, the lip elevates, and the tongue moves toward it. When the finger slides upward along the oronasal groove, the head extends. Upon stimulation of the center of the bottom lip, the lip is lowered and the tongue moves toward it. If the finger slides toward the chin, the mandible is depressed and the neck flexes. The oral reflexes are best elicited when the infant is hungry, just prior to his feeding period.

Tilting Reactions. Tilting reactions are tests for maturation of equilibrium. The center of gravity is changed when the body is in different postures, and protective adaptive responses are observed. There are several levels of performance.

1. The patient is placed *prone* on a flat board with all four limbs fully extended, and the board is tilted to one side. In the presence of a positive tilting response the arm and leg on the raised side go into abduction and extension, the head and thorax are righted, and the arm and leg on the lowered side assume the protective posture. The same test is performed with the child in supine position. The tilting reaction in prone position appears at about six months of age, and in supine position at seven months; both continue throughout life.

2. The child is *seated* on the examining table or on a low chair and tilted to either side. When the response is positive, there are righting of head, neck, and trunk; extension-abduction of the extremities on the raised side; and protective reaction on the lowered side. The positive response appears between seven and nine months of age.

3. The patient is placed *on all fours* and tilted to either side. A positive reaction consists of abduction-extension of the arm and leg on the raised side with extension of head and neck, and protective response of the limbs on the lowered side. The response first appears at about eight months of age and is well established by 12 months. It persists throughout life.

4. The patient, supported from the waist, is held in *standing* position with the feet bearing as much weight as possible. Moved first to either side, then forward and backward, he hops to maintain his balance (Fig. 1–47). The hopping reaction appears between 12 and 18 months.

Motor Evaluation

In the diagnosis and management of disorders of the neuromusculoskeletal system in children, an evaluation of the motor development is imperative. Gesell, Shirley, McGraw, and Zausmer have studied the subject intensively and the reader is referred to their publications.* The importance of determining the quality of motor performance while recording the level of achievement has been emphasized by Zausmer. In its assessment, one has to consider independence and correctness of execution, coordination, rhythm, speed, and endurance.

Zausmer has described the following scale:

O— No attempt has been made.

T— An attempt has been made, thus expressing a certain amount of motivation and understanding of the test situation; however, the additional motivation, understanding, or capacity to perform the act is still missing.

TT— A higher level of motivation and perseverance has been attained. The patient, however, still shows the lack of capacity to achieve the goal even partially.

P— In this category the quality of performance is analyzed. Complete independence has not yet been reached; the patient performs partially, though correctness, coordination, and rhythm have not yet been attained. The pattern is executed poorly.

F— Independence has been reached without assistance. The patient fully achieves the goal. The quality of performance has improved, but it is not yet consistently good.

G— Endurance and speed are stressed, and there are a great number of repetitions and greater speed. The patient shows consistent correctness, coordination, and rhythm—a good pattern.

N— While the preceding grade (G) expressed a still existing need and possibility for growth

---

*See references 72–74, 85, 93, 100–102.

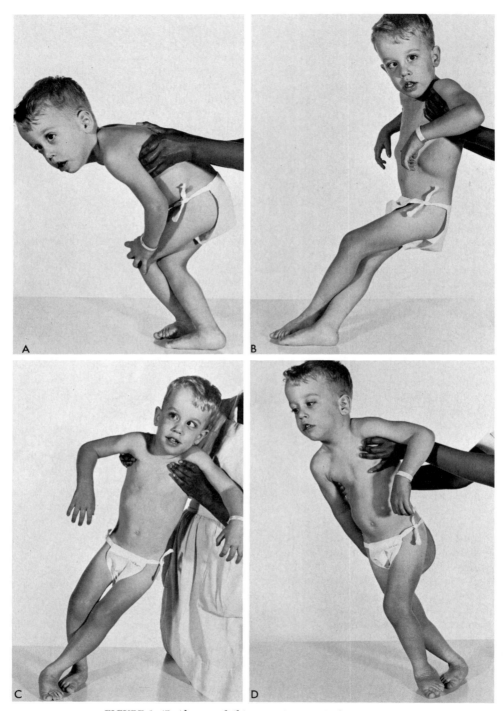

FIGURE 1–47. *Absence of tilting reactions in standing position.*

Normally they should appear between 12 and 18 months. In this six-year-old child with cerebral palsy they are absent: **A** and **B**, on moving forward and backward; **C** and **D**, on moving sideways.

and perfection in all areas of the performance, the N represents the top grade for the performance expected at a given age.[101, 102]

Motor development levels are given in Table 1–9 in the appendix to this chapter.

Zausmer and Tower have also described a quotient for evaluation of motor development that is not widely used.[102] It has definite advantages, as it serves to compare a patient's motor development with that in normal children. It detects and analyzes differences of behavior in separate areas of motor development, observing and recording objectively the course, character, and rate of changes. It requires a therapist, however, who is specially trained to administer such a motor quotient test.

References

1. Hoppenfeld, S.: Physical Examination of the Spine and Extremities. New York, Appleton-Century-Crofts, 1976.
2. McRae, R.: Clinical Orthopaedic Examination. Edinburgh, London, New York, Churchill-Livingstone, 1976.
3. Nicholson, J. T., and Qualls, D. M.: Early evaluation of musculoskeletal lesion by the pediatrician. Pediatr. Clin. North Am., 6:1163, 1959.
4. Salter, R. B.: Textbook of Disorders and Injuries of the Musculoskeletal System. 2nd Ed. Baltimore, Williams & Wilkins, 1983.
5. Wightman, K. J. R.: Patient Examination and History Taking. Canada, Collier-Macmillan, 1977.
6. Zeide, M. S., and Robbins, H.: Glossary of eponyms: Orthopaedic signs, lines and tests. Bull. Hosp. J. Dis., 36:177–206, 1975.
7. Zohn, D. A., and McMannell, J.: Musculoskeletal Pain: Diagnosis and Physical Treatment. Boston, Little, Brown, 1976.

GAIT

8. Anderson, M. J., Bray, J. J., and Hennessy, C. A.: Prosthetic Principles—Above Knee Amputations. Springfield, Ill., Thomas, 1960.
9. Bowker, J. B., and Hall, C. B.: Normal human gait. *In* American Academy of Orthopedic Surgeons: Atlas of Orthotics. St. Louis, Mosby, 1975, p. 134.
10. Burnett, C. N., and Johnson, E. W.: Development of gait in childhood. Part I: Method. Dev. Med. Child Neurol., 13:196, 1971.
11. Burnett, C. N., and Johnson, E. W.: Development of gait in childhood. Part II. Dev. Med. Child Neurol., 13:207, 1971.
12. Close, J. R., Inman, V. T., Poor, P. M., and Todd, F. N.: The function of the subtalar joint. Clin. Orthop., 50:159, 1967.
13. Elftman, H.: The transverse tarsal joint and its control. Clin. Orthop., 16:41, 1960.
14. Hargreaves, P., and Scales, J. T.: Clinical assessment of gait using load measuring footwear. Acta Orthop. Scand., 46:877, 1975.
15. Holt, K. S.: Facts and fallacies about neuromuscular function in cerebral palsy as revealed by electromyography. Dev. Med. Child Neurol., 8:2255, 1966.
16. Inman, V. T.: Conservation of energy in ambulation. Bull. Prosthet. Res., 10–9:26, 1968.
17. Jacobs, N. A., Skorecki, J., and Charnley, J.: Analysis of the vertical component of force in normal and pathological gait. J. Biomech., 5:11, 1972.
18. Levans, A. S., Inman, V. T., and Blosser, J. A.: Transverse rotation of the segments of the lower extremity in locomotion. J. Bone Joint Surg., 30-A:859, 1948.
19. Peizer, E., Wright, D. W., and Mason, C.: Human locomotion. Bull. Prosthet. Res., 10–12:48, 1969.
20. Perry, J., and Hoffer, M. M.: Preoperative and postoperative dynamic electromyography as an aid in planning tendon transfers in children with cerebral palsy. J. Bone Joint Surg., 59–A:531, 1977.
21. Saunders, J. B. M., Inman, V. T., and Eberhart, H. D.: The major determinants in normal and pathological gait. J. Bone Joint Surg., 35–A:543, 1953.
22. Sheridan, M. D.: The developmental progress of infants and young children. H.M.S.O. (London), Ministry of Health Report No. 102, 1960.
23. Shirley, M.: The First Two Years. Minneapolis, University of Minnesota Monogram Series No. 4, 1931, No. 7, 1933.
24. Smidt, G. L., and Wadsworth, J. B.: Floor reaction forces during gait: Comparison of patients with hip disease and normal subjects. Phys. Ther., 53:1056, 1973.
25. Steindler, A.: The pathomechanics of the gait: *In* Kinesiology of the Human Body. Springfield, Ill., Thomas, 1970, Lecture 28, pp. 665–691.
26. Stott, J. R. R., Hutton, W. C., and Stokes, I. A. F.: Forces under the foot. J. Bone Joint Surg., 55–B:335, 1973.
27. Sutherland, D. H.: Gait Disorders in Children and Adolescents. Baltimore, Williams & Wilkins, 1984.
28. Sutherland, D. H., Olshen, R., Cooper, L., and Woo, S. L.–Y.: The development of mature gait. J. Bone Joint Surg., 62–A:336, 1980.

DEFORMITIES

29. Houston, C. S.: Varus and valgus. No wonder they are confused. N. Engl. J. Med., 302:471, 1980.
30. Ober, F. R.: The role of the iliotibial band and fascias: A factor in the causation of low back disabilities and sciatica. J. Bone Joint Surg., 18:185, 1936.
31. Thomas, H. O.: Diseases of the Hip, Knee, and Ankle Joints with Their Deformities Treated by a New and Efficient Method. Liverpool, J. Dobb & Co., 1875; Boston, reproduced by Little, Brown, 1962.
32. Trendelenburg, F.: Ueber den Gang bei Angeborener Huftgelenksluxation. Deutsch. Med. Wochenschr., 21:21, 1895.

RANGE OF MOTION OF JOINTS

33. Allander, E., Björnsson, O. J., Olafsson, O., Sigfusson, N., and Thorsteinsson, J.: Normal range of joint movements in shoulder, hip, wrist and thumb with special reference to side: A comparison between two populations. Int. J. Epidemiol., 3:253, 1974.
34. American Academy of Orthopedic Surgeons, Committee for the Study of Joint Motion: Method of Measuring and Recording Joint Motion. Chicago, American Academy of Orthopedic Surgeons, 1965.
35. Boone, D. C., and Azen, S. P.: Normal range of motion of joints in male subjects. J. Bone Joint Surg., 61–A:756, 1979.
36. Boone, D. C., Azen, S. P., Lin, C.–M., Spence, C., Baron, C., and Lee, L: Reliability of goniometric measurements. Phys. Ther., 58:1355, 1978.
37. Cave, E. F., and Roberts, S. M.: A method for measuring and recording joint function. J. Bone Joint Surg., 18:455, 1936.

38. Coon, V., Donato, G., Houser, C., and Bleck, E. E.: Normal ranges of hip motion in infants six weeks, three months and six months of age. Clin. Orthop., *110*:256, 1975.

39. Darcus, H. D., and Salter, N.: The amplitude of pronation and supination with the elbow flexed to a right angle. J. Anat., *87*:169, 1953.

40. Esch, D., and Lepley, M.: Evaluation of Joint Motion: Methods of Measurement and Recording. Minneapolis, University of Minnesota Press, 1975.

41. Freedman, L., and Munro, R. R.: Abduction of the arm in the scapular plane: Scapular and glenohumeral movements. A roentgenographic study. J. Bone Joint Surg., *48–A*:1503, 1966.

42. Haas, S. S., Epps, C. H., Jr., and Adams, J. P.: Normal ranges of hip motion in the newborn. Clin. Orthop., *91*:114, 1973.

43. Kapandji, I. A.: The Physiology of the Joints. 2nd Ed. Edinburgh, Livingstone, 1970.

44. Mitchell, W. S., Millar, J., and Sturrock, R. D.: An evaluation of goniometry as an objective parameter for measuring joint motion. Scott. Med. J., *20*:57, 1975.

45. Mundale, W. O., Hislop, H. J., Rabideau, R. J., and Kottke, F. J.: Evaluation of extension of the hip. Arch. Phys. Med. Rehabil., *37*:75, 1956.

46. Nemethi, C. E.: Normal wrist motions. Ind. Med. Surg., *22*:230, 1953.

47. Russe, O., Gerhardt, J. J., and King, P. S.: ISOM—International standard orthopedic measurements: S.F.T.R. measuring and recording method. *In* Russe, O. (ed.): An Atlas of Examination. Baltimore, Williams & Wilkins, 1972, pp. 45.

48. Salter, N.: Methods of measurement of muscle and joint function. J. Bone Joint Surg., *37–B*:474, 1955.

49. Salter, N., and Darcus, H. D.: The amplitude of forearm and humeral rotation. J. Anat., *87*:407, 1953.

50. Sammarco, G. J., Burstein, A. H., and Frankel, V. H.: Biomechanics of the ankle: A kinematic study. Orthop. Clin. North Am., *4*:75, 1973.

51. Smahel, Z.: Joint motion of the child hand. Acta Chir. Plast. (Prague), *17*:113, 1975.

52. Spilman, H. W., and Pinkston, D.: Relation of test positions to radial and ulnar deviation. Phys. Ther., *49*:837, 1969.

53. Weseley, M. S., Koval, R., and Kleiger, B.: Roentgen measurement of ankle flexion-extension motion. Clin. Orthop., *65*:167, 1969.

MOTOR POWER—MUSCLE TESTING

54. Daniels, L., Williams, M., and Worthingham, C.: Muscle Testing: Techniques of Manual Examination. 3rd Ed. Philadelphia, Saunders, 1972.

55. Johnson, E. W.: Examination for muscle weakness in infants and small children. J.A.M.A., *168*:1306, 1958.

56. Johnson, M. K., Zuck, F. N., and Wingate, K.: The motor age test: Measurement of motor handicaps in children with neuromuscular disorders such as cerebral palsy. J. Bone Joint Surg., *33–A*:698, 1951.

57. Kendall, H. W., and Kendall, F. P.: Muscles: Testing and Function. 3rd Ed. Baltimore, Williams & Wilkins, 1983.

58. Kop, C. B.: Fine motor abilities of infants. Dev. Med. Child Neurol., *16*:629, 1974.

59. Lovett, R. W., and Martin, E. G.: Certain aspects of infantile paralysis; with a description of a method of muscle testing. J.A.M.A., *66*:729, 1916.

NEUROLOGIC ASSESSMENT

60. Amiel-Tison, C.: A method for neurologic evaluation within the first year of life. Curr. Probl. Pediatr., *7*:2, 1976.

61. Byers, R. K.: The functional significance of persistent tonic neck reflexes in fixed brain lesions. Trans. Am. Neurol. Assoc., *78*:207, 1953.

62. Cahuzac, M., Nichil, J., and Ousset, A.: Principles d'examen d'un infirme moteur cérébral. Rev. Chir. Orthop., *52*:375, 1966.

63. Dargassies, S. S. A.: Neurodevelopmental symptoms during the first year of life. Parts I and II. Dev. Med. Child Neurol., *14*:235, 1972.

64. DeJong, R. N.: The Neurological Examination. 4th Ed. New York, Hoeber Medical Division, Harper & Row, 1979.

65. Dekaban, A.: Neurology of Early Childhood. Baltimore, Williams & Wilkins, 1970.

66. Denny-Brown, D.: Handbook of Neurological Examination and Case Recording. Revised edition. Cambridge, Harvard University Press, 1957.

67. Dohrmann, G. J., and Nowack, W. J.: The upgoing great toe. Optimal method of elicitation. Lancet, *1*:339, 1973.

68. Farmer, T. W.: Pediatric Neurology. 3rd Ed. New York, Hoeber Medical Division, Harper & Row, 1983.

69. Fiorentino, M. R.: Reflex Testing Methods for Evaluating C. N. S. Development. 2nd Ed. Springfield, Ill., Thomas, 1981.

70. Ford, F.: Diseases of the Nervous System in Infancy, Childhood and Adolescence. 6th Ed. Springfield, Ill., Thomas, 1973.

71. Gamstorp, I.: Pediatric Neurology. New York, Appleton-Century-Crofts, 1979.

72. Gesell, A.: How a Baby Grows. New York, Harper, 1945.

73. Gesell, A., and Amatruda, C. S.: Developmental Diagnosis. 3rd Ed., Knobloch, H. and Pasamanick, B. (eds.), Hagerstown, Md. Harper & Row, 1974.

74. Gesell, A., and Amatruda, C.S.: The First Five Years of Life. New York, Harper, 1940.

75. Goldstein, K., Landis, C., Hunt, W. A., et al: Moro reflex and startle pattern. Arch. Neurol. Psychiatr., *40*:322, 1938.

76. Hogan, G. R., and Milligan, J. E.: The plantar reflex of the newborn. N. Engl. J. Med., *285*:502, 1971.

77. Hoppenfeld, S.: Orthopaedic Neurology: A Diagnostic Guide to Neurologic Levels. Philadelphia, Lippincott, 1977.

78. Illingworth, R. S.: The Development of the Infant and Young Child—Normal and Abnormal. 7th Ed. New York, London, Churchill-Livingstone, 1980.

79. Landau, W. M., and Eliasson, S. G.: Disturbances of peripheral nerve function. *In* Eliasson, S. G. (ed.): Neurological Pathophysiology. New York, Oxford University Press, 1974, pp. 49–62.

80. Macht, M. B., and Kuhn, R. A.: The occurrence of extensor spasm in patients with complete transection of the spinal cord. N. Engl. J. Med., *328*:311, 1948.

81. Magnus, R., and deKleijn, A.: Die Abhangigkeit des Tonus der Extremitatenmuske von der Kopfstellung. Pflüger. Arch. Ges. Physiol., *145*:455, 1912.

82. Marshall, J.: Observations on reflex changes in the lower limbs in spastic paraplegia in man. Brain, *77*:290, 1954.

83. McGraw, M. B.: From reflex to muscular control in the assumption of an erect posture and ambulation. Child Dev., *1–3*:291, 1930–1932.

84. McGraw, M. B.: The Moro reflex. Am. J. Dis. Child., *54*:240, 1937.

85. McGraw, M. B.: The Neuromuscular Maturation of the Human Infant. New York, Columbia University Press, 1943; reprint, New York, London, Hafner, 1963.

86. Menkes, J. H.: Textbook of Child Neurology. 2nd Ed. Philadelphia, Lea & Febiger, 1980.

87. Milani-Comparetti, A., and Gidoni, E. A.: Routine developmental examination in normal and retarded children. Dev. Med. Child Neurol., *9*:631, 1967.

88. Mitchell, R. G.: The Moro reflex. Cerebral Palsy Bull., 2:135, 1960.
89. Moro, E.: Das erste tremenon. Munchen. Med. Wochenschr., 65:1147, 1918.
90. Paine, R. S., and Oppe, T. E.: Neurological Examination of Children. London, Spastics Society/Heinemann, 1966.
91. Peterson, H. C.: Neurologic examination of the young child. Pediatr. Ann., 4:8, 1975.
92. Ross, E. D., Velez-Borras, J., and Rossman, N. P.: The significance of the Babinski sign in the newborn—a reappraisal. Pediatrics, 57:13, 1976.
93. Shirley, M.: The First Two Years. Minneapolis, University of Minnesota Monogram Series No. 4, 1931, No. 7, 1933.
94. Thomas A., Chesni, Y., and Saint-Anne, D.: The Neurological Examination of the Infant. London, National Spastics Society, 1960.
95. Volpe, J. J.: Neurology of the Newborn. Philadelphia, Saunders, 1981.
96. Watson, E. H., and Lowrey, G. H.: Growth and Development of Children. 6th Ed. Chicago, Year Book, 1973.
97. Weddell, G., Feinstein, B., and Pattle, R. E.: Electrical activity of voluntary muscle in man under normal and pathological conditions. Brain, 67:178, 1944.
98. Zappella, M.: The placing reaction in the newborn. Dev. Med. Child Neurol., 5:497, 1963.
99. Zappella, M., Foley, J., and Cookson, M.: The placing and supporting reactions in children with mental retardation. J. Ment. Defic. Res., 8:1, 1964.
100. Zausmer, E.: Evaluation of strength and motor development in infants. Phys. Ther. Rev., 33:575, 1953.
101. Zausmer, E.: The evaluation of motor development in children. J. Am. Phys. Ther. Assoc., 44:247, 1964.
102. Zausmer, E., and Tower, G.: A quotient for the evaluation of motor development. Phys. Ther., 46:725, 1966.

RADIOGRAPHY AND OTHER DIAGNOSTIC TOOLS

Radiograms are essential for evaluation of the neuromusculoskeletal system, but they should be taken discriminatively. A conscious effort should be made to minimize irradiation, as is set forth in the monograph on Radiation Protection in Pediatric Radiology published by the National Council on Radiation Protection and Measurements.[36] A meticulous history and a thorough physical examination should determine the area to be x-rayed and the particular views required. On occasion, such as in injuries to joints in children, the contralateral normal side should be radiographed for comparison. Often special views are required, and for these, one may have to use the image intensifier for proper orientation. Average ages of appearance of centers of ossification and fusion of epiphyses in the upper and lower limbs in males and females are shown in Figures 1–48, 1–49, 1–50, and 1–51.

Bone imaging with radionuclides is of tremendous value in early diagnosis of osteomyelitis, stress fracture, the battered child syndrome, and neoplastic and tumorous lesions.

These lesions appear on the scan as an area of increased radionuclide uptake—a "hot spot." In avascular necrosis of bone, especially in its early stages, there is decreased radionuclide uptake—a "cold spot." Bone scans reflect changes in the local blood flow in bone and local metabolic activity.*

Computed tomography is of great value in delineating pathologic changes in various hip conditions, such as femoral antetorsion and concentricity of reduction in congenital dislocation of the hip, in detecting tumors in bone, and in determining the exact site and extent of involvement in intraspinal lesions (especially if combined with myelography) and complex fractures of the spine and pelvis.†

Ultrasound is a noninvasive method of distinguishing fluid-filled cystic lesions from solid lesions such as in popliteal cysts. The Doppler phenomenon uses the ultrasound to assess arterial blood flow in a limb.[20]

Arthroscopy, which has revolutionized the diagnosis and treatment of joint disorders, is discussed in the chapter on joints. Arthroscopic surgery has become a common practice for removal of loose bodies, drilling defects in the articular surface of osteochondritis dissecans, shaving of chondromalacia and partial or total meniscectomy.[12, 25, 26, 28] Intrauterine diagnosis by amniocentesis and fetoscopy has made possible the prenatal diagnosis of major congenital malformations of the musculoskeletal system such as myelomeningocele and Down's syndrome.

Details of these special radiographic and imaging examinations are to be found in the appropriate sections of this book.

Normal values for blood count, blood chemistries, and cerebrospinal fluid are shown in Tables 1–10, 1–11, and 1–12 in the Appendix to Chapter 1.

Electrodiagnosis

A meticulous and thorough clinical appraisal of the neuromusculoskeletal system will often lead to correct diagnosis. On occasion, however, various electrical procedures may be utilized to bring out minimal changes of function. This is particularly true in the diagnosis, localization, and prognosis of lower motor lesions. Electrodiagnostic methods may also aid in the discrim-

---

*See references 1–3, 7–9, 11, 13, 14, 24, 27, 32, 34, 38, 39, 43.
†See references 4, 5, 16–19, 21–23, 29, 35, 37, 40, 44–46.

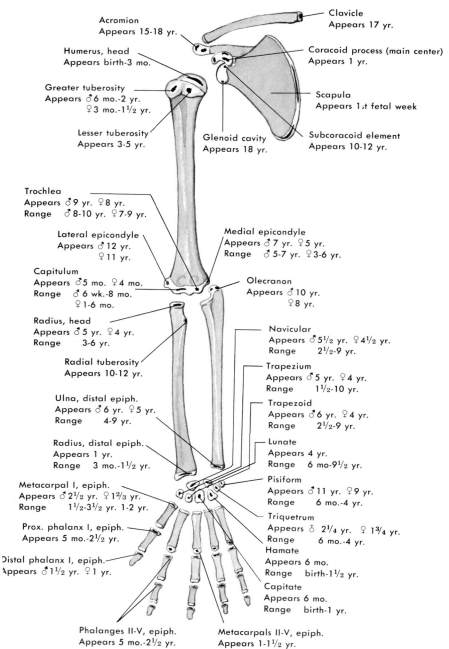

FIGURE 1–48. *Average age of appearance of centers of ossification of epiphyses in the upper limb in males and females.*

(Adapted from von Lanz, T., and Wachsmuth, W.: Praktische Anatomie. Berlin, Julius Springer, 1938, p. 28.)

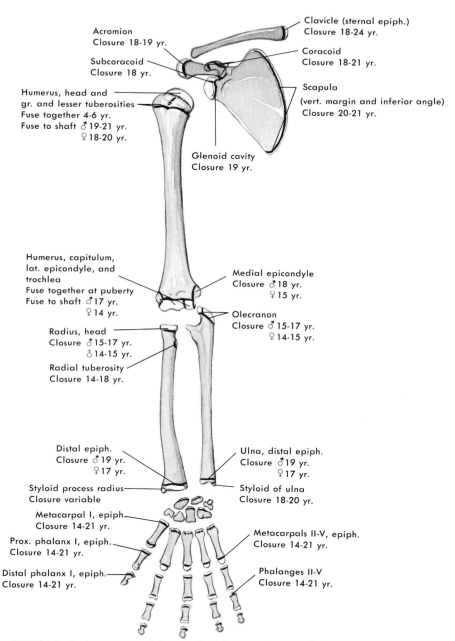

Acromion
Closure 18-19 yr.

Subcoracoid
Closure 18 yr.

Humerus, head and
gr. and lesser tuberosities
Fuse together 4-6 yr.
Fuse to shaft ♂19-21 yr.
♀18-20 yr.

Clavicle (sternal epiph.)
Closure 18-24 yr.

Coracoid
Closure 18-21 yr.

Scapula
(vert. margin and inferior angle)
Closure 20-21 yr.

Glenoid cavity
Closure 19 yr.

Humerus, capitulum,
lat. epicondyle, and
trochlea
Fuse together at puberty
Fuse to shaft ♂17 yr.
♀14 yr.

Radius, head
Closure ♂15-17 yr.
♂14-15 yr.

Radial tuberosity
Closure 14-18 yr.

Medial epicondyle
Closure ♂18 yr.
♀15 yr.

Olecranon
Closure ♂15-17 yr.
♀14-15 yr.

Distal epiph.
Closure ♂19 yr.
♀17 yr.

Styloid process radius
Closure variable

Metacarpal I, epiph.
Closure 14-21 yr.

Prox. phalanx I, epiph.
Closure 14-21 yr.

Distal phalanx I, epiph.
Closure 14-21 yr.

Ulna, distal epiph.
Closure ♂19 yr.
♀17 yr.

Styloid of ulna
Closure 18-20 yr.

Metacarpals II-V, epiph.
Closure 14-21 yr.

Phalanges II-V
Closure 14-21 yr.

FIGURE 1–49. *Average age of closure of epiphyses in the upper limb in males and females.*

(Adapted from von Lanz, T., and Wachsmuth, W.: Praktische Anatomie. Berlin, Julius Springer, 1938, p. 28.)

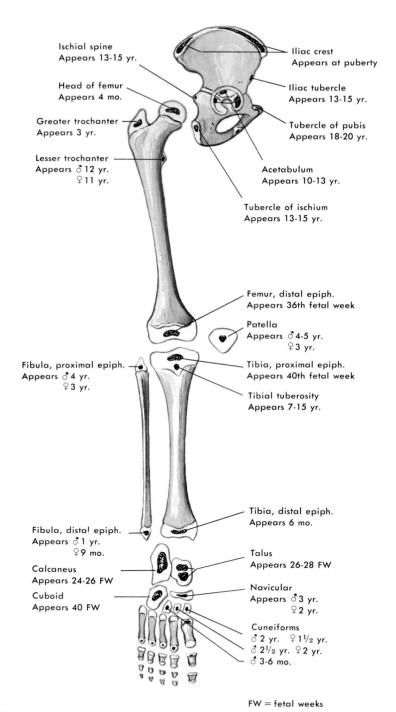

Ischial spine
Appears 13-15 yr.

Iliac crest
Appears at puberty

Head of femur
Appears 4 mo.

Iliac tubercle
Appears 13-15 yr.

Greater trochanter
Appears 3 yr.

Tubercle of pubis
Appears 18-20 yr.

Lesser trochanter
Appears ♂12 yr.
♀11 yr.

Acetabulum
Appears 10-13 yr.

Tubercle of ischium
Appears 13-15 yr.

Femur, distal epiph.
Appears 36th fetal week

Patella
Appears ♂4-5 yr.
♀3 yr.

Fibula, proximal epiph.
Appears ♂4 yr.
♀3 yr.

Tibia, proximal epiph.
Appears 40th fetal week

Tibial tuberosity
Appears 7-15 yr.

Fibula, distal epiph.
Appears ♂1 yr.
♀9 mo.

Tibia, distal epiph.
Appears 6 mo.

Talus
Appears 26-28 FW

Calcaneus
Appears 24-26 FW

Navicular
Appears ♂3 yr.
♀2 yr.

Cuboid
Appears 40 FW

Cuneiforms
♂ 2 yr.   ♀ 1½ yr.
♂ 2½ yr. ♀2 yr.
♂ 3-6 mo.

FW = fetal weeks

FIGURE 1–50. *Average age of appearance of centers of ossification of epiphyses in the lower limb in males and females.*

(Adapted from von Lanz, T., and Wachsmuth, W.: Praktische Anatomie. Berlin, Julius Springer, 1938, p. 28.)

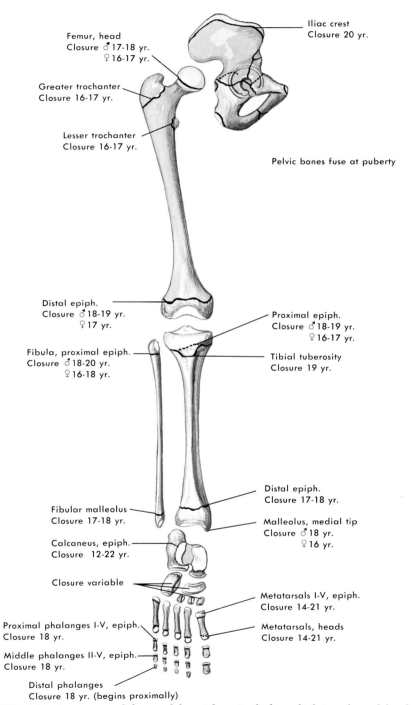

FIGURE 1–51. Average age of closure of the epiphyses in the lower limb in males and females.

(Adapted from von Lanz, T., and Wachsmuth, W.: Praktische Anatomie. Berlin, Julius Springer, 1938, p. 29.)

ination between organic and hysterical paralysis.

It is imperative that one evaluate the results of the various electrical tests as they relate to the total clinical picture. The electrical examination should not be considered a routine procedure in the diagnosis of disorders of the neuromusculoskeletal system.

The electrodiagnostic methods fall into three main groups: tests of neuromuscular excitability by percutaneous stimulation of nerves and muscles; electromyographic studies of motor unit or other muscle action potentials at rest or in action; and nerve conduction velocity studies using both stimulating and recording techniques. In this text, only general principles will be outlined. Current references are listed for more detailed information.*

TESTS OF NEUROMUSCULAR EXCITABILITY

Electrical stimulation of nerves and muscles, as described by Erb in 1883, was until just recently, the universal method of electrodiagnosis.[52] Though used less frequently now, its importance should not be minimized. Two types of current are used. *Galvanic current* (direct or continuous) stimulates both nerves and muscles, and normally produces momentary unsustained contraction of a muscle upon "making" or "breaking" of the circuit. Muscular contraction is induced through either nerve conduction or direct muscle stimulation. *Faradic current* is induced, interrupted, and rapidly alternating. An induction coil, acting as an interruptor through which a contact is repeatedly made and broken, is used to produce a faradic current. Ordinarily, the faradic current is used only in nerve stimulation, and the normal response is a tetantic contraction caused by the rapidly repeated stimuli.

For the electrical examination, the parts of the body to be tested should be relaxed. The limbs should be placed in a proper position for electrical stimulation of the muscle. The stimuli are applied to the *motor nerves* where they are close to the surface of the body and at the *muscle* or *motor points*, the most excitable parts of the muscles. Motor nerves are usually located over the area where the motor nerve enters the muscle belly or at the site of the greatest concentration of nerve endings. Upon stimulation of a nerve, all the muscles supplied by that nerve do contract. Contraction of the muscle is observed by movement of the part it supplies,

by palpation of the muscle belly, or by direct inspection.

In lower motor neuron lesions 10 to 14 days after injury, characteristic electrical changes develop that are known as "reaction of degeneration." In complete reaction of degeneration, no response is obtained from faradic or galvanic stimulation of the motor nerve; whereas, galvanic stimulation of the muscle produces a slow, vermicular, long-drawn contraction that passes into a continuous tetanus, lasting for the entire duration of the current.

Certain disease syndromes are characterized by specific changes in the electrical reactions: in *Thomsen's disease* (myotonia congenita) and *myotonia dystrophica*, the threshold for faradic current is normal, but the contraction obtained is *persistent* and prolonged with delayed reaction. After administration of quinine, this change in the electrical reaction may decrease. In *tetany* there is increased excitability of both nerves and muscles. In *myasthenia gravis*, there is increased fatigability with gradual exhaustion on repeated stimulation. In *familial periodic paralysis* there is cadaveric response with loss of irritability to both faradic and galvanic stimulation during the period of paralysis.

In diseases of the pyramidal, extrapyramidal, or cerebellar systems, and in the paralysis of hysteria or malingering, there are no changes in the electrical reaction. Negative findings in the conditions just mentioned are helpful in differential diagnosis.

Strength-Duration Curve. The curve is obtained by plotting the current in milliamperes necessary to produce a minimal contraction with decreasing duration of stimulus down to 0.1 msec. In the presence of degeneration, the muscle will be stimulated directly and will require more current to produce a response with pulses of shorter than normal duration. This test will give the earliest possible evidence of impending or actual denervation.

Electromyography. A concentric needle electrode inserted into muscle will pick up the action potentials generated by volitional contraction of neighboring motor units, which can then be amplified and visualized on an oscilloscope, then photographed and recorded. A normal muscle at rest shows no electrical activity, but with volitional contraction, it exhibits a series of action potentials. The muscle fibers supplied by a single anterior horn cell and nerve fiber act together, and their action potentials combine to produce the larger action potentials of the motor unit. In general, normal motor unit discharges are spikelike diphasic or triphasic waves, lasting from 5 to 10 msec. They

---

*See References 47–51, 53–56, 58, 60, 63, 64.

occur at a rate of 10 to 30 per second, and at an amplitude of up to 4 millivolts. The shape, duration, amplitude, and rate of discharge vary with the choice of muscle and the intensity of volitional activity.

In children, the multiple needle punctures used in electromyography are not often well tolerated, and cooperation may be poor. Experience and rapid analysis are essential for proper interpretation of the findings. In neuromuscular disorders, several types of electrical activity are found. Electromyography is of most use in the diagnosis and prognosis of peripheral nerve lesions.

About one to two weeks after complete denervation of a muscle, spontaneous discharges occur, even at rest, a result of independent, rhythmic contractions of individual muscle fibers. These contractions are potentials of *fibrillations* that are extremely small, of low voltage (rarely more than 50 mv.), of short duration (less than 1 or 2 msec.), and at a rate of two to ten per second. Fibrillation potentials are present as long as the muscle is not completely degenerated or fibrosed, or until it becomes reinnervated. Polyphasic or complex wave forms appear when a nerve is regenerating. Electromyographic signs of nerve regeneration manifest themselves before it becomes clinically apparent.

Fasciculations, irregular polyphasic discharges, are larger than fibrillations; they are from 0.5 to 1 mv., of 8 to 12 msec. in duration, and occur involuntarily while the muscle is at rest, at a rate of 1 to 30 per minute. With *anterior horn cell degeneration*, such as that in progressive muscular atrophy, the fibrillation potentials are present, but there are also fasciculations. On voluntary muscular contraction, there are isolated motor unit action potentials, which are reduced in number but increased in amplitude. Denervation potentials are seen in poliomyelitis.

In various diseases of muscle there are certain changes in the electromyography both at rest and on activity. In *myotonia*, immediately upon insertion of the needle electrode into the myotonic muscle, there is a rapid shower of high-frequency action potentials that may continue for a period after relaxation. The sounds emanating from the electromyographic loudspeaker exhibit a crescendo and decrescendo quality. This shower of activity can be reproduced by tapping the electrode or by moving it further into the muscle substance. In muscular dystrophy, the action potentials are polyphasic and are of smaller amplitude and shorter than nomal. In *myositis*, there may be fibrillation potentials at rest, and the potentials with voluntary contraction are often polyphasic and are decreased in amplitude and duration.

In the case of upper motor lesions, electromyography is of little assistance in diagnosis.

Nerve Conduction Velocity Determinations. Combined stimulation and recording techniques are used for the determination of motor nerve conduction time. A motor nerve is stimulated at two points, thus determining the latent period between each stimulus and the ensuing muscular contraction. The latency for the propagation of the nerve impulse between the two points stimulated is obtained by subtracting one latency from the other, and hence, the nerve conduction velocity is determined. The nerves most often tested are the peroneal, posterior tibial, median, ulnar, and facial. The average conduction time for these nerves has been determined, varying according to the age of the subject. The normal values are 45 to 65 m./sec. in children over the age of five years. At birth the motor nerve conduction velocity may be as low as 25 m./sec., which gradually increases to 45 m./sec. by the age of three.

In diffuse peripheral neuritis, there is a slowing of conduction velocity—an important finding in differentiation of the lesions of the nerves themselves and diseases of the muscles or anterior horn cells. In locally damaged nerve segments, velocity studies are helpful in localizing the site of the lesion (e.g., as in compression of the ulnar nerve at the elbow). Successive examinations of nerve conduction velocity may give a useful quantitative estimation of the course of the disease.

References

RADIOGRAPHY

1. Alexander, G. W., and Muroff, L. (eds.): Bone Imaging with ^{99m}Tc. New York, Medcom, 1974, p. 16.
2. Batillas, J., Vasilas, A., Pizzi, W. F., et al.: Bone scanning in the detection of occult fractures. J. Trauma, 21:564, 1981.
3. Bauer, G.: Progress in the use of radionuclides in orthopaedics. Acta Orthop. Scand., 46:315, 1975.
4. Brasch, R. C., and Cann, C. E.: Computed tomographic scanning in children: II. An updated comparison of radiation dose and resolving power of commercial scanners. A.J.R., 138:127, 1982.
5. Bull, J.: The history of computed tomography. *In* Caille, J. M., and Salamon, G. (eds.): Computerized Tomography. Berlin, Springer, 1980, pp. 3–6.
6. Caffey, J.: Pediatric X-ray Diagnosis—A Textbook for Students and Practitioners of Pediatrics, Surgery and Radiology. 7th Ed. Chicago, Year Book, 1978.
7. Castronovo, F. P., Guiberteau, M. J., and Berg, G.: Pharmacokinetics of technetium-99m diphosphonate. J. Nucl. Med., 18:809, 1977.
8. Crass, J. R., and L'Heureux, P.: Bone scan appearance of stress fractures. Differentiation from osteosarcoma. Minn. Med., 64:535, 1981.

9. Conway, J. J.: Radionuclide bone imaging in pediatrics. Pediatr. Clin. North. Am., *24*:701, 1977.

10. Curless, R. G., and Nelson, M. B.: Needle biopsies of muscle in infants for diagnosis and research. Dev. Med. Child Neurol., *17*:592, 1975.

11. D'Ambrosia, R. D., Shoji, H., Riggins, R. S., et al.: Scintigraphy in the diagnosis of osteonecrosis. Clin. Orthop., *130*:139, 1978.

12. Dandy, D. J.: Arthroscopic surgery of the knee. *In* Current Problems in Orthopaedics. Edinburgh, Churchill-Livingstone, 1981.

13. Deutsch, S. D., and Gandsman, E. J.: The use of bone scanning for the diagnosis and management of musculoskeletal trauma. Surg. Clin. North Am., *63*:567, 1983.

14. Deutsch, S. D., Gandsman, E. J., and Spraragen, S. C.: Quantitative regional blood-flow analysis and its clinical application during routine bone-scanning. J. Bone Joint Surg., *63-A*:295, 1981.

15. Gelfand, M. J., Thomas, S. R., and Kereiakes, J. G.: Absorbed radiation dose from routine imaging of the skeleton in children. Ann. Radiol. (Paris), *26*:421, 1983.

16. Genant, H. K., Cann, C. E., Chafetz, N. I., et al.: Advances in computed tomography of the musculoskeletal system. Radiol. Clin. North Am., *19*:645, 1981.

17. Genant, H. K., Wilson, J. S., Bovill, E. G., Brunelle, F. O., Murray, W. R., and Rodrigo, J. J.: Computed tomography of the musculoskeletal system. J. Bone Joint Surg., *62-A*:1088, 1980.

18. Gilula, L. A., Murphy, W. A., Tailor, C. C., et al.: Computed tomography of the osseous pelvis. Radiology, *132*:107, 1976.

19. Griffiths, H. J., Hamlin, D. J., Kiss, S., and Lovelock, J.: Efficacy of CT scanning in a group of 174 patients with orthopedic and musculoskeletal problems. Skeletal Radiol., *7*:87, 1981.

20. Haller, O. J., and Shkolnik, A. (eds.): Ultrasound in Pediatrics. Edinburgh, Churchill-Livingstone, 1981.

21. Handel, S. F., and Lee, Y. Y.: Computed tomography of spinal fractures. Radiol. Clin. North Am., *19*:69, 1981.

22. Hubbard, L. F.: Computed tomography in orthopedics. Surg. Clin. North Am., *63*:587, 1983.

23. Hubbard, L. F., McDermott, J. H., and Garrett, G.: Computed axial tomography in musculoskeletal trauma. J. Trauma, *2*:388, 1982.

24. Hughes, S. P. F.: Radionuclides in orthopaedic surgery. J. Bone Joint Surg., *62-B*:141, 1980.

25. Ireland, J., Trickey, E. L., and Stoker, D. J.: Arthroscopy and arthrography of the knee: Critical review. J. Bone Joint Surg., *62-B*:3, 1980.

26. Jackson, R. W., and Danby, D. J.: Arthroscopy of the Knee. New York, Grune & Stratton, 1976.

27. Kirchner, P. T., and Simon, M. A.: Current concepts review: radioisotopic evaluation of skeletal disease. J. Bone Joint Surg., *63-A*:673, 1981.

28. McGinty, J. B.: Arthroscopy, a modality of diagnosis or treatment (Abraham Colles Lecture). J. Irish Coll. Phys. Surg., *11*:63, 1981.

29. McLeod, R. A., Stephens, D. H., Beabout, J. W., Sheedy, P. F., and Hattery, R. R.: Computed tomography of the skeleton. Semin. Roentgenol., 13, 1970.

30. Murray, R. O.: Orthopaedic radiology: An expanding discipline. J. R. Soc. Med., *73*:320, 1980.

31. Murray, R. O., and Jacobson, H. G.: The Radiology of Skeletal Disorders: Exercises in Diagnosis. 2nd Ed. Edinburgh, Churchill-Livingstone, 1977.

32. Nicholas, J. A., and Holder, L. E. (eds.): Bone Imaging in Orthopedic Medicine. A Clinical Casebook. New York, Pro Clinica, 1980.

33. Ozonoff, M. B.: Pediatric Orthopaedic Radiology. Philadelphia, Saunders, 1979.

34. Paul, D. J., and Gilday, D. L.: Polyphosphate bone scanning of non-malignant bone disease in children. J. Can. Assoc. Radiol., *26*:285, 1975.

35. Paul, D. F., Morrey, B. F., and Helms, C. A.: Computerized tomography in orthopaedic surgery. Clin. Orthop., *139*:142, 1979.

36. Poznanski, A. K.: Radiation Protection in Pediatric Radiology. Washington, D.C., National Council on Radiation Protection and Measurements. No. 68, 1981.

37. Schumacher, T. M., Genant, H. K., Korokbin, M., and Bovill, E. G.: Computed tomography: Its use in space occupying lesions of the musculoskeletal system. J. Bone Joint Surg., *60-A*:600, 1978.

38. Smith, F. W., and Gilday, D. L.: Scintigraphic appearances of osteoid osteoma. Radiology, *137*:191, 1980.

39. Sullivan, A. J., Vasileff, T., and Leonard, J. C.: An evaluation of nuclear scanning in orthopaedic infections. J. Pediatr. Orthop., *1*:73, 1981.

40. Ter-Pogossian, M. M.: The challenge of computed tomography. A.J.R., *127*:1, 1976.

41. Thomas, S. R., Gelfand, M. J., Burns, G. S., Purdom, R. C., Kereiakes, J. G., and Maxon, H. R.: Radiation absorbed-dose estimates for the liver, spleen, and metaphyseal growth complexes in children undergoing gallium-67 citrate scanning. Radiology, *146*:817, 1983.

42. Thomas, S. R., Gelfand, M. J., Kereiakes, J. G., Ascoli, F. A., Maxon, H. R., Saenger, E. L., Feller, P. A., Sodd, V. J., and Paras, P.: Dose to the metaphyseal growth complexes in children undergoing ^{99m}Tc-EDPH bone scans. Radiology, *126*:193, 1978.

43. Tyson, I. B., Deutsch, S. D., Gandsman, E. J., et al.: Dynamic bone scanning in the differential diagnosis of skeletal lesions. *In* Hofer, R. (ed.): Radioactive Isotope in Klinik und Forschung. Vienna, Egerman, 1982, p. 331.

44. Watson, R. C.: CT scan—its use and abuse. CA, *28*:100, 1978.

45. Weiner, D. S., Cook, A. J., Hoyt, W. A., Jr., and Drovec, C. E.: Computed tomography in measurement of femoral antetorsion. Orthopedics, *1*:299, 1978.

46. Weis, L., Heelan, R. T., and Watson, R. C.: Computed tomography of orthopaedic traumas of the pelvis and lower extremities. Clin. Orthop., *130*:254, 1978.

ELECTRODIAGNOSTIC METHODS

47. Arieff, A. J., Dobin, N. B., and Tigar, E. L.: Comprehensive electrodiagnosis. J.A.M.A., *181*:1140, 1962.

48. Brazier, M. A. B.: The Electrical Activity of the Nervous System. New York, Macmillan, 1951.

49. Buchthal, F., and Clemmesen, S.: On differentiation of muscle atrophy by electromyography. Acta Psychiatr. Neurol., *16*:143, 1941.

50. Denny-Brown, D.: Interpretation of electromyogram. Arch. Neurol. Psychiatr., *61*:99, 1949.

51. Eaton, L. M., and Lambert, E. H.: Electromyography and electric stimulation of nerves in diseases of motor unit. J.A.M.A., *163*:1117, 1957.

52. Erb, W.: Handbook of Electrotherapeutics. 1883. Trans. by L. Putzel. New York, William Wood, 1883.

53. Gilliatt, R. W.: Electrodiagnosis and electromyography in clinical practice. Br. Med. J., *2*:1073, 1962.

54. Johnson, E. W., and Olsen, K. J.: Clinical value of motor nerve conduction velocity determination. J.A.M.A., *172*:2030, 1960.

55. Kugelberg, E.: Electromyography in muscular dystrophies; differentiation between dystrophies and chronic lower motor neuron lesions. J. Neurol. Neurosurg. Psychiatry, *12*:129, 1949.

56. Licht, S. H.: Practical Electromyography. 4th Ed., E. W. Johnson (ed.). Baltimore, Williams & Wilkins, 1979.

57. Licht, S. (ed.): Electrodiagnosis and Electromyography. 2nd Ed. New Haven, Elizabeth Licht, 1961.

58. Norris, F. H., Jr.: The EMG: A Guide and Atlas for Practical Electromyography. New York, Grune & Stratton, 1963.

59. Pollock, L. J., Golseth, J. G., Mayfield, F., Arieff, A. J., and Oester, Y. T.: Electrodiagnosis of lesions of

peripheral nerves in man. Arch. Neurol. Psychiatr., *60*:1, 1948.

60. Rosenthal, A. M.: Electrodiagnostic testing in neuromuscular disease. J.A.M.A., *177*:829, 1961.
61. Thomas, P. K., Sears, T. A., and Gilliatt, R. W.: The range of conduction velocity in normal motor nerve fibers to the small muscles of the hand and foot. J. Neurol. Neurosurg. Psychiatry, *22*:175, 1959.

62. Wagner, A. L., and Buchthal, F.: Motor and sensory conduction in infancy and childhood. Reappraisal. Dev. Med. Child Neurol., *14*:189, 1972.
63. Watkins, A. L.: An evaluation of electrodiagnostic testing. N. Engl. J. Med., *259*:868, 1958.
64. Wynn-Parry, C. B.: Electrodiagnosis. J. Bone Joint Surg., *43-B*:222, 1961.

Anesthetic Considerations*

Most children undergoing orthopedic operations are basically healthy, but there are some who have special problems that complicate their anesthetic management. Proper preoperative assessment and preparation will lessen the chance of intraoperative or postoperative difficulties and complications. The orthopedic surgeon, by being aware of these potential problems and the need for proper evaluation and treatment, can alert the anesthesiologist to them and assist him with these children.

GENERAL CONSIDERATIONS

The usual minimum laboratory work before surgery is a complete blood count and a urinalysis. A chest radiogram is required in many institutions, but the American Academy of Pediatrics has recently recommended that this practice be discontinued as a general policy. Other laboratory studies such as an electrocardiogram, determination of electrolyte levels, or clotting studies should be done if the clinical findings warrant. For black children, sickle cell preparation should be done. In a child under four months of age, the preparation may be negative and subsequently change to positive. This reversal is due to the replacement of fetal hemoglobin with sickle hemoglobin. If negative in a child under four months of age, the test should be repeated when the child comes for surgery when older than four months. After four months of age, the test does not need to be repeated if negative. If the sickle preparation is positive, a hemoglobin electrophoresis should be done to define the exact hemoglobinopathy. The final laboratory test some institutions perform is a pregnancy test for female teenagers. The use of this test is controversial. At a minimum, recent menstrual history taken in a non-threatening atmosphere by a physician or nurse may be adequate.

Anemia is a relatively common preoperative problem. The anesthesiologist is hesitant to anesthetize a child with anemia because there is less potential delivery of oxygen to the body at a time when the child is stressed, both intraoperatively and postoperatively. There is some statistical evidence that the anemic child is at greater risk of intraoperative cardiac arrest. The cause of the anemia should be determined. If it is due to dietary iron deficiency, this can be corrected by simple administration of iron for a few weeks. The surgery can then be performed when the child has a normal blood count. In contrast, sickle cell anemia does not respond to iron therapy. The only way to raise this patient's red cell count is by transfusion. Here, the need for correction of the anemia must be weighed against the risk of transfusion.

A patient receiving long-term medication should be evaluated to see whether the drugs need to be continued. One taking steroids within the last year will usually require steroid therapy during the operative period. One taking seizure medications should often get his morning dose with a small sip of water. A patient who has had chemotherapy requires close evaluation because many of these drugs can alter cardiac, renal, hepatic, and pulmonary functions as well as blood coagulation.[1] The anesthesiologist needs to know the exact drugs and their total dosages. Children with asthma need to be closely examined to see whether their medications are adequate. Those with mild asthmatic symptoms can often be treated with their usual medication given in the usual morning dose with a sip of water. The more severely affected patient should be evaluated by his pediatrician, and may need to have an aminophylline drip started and adjusted the night before operation. The insulin-dependent diabetic patient should be evaluated by the anesthesiologist and the patient's pediatrician jointly. Depending on the severity and "brittleness" of the diabetes, the patient may need overnight glucose infusions and insulin in divided doses. Regular glucose determinations will be necessary both perioperatively and postoperatively.

*Contributed by Steven Hall, M.D., Attending Anesthesiologist, The Children's Memorial Hospital; Assistant Professor of Anesthesiology, Northwestern University Medical School, Chicago, Illinois.

Special attention should be directed to the infant or child who was premature at birth. These children have a higher incidence of complications, both during their initial hospitalization and later. For instance, for the first six months of life, they tend to have apneic spells after surgery and anesthesia. This means they are not candidates for outpatient surgery during this period.[2] They also have a higher incidence of residual cardiac, pulmonary, and central nervous system problems that can complicate the anesthetic management. The past records of these children must be examined closely. Probably the most common preoperative problem in the child is a possible upper respiratory infection. Diagnosis may be difficult, but *new* coughing, rhinorrhea (especially purulent), fever, congestion, and irritability indicate an infectious process. Often, the parents can give the best information and should be asked whether these symptoms are new for their child. Most anesthesiologists are hesitant to anesthetize a child with an upper respiratory infection because of the increased risk of airway obstruction, laryngospasm, and a stormy anesthetic course. There is evidence that the airway does not return to normal until two weeks after symptoms disappear.[3, 4]

References

1. Chung, F.: Cancer chemotherapy and anesthesia. Can. Anaesth. Soc. J., 29:364, 1982.
2. Gregory, G. A., and Steward, D. J.: Life-threatening perioperative apnea in the ex-"premie." Anesthesiology, 59:495, 1983.
3. McGill, W. A., Coveler, L. A., and Epstein, B. S.: Subacute upper respiratory infection in small children. Anesth. Analg., 58:331, 1979.
4. Steward, D. J., and Sloan, I. A. J.: Recent upper respiratory infection and pulmonary artery clamping in the etiology of postoperative respiratory complications. Can. Anaesth. Soc. J., 16:57, 1969.

SPECIFIC ENTITIES

Muscular Dystrophy

Duchenne's muscular dystrophy and the other dystrophies have many anesthetic implications. Since these patients have poor esophageal motility, they often develop aspiration pneumonitis. This means that the anesthesiologist must evaluate lung function (by chest radiogram and possibly determination of blood gas values). In addition, on induction, he must treat the patient like a child with a full stomach; the trachea should be intubated for protection as rapidly as possible. Poor ventilatory reserves can become apparent in these patients, neces-

sitating intraoperative ventilation and increasing the possibility of needing postoperative ventilation. Any postoperative sedation, especially narcotics, must be used with great care because these children are very susceptible to respiratory depression. Cardiac problems occur frequently in patients with muscular dystrophy. Atrial arrhythmias are very common, but cardiac arrest, mitral valve prolapse, and cardiac dilatation have also been reported.[23] A preoperative electrocardiogram is useful, especially if the child gives a history of palpitations, chest discomfort, or dizziness. If he has a history of significant cardiac symptoms, the patient should be evaluated by a cardiologist before surgery. There is increasing concern that patients with muscular dystrophy are at high risk for malignant hyperthermia.[24] Even in the absence of malignant hyperthermia, the intraoperative use of succinylcholine may be relatively contraindicated because of the risk of massive rhabdomyolysis.[25] It is important to remember that Duchenne's muscular dystrophy is a progressive disease, with greater pulmonary, gastrointestinal, and cardiac debilitation as the child gets older. It is not adequate to depend on prior history, physical examination, and laboratory data. The patient must be re-evaluated each time to ensure that impairment and, therefore, risk have not increased since the patient's last operation.

Myotonias

The same anesthetic problems may arise in patients with myotonia dystrophica as in those with muscular dystrophy. In addition, both the dystrophic and congenital types have a myotonic response to certain stimuli. The commonly used muscle relaxant, succinylcholine, initially causes skeletal muscle to contract ("fasciculations"), then relax. This can lead to severe myotonic muscle contracture that is not relieved by muscle relaxants. Shivering or brisk surgical manipulation can also stimulate such a response. The generalized myotonic contracture can significantly impair ventilation and put the child at great risk. Thus, depolarizing muscle relaxants, especially succinylcholine, are contraindicated in these patients.[29]

Osteogenesis Imperfecta

Mask ventilation and tracheal intubation are often difficult in these patients owing to the combination of short neck, flattened head, and small face. Great care must be taken in their general handling because of the increased risk of fractures, especially once they are anesthetized. A unique aspect of osteogenesis imperfecta is the appearance of hyperthermia intraoperatively. Due to an increased metabolic rate, these children often become hyperthermic during anesthesia. This is not the malignant hyperthermia syndrome, however, and is easily corrected by cooling. In view of this possibility, these patients, as with all children, should have continuous temperature monitoring in the operating room, and intravenous fluids should be given to compensate for fluid loss due to the increased metabolic rate.[9] Newborns with osteogenesis imperfecta are especially prone to serious intraventricular hemorrhage and require special assessment and monitoring.

Arthrogryposis

Arthrogryposis multiplex congenita presents several practical problems to the anesthesiologist. Veins for cannulation are often small, sparse, and difficult to gain access to. Mandibular hypoplasia may make both mask ventilation and intubation extremely difficult. Lateral soft-tissue radiograms of the neck may be useful in patients with a history of difficult intubation. Chest wall and spine deformities may make ventilation difficult, while cardiac abnormalities have also been reported and should be evaluated preoperatively. Contracture of limbs can present positioning problems on the operating table. Careful padding will be necessary to avoid skin damage. The possibility of malignant hyperthermia should be kept in mind during surgery.[32]

Rheumatoid Arthritis

Juvenile rheumatoid arthritis is a systemic disease, and these children may have significant cardiac (pericarditis), lung (restrictive disease), hematologic (pancytopenia), and renal disease. They are often anemic and chronically ill and may also be receiving aspirin (clotting abnormalities), steroids (multiple problems), or chemotherapeutics (hematologic, renal damage). Thus, it is important to review the history and therapy of a patient with rheumatoid arthritis. Because of the multiple problems, preoperative consultation with the patient's managing physician is necessary. Also, these patients with their chronic illness may develop significant psychologic problems and need special care and understanding in their management.

Probably the major problem that anesthesiologists have with the rheumatoid patient is the airway. These children can have temporomandibular joint ankylosis, cricoarytenoid arthritis, and cervical spine instabilty. In patients with symptoms suggestive of impaired airway access, physical examination of the airway is mandatory before the child is anesthetized. Cervical spine radiograms and soft-tissue lateral projections of the neck will help to guide the approach to the airway. Unfortunately, mandibular hypoplasia is also found more frequently in these children, complicating the management of the airway. If the cervical spine is unstable, the orthopedic or neurologic surgeon should be present at induction and should guide any flexion or extension of the neck during the intubation process. Several maneuvers have been used in the intubation of a difficult airway, including awake or fiberoptic intubation, "blind" nasal intubation in the spontaneously breathing patient, tracheostomy, and retrograde intubation of the trachea over a wire inserted through the cricothyroid membrane and advanced into the mouth. The exact technique used depends on the patient and the experience and preferences of the anesthesiologist. In our institution, the advice and assistance of an otolaryngologist are often very helpful.

Myelomeningocele

The child with myelomeningocele often requires repeated orthopedic operations. Because a significant percentage of these patients develop hydrocephalus, the status of their intracranial pressure must be assessed preoperatively. Many of them have a ventriculoperitoneal shunt or other device for drainage of cerebrospinal fluid. Not only should the shunt be functioning well, but the neurosurgeon caring for the patient may request prophylactic antibiotic coverage. General anesthesia in the presence of increased intracranial pressure is very dangerous; there should be no question about the patient's status before surgery. Seizures may be another problem. Antiseizure medication should be continued until operation and restarted as soon as possible postoperatively. Patients with myelomeningocele may develop severe kyphoscoliosis with all its attendant pulmonary and cardiac complications. (See section on kyphoscoliosis.) These patients may have significant urologic difficulties, requiring either diverting operations or frequent catheterizations. If the patient has an ileal conduit or other diverting operation, electrolytes must be checked prior to operation. If the patient is receiving antibiotics, they should be continued in the perioperative period.

Cerebral Palsy

The child with cerebral palsy may have problems with seizure control, malnutrition, recurrent aspiration pneumonitis, or contractures. Proper padding and positioning on the operating table is necessary. Although there has been concern about hyperkalemia after succinylcholine, prospective studies have not confirmed that this is a real problem.

Kyphoscoliosis

The child with kyphoscoliosis may have several abnormalities that are important in his anesthetic management. The underlying cause of the scoliosis may present problems. In the patient with myelomeningocele (hydrocephalus), muscular dystrophy (carditis, aspiration), juvenile rheumatoid arthritis (carditis, lung disease, anemia), or Friedreich's ataxia (sudden death from cardiomyopathy) there may be considerations beyond the scoliosis itself that need to be evaluated before proceeding with surgery. Pulmonary disease in the patient with kyphoscoliosis depends on both the degree of bony deformity and the degree of associated neuromuscular abnormality. In some cases, aspiration pneumonitis will also add to the problem. These patients have decreased vital capacity and, therefore, less ability to cough and breathe deeply. This deficiency makes clearing of secretions difficult, and atelectasis and pneumonia more likely. The patient may also have ventilation-perfusion abnormalities, leading to the need for enriched oxygen, especially in the intraoperative and immediate postoperative periods. In severe cases, long-standing hypoxemia can lead to cor pulmonale and pulmonary hypertension. It should be stressed, though, that the majority of children coming to surgery for kyphoscoliosis have normal pulmonary function tests. Routine preoperative screening should include a good history for exercise tolerance, recurrent pulmonary infections, stridor, dyspnea, and wheezing. During the physical examination, special attention should be paid to the use of accessory muscles. Preoperative pulmonary function testing is useful; a chest radiogram is mandatory. In patients with severe disease, a preoperative blood gas analysis may reveal significant hyperemia. The degree of correction of pulmonary abnormalities required after surgery is not completely clear at this time.[36] It must, however, be anticipated that the patient with severe disease may need overnight mechanical ventilation and subsequent weaning as tolerated. If this is anticipated, both the family and the patient should be advised of this preoperatively. Patients with severe kyphoscoliosis can develop cardiac disease and cor pulmonale with subsequent right ventricular failure can develop late in their course. A preoperative electrocardiogram and echocardiogram will delineate the degree of right ventricular dysfunction. Consultation with the child's cardiologist before surgery is necessary if the patient has any signs of impaired function. In those with significant cardiac disease, central venous or pulmonary artery catheter monitoring in both the operative and the immediate postoperative period can be very useful in gauging fluid and drug management. Intubation may be difficult, especially if there is significant cervical disease or an underlying disorder, such as rheumatoid arthritis, that predisposes to this problem. The presence of halo traction can also complicate the intubation. Preoperative evaluation may include indirect laryngoscopy or neck radiograms. Intraoperative management is very dependent on the proposed operation and the particular needs and preferences of both the surgeon and the anesthesiologist. Hypotensive anesthesia for scoliosis surgery is controversial. Some anesthesiologists feel it is a safe technique and allows less blood loss, whereas other authorities feel the exact opposite.[34, 39] Whether or not hypotension is utilized, blood loss can be significantly reduced by proper attention to positioning (avoidance of abdominal compression), infiltration with 1:500,000 epinephrine solutions, and hyperventilation. Currently, there is interest in hemodilution and autotransfusion techniques when extreme blood loss is likely. Intraoperative evaluation of spinal cord function centers on two diverse approaches. The "wake-up" test evaluates motor function after spinal distraction.[22] For this test, the anesthesiologist has to alter his technique to allow the patient to regain consciousness and motor function gently in the middle of the procedure. Obviously, this has to be planned before the operation begins and must be explained to the patient so that he is not terrified by unexpected awakening. Furthermore, the test may not work adequately in young or uncooperative children. The "wake-up" test is a monitor of motor function, while the second type of test, somatosensory evoked potentials (SSEP), is a test of sensory function. This monitor has the significant advantage of providing continuous testing throughout the operation and the disadvantages of requiring elaborate equipment and experienced personnel. Somatosensory evoked potentials measure sensory function and are adversely affected by changes in anesthetic level and perfusion.[21] The anesthesiologist and surgeon have to plan carefully and cooperate closely during the operation to get useful information from either of these monitors.

Hemophilia

It is not unusual for hemophiliac children to need orthopedic surgery. The management perioperatively is coordinated with the patient's hematologist. Although levels of Factor 8 above 30 per cent are probably adequate for surgery, the child is usually given enough Factor 8 to elevate the level above 50 per cent, and often to 100 per cent. A factor level should be determined shortly before surgery and, later, in the recovery room. In dealing with these patients, it is wise to remember that they are exposed to repeated injections of blood products and have a higher than normal incidence of hepatitis and acquired immune deficiency syndrome (AIDS).

Sickle Cell Disease

About 10 per cent of the American black population has some form of sickle cell disease; its prevalence is less in other, especially Mediterranean, populations. The heterozygote form (Hgb AS) is often associated with a normal hemoglobin and an absence of symptoms, while the homozygotic form (Hgb SS) is associated with anemia and various hemolytic, aplastic, sequestration, and occlusive crises.[11] Hypoxemia, dehydration, poor perfusion, acidosis, cold, increased oxygen consumption, trauma, and many other insults can trigger a crisis. If a patient has a positive sickle cell preparation, a hemoglobin electrophoresis should be performed, and the family should be advised of the findings. If the patient has sickle trait (Hgb A greater than 50 per cent) and is not anemic, the anesthetic can be administered without further work-up. In the patient with sickle cell disease or one of the other variants (sickle cell thalassemia, sickle C), consultation with a hematologist is necessary before proceeding with surgery. Exchange transfusion or hypertransfusion is usually recommended. The anesthetic management will stress maintaining adequate oxygen levels, avoiding acidosis, mildly hyperventilating, and keeping the patient well hydrated. Since overzealous sedation can lead to hypoventilation, acidosis, and hypoxemia, both premedications and postoperative medications should be kept at a minimum. Early awakening and ambulation will help prevent stasis and the attendant risk of sickling.

Malignant Hyperthermia Syndrome

Orthopedic surgeons are more likely than other surgeons to encounter the malignant hyperthermia syndrome in some of their patients. This is because the incidence of malignant hyperthermia is higher than usual in patients with conditions likely to bring them to the attention of an orthopedist. Consequently, orthopedic surgeons need to be aware of the possibility of the syndrome in their patients, asking for a history compatible with the syndrome as part of the routine preoperative evaluation.

Incidence. The syndrome is hereditary and has traditionally been characterized as autosomally dominant with incomplete penetrance and variable expressivity, meaning that the trait would not penetrate to offspring as commonly as expected and would show varying degrees of severity in affected individuals.[5, 14, 20] In some families, however, the pattern of inheritance appears more consistent with an autosomal recessive or multigenic mode of transmission. More importantly, when family members are screened, about half the patients have no other family members with the trait.

Geographically, because of the hereditary nature of the disease, there are clusters of patients with the syndrome. The incidence reported for North America is 1:15,000 for children and 1:50,000 for adults. It has been found in all racial groups and in all age groups, with the highest incidence in young adult men.[4, 6] Overall, there does not seem to be any difference between sexes.

Presumably because of an underlying nonspecific myopathy, patients with this syndrome have a higher than normal incidence of kyphoscoliosis, club foot, winged scapula, and joint hypermobility with repeated dislocations.[4, 6] It is controversial whether there is a greater incidence of malignant hyperthermia syndrome in patients with Duchenne's muscular dystrophy, arthrogryposis, and central core disease.[30, 31]

Pathophysiology. Certain strains of pig (Landrace, Poland, China) have been instrumental in clarifying our understanding of the syndrome. Swine suffer from a similar condition called the porcine stress syndrome. This animal model is similar to the human syndrome, except that nonpharmacologic stresses, e.g., exercise, are much more likely to trigger an attack in pigs.

The primary event in malignant hyperthermia is the triggering of a hypermetabolic state in skeletal muscle. The exact mechanism is still controversial, but the most commonly accepted postulate relates to release of intracellular calcium from the sarcoplasmic reticulum.[18] The sudden rise and continued presence of high myoplasmic calcium levels activates the contracture of the muscle and the accompanying hydrolysis of adenosine triphosphate. There may also be uncoupling of oxidative phosphorylation. Aerobic metabolism, followed by anaerobic metabolism, produces large quantities of carbon dioxide, heat, and lactic acid.[18, 28] Oxygen consumption is vastly accelerated. This process, if allowed to continue, will lead to cell death and lysis.

The sudden increase in carbon dioxide, heat, and lactate, coupled with the decrease in tissue oxygenation, will produce clinical signs such as tachycardia, tachypnea, arrhythmias, hypertension, muscle rigidity, temperature elevation, sweating, cyanosis, dilated pupils, and mottled skin (see Table 1–13 in the appendix to Chapter 1). If the process is allowed to continue, cardiac arrest is likely; if recognized and treated quickly, the overwhelming majority of patients recover without sequelae.

In humans, the most common triggers are anesthetic agents. The depolarizing muscle relaxant, succinylcholine, and the volatile anesthetics, such as halothane, enflurane, isoflurane, and ether, are known triggers.[41] Although there has been concern about the amide-type local anesthetics, e.g., lidocaine and bupivacaine, there is increasing sentiment that these agents are safe to use.[2, 42] Safe anesthetics include the barbiturates, narcotics, benzodiazepines, nitrous oxide, and the nondepolarizing muscle relaxants.

The treatment of an attack is centered on the drug dantrolene sodium. Dantrolene both prevents and aborts attacks of the syndrome. The exact mechanism is debated, but believed to be the result of either a decrease in release of calcium from the sarcoplasmic reticulum or a direct action at the tropinin-tropomyosin complex. Dantrolene releases the contracture of the muscle and restores the metabolic rate to normal. It is the only specific therapy available at this time.

Diagnosis. A knowledgeable surgeon will always ask if there has been difficulty with previous operations or anesthetics—in the patient of the patient's family. Unfortunately, about half the patients who have an intraoperative attack of malignant hyperthermia have had previously uncomplicated operations. Unexplained "difficulty," cardiac arrest, unexpected intensive care unit admission, or prolonged recovery room stay during a previous procedure may be signs of the syndrome. If there is any question, the hospital record should be examined or the physicians involved questioned. A nonanesthetic record of heat intolerance, exercise intolerance, muscle cramps, or sensitivity to caffeine can increase suspicion about someone with other suggestive history. An extensive family history, focusing especially on previous surgery, may reveal other suspicious events.

Laboratory work is usually not helpful in determining susceptibility. Positive creatine phosphokinase determinations are useful only if there is strong suspicion to begin with and have been considered diagnostic only when there is a first-degree relative known to have the syndrome.[1, 6] The only currently accepted test useful in equivocal cases is caffeine-halothane contracture testing of a muscle biopsy.[8, 27] Unfortunately, this is done in only a few medical centers around the country. Newer, noninvasive tests have been proposed but are not yet widely accepted.

Intraoperatively, the diagnosis of malignant hyperthermia is a clinical one. It must be kept in mind that many cases present insidiously or with only a few of the known signs. Tachycardia is usually the first sign of an attack and must be differentiated from "light" anesthesia, hypovolemia, and other problems, such as concurrent infection. Probably the biggest problem in the diagnosis is denial on the part of the anesthesiologist—"This can't be happening to me!" Only by recognizing the possibility of the syndrome in any patient and proceeding accordingly can late diagnosis and morbidity and mortality rates be reduced.

Treatment. Treatment of an attack is both symptomatic and specific (see Tables 1–14 and 1–15 in the appendix to this chapter). Dantrolene is the key to successful management and *must* be immediately available in every hospital, in the operating suite area. Once the initial therapy has succeeded, the patient should continue to receive dantrolene for at least 48 hours and be watched in an intensive care setting.

Along with the specific agent dantrolene, symptomatic therapy with sodium bicarbonate (acidosis), hyperventilation with 100 per cent oxygen (hypercarbia, hypoxemia), diuresis (clogging of renal tubules with myoglobin), procainamide (arrhythmias), cooling, and glucose and insulin (hyperkalemia from cell destruction) may be needed.[2, 17, 18]

Possible late complications include heart failure, renal failure, consumption coagulopathy, cerebral edema, and massive muscle swelling requiring fasciotomy.[40] One of the most dreaded late complications is a recurrence of the syndrome, as late as 36 hours after the initial attack. Thus, the patient must be observed continuously for the first 48 hours.

Surgery for the Susceptible Patient. Patients with malignant hyperthermia can have any surgery they would ever need. The only restriction is that the surgeon and anesthesiologist must prepare ahead of time. Only nontriggering anesthetic drugs may be used, and an anesthetic machine flushed of any vapor should be prepared.[20, 42] Regional anesthesia is a reasonable alternative to general anesthesia in these patients if it is appropriate for the proposed operation.

If a patient is known to be susceptible to malignant hyperthermia, pretreatment with intravenous dantrolene can be given.[17] Flewellen and associates have clearly shown that oral pretreatment doesn't give consistent blood levels of the drug.[15, 16] A dose of 2.5 mg. per kilogram just before surgery is recommended.

Careful preoperative counseling and sedation will lessen the patient's anxiety. The choice between regional and general anesthesia should be based on both the desires of the patient and the expertise of the anesthesiologist.

Counseling the Patient. Once the syndrome has been diagnosed, the patient should be made an "expert" on malignant hyperthermia. Some physicians are still not as well informed on the subject as they should be, so your educational efforts will be a protection for the patient.

The patient should wear a Med-Alert tag at all times. The rest of the family should be evaluated for the syndrome. This sometimes requires a great deal of peristence and work on the surgeon's part. Finally, it is useful to direct the patient to the Malignant Hyperthermia Association of the United States (MHAUS),* a support group of people with the syndrome and other interested persons.

References

1. Amaranth, L., Lavin, T. J., Trusso, R. A., and Boutros, A. R.: Evaluation of creatinine phosphokinase screening as a predictor of malignant hyperthermia. Br. J. Anaesth., 55:531, 1983.
2. Britt, B. A.: Malignant hyperthermia. *In* Orkin, F. K., and Cooperman, L. H. (eds.): Complications in Anesthesiology. Philadelphia, Lippincott, 1983, p. 291.
3. Britt, B. A.: Malignant hyperthermia. Can. Anaesth. Soc. J. 32:666, 1985.
4. Britt, B. A., and Kalow, W.: Malignant hyperthermia: a statistical review. Can. Anaesth. Soc. J., 17:293, 1970.
5. Britt, B. A., Locher, W. G., and Kalow, W.: Hereditary aspects of malignant hyperthermia. Can. Anaesth. Soc. J., 16:89, 1969.
6. Britt, B. A., Endrenyi, L., Scott, E., and Frodis, W.: Effect of temperature, time, and fascicle size on the caffeine contracture test. Can. Anaesth. Soc. J., 27:1, 1980.
7. Britt, B. A., Scott, E., Frodis, W., et al.: Dantrolene—in vitro studies in malignant hyperthermia susceptible (MHS) and normal muscle. Can. Anaesth. Soc. J., 31:130, 1984.
8. Britt, B. A., Endrenyi, L., Peters, P. L., Francis, H.-F., Kwong, and Kadijevic, L.: Screening of malignant hyperthermia susceptible families by creatine phosphokinase measurement and other clinical investigations. Can. Anaesth. Soc. J., 23:263, 1976.
9. Brown, T. C. K., and Fisk, G. C.: Anaesthesia for Children. Oxford, Blackwell, 1979, p. 233.
10. Committee on Hospital Care, American Academy of Pediatrics: Preoperative chest radiographs. Pediatrics, 71:858, 1983.
11. Couley, C. L., and Carache, S.: Mechanisms by which some abnormal hemoglobins produce clinical manifestations. Semin. Hematol., 4:53, 1967.
12. Denborough, M. A., and Lovell, R. R. H.: Anaesthetic deaths in a family. Lancet, 2:45, 1960.
13. Donlon, J. V., Newfield, P., Streter, F., and Ryan, J. F.: Implications of masseter spasm after succinylcholine. Anesthesiology, 49:298, 1978.
14. Ellis, F. R., Cain, P. A., and Harriman, D. G. F.: Multifactorial inheritance of malignant hyperthermia susceptibility. *In* Aldrete, J. A., and Britt, B. A. (eds.): Second International Symposium on Malignant Hyperthermia. New York, Grune & Stratton, 1979, p. 329.
15. Flewellen, E. H., Nelson, T. E., and Jones, M. D.: Dantrolene dose response in awake man: implications for management of malignant hyperthermia. Anesthesiology, 59:275, 1983.
16. Flewellen, E. H., Nelson, T. E., Jones, W. P., Arens, J. F., and Wagner, D. L.: Dantrolene dose response in awake man: Implications for management of malignant hyperthermia. Anesthesiology 59:273, 1983.
17. Frank, J. P., Harati, Y., Butler, I. J., Nelson, T. E., and Scott, C. I.: Central core disease and malignant hyperthermia syndrome. Ann. Neurol., 7:11, 1980.
18. Gronert, G. A.: Malignant hyperthermia. Anesthesiology, 53:395, 1980.
19. Gronert, G. A.: Human malignant hyperthermia: Awake episodes and correction by dantrolene. Anesth. Analg., 59:377, 1980.
20. Gronert, G. A.: Malignant hyperthermia. Semin. Anesth., 2:197, 1983.
21. Grundy, B. L., Nash, C. L., and Brown, R. H.: Deliberate hypotension for spinal fusion: prospective randomized study with evoked potential monitoring. Can. Anaesth. Soc. J., 29:452, 1982.
22. Hall, J. E., Levine, C. R., Sudhir, K. G.: Intraoperative awakening to monitor spinal cord function during Harrington instrumentation and spine fusion. J. Bone Joint Surg., 60-A:533, 1978.
23. Katz, J., Benumof, J., and Kadis, L. B.: Anesthesia and uncommon diseases. Philadelphia, Saunders, 1981, p. 531.
24. Kelfer, H. M., Singer, W. D., Reynolds, R. N.: Malignant hyperthermia in a child with Duchenne muscular dystrophy. Pediatrics, 71:118, 1983.
25. Miller, E. D., Sanders, D. B., Rowlinson, J. C., Berry, F. A., Sussman, M. D., and Epstein, R. M.: Anesthesia-induced rhabdomyolysis in a patient with Duchenne's muscular dystrophy. Anesthesiology, 48:146, 1978.
26. Nelson, T. E., and Flewellyn, F. H.: The malignant

*Malignant Hyperthermia Association of the United States, P.O. Box 3231, Darien, Connecticut 06820. 24 Hour Hotline: (209) 634-4917.

hyperthermia syndrome. N. Engl. J. Med., *309*:416, 1983.

27. Nelson, T. E., Flewellen, E. H., and Gloyna, D. F.: Spectrum of susceptibility to malignant hyperthermia— diagnostic dilemma. Anesth. Analg., *62*:545, 1983.

28. Okumura, F., Crocker, B. D., and Denborough, M. A.: Site of the muscle cell abnormality in swine susceptible to malignant hyperthermia. Br. J. Anaesth., *52*:377, 1980.

29. Patterson, I. S.: Generalized myotonia following suxamethonium. Br. J. Anaesth., *34*:340, 1962.

30. Relton, J. E. S.: Hyperpyrexia in association with general anesthesia in children. Can. Anaesth. Soc. J., *13*:419, 1966.

31. Rosenberg, H., and Heiman-Patterson, T.: Duchenne's muscular dystrophy and malignant hyperthermia: Another warning. Anesthesiology, *59*:362, 1983.

32. Salem, M. R.: Anesthesia for orthopedic surgery. *In* Gregory, G. A. (ed.): Pediatric Anesthesia. New York, Churchill-Livingstone, 1983, p. 878.

33. Salem, M. R., Bennett, E. J., and Schweiss, J. F.: Cardiac arrest related to anesthesia: contributing factors in infants and children. J.A.M.A., *233*:238, 1975.

34. Salem, M. R., Toyama, R., and Wong, A. Y.: Haemodynamic responses to induced hypotension in children. Br. J. Anaesth., *50*:489, 1976.

35. Schulte-Sasse, U., Hess, W., and Eberlein, H. J.: Postoperative malignant hyperthermia and dantrolene therapy. Can. Anaesth. Soc. J., *30*:635, 1983.

36. Shannon, D. C., Riseborough, E. J., and Valenca, L. M.: The distribution of abnormal lung function in kyphoscoliosis. J. Bone Joint Surg., *52*-A:131, 1970.

37. Solomons, C. C., and Masson, N. C.: Platelet model for halothane-induced effects on nucleotide metabolism applied to malignant hyperthermia. Acta Anaesthesiol. Scand., *28*:185, 1984.

38. Gronert, G. A., Mott, J., and Lee, J.: Aetiology of malignant hyperthermia. Br. J. Anaesth., *60*:253, 1988.

39. Steward, D. J.: Outpatient pediatric anesthesia. Anesthesiology, *43*:268, 1975.

40. Wade, J. G.: The late treatment of malignant hyperthermia. *In* Gordon, A., Britt, B. A., and Kalow, W., (eds.): International Symposium on Malignant Hyperthermia. Springfield, Ill., Thomas, 1973, p. 44.

41. Wingard, D. W.: Malignant hyperthermia: acute stress syndrome of man? *In* Henschel, E. O. (ed.): Malignant Hyperthermia—Current Concepts. New York, Appleton-Century-Crofts, 1977, p. 70.

42. Wingard, D. W., and Bobko, S.: Failure of lidocaine to trigger porcine malignant hyperthermia. Anesth. Analg., *58*:99, 1979.

PREOPERATIVE CONSULTATION

Obviously, close cooperation and discussions between the orthopedic surgeon and the anesthesiologist will lead to expedient preparation of the child for surgery. It is to no one's interest to have an operation cancelled at 8:00 A.M. on the morning it is scheduled because other laboratory work is needed, the child has a cold, or a hematologist's evaluation for sickle cell anemia must be done.

One of the harder questions to answer about preoperative evaluation is When does another physician, such as the child's pediatrician, cardiologist, or hematologist, need to be consulted

prior to surgery? In some institutions, all children who are to undergo operations come with a note from their pediatrician or a family practitioner stating that the child is suitable for surgery. In healthy children, this probably is not necessary. In the chronically ill child, however, the primary physician may have to expend considerable effort to get the child in the best possible shape for operation. In these cases, they should be notified of impending surgery well in advance of the actual day. When a specialist is consulted, the anesthesiologist is looking for the answer to three basic questions. *What are the underlying problems in this particular child?* The basic problems, especially physiologic abnormalities, may significantly affect the anesthetic management. For instance, a patient who has received large quantities of doxorubicin (Adriamycin) chemotherapy is likely to be subject to cardiomyopathy.[1] Anesthetics that depress myocardial function, such as halothane, are used in very small quantities if at all. *Is the patient in the best physical condition possible?* If the answer is no, then elective surgery should be postponed until after further treatment. If the answer is yes, then one should proceed with anesthesia. *Does the patient have any known idiosyncrasies?* Some patients show abnormal drug reactions, benign arrhythmias, prolonged sedation after certain drugs, or other reactions that are known to their primary physicians. These are useful to learn ahead of time.

Reference

1. Chung, F.: Cancer chemotherapy and anesthesia. Can. Anaesth. Soc. J., *29*:364, 1982.

OUTPATIENT SURGERY

Outpatient surgery is becoming increasingly popular, especially in pediatric hospitals. Doing minor procedures such as spica cast application, pin removal, or soft-tissue biopsies saves time, cost, and the psychologic trauma of overnight hospitalization. It has been demonstrated that the outpatient is exposed to fewer hospital-acquired infections.[1] Only patients who are in stable condition, are in relatively good health, and have responsible parents are candidates for outpatient surgery. Any records of past hospitalizations, medications, or complications should be available. It speeds the day of surgery if laboratory work is done ahead of time. Complicated cases or patients who are marginally acceptable for outpatient surgery should be discussed with the anesthesiologist ahead of the day of the procedure.

Reference

1. Steward, D. J.: Manual of Pediatric Anesthesia. New York, Churchill-Livingstone, 1979, p. 203

RISK OF ANESTHESIA

There are no good studies on the risk of surgery for children undergoing orthopedic procedures. Extrapolating from other work, however, it can be anticipated that otherwise healthy children have an exceedingly low risk of death. Many would claim there is none, but the rare occurrence of drug allergy, malignant hyperthermia, equipment failure, and the like probably produces a finite, though very small, risk. The risk of morbidity and death increases as the extent of surgery increases and the underlying medical problems of the patient increase. Complications can be kept to a minimum with proper evaluation and preparation by both the orthopedic surgeon and the anesthesiologist and their continued communication in the perioperative period.

Appendix to Chapter 1

Table 1–1. *Normal Measurements in Relation to Age**
Male

Age	Height (cm.)	Weight (kg.)	Span	Upper Meas.	Lower Meas.	Ratio U/L	Head (cm.)	Chest (cm.)	Abdomen (cm.)
Birth	51.3	3.36	48.5	32.3	19.1	1.69	35.3	35.1	34.0
1 mo.	55.6	4.72	53.6	34.8	20.8	1.67	38.6	36.3	35.1
2 mo.	58.7	5.44	55.9	36.6	22.1	1.65	40.6	39.6	38.6
3 mo.	61.2	6.17	58.4	38.1	23.1	1.65	42.2	41.7	40.6
4 mo.	63.5	6.80	61.0	39.4	24.1	1.63	43.2	42.9	41.9
5 mo.	65.3	7.17	62.0	40.4	24.9	1.62	44.2	43.7	42.7
6 mo.	67.1	7.85	64.5	41.4	25.7	1.61	45.0	44.5	43.4
7 mo.	68.8	8.16	65.8	42.4	26.4	1.61	45.5	45.0	43.9
8 mo.	70.1	8.48	67.1	42.9	27.2	1.58	46.0	45.5	44.5
9 mo.	71.4	8.80	68.3	43.7	27.7	1.58	46.2	45.7	44.7
10 mo.	72.6	9.07	69.3	44.2	28.4	1.55	46.7	46.2	45.0
11 mo.	73.9	9.39	70.6	44.7	29.2	1.53	47.0	46.5	45.2
12 mo.	74.9	9.71	71.9	45.5	29.5	1.54	47.2	47.0	45.5
15 mo.	78.0	10.29	74.4	47.0	31.0	1.52	48.0	47.8	46.2
18 mo.	81.0	11.2	78.2	48.8	32.3	1.51	48.5	48.5	47.0
21 mo.	83.6	11.8	80.8	49.8	33.8	1.47	49.0	49.3	47.5
24 mo.	86.1	12.4	83.1	50.8	35.3	1.44	49.3	50.0	48.0
30 mo.	90.7	13.2	86.9	52.8	37.8	1.40	49.8	51.3	48.8
36 mo.	94.7	14.5	91.9	54.1	40.6	1.33	50.3	52.3	49.5
42 mo.	98.6	15.4	95.8	55.9	42.7	1.31	50.8	53.3	50.3
48 mo.	102.1	16.1	98.6	57.2	45.0	1.27	51.1	54.4	50.8
54 mo.	105.4	17.1	102.4	58.2	47.2	1.23	51.6	55.1	51.3
60 mo.	108.5	17.8	105.2	59.4	49.0	1.21	51.8	56.1	51.8
5½ yr.	111.5	19.0	109.0	60.2	51.3	1.17	51.8	56.9	52.3
6 yr.	114.3	19.9	111.8	61.0	53.3	1.14	52.1	57.7	53.1
6½ yr.	117.1	20.8	114.6	61.7	55.4	1.11	52.1	58.4	53.6
7 yr.	119.9	21.8	117.3	62.7	57.2	1.10	52.3	59.2	54.1
7½ yr.	122.4	22.9	120.1	63.2	59.2	1.07	52.6	60.2	54.6
8 yr.	125.0	23.9	123.4	64.3	60.7	1.06	52.6	61.0	55.4
8½ yr.	127.5	25.1	126.5	65.3	62.2	1.05	52.8	61.7	55.9
9 yr.	130.0	26.3	129.5	66.0	64.0	1.03	53.1	62.5	56.6
9½ yr.	132.6	27.7	132.6	67.1	65.5	1.02	53.1	63.5	57.2
10 yr.	135.1	29.2	135.6	68.1	67.1	1.02	53.3	64.3	57.9
10½ yr.	137.7	30.7	138.4	68.8	68.8	1.00	53.3	65.3	58.4
11 yr.	140.2	32.3	141.2	69.9	70.4	0.99	53.6	66.3	59.2
11½ yr.	142.7	33.9	144.0	70.9	71.9	0.99	53.8	67.6	59.9
12 yr.	145.0	35.5	147.1	71.9	73.2	0.98	53.8	68.6	60.7
12½ yr.	147.3	37.2	150.1	72.9	74.4	0.98	54.1	69.9	61.5
13 yr.	149.6	38.9	152.9	73.9	75.7	0.98	54.4	71.1	62.5
13½ yr.	151.9	40.7	155.7	74.9	77.0	0.97	54.6	72.6	63.5

*From Johns Hopkins Hospital: Harriet Lane Handbook, 5th edition. Copyright © 1969, Year Book Medical Publishers, Inc. Reprinted by permission.

Table 1–2. *Normal Measurements in Relation to Age**
Female

Age	Height (cm.)	Weight (kg.)	Span	Upper Meas.	Lower Meas.	Ratio U/L	Head (cm.)	Chest (cm.)	Abdomen (cm.)
Birth	50.5	3.40	48.3	32.0	18.5	1.73	34.5	34.5	33.5
1 mo.	54.6	4.40	52.1	34.3	20.3	1.69	37.8	35.8	34.5
2 mo.	57.7	5.08	54.4	36.1	21.6	1.67	39.9	38.9	38.1
3 mo.	60.2	5.76	56.9	37.6	22.6	1.66	41.4	40.6	39.9
4 mo.	62.5	6.39	59.2	38.6	23.9	1.62	42.4	41.9	41.1
5 mo.	64.3	7.03	61.7	39.6	24.6	1.61	43.4	42.7	41.9
6 mo.	66.0	7.35	63.0	40.6	25.4	1.60	43.9	43.2	42.7
7 mo.	67.6	7.66	64.3	41.4	26.2	1.58	44.4	43.7	43.2
8 mo.	68.8	7.98	65.5	42.2	26.7	1.58	45.0	44.2	43.7
9 mo.	70.1	8.25	66.5	42.7	27.4	1.56	45.2	44.7	43.9
10 mo.	71.4	8.53	67.8	43.2	28.2	1.53	45.7	45.2	44.2
11 mo.	72.6	8.84	69.1	43.9	28.7	1.53	46.0	45.5	44.4
12 mo.	73.7	9.12	70.4	44.4	29.2	1.52	46.2	46.0	44.7
15 mo.	76.7	9.66	72.9	46.0	30.7	1.50	47.0	46.7	45.5
18 mo.	79.8	10.5	76.4	47.5	32.3	1.47	47.5	47.5	46.2
21 mo.	82.3	11.1	79.0	48.8	33.5	1.45	48.0	48.3	46.7
24 mo.	84.8	11.7	81.5	49.9	35.0	1.42	48.3	48.8	47.2
30 mo.	89.2	12.6	85.3	51.8	37.3	1.39	48.8	49.8	48.0
36 mo.	93.2	13.5	89.1	53.1	40.1	1.32	49.3	50.8	48.5
42 mo.	97.0	14.5	93.0	54.6	42.4	1.29	49.8	51.8	49.0
48 mo.	100.6	15.4	96.8	55.9	44.7	1.25	50.0	52.6	49.5
54 mo.	103.9	16.4	100.8	56.9	47.0	1.21	50.5	53.3	50.0
60 mo.	107.2	17.1	103.4	58.2	49.0	1.19	50.8	54.4	50.5
5½ yr.	110.2	18.2	107.4	58.9	41.3	1.15	51.0	55.1	50.8
6 yr.	113.3	19.0	110.0	60.2	53.1	1.13	51.0	55.9	51.3
6½ yr.	116.1	20.0	112.8	61.2	54.9	1.12	51.3	56.6	51.8
7 yr.	118.9	21.4	116.8	62.0	56.9	1.09	51.6	57.0	52.1
7½ yr.	121.7	22.4	119.6	62.7	58.9	1.06	51.6	58.4	52.6
8 yr.	124.2	23.6	122.4	63.5	60.7	1.05	51.8	59.4	52.8
8½ yr.	126.7	24.8	125.2	64.5	62.2	1.04	52.1	60.4	53.3
9 yr.	129.3	26.0	128.0	65.3	64.0	1.02	52.1	61.5	53.8
9½ yr.	131.8	27.5	130.8	66.3	65.5	1.01	52.3	62.5	54.6
10 yr.	134.6	28.8	133.6	67.8	66.8	1.01	52.6	63.5	55.4
10½ yr.	137.4	30.5	136.4	69.1	68.3	1.01	52.8	64.8	56.1
11 yr.	140.5	32.8	140.5	70.4	70.1	1.00	53.1	66.3	56.9
11½ yr.	143.5	34.6	143.0	71.6	71.9	1.00	53.1	67.6	57.9
12 yr.	146.3	36.6	146.1	72.9	73.4	0.99	53.3	68.8	58.9
12½ yr.	149.1	38.6	148.6	74.2	74.9	0.99	53.6	70.1	59.9
13 yr.	151.6	40.8	151.6	75.4	76.2	0.99	53.8	71.4	60.7
13½ yr.	153.9	43.3	154.4	77.0	77.0	1.00	54.1	72.4	61.5

*From Johns Hopkins Hospital: Harriet Lane Handbook, 5th edition. Copyright © 1969, Year Book Medical Publishers, Inc. Reprinted by permission.

Table 1–3. *Chart for Muscle Examination in Spastic Paralysis*

MUSCLE EXAMINATION
CHILDREN'S MEMORIAL HOSPITAL

Patient Name _____   Chart No. _____

Attending Physician _____   Patient Date of Birth _____

			LEFT						EXAMINER'S INITIALS							RIGHT				
									DATE												
IP	CC	IP	CC	IP	CC	IP	CC				CC	IP	CC	IP	CC	IP	CC	IP			
								NECK	FLEXORS	STERNOCLEIDOMASTOID											
									EXTENSOR GROUP												
								TRUNK	FLEXORS	RECTUS ABDOMINIS											
									RT. EXT. OBL. / LT. INT. OBL. ROTATORS	LT. EXT. OBL. / RT. INT. OBL.											
									TRANSVERSUS ABDOMINUS												
									EXTENSORS	THORACIC GROUP / LUMBAR GROUP											
									PELVIC ELEV.	QUADRATUS LUMB.											
								HIP	FLEXORS	ILIOPSOAS											
									EXTENSORS	GLUTEUS MAXIMUS											
									ABDUCTORS	GLUTEUS MEDIUS											
									ADDUCTOR GROUP												
									EXTERNAL ROTATOR GROUP												
									INTERNAL ROTATOR GROUP												
									SARTORIUS												
									TENSOR FASCIAE LATAE												
								KNEE	FLEXORS	BICEPS FEMORIS / INNER HAMSTRINGS											
									EXTENSORS	QUADRICEPS											
								ANKLE	PLANTAR FLEXORS	GASTROCNEMIUS / SOLEUS											
								FOOT	INVERTORS	TIBIALIS ANTERIOR / TIBIALIS POSTERIOR											
									EVERTORS	PERONEUS BREVIS / PERONEUS LONGUS											
								TOES	M.P. FLEXORS	LUMBRICALES	1										
											2										
											3										
											4										
									I.P. FLEXORS (1ST)	FLEX. DIGIT. BR.	1										
											2										
											3										
											4										
									I.P. FLEXORS (2ND)	FLEX. DIGIT. L.	1										
											2										
											3										
											4										
									M.P. EXTENSORS	EXT. DIGIT. BR.	1										
											2										
											3										
											4										
									I.P. EXTENSORS	EXT. DIGIT. L.	1										
											2										
											3										
											4										
								HALLUX	M.P. FLEXOR	FLEX. HALL. BR.											
									I.P. FLEXOR	FLEX. HALL. L.											
									M.P. EXTENSOR	EXT. HALL. BR.											
									I.P. EXTENSOR	EXT. HALL. L.											
								CHEST	INSPIRATION	(MEASUREMENTS)											
									EXPIRATION												
								ABDOMEN	UMBILICUS TO ANT. SUP. SPINE												
								LOWER	CIRCUMFERENCE — MID CALF												
								EXTREMITY	CIRCUMFERENCE — MID THIGH												
									ANT. SUP. SPINE TO INT. MALLEOLUS												
									UMBILICUS TO INTERNAL MALLEOLUS												

X	Present	Unable to be graded	F–	Fair Minus	Incomplete range of motion against gravity
N	Normal	Complete range of motion against gravity with full resistance	P	Poor	Complete range of motion with gravity eliminated
G	Good	Complete range of motion against gravity with moderate resistance	P–	Poor Minus	Incomplete range of motion with gravity eliminated
F+	Fair Plus	Complete range of motion against gravity with slight resistance	T	Trace	Contraction is felt but there is no visible joint movement
F	Fair	Complete range of motion against gravity	0	Zero	No contraction felt in the muscle

IP = In Pattern   CC = Cerebral Control

Table continued on following page

Table 1–13. Orthopedic History and Physical Examination Continued

LEFT												RIGHT							
								EXAMINER'S INITIAL											
								DATE											
IP	CC	IP	CC	IP	CC	IP	CC					CC	IP	CC	IP	CC	IP	CC	IP
								SCAPULA	ABDUCTOR	SERRATUS ANTERIOR									
									ELEVATOR	UPPER TRAPEZIUS									
									DEPRESSOR	LOWER TRAPEZIUS									
									ADDUCTORS	MIDDLE TRAPEZIUS / RHOMBOIDS									
								SHOULDER	FLEXOR	ANTERIOR DELTOID									
									EXTENSORS	LATISSIMUS DORSI / TERES MAJOR									
									ABDUCTOR	MIDDLE DELTOID									
									HORIZ. ABD.	POSTERIOR DELTOID									
									HORIZ. ADD.	PECTORALIS MAJOR									
								EXTERNAL ROTATOR GROUP											
								INTERNAL ROTATOR GROUP											
								ELBOW	FLEXORS	BICEPS BRACHI / BRACHIORADIALIS									
									EXTENSOR	TRICEPS									
								FOREARM	SUPINATOR GROUP										
									PRONATOR GROUP										
								WRIST	FLEXORS	FLEX. CARPI RAD.									
										FLEX. CARPI ULN.									
										PALMARIS LONGUS									
									EXTENSORS	EXT. CARPI RAD.L & BR. / EXT. CARPI ULN.									
								FINGERS	M.P. FLEXORS	LUMBRICALES	1								
											2								
											3								
											4								
									I.P. FLEXORS (1ST)	FLEX. DIGIT. SUB.	1								
											2								
											3								
											4								
									I.P. FLEXORS (2ND)	FLEX. DIGIT. PROF.	1								
											2								
											3								
											4								
									M.P. EXTENSOR.	EXT. DIGIT. COM.	1								
											2								
											3								
											4								
									ADDUCTORS	PALMAR INTEROSSEI	1								
											2								
											3								
											4								
									ABDUCTORS	DORSAL INTEROSSEI	1								
											2								
											3								
											4								
								ABDUCTOR DIGITI QUINTI											
								OPPONENS DIGITI QUINTI											
								THUMB	M.P. FLEXOR	FLEX. POLL. BR.									
									I.P. FLEXOR	FLEX. POLL. L									
									M.P. EXTENSOR	EXT. POLL. BR.									
									I.P. EXTENSOR	EXT. POLL. L.									
									ABDUCTORS	ABD. POLL. BR. / ABD. POLL. L.									
								ADDUCTOR POLLICIS											
								OPPONENS POLLICIS											
								FACE											

ADDITIONAL DATA:

SIGNATURE _____

Table 1–4. *Chart for Muscle Examination in Flaccid Paralysis*

Muscle Examination
Children's Memorial Hospital

Patient Name _____   Chart No. _____

Attending Physician _____   Patient Date of Birth _____

Left — ★ Enter initials of examiner / + Enter date of examination. Right — ★ Enter initials of examiner / + Enter date of examination.

Region	Group	Muscle	$(C)_{123}$	T_{1234}	T_{56}	T_{78}	$T_{9\,10\,11}$	T_{12}	L_1	L_2	L_3	L_4	L_5	S_1	S_2	S_3
Neck	Flexors	Sternocleidomastoid $C_{12345678}\,T_1$	•													
	Extensor Group															
Trunk	Extensors	Thoracic Group		•	•	•	•									
		Lumbar Group		•	•	•	•									
	Flexors	Rectus Abdominis			•	•	•									
	Rotators	⌐Lt. Int. Obl. ⌐Rt. Int. Obl. / ⌐Rt. Ext. Obl. ⌐Lt. Ext. Obl.				•	•	(•)								
							•	•	1	(2)						
	Pelvic Elev.	Quadratus Abdom.						•	1	2	3					
Hip	Flexors	Iliopsoas							1	2	3	4				
		Sartorius								2	3	(4)				
	ADDuctor Group									2	3	4				
Knee	Extensors	Quadriceps								2	3	4				
Hip	ABDuctors	Gluteus Medius											5	1		
		Tensor Fasciae Latae										4	5	1		
	IR Group											4	5	1		
Foot	Inv. & Drsfl	Tibialis Anterior										4	5	1		
	Evertors	Peroneus Brevis										4	5	1		
		Peroneus Longus										4	5	1		
Hallux	M.P. Ext	Ext. Hall. Br.										4	5	1		
	I.P. Ext	Ext. Hall. L.										4	5	1		
	M.P. Flexor	Flex. Hall. Br.										4	5	1		
Toes	I.P. Flexors	Flex. Digit. Br. 1										4	5	1		
		2										4	5	1		
		3										4	5	1		
		4										4	5	1		
	M.P. Extensors	Ext. Digit. Br. 1										4	5	1		
		2										4	5	1		
		3										4	5	1		
		4										4	5	1		
	I.P. Extensors	Ext. Digit. L. 1										4	5	1		
		2										4	5	1		
		3										4	5	1		
		4										4	5	1		
Foot	Invertor	Tibialis Posterior										(4)	5	1		
Toes	M.P. Flexors	Lumbricales 1										4	5	1		
		2										(4)	(5)	1	2	
		3										(4)	(5)	1	2	
		4										(4)	(5)	1	2	
Knee	M. Flexors	Inner Hamstrings										(4)	(5)	1	2	
Hip	E.R. Group											4	5	1	2	(3)
Toes	I.P. Flexors	Flex. Digit. L. 1											5	1	(2)	
		2											5	1	(2)	
		3											5	1	(2)	
		4											5	1	(2)	
Hip	Extensor	Gluteus Maximus											5	1	2	
Ankle	Plantar Flexors	Soleus											5	1	2	
		Gastrocnemius												1	2	
Hallux	I.P. Flexors	Flex. Hall. L.											5	1	2	
Knee	L. Flexor	Biceps Femoris											5	1	2	3

X	Present	Unable to be graded
N	Normal	Complete range of motion against gravity with full resistance
G	Good	Complete range of motion against gravity with moderate resistance
F+	Fair Plus	Complete range of motion against gravity with slight resistance
F	Fair	Complete range of motion against gravity
F-	Fair Minus	Incomplete range of motion against gravity
P	Poor	Complete range of motion with gravity eliminated
P-	Poor Minus	Incomplete range of motion with gravity eliminated
T	Trace	Contraction is felt but there is no visible joint movement
0	Zero	No contraction felt in the muscle

Form No. 77053

Table continued on following page

Table 1–4. Chart for Muscle Examination in Flaccid Paralysis Continued

* Enter initials of examiner

+ Enter date of examination

Region	Action	Muscle	#	C1	C2	C3	C4	C5	C6	C7	C8	T1
Scapula	Elevator	Upper Trapezius			2	3	4					
	Depressor	Lower Trapezius			2	3	4					
	ABDuctors	Middle Trapezius			2	3	4					
		Rhomboids					4	5				
Shoulder	ABDuctors	Middle Deltoid					4	5	6			
		Supraspinatus					4	5	6			
	Ext. Rotators	Infraspinatus					(4)	5	6			
		Teres Minor					(4)	5	6			
	Flexor	Anterior Deltoid						5	6			
		Posterior Deltoid						5	6			
Elbow	Flexors	Biceps Brachii						5	6			
		Brachioradialis						5	6			
Shoulder	Extensor	Teres Major						5	6	7		
	Horiz. Add.	Pectoralis Major						5	6	7		
	Internal Rotator	Subscapularis						5	5	7		
Forearm	Supinator	Supinator						5	6	7		
Scapula	ABDuctor	Serratus Anterior						5	6	(7)	8	
Wrist	Extensor	Ext. Carpi Rad. L. & Br.						5	6	7	8	
Forearm	Pronation	Pronator Group							6	7		
Shoulder	Extensor	Latissimus Dorsi							6	7	8	
Wrist	Flexors	Flex. Carp. Rad.							6	7	8	
	Extensor	Ext. Carp. Uln.							6	7	8	
Finger	M.P. Extensor	Ext. Digit. Com.	1						6	7	8	
			2						6	7	8	
			3						6	7	8	
			4						6	7	8	
Thumb	M.P. Extensor	Ext. Poll. Br.							6	7	8	
	I.P. Extensor	Ext. Poll. L.							6	7	8	
	ABDuctor	ABD. Poll. L.							6	7	8	
Elbow	Extensor	Triceps							6	7	8	1
Wrist	Flexors	Palmaris Longus							(6)	7	8	1
Fingers	M.P. Flexors	Lumbricales	1						(6)	7	8	1
			2									
Thumb	M.P. Flexor	Flex. Poll. Br.							6	7	8	1
	I.P. Flexor	Flex. Poll. L.							(6)	7	8	1
	ABDuctor	ABD. Poll. Br.							6	7	8	1
	Opponent	Opponens Poll.							6	7	8	1
Wrist	Flexor	Flex. Carpi Uln.								7	8	1
Fingers	M.P. Flexors	Lumbricales	3							(7)	8	1
			4							(7)	8	1
	I.P. Flexors (1st)	Flex. Digit. Sub.	1							7	8	1
			2							7	8	1
			3							7	8	1
			4							7	8	1
	I.P. Flexors (2nd)	Flex. Digit. Prof.	1							7	8	1
			2							7	8	1
			3							7	8	1
			4							7	8	1
	ADDuctors	Palmar Interossei	1								8	1
			2								8	1
			3								8	1
			4								8	1
	ABDuctors	Dorsal Interossei	1								8	1
			2								8	1
			3								8	1
			4								8	1
Thumb	ADDuctors	ADDuctor Pollicis									8	1

Table 1–5. *Grading of Muscle Strength**

Grade	Definition
0	No palpable contraction of muscle
Trace	Palpable contraction of muscle, no motion of part that muscle should move
Poor	Muscle moves part through its range, but not against gravity
Fair	Muscle carries part through its range of motion against gravity, but not against added resistance
Good	Muscle lifts part against gravity and added resistance (good minus and good plus used to indicate variations in resistance)
Normal	Normal strength
In practice, certain modified grades may be added:	
Poor minus	Muscle moves part, but not against gravity and not through full range
Fair minus	Muscle moves part against gravity, but not through full range

*For the technique of testing the strength of individual muscles, the reader is referred to Daniels, Williams, and Worthingham, and to Kendall and Kendall.[54, 57] The charts used by the author are shown in Tables 1–3 and 1–4.

The segmental and peripheral nerve innervation of muscles for movements of the shoulder girdle and upper extremity is given in Table 1–6 and that of the lower extremity in Table 1–7.

Table 1–6. *Innervation of Muscles Responsible for Movements of the Shoulder Girdle and Upper Extremity**

Muscle	Segmental Innervation	Peripheral Nerve
Trapezius	Cranial XI; C(2) 3–4	Spinal accessory nerve
Levator anguli scapulae	{ C 3–4	Nerves to levator anguli scapulae
	{ C 4–5	Dorsal scapular nerve
Rhomboideus major	C 4–5	Dorsal scapular nerve
Rhomboideus minor	C 4–5	Dorsal scapular nerve
Serratus anterior	C 5–7	Long thoracic nerve
Deltoid	C 5–6	Axillary nerve
Teres minor	C 5–6	Axillary nerve
Supraspinatus	C (4) 5–6	Suprascapular nerve
Infraspinatus	C (4) 5–6	Suprascapular nerve
Latissimus dorsi	C 6–8	Thoracodorsal nerve (long subscapular)
Pectoralis major	C 5–T 1	Lateral and medial anterior thoracic
Pectoralis minor	C 7–T 1	Medial anterior thoracic
Subscapularis	C 5–7	Subscapular nerves
Teres major	C 5–7	Lower subscapular nerve
Subclavius	C 5–6	Nerve to subclavius
Coracobrachialis	C 6–7	Musculocutaneous nerve
Biceps brachii	C 5–6	Musculocutaneous nerve
Brachialis	C 5–6	Musculocutaneous nerve
Brachioradialis	C 5–6	Radial nerve
Triceps brachii	C 6–8 (T 1)	Radial nerve
Anconeus	C 7–8	Radial nerve
Supinator brevis	C 5–7	Radial nerve
Extensor carpi radialis longus	C (5) 6–7 (8)	Radial nerve
Extensor carpi radialis brevis	C (5) 6–7 (8)	Radial nerve
Extensor carpi ulnaris	C 6–8	Radial nerve
Extensor digitorum communis	C 6–8	Radial nerve
Extensor indicis proprius	C 6–8	Radial nerve
Extensor digiti minimi proprius	C 6–8	Radial nerve
Extensor pollicis longus	C 6–8	Radial nerve
Extensor pollicis brevis	C 6–8	Radial nerve
Abductor pollicis longus	C 6–8	Radial nerve
Pronator teres	C 6–7	Median nerve
Flexor carpi radialis	C 6–7 (8)	Median nerve
Pronator quadratus	C 7–T 1	Median nerve
Palmaris longus	C 7–T 1	Median nerve
Flexor digitorum sublimis	C 7–T 1	Median nerve
Flexor digitorum profundus (radial half)	C 7–T 1	Median nerve
Lumbricales 1 and 2	C 7–T 1	Median nerve
Flexor pollicis longus	C 8–T 1	Median nerve
Flexor pollicis brevis (lateral head)	C 8–T 1	Median nerve
Abductor pollicis brevis	C 8–T 1	Median nerve
Opponens pollicis	C 8–T 1	Median nerve
Flexor carpi ulnaris	C 7–T 1	Ulnar nerve
Flexor digitorum profundus (ulnar half)	C 7–T 1	Ulnar nerve
Interossei	C 8–T 1	Ulnar nerve
Lumbricales 3 and 4	C 8–T 1	Ulnar nerve
Flexor pollicis brevis (medial head)	C 8–T 1	Ulnar nerve
Flexor digiti minimi brevis	C 8–T 1	Ulnar nerve
Abductor digiti minimi	C 8–T 1	Ulnar nerve
Opponens digiti minimi	C 8–T 1	Ulnar nerve
Palmaris brevis	C 8–T 1	Ulnar nerve
Adductor pollicis	C 8–T 1	Ulnar nerve

*From Dejong, R. N.: The Neurological Examination. New York, Hoeber Medical Division, Harper & Row, 1967, pp. 456–457.

Table 1–7. *Innervation of Muscles Responsible for Movements of the Lower Extremities**

Muscle	Segmental Innervation	Peripheral Nerve
Psoas major	L (1) 2–4	Nerve to psoas major
Psoas minor	L 1–2	Nerve to psoas minor
Iliacus	L 2–4	Femoral nerve
Quadriceps femoris	L 2–4	Femoral nerve
Sartorius	L 2–4	Femoral nerve
Pectineus	L 2–4	Femoral nerve
Gluteus maximus	L 5–S 2	Inferior gluteal nerve
Gluteus medius	L 4–S 1	Superior gluteal nerve
Gluteus minimus	L 4–S 1	Superior gluteal nerve
Tensor fasciae latae	L 4–S 1	Superior gluteal nerve
Piriformis	S 1–2	Nerve to piriformis
Adductor longus	L 2–4	Obturator nerve
Adductor brevis	L 2–4	Obturator nerve
Adductor magnus	{ L 2–4	Obturator nerve
	{ L 4–5	Sciatic nerve
Gracilis	L 2–4	Obturator nerve
Obturator externus	L 2–4	Obturator nerve
Obturator internus	L 5–S 3	Nerve to obturator internus
Gemellus superior	L 5–S 3	Nerve to obturator internus
Gemellus inferior	L 4–S 1	Nerve to quadratus femoris
Quadratus femoris	L 4–S 1	Nerve to quadratus femoris
Biceps femoris (long head)	L 5–S 1	Tibial nerve
Semimembranosus	L 4–S 1	Tibial nerve
Semitendinosus	L 5–S 2	Tibial nerve
Popliteus	L 5–S 1	Tibial nerve
Gastrocnemius	L 5–S 2	Tibial nerve
Soleus	L 5–S 2	Tibial nerve
Plantaris	L 5–S 1	Tibial nerve
Tibialis posterior	L 5–S 1	Tibial nerve
Flexor digitorum longus	L 5–S 1	Tibial nerve
Flexor hallucis longus	L 5–S 1	Tibial nerve
Biceps femoris (short head)	L 5–S 2	Common peroneal nerve
Tibialis anterior	L 4–S 1	Deep peroneal nerve
Peroneus tertius	L 4–S 1	Deep peroneal nerve
Extensor digitorum longus	L 4–S 1	Deep peroneal nerve
Extensor hallucis longus	L 4–S 1	Deep peroneal nerve
Extensor digitorum brevis	L 4–S 1	Deep peroneal nerve
Extensor hallucis brevis	L 4–S 1	Deep peroneal nerve
Peroneus longus	L 4–S 1	Superficial peroneal nerve
Peroneus brevis	L 4–S 1	Superficial peroneal nerve
Flexor digitorum brevis	L 4–S 1	Medial plantar nerve
Flexor hallucis brevis	L 5–S 1	Medial plantar nerve
Abductor hallucis	L 4–S 1	Medial plantar nerve
Lumbricales (medial 1 or 2)	L 4–S 1	Medial plantar nerve
Quadratus plantae	S 1–2	Lateral plantar nerve
Adductor hallucis	L 5–S 2	Lateral plantar nerve
Abductor digiti quinti	S 1–2	Lateral plantar nerve
Flexor digiti quinti brevis	S 1–2	Lateral plantar nerve
Lumbricales (lateral 2 or 3)	S 1–2	Lateral plantar nerve
Interossei	S 1–2	Lateral plantar nerve

*From DeJong, R. N.: The Neurological Examination. New York, Hoeber Medical Division, Harper & Row, 1967, pp. 483–484.

Table 1–8. Reflexes of Neurophysiologic Maturation

Reflex	Test Position	Stimulus	Response
Palmar (hand) grasp (Fig. 1–35)	Supine. Head must be in midline	Introduction of a pencil or rod into palm from ulnar side; object pulled on after grasp	Fingers will flex and grasp object Thumb will not oppose but will flex if extended If response marked, infant can be suspended by object he is holding
Plantar (foot) grasp (Fig. 1–36)	Supine	Light digital pressure on plantar aspect of foot	Tonic flexion and adduction of toes
Moro (Fig. 1–37)	Supine with both upper and lower limbs in natural extension	Sudden extension of neck by raising the head off the table, supporting head on palm of hand, then suddenly dropping hand Raising the infant by holding the hands and then rapidly releasing Sharp bang on table or sudden tap on abdomen	*First phase*—abduction and extension of all four limbs and extension of spine; extension and fanning of digits; followed by: *Second phase*—adduction and flexion of all four limbs as if embracing
Startle	Supine with all four limbs in natural extension	Sudden loud noise Tapping sternum	Flexion of elbows and knees, hands closed
Placing reaction			
Lower limb (Fig. 1–38)	Vertical suspension by holding at waist	Touching anterior aspect of legs and dorsum of feet on edge of table	Foot placed on table by spontaneous flexion of hip and knee and dorsiflexion of ankle
Upper limb (Fig. 1–39)	Vertical suspension (feet down) by holding at waist	Bringing dorsum of ulna against edge of table	Hand placed on table by flexion of elbow
Walking or stepping (Fig. 1–40)	Upright. Hold supporting trunk	Pressing (touching) soles of feet on hard surface and gently inclining and moving child forward	Alternating flexion and extension of lower limbs simulating walking (rhythmical, coordinated, needs only forward movement, no propulsion)
Crossed extension (Phillippson's reflex) (Fig. 1–41)	Supine, lower limbs in midline and extended at hip and knee	Firm pressure to sole of one foot by rubbing or stroking Strong pressure in inguinal region	Opposite free lower limb flexes, adducts, then extends
Withdrawal	Supine, lower limbs in midline and natural extended posture	Pinprick to sole	Dorsiflexion of ankle, flexion of hip and knee (withdraws limb from noxious stimulus)
Positive support or leg straightening	Upright, supported under axillae and around chest	Press soles of feet to the ground or table several times	Lower limbs and trunk go into extension, serving as strong pillars for weight-bearing
Extensor thrust	Lower limbs held in flexed position	Apply pressure to the sole of the foot	Sudden—extension of entire lower limb (sometimes followed by flexion)
Trunk incurvation (Galant's reflex) (Fig. 1–42)	Prone	Strike lumbar region of back with index finger—10th rib to iliac crest—in the paravertebral area about 3 cm. from midline. Alternate method—prick outer side of gluteal area	Lateral flexion (incurvation) of trunk toward side of stimulus
Tonic neck			
Asymmetric (Fig. 1–43)	Supine with head in midline	Rotate head to one side (without flexion of neck) to the count of 10 seconds, then rotate to the opposite side	Limbs on *chin side*—become rigid and elbow and knee go into extension Limbs on *occiput side*—elbow and knee become flexed
Symmetric (Fig. 1–44)	Quadriped position	Extend head-neck Flex head-neck	Upper limbs extend and lower limbs go into flexion Upper limbs flex and lower limbs extend

***Table 1–8.** Reflexes of Neurophysiologic Maturation* Continued

Appears	Disappears	Significance of Absence	Significance of Abnormal Persistence
Birth	2–4 mo.	Flaccid paralysis	Flexor hypertonicity as in spastic cerebral palsy Asymmetric in hemiplegia
Birth	9–12 mo.	Flaccid paralysis	Spasticity of leg and foot muscles
Birth	3–6 mo.	In flaccid paralysis, may be asymmetric in obstetric brachial plexus paralysis In generalized hypotonia or weakness of muscles, as amyotonia congenita In severe hypertonicity increased flexor muscle tone prevents extension of limbs	After six months, delayed maturation of central nervous system as in cerebral palsy
Birth	Present through life	Severe hypotonia Asymmetric obstetric brachial plexus paralysis	—
Birth	2–4 mo. and may persist	Brain damage if absent at birth	—
Birth	1–2 mo. and may persist	Brain damage if absent at birth	—
Birth	1–2 mo.	Flaccid paralysis if absent at birth	Brain damage if persists after 3–4 months
Birth	1–2 mo.	Flaccid paralysis if absent at birth	Partial or incomplete cord lesions Brain damage
Birth	1–2 mo.	Flaccid paralysis as in myelomeningocele or intraspinal lesions	Spasticity of lower limbs as in cerebral palsy
Birth	4 mo.	—	Reciprocal leg movements cannot appear, infant cannot walk
Birth	2 mo.	Flaccid paralysis	Brain damage and delayed maturation of central nervous system
Birth	2–2½ mo	?	May cause scoliosis if dominant unilaterally
Birth	4–6 mo.	Flaccid paralysis Severe hypotonia	Severe brain damage as in cerebral palsy
5–8 mo.	No absolute time (one year)	Cannot assume "four-point" kneeling position	Prevents reciprocal lower limb motion, hinders ambulation Prevents crawling Causes adduction, medial rotation flexion gait pattern

Table continued on following page

Table 1–8. Reflexes of Neurophysiologic Maturation Continued

Reflex	Test Position	Stimulus	Response
Landau	Prone, supported under abdomen and lower thorax	First passively flex and then extend the neck-head	On flexion of neck-head, the trunk and lower and upper limbs go into flexion. On extension of head-neck, the limbs and trunk extend
Parachute (protective extension of arms) Forward (Fig. 1–45)	Prone, suspended in the air by waist	Move head suddenly toward floor by tipping or plunging downward	Sudden extension of arms and wrists to protect head
Backward	Sitting or standing in neutral position	Sudden tip or push backward with enough force to offset balance	Backward extension of both upper limbs. Fingers extended and abducted—and weight is born on hands
Tilting			
Prone and supine	Prone (or supine) on tilt table (flat board) with all four limbs in neutral extension	Tilt table slowly to one side	Lateral flexion of trunk with concavity upwards. The arm and leg on upper side go into abduction and extension. Arm and leg on lower side go into protection.
On all fours	Placed on all fours on tilt table	Tilt to either side	As above
Standing	Supported from waist, standing on tilt board	Movement first to either side and then forward and backward	As above
Righting			
Neck	Supine, head in midline and all four limbs fully extended	Flexion and rotation of head to one side, maintaining position to count of ten	Body rotates *as a whole* in same direction as head
Body	As for neck righting	Rotation of shoulder to one side, maintained to count of ten	Sequential rotation of trunk
Labyrinthine Prone	Blindfolded (to rule out optical righting reflexes) Suspended prone in space by support to abdomen	Posture in space	Extension of neck, bringing face horizontal to floor
Supine	Same as prone but *supine*	Posture in space	Flexion of head-neck bringing face horizontal to floor
Upright	Blindfolded, held at pelvis and suspended vertically in space	Tilt to either side	Head will automatically right to vertical position with the mouth horizontal
Optical (Fig. 1–46)	Same as labyrinthine but eyes *open*	Same as labyrinthine	Same as above

***Table 1–8.** Reflexes of Neurophysiologic Maturation* Continued

Appears	Disappears	Significance of Absence	Significance of Abnormal Persistence
6 mo.	24–30 mo	Motor weakness	Delayed reflex maturation, usually breaks up predominant flexion pattern
6 mo.	Present through life	Brain damage Delayed maturation	—
9 mo.	Present through life	Delayed maturation	—
6 mo.	Present through life	—	—
12 mo.	Present through life	—	
Birth	6 mo.	Delayed maturation	Brain damage
6 mo.	5 yr. to life	—	—
1–2 mo.	Present through life	Delayed maturation	—
6 mo.	Present through life	Delayed maturation	—
6–8 mo.	Present through life	Delayed maturation	—
6–8 mo.	Present through life	Delayed maturation	—

Table 1–9. Motor Development Evaluation*

Developmental Age	Skill	Developmental Age		Skill
Locomotion		Manipulation, Upper Extremity Function, and Language		
3 months	Lifts head up when prone	3 months	Hand skills	Symmetrical head and arm posture (supine)
6 months	Head held steady when sitting			Active arm motion on sight of toy
	Turns head side to side		Feeding	Lip pressure
	No head lag when pulled to sitting			Coordination of sucking and swallowing
	Rolls over		Language	Vocalizes without crying
9 months	Sits without support, legs extended	6 months	Hand skills	Purposefully reaches out and touches object
	Sits "tailor fashion"–external rotation			Palmar grasp of rattle
	Sits with legs in internal rotation			Involuntary release of rattle
	Pulls self to stand		Feeding	Hand to mouth
	Stands with two-hand support		Language	Laughs and smiles
12 months	Leans and recovers balance when sitting	9 months	Hand skills	Transfers object both ways
	Walks with one-hand support			Extended reach and grasp
				Uses finger and thumb to grasp object
14 months	Stands without support			Releases object with flexed wrist
	Walks forward without support		Feeding	Can protrude tongue
	Stoops and recovers balance			Feeds self cookies
18 months	Ascends stairs with two-hand support		Language	Da-da, ma-ma (non-specific)
2 years	Ascends stairs with no support, one foot at a time	1 year	Hand skills	Attempts to stack one block on another (brings over and drops)
	Runs forward			Hits two objects together
	Kicks ball forward			Voluntary release of object
3 years	Ascends stairs without support, foot over foot			Rolls ball imitatively
	Descends stairs with support, one foot at a time			Puts round block into round hole
	Jumps in place			Puts cube into container
	Pedals tricycle			Can hold crayon and imitate scribbling
4 years	Descends stairs without support, foot over foot		Feeding	Picks spoon up from table
	Beginning to balance on one foot			Chews cookies or toast
5 years	Hops on one foot without support			Drooling controlled at all times
	Heel-toe walk			Drinks milk from cup, if held
6 years	Skips one foot at a time		Dressing	Cooperates (extends arm for sleeve)
	Backward heel-toe walk		Language	Two or more words (other than ma-ma or da-da)
	Throws ball up and catches it with one hand			
	Hits small target from 12" distance	18 months	Hand skills	Builds three-block tower (1" cube)
				Turns pages (two or three at a time)
				Puts pegs into hole (1" diameter)
				Pounds

*Development is rated according to the Zausmer scale discussed on page 55: O, no attempt made; T, attempt made, but fails; P, poor or partial completion; F, fair performance, fluctuates; G, good, attaining speed; N, normal skill and speed; NT, not tested.

***Table 1–9.** Motor Development Evaluation* Continued

Developmental Age		Skill	Developmental Age		Skill
Manipulation, Upper Extremity Function, and Language Continued			*Manipulation, Upper Extremity Function, and Language* Continued		
		Hurls Ball	4 years	Hand skills	Overhand throw of ball
		Points to nose, eyes, ears		Feeding	Drinks through straw without mashing it
	Feeding	Drinks from cup (one- or two-handed)		Dressing	Puts shoes on correct feet
		Feeds self with spoon, but messy			Laces shoes, but does not tie bow
	Dressing	Removes socks, shoes			Dresses, knows back and front of clothes
	Language	Vocabulary of 10 words including names			Washes and dries face
2 years	Hand skills	Six-block tower			Brushes or combs hair
		Turns pages one at a time			Brushes teeth
		Throws bean bags			Manages buttons on self
		Strings beads (1″)		Language	Counts three objects correctly
		Throws 3″ ball, but inaccurately		Writing	Copies cross
	Feeding	Feeds self semi-solid food with spoon	5 years	Hand skills	Bounces ball and catches it
		Drinks from cup or glass (1 handed)			Performs three simple directions in sequence
		Drinks from straw		Dressing	Dresses self completely except for back fasteners
	Language	Three-word sentences		Language	Names four colors
	Writing	Imitates vertical, horizontal and circular strokes; cannot initiate himself			Names penny, nickel, dime
					Counts 10 objects correctly
		Matches colors		Writing	Draws recognizable man
2½ years	Dressing	Unlaces and removes shoes			Colors within 1″ area
		Takes off pants			Uses scissors, follows line
	Writing	Holds crayon with fingers	6 years	Feeding	Cuts with knife and fork
3 years	Hand skills	Creases paper neatly		Dressing	Buttons small buttons on shirt
		Nine-block tower			Ties bows on shoes
		Rides tricycle			Combs and brushes hair
	Feeding	Feeds self with fork		Writing	Copies printing (A, B, C)
	Dressing	Dresses self with supervision			
		Learning to lace shoes			
		Puts on shoes, not necessarily on correct foot			
		Tries to wash and dry hands			
	Language	Knows whether boy or girl			
	Writing	Copies circles, cannot copy cross			
		Tries to use scissors, but cannot follow line			

*Development is rated according to the Zausmer scale discussed on page 55: O, no attempt made; T, attempt made, but fails; P, poor or partial completion; F, fair performance, fluctuates; G, good, attaining speed; N, normal skill and speed; NT, not tested.

Table 1–10. Hematology*

	Gm. Hgb.	Per Cent Hct.	WBC/mm.³	Per Cent Polys	Per Cent Rectics
1 day	16–22†	53–73†	18,000 (7–35,000)	45–85	2.5–6.5
1 week	13–20†	43–66†	10,000 (4–20,000)	30–50	0.1–4.5
1 mo	16	53	10,000 (6–18,000)	30–50	0.1–1.0
3 mo.	11.5	38	10,000 (6–17,000)	30–50	0.7–3.0
6 mo.	12	40	10,000 (6–16,000)	30–50	0.7–2.3
1 yr.	12	40	10,000 (6–15,000)	30–50	0.6–1.7
2–6 yr.	13	43	9,000 (7–13,000)	35–55	0.5–1.0
7–12 yr.	14	46	8,500 (5–12,000)	40–60	0.5–1.0

Absolute eosinophil count: 100–600/mm.³, average 250

†Under the age of 1 month capillary Hgb. and Hct. exceed venous:

1 hour: 3.6 gm. av. difference

5 days: 2.2 gm. av. difference

3 weeks: 1.1 gm. av. difference

Table 1–11. *Blood Chemistries**

Alkaline phosphatase: infants	5–10 Bodansky units
1–10 yr	3–14 B.U. (average 7)
11–17 yr	10–14 B.U.
Over 17 yr	3–7 B.U.
Amylase	90–300 mg./100 ml.
Ascorbic acid	over 0.3 mg./100 ml.
Bicarbonate (CO_2 capacity or combining power)	22–30 mEq./L.
Bilirubin: cord	up to 1.8 mg./100 ml.
2–4 days	mean peak 7 mg./100 ml., range 2–12 mg./100 ml.
after newborn period	less than 0.8 mg./100 ml. Total
Bromsulphalein retention (at 45 minutes)	less than 5% after the newborn period, when up to 20% is normal
Calcium	9.0–11.5 mg./100 ml.
Carotene: newborn	25 mcg./100 ml.
thereafter	60–180 mcg./100 ml.
Cephalin flocculation infants	erratic
thereafter	0 to 1+ (3+ is maximum)
Chloride	94–106 mEq./L.
Cholesterol	150–275 mg./100 ml., 65–75% esterified
Copper: 1 mo.	50–100 mcg./100 ml.
1 yr	110–175
5–17 yr	80–280
adult	80–180
Corticosteroids (plasma)	8–20 mcg./100 ml. (av. 15), lower in newborn.
(Determine 8–9 A.M.	Marked diurnal variation)
Creatinine	0.9–1.9 mg./100 ml.
Glucose (fasting)	55–100 mg./100 ml.
Iodine, protein bound: newborn	6–10.7 mcg./100 ml.
1 wk.	9–14
1–12 wk	5.6–9.2
3–12 mo.	5.3–7.3
thereafter	3.5–8.0

Butanol extractable iodine averages 0.5 mcg. lower

Iron	Mean serum Fe	Total Fe binding capacity	Per cent saturation
1 wk.	148 mcg./100 ml.	262 mcg./100 ml.	65
3 mo.	50	350	15
6–12 mo.	106	429	25
1–2 yr	95	414	22
2–6 yr	116	395	28
6–12 yr	127	340	38

Ketones	up to 3 mg./100 ml.
Lactic acid (fasting)	up to 10 mg./100 ml. if precipitated stat, otherwise up to 20 mg./100 ml.
Lactic dehydrogenase	200–600 units/ml.
Lead	under 0.06 mg./100 ml.
Lipids: total	400–900 mg./100 ml.
phospholipids	mean 225 mg./100 ml. (usually slightly higher than cholesterol)
Magnesium	1.9–2.3 mEq./L. (av. 2.0)
Mucoproteins (as tyrosine)	1.9–4.5 mg./100 ml.
pH (arterial whole blood)	7.35–7.45 (0.03 lower in venous blood)
Pco_2 (arterial)	35–45 mm. Hg
Po_2 (arterial)	85–100 mm. Hg
Phosphorus, in organic: 1st yr.	4–7 mg./100 ml.
1–12 yr	5–6 mg./100 ml.
adult	3–4 mg./100 ml.
Potassium: 0–10 days	up to 7 mEq./L.
thereafter	3.2–6.0 mEq./L.
Proteins: total	6–8 gm./ml.
albumin	4.7–5.7
globulin	1.3–2.5

*From Johns Hopkins Hospital: Harriet Lane Handbook, 5th edition. Copyright © 1969. Year Book Medical Publishers, Inc. Reprinted by permission.

Table continued on following page

Table 1–11. *Blood Chemistries** Continued

Proteins: average (range)	Total	Albumin	Globulin	Gamma globulin
premature	5.5	3.7	1.8	0.7
	(4–6)	(2.5–4.5)	(1.2–2)	(0.5–0.9)
FT newborn	6.4	3.4	3.1	0.8
	(5–7.1)	(2.5–5)	(1.2–4)	(0.7–0.9)
1–3 mo.	6.6	3.8	2.5	0.3
	(4.7–7.4)	(3–4.2)	(1–3.3)	(0.1–0.5)
3–12 mo.	6.8	3.9	2.6	0.6
	(5–7.5)	(2.7–5)	(2–3.8)	(0.4–1.2)
1–15 yr	7.4	4.0	3.1	0.9
	(6.5–8.6)	(3.2–5)	(2–4.4)	(0.6–1.2)

Plasma fibrinogen: 0.28 (0.22–0.32) at all ages

Sodium . . . . .134–151 mEq./L.
Thymol turbidity . . . . .0–5 units
Tocopherol (vitamin E): Premature . . . . .0.05–0.35 mg./ml.
                FT newborn. 0.1–0.35
                2–5 mo. 0.2–0.6
                6–24 . . . . .0.35–0.8
                2–12 yr. 0.55–0.9
                adults and breast-fed babies . .0.6–1.1

Transaminases: SGOT   SGPT
  1st wk . . . . .10–120 u.   10–90 u.
  thereafter . . . . .5–45 u.   5–45 u.
Urea nitrogen. . . . . .5–20 mg./100 ml.
  nonprotein nitrogen. . . . . .22–40 mg./100 ml.
Uric acid . . . . .2–6 mg./100 ml.
Vitamin A . . . . .over 40 mcg./100 ml.
Zinc turbidity: newborn. . . . . .less than 10
               1–8 mo. . . . . .less than 3
               9–12 mo. . . . . .less than 5
               thereafter. . . . . .less than 8

*From Johns Hopkins Hospital: Harriet Lane Handbook, 5th edition. Copyright © 1969. Year Book Medical Publishers, Inc. Reprinted by permission.

Table 1–12. *Cerebrospinal Fluid**

Amount (obtainable by LP): newborn: up to 5 ml.
                      adult: 100–150 ml
Initial pressure: newborn 50–80 mm. CSF
                infant 40–150 mm.
                child 70–200 mm.
Sp. gr. 1.005–1.009
pH 38°C 7.33–7.42
Calcium: 4.5–5.5 mg./100 ml. (approximates ionized
         serum Ca)
Cell count: Up to 25 WBC's (av. 8) and up to 650
         RBC's/mm.[3]
         after first mo. Up to 7 lymphocytes

Glucose 40–80 mg./100 ml. (at least ½ of blood sugar)
Pandy test (mainly globulin) 0 (may be positive in
  newborn)
Protein (80% albumin): ventricular 5–15 mg./100 ml.
                   cisternal 5–25 mg./100 ml.
                   lumbar 5–40 mg./100 ml.
                   up to 150 mg./100 ml. in
                   newborn†
GOT 4–14 units, often about ½ of SGOT

*Data from Wyers, H. J. G., and Bakker, J. C. W.: Maandschrift voor Kindergeneskunde, 1954, p. 253.
†There is too little data available on newborn CSF to define normal limits or to allow fine diagnostic distinctions.

Table 1–13. Orthopedic History and Physical Examination

ORTHOPEDIC HISTORY AND PHYSICAL EXAMINATION

DATE:

INFORMANT:

CHIEF COMPLAINT:

PRESENT ILLNESS:

PRENATAL HISTORY:

Threatened Abortion - Any Bleeding:

Toxemia:

Infections:

Herpes:

Medications:

Trauma:

Radiation

Fetal Movements - Which Month of Pregnancy?:

BIRTH HISTORY:

Length of Pregnancy:

Spontaneous or Induced Labor:

Duration of Labor:

Obstetrical Anesthesia - General, Block or None:

Table continued on following page

Table 1–13. Orthopedic History and Physical Examination Continued

CONDITION OF NEWBORN:

Birth Weight: Birth Length:

Cyanosis: Jaundice:

Convulsions:

Any Respiratory Problems?:   Was Oxygen Required?:

Was Resuscitation Necessary?:

Any Injuries or Evidence of Trauma?:

Any Deformities of Limbs?:

Length of Hospital Stay?:

DEVELOPMENTAL MILESTONES:

Posture and Locomotion - Age

    Held Up Head: Rolled Over - 1. Front to Back:

                                              2. Back to Front:

    Sat: Crawled: Stood: Walked:

Upper Limb Function - Age

    Held Bottle: Reached for and Grasped Toy:

    Transferred Objects from   Showed Hand Preference:
    Hand to Hand:

Social Development:

    Language - Commenced to Talk:

    Toilet Training - 1. Stool:

                  2. Urine:

    School History:

PAST HISTORY:

General Health:

Previous Illnesses:

Previous Hospitalizations:

Date: Diagnosis: Hospital:

_____   _____   _____   _____

_____   _____   _____   _____

_____   _____   _____   _____

_____   _____   _____   _____

Table 1–13. Orthopedic History and Physical Examination Continued

Recent Exposure to Contagious Disease:

Medications - Previous: **Present:**

Unusual Bleeding: **Easy Bruising:**

Allergies: **Hives, Eczema, Asthma:**

Adverse Reaction to Anesthesia: **Problems with Temperature Control:**

IMMUNIZATIONS:	**Date:**	**Booster:**	**Reaction:**
DPT	_____	_____	_____
Oral Polio	_____	_____	_____
Smallpox	_____	_____	_____
Rubeola	_____	_____	_____
Mumps	_____	_____	_____
Other	_____	_____	_____
TBC Test	_____	_____	_____

REVIEW OF SYSTEMS:

Respiratory:

Cardiovascular:

Gastrointestinal:

Genitourinary:

Endocrine:

Nervous System:

Musculoskeletal:

FAMILY HISTORY:

Father: Mother:

Siblings: Grandparents and Other Relatives:

Any Anesthetic Difficulties in Family?:

Malignant Hyperthermia?:

Table continued on following page

Table 1–13. *Orthopedic History and Physical Examination* Continued

PHYSICAL EXAMINATION:

Height-Standing: Height-Sitting:

B.P.:   Pulse: Respiration: Temp.:

General Appearance:

Skin: Nails: Hair:

Head: Circumference: Fontanelles-Anterior:

                                                        Posterior:

Eyes: Ears: Nose:

Mouth: Palate: Throat:

Neck: Lymph Nodes:

Lungs:

Heart: Vessels:

Abdomen: Liver: Spleen: Bowel Sounds: Hernia:

Kidneys: Bladder: Genitalia:

EXAMINATION OF NEUROMUSCULOSKELETAL SYSTEM (ORTHOPEDIC)

Appliances – Orthoses: Night Splints:

Shoes: Abnormal Wear:

Stance – Posture

PA/AP – Scoliosis:

        Rotation of Vertebrae-Symmetry of Flank Creases:

        Level of Shoulders:

Lateral – Lordosis: Kyphosis:

Motion of Spine

Balance of Shoulders Over Pelvis:

        PA:

        Lateral:

Level of Iliac Crests: Lift Under Foot:
                             – To Level Iliac Crests: Right: Left:
                             – To Balance Head-Shoulders
                               Over Pelvis: Right: Left:

Table 1–13. Orthopedic History and Physical Examination Continued

Trendelenburg Test   Immediate: Delayed:

Lower Limb Alignment   Line of Weight-Bearing:

Feet: Longitudinal Arch:

Upper Limb Alignment

Gait

    Pathologic – Describe: Foot Progression Angle:

Deformities

    Hip Flexion-Thomas Test:

    Hip Abduction – Ober Test:

Lower Limb Lengths:

Actual	Right:	Left:	Inequality:
Apparent	Right:	Left:	Inequality:
Length of Femora	Right:	Left:	Inequality:
Galeazzi Test	Right:	Left:	Inequality:
Length of Tibiae	Right:	Left:	Inequality:
Ellis Test	Right:	Left:	Inequality:

Upper Limb Lengths:

Total Length	Right:	Left:	Inequality:
Arm Length	Right:	Left:	Inequality:
Forearm Length	Right:	Left:	Inequality:

Circumference:

Calves	Right:	Left:
Thighs	Right:	Left:
Arms	Right:	Left:
Forearms	Right:	Left:

Genu Valgum

Distance Between Medial Malleoli with Medial Femoral Condyles Touching:

Angle Between Lateral Surfaces of Thigh and Leg   Right: Left:

Deformity Below Knee?   Tibia Valga?   Right: Left:

Table continued on following page

Table 1–13. Orthopedic History and Physical Examination Continued

Ankle

     Plantar flexion (flexion)   Right: Left:

     Dorsiflexion (extension)   Right: Left:

Foot

     Inversion   Right: Left:

     Eversion   Right: Left:

Forefoot

     Abduction   Right: Left:

     Adduction   Right: Left:

Toes – Describe:

Shoulder

     Flexion (or forward flexion)   Right: Left:

     Extension   Right: Left:
     (or backward extension)

     Elevation–Total   Right: Left:

              Glenohumeral   Right: Left:

     Horizontal Abduction   Right: Left:

     Horizontal Adduction   Right: Left:

     Rotation–arm at side of body

     Medial   Right: Left:

     Lateral   Right: Left:

     Rotation–arm at 90° elevation
       and 90° of abduction
       Downward (Medial)   Right: Left:

       Upward (Medial)   Right: Left:

Elbow

     Flexion   Right: Left:

     Extension   Right: Left:

Forearm

     Pronation   Right: Left:

     Supination   Right: Left:

Table 1–13. *Orthopedic History and Physical Examination* Continued

<u>Genu Varum</u>

　Distance between medial condyles of femur with medial malleoli touching:

　Angle between medial surface of thigh-leg　　　Right:　　　　Left:

　Deformity Below Knee?　　Tibia vara?　　　Right:　　　　Left:

<u>Upper Limb</u>

　Cubitus Varus?　　　　Valgus?

<u>Rotational Deformity</u>

　Femoral Torsion – Ryder Test:　　Antetorsion° :　　Retrotorsion°:

　Tibiofibular Torsion:　　　Lateral:　　　Medial:

　Thigh-Foot Angle:　　　Right:　　Left:

<u>Range of Motion of Joints:</u>

　<u>Hip</u>

　　Flexion　　　　　　Right:　　　　Left:

　　Extension　　　　　Right:　　　　Left:

　　Abduction (in extension)　　Right:　　　　Left:

　　Abduction (in 90° flexion)　　Right:　　　　Left:

　　Rotation in extension

　　　　Medial　　　　Right:　　　　Left:

　　　　Lateral　　　　Right:　　　　Left:

　　Rotation in 90° flexion

　　　　Medial　　　　Right:　　　　Left:

　　　　Lateral　　　　Right:　　　　Left:

　<u>Knee</u>

　Flexion　　　　　　Right:　　　　Left:

　Extension　　　　　Right:　　　　Left:

Table continued on following page

Table 1–13. Orthopedic History and Physical Examination Continued

---

<u>Wrist</u>

  Palmar Flexion   Right: Left:

  Dorsiflexion   Right: Left:

  Radial Deviation   Right: Left:

  Ulnar Deviation   Right: Left:

<u>Hand</u>

  Thumb–Fingers – Describe

<u>Motor Power – Muscle Testing</u>

  (See Muscle Testing Chart)

<u>Neurologic Assessment</u>

<u>Reflex Maturation Level</u>

<u>Motor Developmental Level</u>

<u>Roentgenographic Findings</u>

<u>Other Laboratory Findings</u>

Table 1–13. Orthopedic History and Physical Examination Continued

<u>Diagnosis</u>

      Primary:

      Secondary:

<u>Treatment Plan</u>

<u>Details of Post-Operative Care</u> - Discussed with Parents - Is it Adequate?

<u>Problems and Complications</u> - Discussed with Parents

Table 1–14. Signs of an Attack of Malignant Hyperthermia Syndrome

Clinical

Tachycardia—usually the first sign!
Tachypnea
Arrhythmias—usually premature ventricular contractions (PVCs)
Rigidity—not always present
Hyperthermia—often a late sign
Unstable blood pressure
Sweating, mottled skin
Cyanosis, dark venous blood
Dilated pupils

Laboratory

Arterial blood gas
    Acidosis (metabolic and respiratory)
    Hypercarbia
    Hypoxemia
Venous blood gas
    Acidosis, hypercarbia, hypoxemia may be *more* profound
    Elevated creatine phosphokinase (CPK) levels
    Hyperkalemia
    Myoglobinuria ("brown urine")

Table 1–15. Treatment of an Attack of Malignant Hyperthermia

Stop anesthetics and surgery
Hyperventilate with 100% oxygen
Call for help!
Dantrolene—2.5 mg./kg. initially, up to 10 mg./kg.
    —The definitive therapy
    —Give repeat doses for tachycardia, acidosis, elevated temperature
Sodium bicarbonate—2 mg./kg. initially, then as needed
Cooling—Iced intravenous, intragastric fluids, skin cooling (don't overcool)
Diuresis—Furosemide or mannitol, as needed
Control arrhythmias—procainamide
Monitors—ECG, $ETCO_2$, pulse oximetry, urine output, core temperature, arterial blood pressure, CVP
Don't transfer patient to an intensive care unit until the patient is stable.

2. Congenital Deformities

Physical variation in human beings is the rule but is ordinarily of little consequence. When, however, a variation departs from normal to such an extent that natural function or appearance is impaired, it is classified as a deformity. The term *congenital* implies that this anomaly is present at or before birth.

In recent years, great strides have been made in studying the causation of congenital deformities. A detailed description of the principles of genetics is, however, beyond the scope of this book; therefore, they are not discussed here.

The significance of a congenital deformity varies with its type; it may be minor, as in webbing of the toes, for example, or serious and disabling, as in absence of the proximal femur.

To obtain optimum results, early recognition and early treatment are essential. If a deformity is present, it should be carefully studied and evaluated as to its type and severity, the degree of disability anticipated, and the course of treatment to be followed. In severe deformities, treatment may extend over a long span of time. Supervision throughout the period of growth is often necessary. The child should be evaluated as a whole, his educational potential should be determined, and he should be given vocational guidance in fields that his physical disability permits.

CLASSIFICATION

Congenital malformations of the musculoskeletal system encompass a broad spectrum of deformities. Precise classification of congenital limb deficiencies has been difficult, and until recently a universally adopted nomenclature has been lacking. Instead a semantic jumble of Greek and Latin words has been used to describe congenital limb malformations. In 1837, Geoffrey Saint-Hilaire published a classification of congenital anomalies and introduced the terms *phocomèle, hemimèle,* and *ectromèle.*[19] Such terms derived from Greek and Latin roots created a confusing conglomeration of terminology. Frantz and O'Rahilly, in 1961, proposed a concise and comprehensive classification based on embryologic and teratologic considerations. It was designed to delineate the functional handicap of the child with a limb deficiency and assist in fitting him with a prosthesis.[10] The subcommittee on Children's Prosthetics of the National Academy of Science–National Research Council modified the Frantz-O'Rahilly classification. Further changes were made by the American Society of Surgery of the Hand, the International Federation of Hand Societies, and the International Society for Prosthetics and Orthotics. This classification is explained in detail by Swanson.[20–24] The classification divides congenital malformation of the limbs into seven categories based on the embryologic failure that has malformed the part: failure of formation of parts (arrest of development), failure of differentiation (separation of parts), duplication, overgrowth (gigantism), undergrowth (hypoplasia), congenital constriction band syndrome, and generalized skeletal abnormalities (Table 2–1). Eponyms are deleted. Greek and Latin terms are replaced by simple descriptive terminology. The term *hemimelia* is deleted because in some ways it implies absence of half a limb, although there are cases in which a greater or lesser portion of a limb is missing. Terms such as *ectromelia* and *phocomelia* are eliminated. With this classification, common malformations can be recorded with minimal confusion, and complex deficiencies can be categorized. The anomaly can be subclassified, and the degree of deformation can be expressed. In the literature, however, Greek and Latin words still do appear, and the reader should be knowledgeable. Therefore a glossary of words used to describe congenital limb deficiencies is given in Table 2–2. The Latin prefix *a*, meaning "without," refers to an absence of a part of the body, hence *amelia* (melos meaning "a limb") denotes absence of a limb, *acheiria* of a hand, *apodia* of a foot, *adactylia* of a digit, *aphalangia* of one or more phalanges. The Greek prefix *hemi*, or "half," is used as in "hemimelia," meaning "half a limb." The prefix *phoco*, derived from the Greek word *phoke*, "a seal," pertains to a limb that is attached directly to the trunk, as in *phocomelia* (a flipper-like limb). *Meros* in Greek means partial. The term *ray* is used to describe a digit, including its metacarpal (or metatarsal) and in some instances, as in the thumb or great toe, the associated carpal or tarsal bone. The word *limb* is used in preference to *extremity* because the latter term is not accurately descriptive.

Failure of Formation of Parts (Arrest of Development)

This may be complete or partial with the deficiency involving bony as well as soft-tissue structures either separately or together. This category can be subdivided into two types—transverse and longitudinal. The *transverse* defect involves the entire width of the limb, as in congenital amputations, whereas in the *longitudinal* deficiency only the preaxial (as in congenital absence of the radius) or postaxial (as when the ulna or fibula is absent) is involved. The word *terminal* is used when all the parts

distal to and in line with the deficient portion are affected; the term *intercalary* denotes the absence of a middle part with the proximal and distal portions being present. The intercalary deficiencies are classified with the longitudinal defects.

TERMINAL TRANSVERSE DEFICIENCIES (CONGENITAL AMPUTATIONS)

Transverse deficiencies result from arrest of formation in the limb anlage, with amputations taking place at any level along the limb axis and with a spectrum ranging from absence of an entire limb to that of a toe or finger (Fig. 2–1). The transverse deficiencies are classified by naming the level at which the remainder of the limb terminates. Abbreviations are given to denote the level, and the limb is identified as upper or lower and right or left.

Most cases of congenital amputations occur sporadically. The incidence varies with the level of amputation, for example, one forearm amputation occurs in 20,000 live births, whereas one congenital amputation of the arm occurs in 270,000 live births.[3]

LONGITUDINAL DEFICIENCIES

Longitudinal deficiencies comprise all failures of formation of parts other than the transverse type. They are named according to the bones that are completely or partially absent; any bones not named are assumed to be present. Involvement may be preaxial, postaxial, or central. The *preaxial* longitudinal deficiencies include those of the radius and the tibia, while the *postaxial* group includes those of the ulna and the fibula (Figs. 2–2 and 2–3). In the *central* deficiencies the second, third, or fourth ray of the hand or foot, with or without the associated carpals or tarsals, is absent (Fig. 2–4). In the lobster-claw or cleft hand or foot the middle ray may be missing. In the more severe form of central deficiency, nubbins may represent the central three digits. Phocomelia is the most severe form of longitudinal limb deficiency, with failure of development in the proximodistal direction (Fig. 2–5).

Failure of Differentiation (Separation) of Parts

In this category are included all defects in which the basic anatomic units (bony, dermatomyofascial, and neurovascular) are developed but not separated.

Text continued on page 110

Table 2–1. *Classification of Congenital Deficiency of the Limbs*

Failure of Formation of Parts (Arrest of Development)	Failure of Formation of Parts (Arrest of Development) *(Continued)*
Transverse deficiency	Metacarpals (Mc) 1 2 3 4 5 ray
Upper limb (UL) Right (R) Left (L)	Total
Shoulder (Sh)—total	Partial
Arm (Arm)	Phalanges (Ph) 1 2 3 4 5 ray
Total	Total
Upper ⅓	Partial
Middle ⅓	Lower limb (LL) Right (R) Left (L)
Lower ⅓	Pelvis (Pe)
Forearm (Fo)	Total
Total	Partial
Upper ⅓	Ilium
Middle ⅓	Pubis
Lower ⅓	Ischium
Carpal (Ca)	Femur (Fe)
Total	Total
Partial	Partial
Metacarpal (Mc)	Tibia (Ti)
Total	Total
Partial	Partial
Phalangeal (Ph)	Fibula (Fi)
Total	Total
Partial	Partial
Lower limb (LL) Right (R) Left (L)	Tarsal (Ta)
Hip (H)	Total
Total	Partial
Thigh (Th)	Metatarsal (Mt) - 1 2 3 4 5 ray
Total	Total
Upper ⅓	Partial
Middle ⅓	Phalanges (Ph) - 1 2 3 4 5 ray
Lower ⅓	Total
Leg (Leg)	Partial
Total	Failure of Differentiation (Separation of Parts)
Upper ⅓	Upper limb (UL) Right (R) Left (L)
Middle ⅓	Shoulder
Lower ⅓	Congenital high scapula (Sprengel's
Tarsal (Ta)	deformity)
Total	Arm—elbow
Partial	Elbow synostosis—radiohumeral
Metatarsal (Mt)	Forearm
Total	Synostosis of proximal radius and ulna
Partial	With radial head dislocation
Phalangeal (Ph)	Without radial head dislocation
Total	Hand
Partial	Carpal
Longitudinal deficiency	Synostosis
Upper limb (UL) Right (R) Left (L)	Other deformities
Scapula (Sc)	Metacarpals
Total	Synostosis
Partial	Other deformities
Clavicle (Cl)	Digital
Total	Symphalangia
Partial	Syndactyly
Humerus (Hu)	Simple
Total	Complicated
Partial	Soft tissue
Radius (Ra)	Nails (synonychia)
Total	Other
Partial	Skeletal
Ulna (Ul)	Fusions
Total	Phalanges
Partial	Acrosyndactyly
Carpal (Ca)	Apert's syndrome
Total	Disarray
Partial	Brachysyndactyly

Table continued on opposite page

Table 2–1. *Classification of Congenital Deficiency of the Limbs* (Continued)

Failure of Differentiation (Separation of Parts) *(Continued)*
  Contracture—resulting from failure of
    differentiation of muscle, ligaments, and
    capsular structures
    Soft-tissue
      Arthrogryposis
      Pterygium cubitale or
      Windblown hand or foot
      Thumb-web space contracture
      Camptodactyly
      Trigger thumb
    Skeletal
      Clinodactyly
      Kirner's deformity
      Delta phalanx
  Lower limb (LL) Right (R) Left (L)
    Hip (Hi)
    Thigh—knee
      Synostosis of knee
    Leg
      Synostosis of tibia to fibula
    Ankle–foot
      Tarsal
        Synostosis
        Other deformities
      Metatarsals
        Synostosis
        Other deformities
      Digital
        Symphalangia
        Syndactyly
          Simple
          Complicated

  Contracture—resulting from failure of
    differentiation of muscle, ligaments, and
    capsular structures
Duplication
  Upper limb (UL) Right (R) Left (L)
    Whole limb
    Partial limb
    Mirror hand (ulnar dimelia)
    Polydactyly
      Thumb (preaxial)
      Little finger (postaxial)
      Central
      Polysyndactyly
  Lower limb (LL) Right (R) Left (L)
    Whole limb
    Partial limb
    Mirror foot (fibular dimelia)
    Polydactyly
      Hallux (preaxial)
      Little toe (postaxial)
      Central
      Polysyndactyly
Overgrowth (Gigantism)—all or part of a limb
  Macrodactyly
Undergrowth (Hypoplasia)
Congenital Constriction Band Syndrome
Generalized Skeletal Abnormalities—Manifestation of a
  generalized skeletal development defect; deformities
  encountered are unique to each syndrome

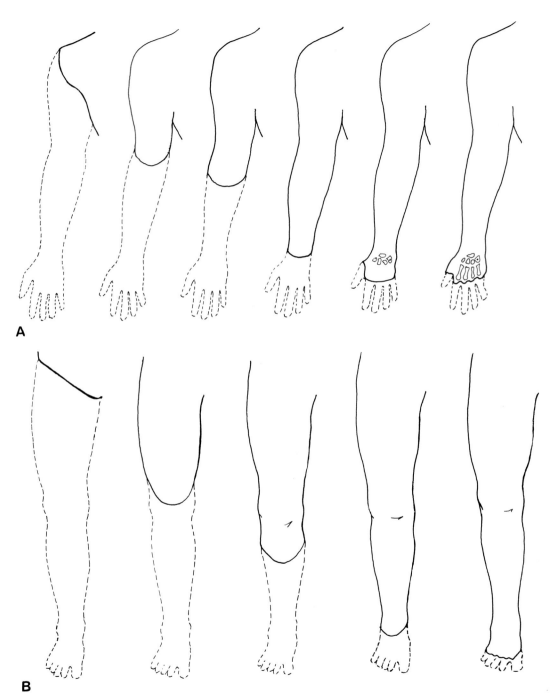

FIGURE 2–1. Spectrum of terminal transverse deficiencies.

A. In the upper limb. **B.** In the lower limb.

Table 2–2. Glossary

acheiria (achiria)—absence of hand
acheriopodia—absence of hands and feet
acro- —peak or end
acromelia—shortening of the hand
acrosyndactyly—fusion of terminal portion of two or more digits with proximal epithelial line clefts or sinuses between digits
adactylia or adactyly—absence of all fingers or toes
agenesis—absence or no development
amelia—absence of limb
amelia totalis—absence of all four limbs
amputation—absence of a distal part of a limb
aphalangia—absence of phalanges
aplasia—absence of a specific bone or bones
apodia—absence of foot
arachnodactyly—long, slender digits
ateliosis—incomplete or imperfect development
basi- (basio-)—basal or proximal
brachy- —short
brachybasophalangia—short proximal phalanx
brachydactyly—short fingers (usually refers to short phalanges)
brachymegalodactyly—short broad digit (stub thumb or type D brachydactyly)
brachymelia—short limb without absence of bony elements
brachymesophalangia—short middle phalanx
brachymetacarpia (brachymetacarpalia)—short metacarpals
brachymetapodia—short metacarpals and metatarsals
brachymetatarsia—short metatarsals
brachyphalangia—short phalanx
brachytelephalangia—short distal phalanx
camptodactyly—curvature of finger in plane of flexion of the digit
central defect (cleft or lobster claw hand)—absence of one or more of central rays of hand, the second, third, or fourth or any combination thereof
cheiria (chiria)—with reference to hand or cheir- (cheiro-) —relationship to
cleft hand—central ray deficiency
clinarthrosis—oblique or lateral angular deviation in alignment of joints
clinodactyly—deviation of a finger in the plane of the hand
dactylia—with reference to digit or dactyl- (dactylo-)— relationship to
delta phalanx—triangular ossicle
di- —double
dicheiria (dichiria)—double or mirror hand
dimelia—double or mirror limb
dys- —deformed, ill, bad
dystelephalangia—deformed terminal phalanx (Kirner deformity)
ectro- —absence (from Greek *ektroma*, "abortion")
ectrocheiria—total or partial absence of hand
ectrodactyly—total or partial absence of fingers or hand
ectromelia—total or partial absence of fingers or hand
ectrophalangia—absence of one or more phalanges
ectropodia—total or partial absence of foot
hemimelia—absence or part of limb
hyper- —above or increased
hyperphalangia—presence of more than normal number of phalanges in transverse direction
hypo- —below or decreased
hypodactyly—fewer than normal number of fingers

hypogenesis—incomplete development
hypophalangia—fewer than normal number of phalanges
hypoplasia—incomplete development of specific part
intercalary deficiency—absence of middle portion of limb while proximal and distal portions are present
longitudinal deficiency—absence of limb extending parallel to long axis; may be preaxial, postaxial, or central
macro- —excessive size
macrodactyly—hyperplasia of digit
manus—hand
megalodactyly—hyperplasia of digit
melia—referring to the limb
mero- —part or partial
meromelia—partial absence of limb
meso- —middle
micro —small size
microcheiria (microchiria)—hypoplasia of all parts of hand
micromelia—short limbs without absence of bone elements
oligo- —few or little
oligodactyly—absence of some of the fingers
parastremma—distorted limb
pero- —deformed or defective
perodactyly—deformed fingers
peromelia—hemimelia, especially for hands ending in a stump
phoco- —short (from Greek *phoke*, "seal")
phocomelia (derived from Greek *phoke*, meaning "seal," and *melos*, "limb") In complete form, the hands and feet sprout directly from the trunk—the arm and forearm are absent in the upper limb, and the thigh and leg are absent in the lower limb. The deficiency may be proximal (arms and thighs missing) or distal (forearms and legs missing)
pod- (podio-)—related to the foot
poikilodactyly—irregular or varied digit
poly- —many or increased number
polydactyly—more than normal number of digits
polyphalangia—more than normal number of phalanges in transverse direction
postaxial—pertaining to ulnar side of upper limb, fibular side of lower limb
preaxial—pertaining to the radial side of upper limb or thumb, tibial side of lower limb
streblo- —twisted
syn- (sym-)—fusion or together
symbrachydactyly—short digits with syndactyly
symphalangia—bony fusion of phalanges (end-to-end) or clinically rigid digits
syndactyly—fusion of adjacent digits. May be complete or incomplete with reference to cutaneous involvement, simple or complex with reference to bony involvement
synonychia—fusion of fingernail common to two or more digits
synostosis—bony fusion
tele- —distant or end
terminal deficiency—absence of bones distal to proximal limit of deficiency, may be either transverse or longitudinal
transverse deficiency—absence or part of limb (across width of limb)

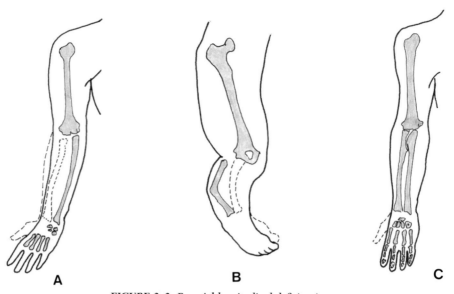

FIGURE 2–2. Preaxial longitudinal deficiencies.

A. Of the radius. **A.** Of the tibia. **C.** Of the thumb.

Duplication

Duplication results from splitting of the original embryonic part due to an insult to the limb bud and its ectodermal cap at a very early stage of their development. Duplication may involve a single bone or an entire limb. Polydactyly is the most common form of duplication.

Overgrowth (Gigantism)

In this category are included conditions in which the whole limb or a part of it (digit, hand, or forearm; or toe, foot, or leg) is disproportionately large. The overgrowth may involve only the skeleton, the soft-tissue parts appearing normal; or the soft-tissue components may

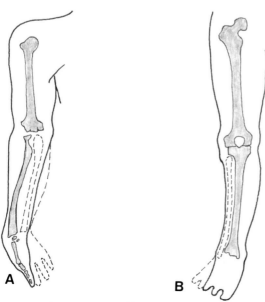

FIGURE 2–3. Postaxial longitudinal deficiencies.

A. Of the ulna. **ₚ** Of the fibula.

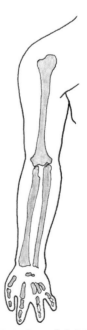

FIGURE 2–4. Central deficiency of the long finger.

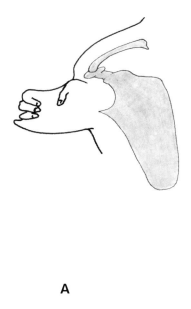
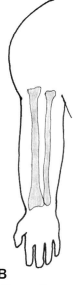
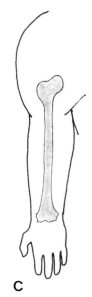

A   **B**   **C**

FIGURE 2–5. Phocomelia.

A. Complete. **B.** Proximal. **C.** Distal.

be enlarged by fat, lymphangioma, or angioma. Macrodactyly is a typical example of overgrowth.

Undergrowth (Hypoplasia)

In this category are included all incomplete developments of the parts. The defect may include the entire upper or lower limb or its components. It may involve the entire system or any part of it—skin, nails, muscle and tendons, ligaments, nerves, vessels, or bones.

Congenital Constriction Band Syndrome

This defect may manifest itself as a constriction band, in utero amputation of a limb or any of its distal parts, or acrosyndactyly.

Generalized Skeletal Developmental Defects

(This topic is discussed in the section on bone, Chapter 3.)

References

1. Bagg, H. J.: Etiology of certain congenital structural defects. Am. J. Obstet. Gynecol., 8:131, 1924.
2. Barsky, A. J.: Congenital Anomalies of the Hand and Their Surgical Treatment. Springfield, Ill., C. Thomas, 1958.
3. Birch-Jensen, A.: Congenital deformities of the upper extremities. (Translated by E. Aagesen.) Odense, Denmark, Andelsbogtrykkeriet and Det Danske Forlag, 1949, pp. 15–36.
4. Boyes, J. H.: Bunnell's Surgery of the Hand. Philadelphia, Lippincott, 1956.
5. Burtch, R. L.: Nomenclature for congenital skeletal limb deficiencies, a revision of the Frantz and O'Rahilly classification. Artif. Limbs, 10:24, 1966.
6. Duraiswami, P. K.: Experimental causation of congenital skeletal defects and its significance in orthopaedic surgery. J. Bone Joint Surg., 34-A:646, 1952.
7. Entin, M. A., Barsky, A. J., and Swanson, A. B.: Committee report to American Society for Surgery of the Hand, 1966.
8. Flatt, A. E.: A test of a classification of congenital anomalies of the upper extremity. Surg. Clin. North Am., 50:509, 1970.
9. Frantz, C. H.: Increased incidence of malformed infants in West Germany during 1959–62. Ill. Med. J., 123:27, 1963.
10. Frantz, C. H., and O'Rahilly, R.: Congenital skeletal limb deficiencies. J. Bone Joint Surg., 43-A:1202, 1961.
11. Hall, C. B., Brooks, M. B., and Dennis, J. F.: Congenital skeletal deficiencies of the extremities: Classification and fundamentals of treatment. J.A.M.A., 180:590, 1962.
12. Henkel, H. L., and Willert, H. G.: Dysmelia, a classification and a pattern of malformation of congenital limb deficiencies. J. Bone Joint Surg., 51-B:399, 1969.
13. International Society for Prosthetics and Orthotics, Working Group: The proposed international terminology for classification of congenital limb deficiencies. London, Spastics International Medical Publications in association with Heinemann Medical Books, and Lippincott, 1975.
14. Kanavel, A. B.: Malformations of the hand. Arch. Surg., 24:153, 1932.
15. Kay, H. W.: A proposed international terminology for the classification of congenital limb deficiencies. Orthop. Prosthet. Appl. J., 28:33, 1974.

16. Kelikian, H.: Congenital Deformities of the Hand and Forearm. Philadelphia, Saunders, 1974, pp. 51–88.
17. O'Rahilly, R.: Morphological patterns in limb deficiencies and duplications. Am. J. Anat., 89:135, 1951.
18. Patterson, T. J. S.: Congenital deformities of the hand. Hunterian Lecture delivered at Royal College of Surgeons of England, April 1959.
19. Saint-Hilaire, I. G.: Histoire générale et particulière des anomalies de l'organisation chez d'homme et les animaux . . . , Avec Atlas, 4 volumes. Paris, Baillière, 1832–1837.
20. Swanson, A. B.: A classification for congenital malformations of the hand. Bull. N.Y. Acad. Med., 10:166, 1964.
21. Swanson, A. B.: Classification of limb malformations on the basis of embryological failures: A preliminary report. N.Y. Univ. Interclin. Info. Bull., 6:1, 1966.
22. Swanson, A. B.: Severe congenital anomalies of the upper limb, considerations for classifications and treatment. *In* Cramer, L. M., and Chase, R. A. (eds.): Symposium on the Hand, Vol. 5. St. Louis, Mosby, 1971, pp. 132–149.
23. Swanson, A. B.: A classification for congenital limb malformations. J. Hand Surg., 1:8, 1976.
24. Swanson, A. B., Barsky, A. J., and Entin, M. A.: Classification of limb malformations on the basis of embryological failures. Surg. Clin. North Am., 48:1169, 1968.

CONGENITAL MUSCULAR TORTICOLLIS

Unilateral contracture of the sternocleidomastoid muscle results in congenital muscular torticollis, an asymmetrical deformity of the head and neck in which the head is tilted toward the side with the shortened muscle and the chin rotated toward the opposite side. The term *torticollis* is derived from two Latin words, *tortus*, meaning "twisted," and *collum*, meaning "neck." *Wryneck*, a lay term, is used to describe torticollis arising from any cause. The condition is more common in girls than in boys.

Etiology

The immediate cause of the deformity is fibrosis within the sternocleidomastoid muscle, which subsequently contracts and shortens. The exact pathogenesis of the fibrosis is unknown. It has, however, been the subject of considerable investigation through the years and has been comprehensively reviewed by Lidge, Bechtol, and Lambert.[71]

Brooks, in 1922, in experimental work on dogs, studied the pathologic changes produced in muscles as a result of vascular disturbances. He completely occluded the vein leading from a muscle but left the artery intact. This resulted in edema, degeneration of muscle fibers, acute inflammation, and eventual fibrosis of the muscle—a pathologic picture similar to that seen in congenital muscular torticollis. Brooks also found that permanent occlusion of only the

arterial supply of the muscle resulted in extreme atrophy and necrosis of the muscle but did not cause fibrosis and replacement with fibrous tissue. Intramuscular hemorrhage with or without interference with the nerve or arterial supply did not produce fibrosis.[12] Jepson, in 1926, and Middleton, in 1930, did similar experimental work and arrived at essentially the same conclusions as Brooks.[59, 81]

Breech and difficult forceps deliveries are very prevalent in the birth histories of patients with congenital muscular torticollis.[19, 20] It has been proposed that traumatic rupture of the muscle forms a hematoma, which subsequently organizes to produce a band of fibrous tissue within the muscle. But microscopic examination of surgical specimens reveals no evidence of hemorrhage or hemosiderin and no suggestion of reaction to trauma. Thus the question is raised whether breech presentation is a predisposing factor in congenital muscular torticollis or whether the torticollis tends to cause breech presentation and intrauterine malposition.

In about 75 per cent of cases of torticollis the right side was involved.[75] Congenital dysplasia of the hip was found in one of five of the children with congenital muscular torticollis by Hummer and MacEwen.[52] The frequency with which congenital dislocation of the hip is associated with congenital muscular torticollis has also been observed by Weiner.[113] That hereditary malformation or congenital defect of the sternocleidomastoid muscle is involved is suggested by the presence of other congenital malformations in some children with torticollis. A familial history is usually unobtainable, but torticollis has been reported in identical twins.[103]

The exact cause of fibrosis of the sternocleidomastoid muscle in congenital muscular torticollis is not known. As fibrotic changes in muscles of animals can be produced by venous occlusion, and as intrauterine malposition is commonly associated with the deformity, one may adduce that possibly it is due to a local ischemic process resulting from intrauterine malposition.

Pathology

On section, the "tumor" appears white and glistening, in gross appearance resembling a soft fibroma. Microscopic study shows that it consists of dense fibrous tissue. There is no evidence of hemorrhage or hemosiderin. In an older child, after the disappearance of the tumor, tissue excised from the sternocleidomastoid muscle shows that the muscle has been replaced by fibrous tissue. Other findings in the muscle consist of muscle giant cells, loss of transverse striations, vacuolization, and disruption of endomysial sheaths.[21] Reye studied longitudinal sections of autopsy material from one-, three-, and five-month-old infants with congenital muscular torticollis.[94] He found that a regular arrangement of fibrous tissue had replaced the affected muscle and that there was no line of demarcation between the fibrous tissue and the tendinous attachment of the muscle. Electron microscopic studies have shown nonspecific changes consistent with degeneration of immobilization, probably secondary to the extensive fibrosis in the muscle. There are marked increases in interstitial collagen deposition and scattered areas of amorphous ground substance with electron-dense deposits, but no vascular abnormalities.[80]

Clinical Findings

The deformity may be present at birth or it may become evident about the second or third week. The head is tilted toward the side of the affected muscle, and the chin is rotated to the opposite side (Fig. 2–6). Rotation of the neck to the side of the deformity and lateral motion to the opposite side are limited. Palpation will usually reveal a hard, nontender, fusiform swelling, or "tumor," in the sternocleidomastoid muscle. Usually both the sternal and clavicular heads are involved. Occasionally only the sternal head is affected. The superior portion of the muscle close to its mastoid attachment is rarely, if ever, involved. It gradually enlarges during the ensuing two to four weeks, reaching the size of the distal phalanx of the adult thumb. Then it begins to regress and gradually disappears in two to six months.

If the contracture is not treated, secondary deformities of the face and head develop. The face on the side of the contracted muscle becomes flattened because of external pressure. The infant usually sleeps in prone posture. Spontaneously, as it is more comfortable, the neck is rotated so that the affected side is down. Ipsilaterally, the face is flattened by remodeling to conform to the bed. A word of caution is appropriate—plagiocephaly can be congenital owing to synostosis of the coronal fissures; this is ruled out by radiograms of the skull.

With skeletal growth, asymmetry of the face increases (Fig. 2–7). The levels of the eyes and ears change, defects that are less noticeable when the head is tilted to one side and more obvious when the head and neck are straight in the midline. Eyestrain may result from ocular

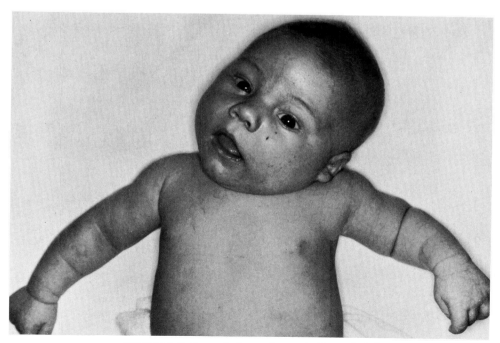

FIGURE 2–6. *Congenital muscular torticollis on the left.*

The head is tilted to the left and the chin rotated to the right.

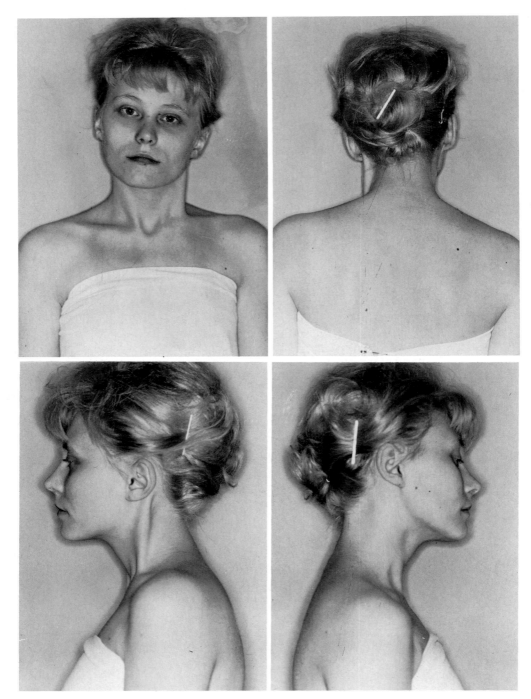

FIGURE 2–7. Untreated left congenital muscular torticollis in an 18-year-old girl.

Note the asymmetry of the face. On the affected side it is shortened from above downward and it is relatively wide from side to side. The levels of the eyes and the ears are asymmetrical.

imbalance. A lower cervical–upper dorsal scoliosis with concavity toward the affected side may develop.

If the deformity is not corrected, the soft tissues of the affected side undergo adaptive shortening as growth proceeds. The deep cervical fascia becomes thickened and contracted. The scalenus anterior and medius muscles become shortened. Later, the carotid sheath and the enclosed vessels contract.

In rare cases of double torticollis, in which both sternocleidomastoid muscles are affected, the neck is in the midline but appears short, the chin is elevated, and the face is tilted upward.

Diagnosis

Recognition of congenital muscular torticollis is not usually difficult because of the characteristic cordlike contracture of the sternocleidomastoid muscle. The early fusiform "tumor" may escape notice. Postural torticollis should be distinguished from congenital muscular torticollis. The postural deformation is caused by intrauterine malposture, and the deformity is less severe. Although the sternocleidomastoid muscle is shortened, there is no true fibrotic replacement of the muscle. Often there are other findings associated with intrauterine malposture such as pelvic obliquity with abduction-adduction contracture of the hips, or postural metatarsus varus or valgus. Postural torticollis responds quickly to passive manipulative stretching. In the literature there is a tendency to lump postural and true congenital muscular torticollis together; the so-called spontaneous cures of torticollis are those that are in cases of postural and not true congenital muscular torticollis.

Torticollis may be caused by contracture of muscles other than the sternocleidomastoid, such as the scalenus anterior and the omohyoid.[66, 92] Pirsing reported torticollis in a boy in whom it was caused by contracture of one omohyoid muscle with lateral displacement of the larynx and trachea and asymmetry of the face. When surgical release corrected the torticollis, the larynx returned to midline position and the asymmetrical face returned to normal.[92] Every patient should have radiograms of the cervical spine made to exclude congenital anomalies of the vertebrae, such as hemivertebrae, unilateral atlanto-occipital fusion, and the Klippel-Feil syndrome. In the differential diagnosis, one should also consider traumatic disorders of the cervical spine, such as fracture or rotary

Table 2–3. *Differential Diagnosis of Congenital Muscular Torticollis*

Congenital Anomalies
Postural torticollis
Hemivertebra, cervical–superior dorsal spine
Unilateral atlanto-occipital fusion
Klippel-Feil syndrome
Unilateral congenital absence of sternocleidomastoid muscle
Pterygium colli
Trauma—particularly C-1, C-2
Rotatory subluxation
Fracture
Inflammatory Conditions—unilateral
Cervical lymphadenitis
Spontaneous hyperemic subluxation of the atlas
Rheumatoid arthritis
Neurologic Disorders
Visual disturbances
Syringomyelia
Cervical spinal cord tumor
Brain tumor, posterior fossa
Acute Calcification of Cervical Disc

subluxation, particularly of C-1 and C-2; unilateral inflammatory conditions such as cervical lymphadenitis; spontaneous hyperemic subluxation of the atlas; rheumatoid arthritis; visual disturbances in which a child sees objects in a normal fashion only when the head is tilted; acute calcification of a cervical disc; tumors of the cervical spinal cord or of the brain (posterior fossa); syringomyelia; and spasmodic torticollis. Unilateral congenital absence of the sternocleidomastoid muscle may cause torticollis (Table 2–3).[77]

Treatment

Treatment should be begun as soon as the diagnosis is made. Manipulations consisting of passive stretching of the contracted sternocleidomastoid muscle should be performed by the parents after adequate instruction (Fig. 2–8). First, the head is bent laterally so that the ear on the side opposite the shortened muscle approaches the shoulder, as shown in Figure 2–8 B; then the head is rotated so that the chin approaches the shoulder of the affected side as in Figure 2–8 C. During these manipulations, in order to obtain maximum stretching of the sternocleidomastoid muscle, the neck should be in comfortable hyperextended position and counter traction should be applied by holding the ipsilateral shoulder and chest. An additional method of stretching the sternocleidomastoid muscle is to make use of gravity by placing the infant supine on the mother's lap with the head hanging into hyperextension. One hand stabi-

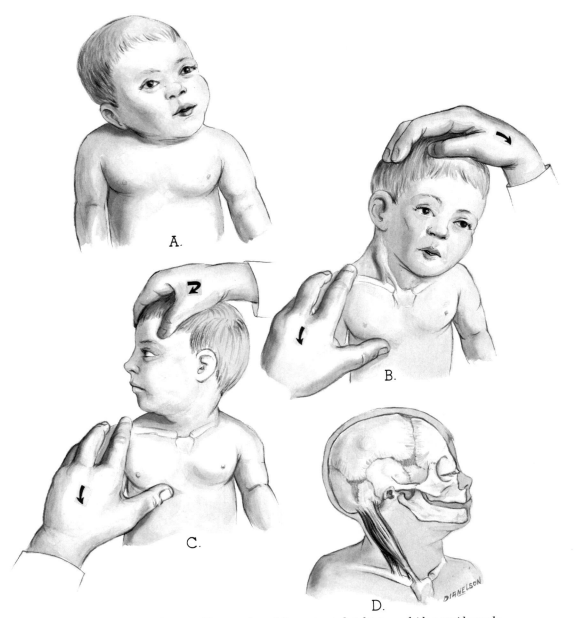

FIGURE 2–8. *Passive stretching exercises of the contracted right sternocleidomastoid muscle in congenital muscular torticollis.*

A. The deformity. **B.** The head is bent laterally so that the ear on the left side touches the left shoulder. Note the "tumor" in the sternocleidomastoid muscle. **C.** The head is rotated to the right so that the chin approaches the right shoulder. **D.** The anatomy of the sternocleidomastoid muscle.

lizes the shoulders and chest, and the other hand tilts the head laterally away from the contracted muscle so that the contralateral ear touches the opposite shoulder. The chin is then rotated toward the contracted muscle.

It is important to hold the muscle stretched to the count of 10. The exercises should be performed 15 to 20 times in each direction, 4 to 6 times a day. In addition, the crib should be turned so that the infant's unaffected side is against the wall and he will rotate his head to look toward the involved side when his attention is attracted, actively stretching the muscle when reaching and grasping for toys. Prone posture during sleep should be avoided, as it will aggravate the facial deformities and the contracture. Ordinarily, if the stretching exercises are begun at a very early age and performed faithfully and correctly every day, the contracture of the sternocleidomastoid muscle will be corrected and surgery will not be necessary. Coventry and Harris obtained excellent results in 30 of 35 patients (86 per cent) who were treated conservatively at home by the parents.[22] Ferkel and associates obtained good or excellent results in 12 of 14 patients (86 per cent) who were treated nonoperatively before the age of one year.[29] Ling and Low reported 76.8 per cent good response to frequent passive stretching of the sternocleidomastoid muscle.[73] Certain authors, however, still advise excision of the "tumor" in early infancy. Such early surgery should be abandoned, as there is no reason to subject an infant to drastic operative procedures when conservative measures are successful in such a high percentage of cases.

Surgery is indicated when the torticollis does not respond to conservative measures up to one year of age, or in cases in which the condition is neglected until the child is a year old or when the parents have not complied in performing an effective exercise regimen. It is unlikely that the fibrous cord that replaces the sternocleidomastoid muscle can be stretched by manipulation after the age of one year. This is especially true if restriction of rotation of the neck is greater than 30 degrees and there is an established facial asymmetry. This is well supported by the findings of Canale and Ferkel and their associates.[17, 29] Satisfactory results are usually obtained by division or partial excision of the muscle, provided the head is kept in the

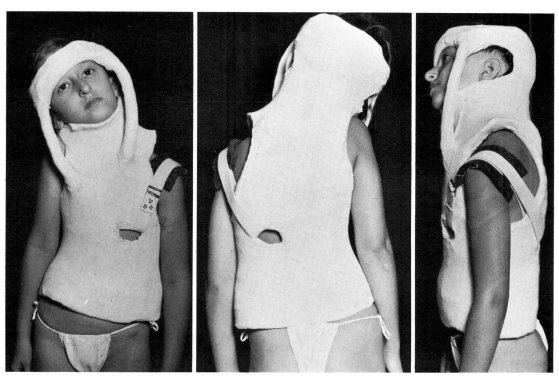

FIGURE 2–9. The cast used following division of the sternocleidomastoid muscle in congenital muscular torticollis.

The head and neck are maintained in the overcorrected position. Note the countertraction with a felt-padded strap on the ipsilateral shoulder.

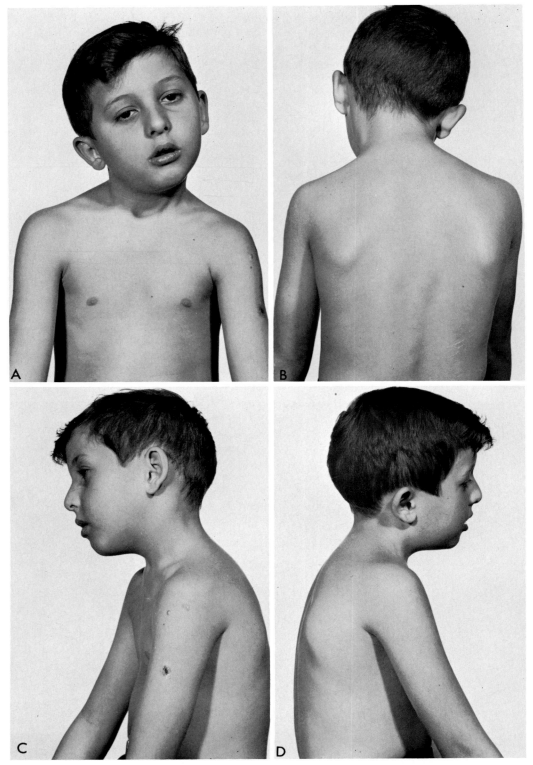

FIGURE 2–10. Congenital muscular torticollis on the right in a ten-year-old boy.

A to D. Preoperative photographs.

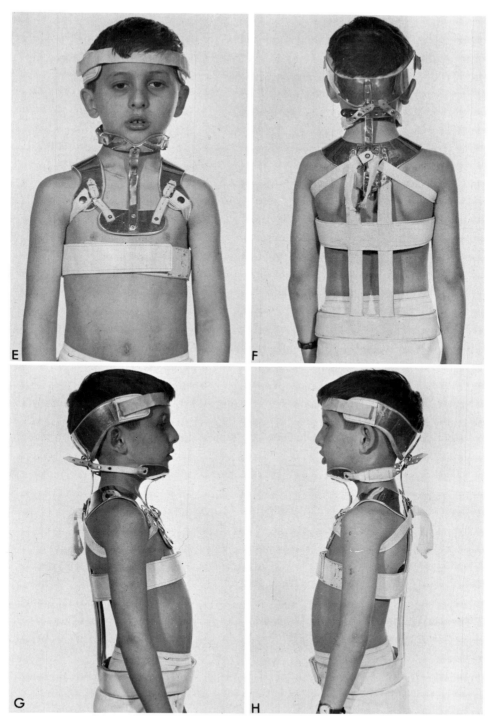

FIGURE 2–10 Continued. Congenital muscular torticollis on the right in a ten-year-old boy.

E to H. Modified Buckminster Brown brace holds the head and neck in the corrected position.

Illustration continued on following page

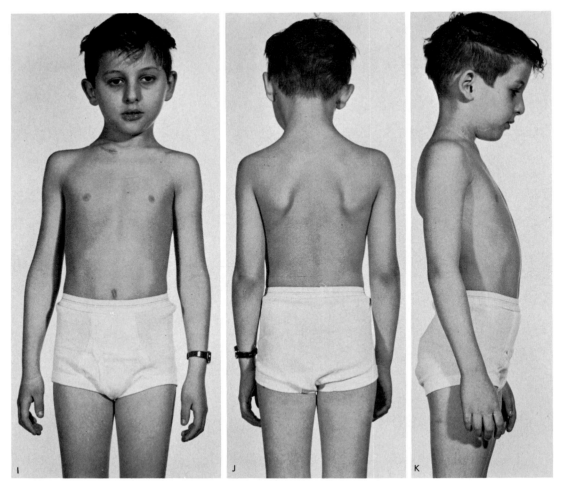

FIGURE 2–10 Continued. Congenital muscular torticollis on the right in a ten-year-old boy.

I to **K.** Postoperative photographs.

corrected position for a sufficient length of time after the operation, and active and passive exercises are carried out to prevent any recurrence of the deformity (Figs. 2–9, 2–10, and 2–11). The muscle may be divided at either end or at both ends.

The technique of division of the distal attachment of the sternocleidomastoid is illustrated in Plate 1. Distal myotomy is easier to perform than division at the proximal end, and the anatomic dissection is simpler. The scar is usually insignificant. Division of the sternal head, however, interrupts the normal **V** contour provided by the sternocleidomastoid muscle and, therefore, is esthetically objectionable.

Division of the muscle at its proximal end, first described by Tillaux and Lange, preserves this contour and leaves a scar that is not usually visible; the actual division of the muscle, how-

ever, is more difficult, requiring accurate anatomic dissection.[106] Also, the spinal accessory nerve may be damaged if lengthening of more than 2.5 cm. is required. Therefore, this author recommends Z-lengthening of the sternal attachment of the sternocleidomastoid muscle; partial excision of its clavicular attachment; and in severe, neglected cases, also bipolar release by sectioning of the mastoid origin.

Some authors have recommended complete excision of the sternocleidomastoid muscle.[14, 82] This is very rarely, if ever, indicated except in the case of an adolescent patient in whom the muscle has become fibrotic and very short. In such an instance, the author performs release at both ends by two separate incisions. Injury to the accessory nerve, the carotid vessels, and the phrenic and hypoglossal nerves should be avoided.

Text continued on page 126

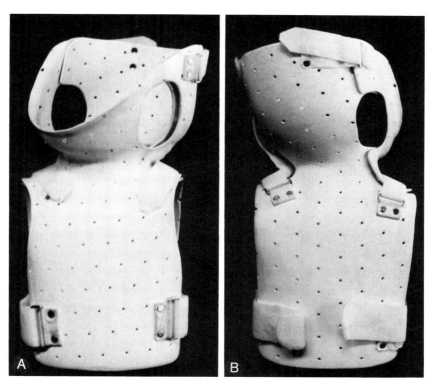

FIGURE 2–11. *Torticollis orthosis.*

The orthosis is manufactured of plastic to maintain the head and neck in corrected position in the postoperative period. **A.** Front. **B.** Back.

Operative Treatment for Congenital Muscular Torticollis

OPERATIVE TECHNIQUE

A. The patient is placed in supine position, and the head and neck are prepared and draped so that they can be manipulated to check correction of the contractural deformity during the operation. A transverse incision 4 to 5 cm. long is made in line with the skin creases and centered over the lower part of the sternocleidomastoid muscle. It should be one fingerbreadth proximal to the clavicle. The skin incision should not be made inferior to the clavicle, as the resulting healed scar will spread and be cosmetically objectionable.

B and **C.** Next, the subcutaneous tissue and the platysma muscle are divided. Injury to the anterior and external jugular veins, the carotid vessels, and other deep structures should be avoided.

D and **E.** By dull dissection, the clavicular and sternal parts of the attachment of the sternocleidomastoid muscle are exposed.

Plate 1. Operative Treatment for Congenital Muscular Torticollis

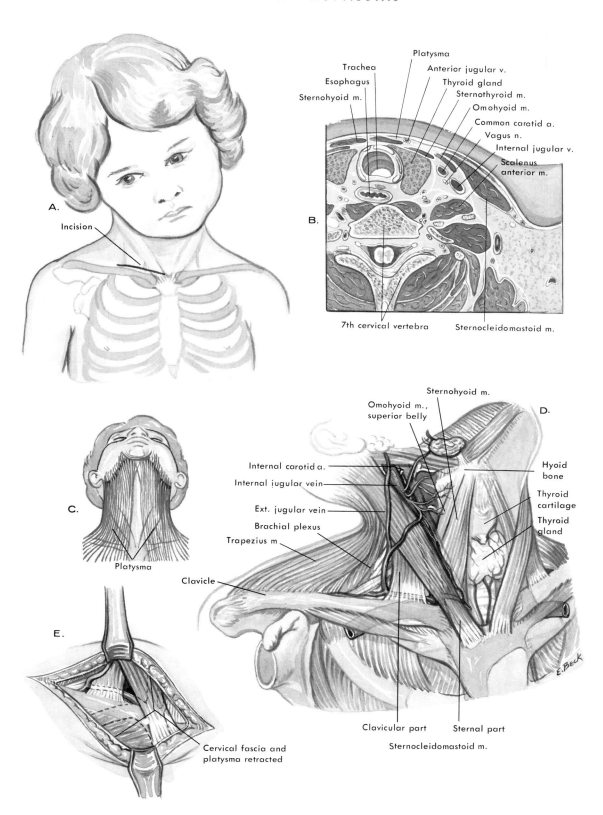

A.

Incision

B.

Trachea
Esophagus
Sternohyoid m.
Platysma
Anterior jugular v.
Thyroid gland
Sternothyroid m.
Omohyoid m.
Common carotid a.
Vagus n.
Internal jugular v.
Scalenus anterior m.

7th cervical vertebra   Sternocleidomastoid m.

C.

Platysma

D.

Omohyoid m., superior belly
Sternohyoid m.
Internal carotid a.
Internal jugular vein
Ext. jugular vein
Brachial plexus
Trapezius m
Clavicle
Hyoid bone
Thyroid cartilage
Thyroid gland

Clavicular part   Sternal part
Sternocleidomastoid m.

E.

Cervical fascia and
platysma retracted

E. Beck

123

Operative Treatment for Congenital Muscular Torticollis
(Continued)

F. A staphylorrhaphy probe is gently passed posterior to the sternocleidomastoid muscle to protect the deep structures. Then a large hemostat is used to clamp both heads of attachment of the sternocleidomastoid muscle, and about 2 cm. of their distal ends are resected with a scalpel. The degree of correction obtained is checked by manipulating the head and neck—rotating the chin toward the affected side and flexing the head laterally so that the opposite ear touches the contralateral shoulder. Often one has to divide contracted bands of deep fascia. The shortened deep structures are explored digitally and sectioned under direct vision. After complete hemostasis is obtained the wound is closed.

G and **H.** If it is desirable to preserve the V contour of the neck, especially in girls, the clavicular attachment of the sternocleidomastoid muscle is divided transversely, but the sternal head is lengthened by an oblique cut, and the muscle ends are sutured.

I. Sometimes, when the deformity is not severe, the sternocleidomastoid muscle can be released at its origin. The resultant scar will be hidden behind the ear. A small transverse incision is made immediately inferior to the mastoid process. The subcutaneous tissue is divided in line with the skin incision, and the muscle is gently divided and elevated near the bone. Caution! Do not damage the spinal accessory nerve.

POSTOPERATIVE CARE

In the child under two years of age, a cast or head-halter traction is not necessary. As soon as the child is comfortable, passive exercises are performed to maintain range of motion. The older patient, when the deformity is quite severe, is placed in head-halter traction immediately after surgery. The chin is directed toward the side of the contracted muscle and the ear tilted toward the opposite shoulder; counter traction is applied by means of longitudinal distal traction on the upper limb of the affected side. On the third or fourth postoperative day, the patient is placed in a Minerva cast, which holds the head in the overcorrected position. There should be distal traction on the shoulder of the side that was operated on as shown in Figure 2–9. In four weeks the cast is removed, and the patient wears a night brace to maintain the head in the corrected position. The brace is worn only at night, and passive and active exercises are performed to restore normal alignment of the head and neck.

Plate 1. Operative Treatment for Congenital Muscular Torticollis

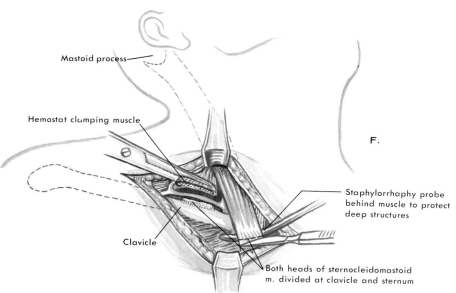

Mastoid process

Hemostat clamping muscle

Clavicle

F.

Staphylorrhaphy probe behind muscle to protect deep structures

Both heads of sternocleidomastoid m. divided at clavicle and sternum

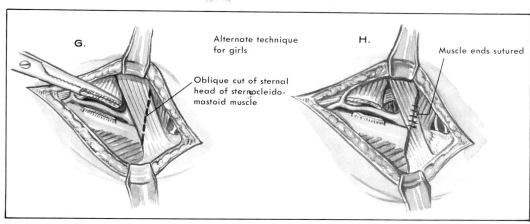

G.

Alternate technique for girls

H.

Oblique cut of sternal head of sternocleido-mastoid muscle

Muscle ends sutured

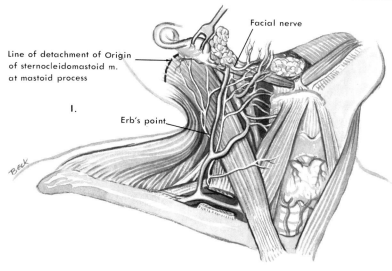

Line of detachment of Origin of sternocleidomastoid m. at mastoid process

Facial nerve

I.

Erb's point

Beck

References

1. Aberle, W.: Aetiologisches zum Schiefhals. Z. Orthop. Chir., 49:27, 1927.
2. Alldred, A.: Congenital muscular torticollis. J. Bone Joint Surg., 53-B:358, 1971.
3. Armstrong, D., Pickrell, K., Fetter, B., and Pitts, W.: Torticollis: An analysis of 271 cases. Plast. Reconstr. Surg., 35:14, 1965.
4. Barcat, J., and Godard, F.: Le traitement du torticolis congénitale par allongement du sterno-cleido-mastoidien. J. Chir. (Paris), 84:335, 1962.
5. Baxter, C. F., Johnson, E. W., Lloyd, R. J., and Chatworthy, H. W., Jr.: Prognostic significance of electromyography in congenital torticollis. Pediatrics, 28:442, 1961.
6. Bianco, A. J., Jr.: Congenital muscular torticollis. Thesis, Graduate School, University of Minnesota, 1958.
7. Biesin, A., and Aldere, M.: Mediating plastic surgery in congenital torticollis. Beitr. Orthop. Traumatol., 17:170, 1970.
8. Böhm, M.: Die Schiefhaltung des Kopfes. Dtsch. Med. Wochenschr., 52:529, 1926.
9. Boltshauser, E.: Differential diagnosis of juvenile torticollis. Schweiz. Med. Wochenschr., 106:1261, 1976.
10. Brackbill, Y., Douthit, T. C., and West, H.: Psychophysiologic effects in the neonate of prone versus supine placement. J. Pediatr., 82:84, 1973.
11. Brackett, E.: Treatment of torticollis. Trans. Am. Orthop. Assoc., 10:105, 1897.
12. Brooks, B.: Pathologic changes in muscle as a result of disturbances of circulation. Arch. Surg., 5:188, 1922.
13. Brown, J. R.: Torticollis successfully treated at the Boston Orthopedic Infirmary. Boston Med. Surg. J., 26:58, 1842.
14. Brown, J. R., and McDowell, F.: Wry-neck facial distortion prevented by resection of fibrosed sternocleidomastoid muscle in infancy and childhood. Ann. Surg., 131:721, 1950.
15. Browne, D.: Congenital deformities of mechanical origin. Proc. R. Soc., 29:1409, 1936.
16. Caillens, J.-P., Jarrousse, Y., and Dimeglio, E.: Le torticolis "congénital" de l'enfant: Rééducation appareillage. In Simon, L. (ed.): Actualités en Réduction Fonctionnelle et Réadaptation. Paris, New York, Masson, 1976, pp. 190–194.
17. Canale, S. T., Griffin, D. W., and Hubbard, C. N.: Congenital muscular torticollis. J. Bone Joint Surg., 64-A:810, 1982.
18. Cattaneo, L., and Defabiani, F.: Congenital hereditofamilial myogenic torticollis. Min. Ortop., 20:650, 1969.
19. Chandler, F. A.: Muscular torticollis. J. Bone Joint Surg., 30-A:566, 1948.
20. Chandler, F. A., and Altenberg, A.: "Congenital" muscular torticollis. J.A.M.A., 125:476, 1944.
21. Clark, R. N.: Diagnosis and management of torticollis. Pediatr. Ann., 5:231, 1976.
22. Coventry, M. B., and Harris, L.: Congenital muscular torticollis in infancy. Some observations regarding treatment. J. Bone Joint Surg., 41-A:815, 1959.
23. Dahmen, G.: Über die Beobachtung eines doppelten Schiefhalses. Z. Orthop., 95:246, 1962.
24. Dethloff, E., and Rack, G.: Muscular torticollis and its significance. Beitr. Orthop. Traumatol., 13:474, 1966.
25. Dunn, P. M.: Congenital sternocleidomastoid torticollis: an intrauterine postural deformity. In Proceedings of the forty-fifth annual meeting of the British Paediatric Association. Arch. Dis. Child., 49:824, 1974.
26. Elowson, S.: Torticolis congénital, causé par des déformations des vertèbres. Acta Orthop. Scand., 1:75, 1930.
27. Estève, P.: Torticolis congénital. Sem. Hôp. Paris, 30:3608, 1954.
28. Faysse, R., Gignolly, M., Spay, G., and Murat, J.: A propos de 87 observations de torticolis congénital. Ann. Chir. Infant., 6:313, 1965.
29. Ferkel, R. D., Westin, G. W., Dawson, E. G., and Oppenheim, W. L.: Muscular torticollis. A modified surgical approach. J. Bone Joint Surg., 65-A:894, 1983.
30. Fitzsimmons, H. J.: Congenital torticollis. Review of the pathological aspects. N. Engl. J. Med., 209:66, 1933.
31. Gallavardin, L., and Savy, P.: Sur un cas de torticolis congénital avec autopsie et examen histologique de système nerveux. Lyon Med., 101:767, 1903.
32. Garceau, G. J.: Congenital muscular torticollis. Hematoma, fact or myth. R. I. Med. J., 45:401, 1962.
33. Gasek, Z.: Pathogenesis of congenital torticollis. Acta Chir. Orthop. Traumatol. Cech., 37:303, 1970.
34. Gilbert, G. J.: Familial spasmodic torticllis. Neurology (Minneap.), 27:11, 1977.
35. Goeminne, L.: Congenital muscular torticollis. Acta Genet. Med. Gemellol. (Roma), 17:439, 1968.
36. Gorlin, R. J., and Pindborg, J. J.: Syndromes of the Head and Neck. New York, McGraw-Hill, 1964.
37. Graveleau, D.: Le torticolis congénital. Concours Med., 79:2029, 1959.
38. Gupta, S. K.: Bilateral torticollis. Indian Med. Gaz., 65:15, 1930.
39. Gvozdev, N. I.: Organization of early detection of dysplasia of the hip joint and muscular torticollis in children. Ortop. Travmatol. Protez., 9:82, 1976.
40. Haike, H., and Wessels, D.: Late results of the treatment of muscular torticollis with special consideration to the growth of the skull. Munch. Med. Wochenschr., 110:851, 1968.
41. Hal, I. van der: The treatment of congenital muscular torticollis. Maandschr. Kindergeneeskd., 40:227, 1972.
42. Hansen, D. A.: Torticollis. S. Afr. Med. J., 46:480, 1972.
43. Harman, J. W.: Significance of local vascular phenomena in production of ischemic necrosis in skeletal muscle. Am. J. Pathol., 24:625, 1948.
44. Hellstadius, A.: Torticollis congenita. Acta Chir. Scand., 62:586, 1927.
45. Hensinger, R. N., and MacEwen, G. D.: Congenital muscular torticollis. In Rothman, R. H., and Simeone, F. A. (eds.): The Spine. Congenital Anomalies of the Spine. Philadelphia, Saunders, 1975, pp. 195–200.
46. Hiatt, R. L., and Cope-Troupe, C.: Abnormal head positions due to ocular problems. Ann. Ophthalmol., 10:881, 1978.
47. Hoffa, A.: Zur Behandlung des hochgradigen Schiefhalses nach Mikulicz. Chir. Kongr., 2:340, 1900.
48. Hohmann, G.: Ueber den Muskulaeren Schiefhals. Verh. Dtsch. Orthop. Ges., 128, pp. 1–144.
49. Horton, C. E., Crawford, H. H., Adamson, J. E., and Ashbell, T. S.: Torticollis. South. Med. J., 60:953, 1967.
50. Hough, G. N.: Congenital torticollis, a review and result study. Surg. Gynecol. Obstet., 58:972, 1934.
51. Hulbert, K. F.: Congenital torticollis. J. Bone Joint Surg., 32-B:50, 1950.
52. Hummer, C. D., Jr., and MacEwen, G. D.: The coexistence of torticollis and congenital dysplasia of the hip. J. Bone Joint Surg., 54-A:1255, 1972.
53. Imhauser, G.: Ist der muskulare Schiefhals angeboren? Z. Orthop., 106:457, 1969.
54. Isigkeit, E.: Untersuchungen über die Heredität orthopadischer Leiden. III. Der angeborene Schiefhals. Arch. Orthop. Unfallchir., 30:459, 1931.

55. Iwahara, T., and Ikeda, A.: On the ipsilateral involvement of congenital muscular torticollis and congenital dislocation of the hip. J. Jpn. Orthop. Assoc., 35:1221, 1962.

56. Jacquemart, M., and Piedallu, P.: Le torticolis "congénital" est-il simplement un torticolis obstetrical? Concours. Med., 86:4867, 1964.

57. Jacquemart, M., and Piedallu, P.: Torticolis congénital. Concours. Med., 87:2949, 1965.

58. Jahss, S. A.: Torticollis. J. Bone Joint Surg., 18:1065, 1936.

59. Jepson, P. N.: Ischemic contracture. Experimental study. Ann. Surg., 84:785, 1926.

60. Jones, P. G.: Torticollis in Infancy and Childhood. Sternomastoid Fibrosis and the Sternomastoid "Tumour." Springfield, Thomas, 1968.

61. Judet, R., Judet, J., Lord, P., Foy-Camille, R., and Letournel, E.: Torticolis congénital. Gaz. Med. Fr., 71:1033, 1964.

62. Kalmar, L., and Papp, L.: Etiology of muscular torticollis. Beitr. Orthop. Traumatol., 20:315, 1973.

63. Kaplan, E. B.: Anatomical pitfalls in the surgical treatment of torticollis. Bull. Hosp. Joint Dis., 15:154, 1954.

64. Kastendieck, H.: Der muskulare Schiefhals beim Neugeborenen. Leipzig, Thieme, 1952.

65. Kiesewetter, W. B., Nelson, P. K., Palladino, V. S., and Koop, C. E.: Neonatal torticollis. J.A.M.A., 157:1281, 1955.

66. Koulalis, G.: Bedeutung des Musculus scalenus anterior fur die Entstehung des Schiefhalses. Z. Orthop., 105:69, 1968.

67. Krogius: Zur Pathogenese des muskularen Schiefhalses. Acta Chir. Scand., 56:497, 1923–1924.

68. Lackum, H. L. von: Torticollis: Removal in early life of the fibrous mass from the sternomastoid muscle. Surg. Gynecol. Obstet., 48:691, 1929.

69. Landgraf, E. von: Torticollis, congenital, early operation. Z. Orthop. Chir., 48:39, 1927.

70. Laurence G.: Le torticolis musculaire de l'enfant. Rev. Prat., 14:669, 1964.

71. Lidge, R. T., Bechtol, R. C., and Lambert, C. N.: Congenital muscular torticollis. Etiology and pathology. J. Bone Joint Surg., 39-A:1165, 1957.

72. Ling, C. M.: The influence of age on the results of open sternomastoid tenotomy in muscular torticollis. Clin. Orthop., 116:142, 1976.

73. Ling, C. M., and Low, Y. S.: Sternomastoid tumor and muscular torticollis. Clin. Orthop., 86:144, 1972.

74. Lipson, E. H., and Robertson, W. C., Jr.: Paroxysmal torticollis of infancy: familial occurrence. Am. J. Dis. Child., 132:422, 1978.

75. MacDonald, D.: Sternomastoid tumor and muscular torticollis. J. Bone Joint Surg., 51-B:432, 1969.

76. MacLennan, J. D.: Streptococcal infection of muscle. Lancet, 1:582, 1943.

77. McKinley, L. M., and Hamilton, L. R.: Torticollis caused by absence of the right sternocleidomastoid muscle. South. Med. J., 69:1099, 1976.

78. Martinie-Dubousquet, J.: Remarques sur le torticolis congénital. Ann. Chir. Infant., 3:195, 1962.

79. Meyerding, H. W.: Congenital torticollis. J. Orthop. Surg., 3:91, 1921.

80. Mickelson, M. R., Cooper, R. R., and Ponseti, I. V.: Ultrastructure of the sternocleidomastoid muscle in muscular torticollis. Clin. Orthop., 110:11, 1975.

81. Middleton, D. S.: The pathology of congenital torticollis. Brit. J. Surg., 18:188, 1930.

82. Mikulicz, J.: Über die Exstirpation des Kopfnickers beim Muskularen Schiefhals, nebst Bemerkungen zur Pathologie dieses Leidens. Zbl. Chir., 22:1, 1895.

83. Morrison, D. L., and MacEwen, G. D.: Congenital muscular torticollis: Observations regarding clinical findings, associated conditions, and results of treatment. J. Pediatr. Orthop., 2:500, 1982.

84. Moseley, T. M.: Treatment of facial distortion due to wryneck in infants by complete resection of the sternomastoid muscle. Am. Surg., 28:698, 1962.

85. Muller, G.: Beobachtung eines doppelten Schiefhalses. Z. Orthop., 93:432, 1960.

86. Murphy, W. J., and Gellis, S. S.: Torticollis with hiatus hernia in infancy. Am. J. Dis. Child., 131:564, 1977.

87. Nagura, S.: Zür Atiologie des angeborenen Schiefhalses. Zbl. Chir., 81:593, 1956.

88. Nagura, S.: Zür Frage der verebung des angeborenen Schiefhalses. Arch. Orthop. Unfallchir., 52:341, 1960.

89. Nagura, S.: Umwelteinflusse und der angeborene Schiefhals. Z. Orthop., 110:52, 1972.

90. Nove-Josserand and Viannay, Ch.: Pathogenie du torticolis congénital (theorie ischemique). Rev. Orthop., 7:397, 1906.

91. Oh, I., and Nowacek, C. J.: Surgical release of congenital torticollis in adults. Clin. Orthop., 131:141, 1978.

92. Pirsing, W.: Kongenitaler Schiefhals mit kemlkopf-trachea-verlagerung durch. Kontraktur des Musculus omohyoideus. Arch. Otorhinolaryngol., 215:335, 1977.

93. Power, D'Arcy: Wry-neck and congenital haematoma of the sternomastoid muscle. Med. Chir. Trans., 76:137, 1893.

94. Reye, R. D. K.: Sterno-mastoid tumour and congenital muscular torticollis. Med. J. Aust., 1:867, 1951.

95. Rossi, D.: Un caso di torticollo congenito in un feto estratto con parto caesareo. Riv. Ostet. Ginecol. Pract., 10:277, 1928.

96. Salmon, M. M.: Discussion of paper of Faysse, R., et al. In Ann. Chir. Infant., 8:318, 1965.

97. Sanerkin, N. G., and Edwards, P.: Birth injury to the sternomastoid muscle. J. Bone Joint Surg., 48-B:441, 1966.

98. Soeur, R.: Treatment of congenital torticollis. J. Bone Joint Surg., 22:35, 1940.

99. Spencer, H. R.: On haematoma of the sterno-mastoid muscle in new-born children. J. Pathol., 1:112, 1892.

100. Staheli, L. T.: Muscular torticollis: Late results of operative treatment. Surgery, 69:469, 1971.

101. Steinbruck, K., Porep, A., and Rompe, G.: Family studies in torticollis—results and difficulties from a clinical point of view. Z. Orthop., 116:566, 1978.

102. Stern, A.: Zur Ätiologie des angeborenen Schiefhalses. Monatsch. Geburts. Gynakol., 65:179, 1924.

103. Stevens, A. E.: Congenital torticollis in identical twins. Lancet, 2:378, 1948.

104. Straus, W. L., Jr., and Howell, A. B.: The spinal accessory nerve and its musculature. Q. Rev. Biol., 11:387, 1936.

105. Tanabe, G.: Operative treatment of congenital muscular torticollis: long-term results of myotomy. Acta Med. Okayama, 31:59, 1977.

106. Tillaux, P. J., and Lange, C.: Quoted in Lange, C.: Zur Behandlung der Schiefhalses. Wochenschr. Orthop. Chir. (Stuttg.), 27:440, 1910.

107. Tönnis, D.: Elektromyographische und histologische Untersuchungen zur Frage der Entstehung des muscularen Schiefhalses und des angeborenen Schulterblatthochstandes. Arch. Orthop. Unfallchir., 56:435, 1964.

108. Turk, G., Torklus, D. von, and Haeusermann, U.: Bedeutung der Fasciitis nodularis der Halsregion (Fibromatosis colli) im Kindesalter. Z. Kinderchir., 14:374, 1974.

109. Vignolo, Q.: Special myoplastic procedure for congenital torticollis. Arch. Ital. Chir., 12:713, 1925.

110. Wachsman, K., and Bazant, B.: Über den Einfluss

der Torticollis muscularis congenita auf die Symmetrie des Gesichts und des Gebisses. Fortschr. Kieferorthop., 23:90, 1962.

111. Warren, J. M.: Division of the sternomastoid muscle for wry neck. Boston Med. Surg. J., 24:121, 1841–1842.

112. Warter, J., Asch, L., Frank, R., Wiederkemr, J. L., and Nicolas, P.: Torticolis musculaire congénital associé à des anomalies dentelles et cardiaque. Sem. Hôp. Paris, 42:237, 1966.

113. Weiner, D. S.: Congenital dislocation of the hip associated with congenital muscular torticollis. Clin. Orthop., 121:163, 1976.

KLIPPEL-FEIL SYNDROME

The Klippel-Feil syndrome (also known as congenital synostosis of the cervical vertebrae, or brevicollis) is a rare malformation in which there is congenital fusion of two or more vertebrae in the cervical region. It is manifested clinically by shortening of the neck with limitation of its motion and low posterior hairline. This triad of findings should warn of the risk of less apparent but serious accompanying abnormalities of the genitourinary, cardiopulmonary, and nervous systems.

The first complete clinical description of this syndrome was given by Klippel and Feil in 1912. The patient was a 46-year-old French tailor who died of renal disease, and the report included detailed postmortem studies.[73] There had been, however, earlier reports by other authors.[25] Feil, in 1919, reported three additional cases of congenital cervical fusion, and distinguished between three morphologic groups. In Type I, there is massive fusion of many cervical and upper thoracic vertebrae with synostosis; in Type II, the fusion is at only one or two interspaces, with hemivertebrae, occipito-atloid fusions, and other anomalies present in some; and in Type III, cervical fusions are associated with lower thoracic or upper lumbar fusions.[41]

Etiology

This disorder results from failure of normal segmentation of the mesodermal somites during the third to the eighth weeks of fetal life. The exact cause is still subject to conjecture. Several instances of more than one case of the Klippel-Feil syndrome in the same family have been recorded. The condition is more preponderant in the female. Gunderson and associates studied the families of 11 probands with congenital cervical fusions. Radiograms of 121 family members were made. In six of the seven families with Type II fusions, relatives of the probands also had cervical fusions. Three specific genetic abnormalities were noted. Fusion of C-2 and C-3 is inherited as an autosomal dominant disorder; variable cervical fusion is a dominantly inherited trait with considerable penetration and expression. In the familes of probands with Type I fusion, Gunderson's group could not find any similarly affected relatives.[57, 58]

Clinical Features and Associated Anomalies

Clinical manifestations vary according to the severity of the deformity. Diagnosis may be made at any age. If only two or three cervical vertebrae are fused, the anomaly may be incidentally discovered on radiographic examination.

In the more involved cases, the neck is short, the head appearing to sit directly on the thorax, and the posterior hairline is low (Figs. 2–12 A to C and 2–13 A and B).[39, 41, 100, 111] There is marked limitation of motion of the cervical spine. Flexion and extension, which take place mostly between the occiput and atlas, are better preserved than lateral motion of the neck. Often, there is webbing of soft tissues on each side of the neck, extending from the mastoid process to the acromion of the shoulders, which is referred to as "pterygium colli." This webbing increases the apparent width of the neck and may involve the muscles and the fascia as well as the skin.

In some patients there is associated *torticollis*, which may be due either to contracture of the sternocleidomastoid muscle or to bony abnormalities. Torticollis is usually associated with facial asymmetry. *Sprengel's deformity* is a common accompaniment to the Klippel-Feil syndrome.[20, 67] This significant relationship of the two anomalies is explained by the embryology of the scapula, which develops at three weeks of gestation from mesodermal tissue high in the neck at the level of the third and fourth cervical vertebrae. The scapula descends to its thoracic region at the eighth week. *Scoliosis* is the most frequently associated skeletal deformity, occurring in about 60 per cent of the patients with Klippel-Feil syndrome.[62, 78] Other congenital anomalies of the musculoskeletal system may occur, such as cervical ribs, congenital fusion of ribs, abnormal costovertebral joints, syndactyly, hypoplastic thumbs, supernumerary digits, hypoplasia of the pectoralis major muscle, hemiatrophy of the upper or lower limbs, talipes equinovarus, and sacral agenesis (Table 2–4).

Urinary tract abnormalities are common—

Table 2–4. *Associated Anomalies in Klippel-Feil Syndrome*

Musculoskeletal System
  Relatively common:
    Scoliosis
    Sprengel's deformity
    Torticollis
    Pterygium colli
  Rare:
    Cervical ribs
    Congenital fusion of ribs
    Abnormally contoured joints
    Syndactyly
    Hypoplastic thumbs
    Supernumerary digits
    Absence or hypoplasia of pectoralis major muscle
    Hemiatrophy of upper or lower limb
Urinary System
  Agenesis of kidney
  Horseshoe kidney
  Hydronephrosis
  Tubular ectasia
  Renal ectopia
  Double collecting system

Genital System
  Ovarian agenesis
  Absence of vagina
Cardiovascular System
  Interventricular septal defect
  Patent ductus arteriosus
  Coarctation of aorta
  Patent foramen ovale
Pulmonary System
  Ectopic lung
  Agenesis of lung
  Mediastinal bronchogenic cyst
Deafness
Nervous System
  Synkinesia
  Spinal cord compression
  Facial nerve palsy
  Rectus palsy
  Ptosis of the eye
Miscellaneous Deformities
  Cleft palate

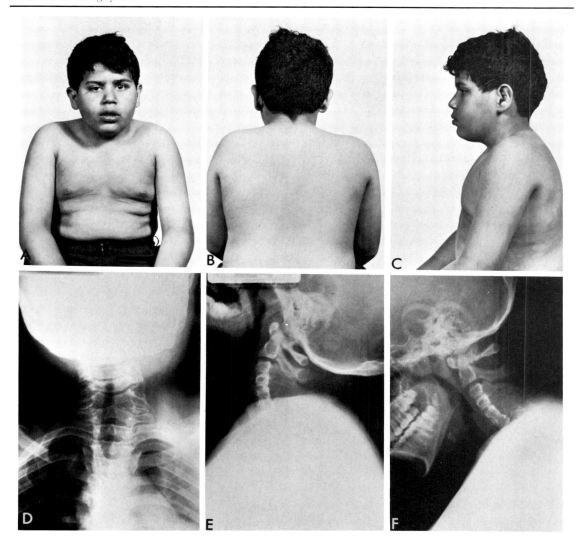

FIGURE 2–12. Klippel-Feil syndrome in a 12-year-old boy.

A to **C.** Clinical appearance of the patient. Note the short neck with the head appearing to sit directly on the thorax. **D** to **F.** Anteroposterior and lateral radiograms of the cervical spine. Note the failure of segmentation and the fusion into a homogeneous mass of bone of the four lower cervical vertebrae.

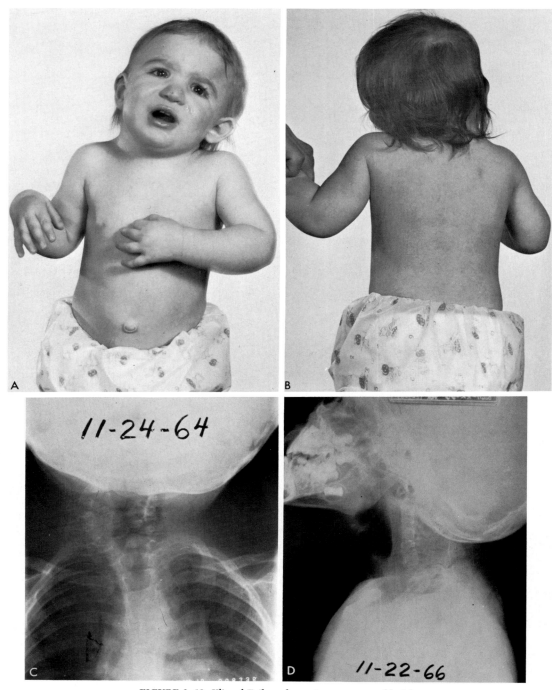

FIGURE 2–13. *Klippel-Feil syndrome in a one-year-old girl.*

A and B. Clinical appearance. C and D. Radiograms of same patient. Note the spina bifida due to failure of development of posterior laminar arches.

they include agenesis of the kidney, horseshoe kidney, hydronephrosis, tubular ectasia, renal ectopia, and double collecting system.[35, 52, 63, 83, 88, 99] Intravenous pyelography is vital in assessment of the Klippel-Feil syndrome. It is important to remember that the patient first described by Klippel and Feil died from renal disease and uremia, not from neurologic problems related to the fused cervical vertebrae.

Cardiovascular abnormalities may be associated with the Klippel-Feil syndrome—4.2 per cent of the cases in the study of Morrison and associates.[59] Interventricular septal defect is the most common cardiac anomaly. Other abnormalities reported are patent ductus arteriosus, coarctation of the aorta, and patent foramen ovale.[40, 72, 92] Other associated visceral abnormalities are ectopic lung, agenesis of lung, mediastinal bronchogenic cyst, ovarian agenesis, and absence of the vagina.[7, 12, 17, 23]

Deafness is common in Klippel-Feil disease.[68, 70, 79, 95, 117, 118] All types of hearing loss have been described. There is no characteristic audiologic anomaly. Hearing loss will retard development of speech and language.

Synkinesia may occur in the Klippel-Feil

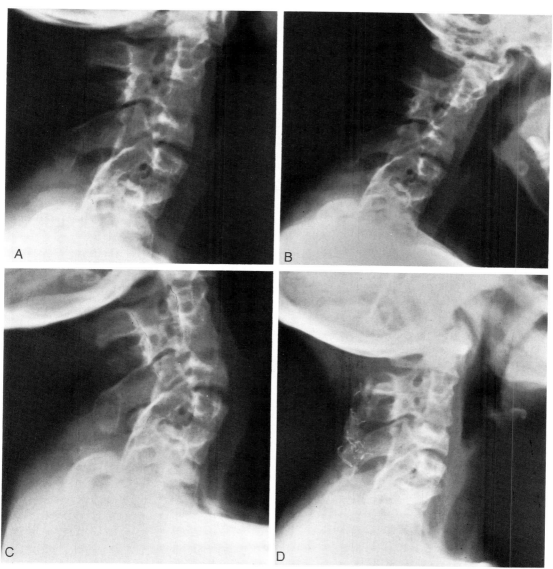

FIGURE 2–14. *Lateral radiograms of cervical spine in Klippel-Feil syndrome.*

Radiograms show instability between the fused segments at the region of C-4 and C-5. **A.** Neutral position. **B.** Flexion. **C.** Extension. **D.** Postoperative view following fusion.

syndrome. It consists of involuntary paired movements of the hands ("mirror motion")—the patient is unable to move the hands independently.

A neurologic deficit due to compression of the spinal cord or nerve roots may occur. Facial nerve palsy, rectus muscle palsy, ptosis of the eye, and cleft palate may accompany the Klippel-Feil syndrome.[116]

Radiographic Features

Roentgenographic examination is important in establishing a diagnosis and in determining the extent of the deformity (see Figs. 2–12 D to F and 2–13 C and D). The cervical vertebrae are often obscured by the overlapping occiput and mandible; not infrequently, one may have to resort to laminography for proper visualiza-

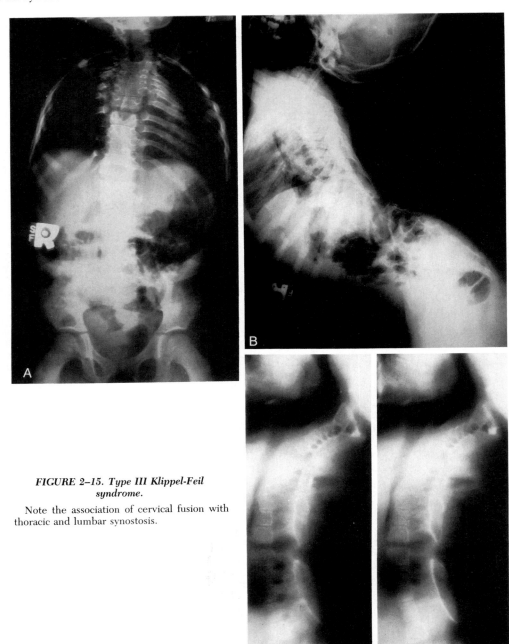

FIGURE 2–15. Type III Klippel-Feil syndrome.

Note the association of cervical fusion with thoracic and lumbar synostosis.

tion. The vertebral bodies are often flattened and widened. The intervertebral discs are narrowed or obliterated. Cervical spina bifida is very common. Hemivertebrae, cervical ribs, and platybasia have been observed in association with the Klippel-Feil syndrome.

In the differential diagnosis, one should consider bilateral Sprengel's deformity, acquired fusion of the vertebrae following fracture healing, and inflammatory conditions such as rheumatoid arthritis or discitis. Lateral flexion-extension radiograms demonstrate vertebral instability and the level of involvement (Fig. 2–14). In early life, posterior fusions of laminae are more apparent than anterior vertebral body synostosis (Fig. 2–15).

Treatment

Treatment consists of passive stretching exercises to obtain the maximum range of motion. These should be started immediately after birth and continued throughout the growth period. The distraction forces provided by a Milwaukee brace may be somewhat beneficial, especially if there is associated kyphoscoliosis.

Instability of the cervical spine is treated by fusion. Surgical efforts are directed toward the improvement of both appearance and function. Webbing of the skin that exaggerates the deformity can often be alleviated by plastic procedures such as a Z-plasty with fascial and muscle release, which will also permit greater freedom of neck movement.

Contracture of the sternocleidomastoid muscle can be corrected by its division or partial excision. If the Klippel-Feil syndrome occurs in association with Sprengel's deformity, the high scapula may be surgically restored to its normal position, thus increasing the apparent length of the neck. "Cervicalization" of the upper thoracic segment by means of bilateral resection of the first four ribs has been described by Bonola.[16] The advantages of the cosmetic improvement afforded by this procedure should be weighed against the potential grave complications inherent in it, such as brachial plexus injury.

References

1. Algom, M., and Schlesinger, Z.: Prolapse of the mitral valve in Klippel-Feil syndrome (Letter). Chest, 79:127, 1981.
2. Allen, W. E., Jr.: Klippel-Feil malformation: report of a case in an adult. Radiology, 44:79, 1945.
3. Avery, L. W., and Rentfro, C. C.: The Klippel-Feil syndrome. Arch. Neurol. Psychiat., 36:1068, 1936.
4. Axeman, K., Cernusakova, V., and Kolar, J.: Dystopische Kuchenniere beim Klippel-Feil Syndrom. Beitrag zur sonographischen Diagnostik. R.O.F.O., 140:617, 1984.
5. Baga, N., Chusid, E. L., and Miller, A.: Pulmonary disability in the Klippel-Feil syndrome. A study of two siblings. Clin. Orthop., 64:105, 1969.
6. Bailey, R. W.: Congenital Deformities of the Cervical Spine. Philadelphia, Lea & Febiger, 1974, pp. 6–9.
7. Baird, P. A., and Lowry, R. B.: Absent vagina and the Klippel-Feil anomaly. Am. J. Obstet. Gynecol., 118:290, 1974.
8. Baird, P. A., Robinson, G. C., and Buckler, W. St. J.: Klippel-Feil syndrome. Am. J. Dis. Child., 113:546, 1967.
9. Bara, F. Z.: Klippel-Feil syndrome with manifestations simulating rheumatoid arthritis. Wiad. Lek., 35:587, 1982.
10. Bauman, G. I.: Absence of the cervical spine. Klippel-Feil syndrome. J.A.M.A., 98:129, 1932.
11. Bell, J. F., Kuhlmann, R. F., and Molloy, M. K.: Congenital defects of shoulder girdle, sternum, spine and pelvis. Pediatr. Clin. North Am., 14:397, 1967.
12. Benesova, A., Balatka, J., and Filip, J.: Agenesis of the left lung in a child with the Klippel-Feil syndrome. Cesk. Pediatr., 33:346, 1978.
13. Berdel, D., and Burmeister, W.: Pickwick and Klippel-Feil syndromes in a boy aged 12 with reciprocal translocation of D. chromosome. Klin. Paediatr., 186:467, 1974.
14. Berke, J. P., and Magee, K. R.: Craniofacial dysostosis with syringomyelia and associated anomalies. Arch. Neurol., 33:63, 1976.
15. Bizarro, A. H.: Brevicollis. Lancet, 2:828, 1938.
16. Bonola, A.: Surgical treatment of the Klippel-Feil syndrome. J. Bone Joint Surg., 38-B:400, 1956.
17. Bracher, A. N., and Koontz, A. R.: Mediastinal bronchogenic cyst and Klippel-Feil syndrome. J.A.M.A., 150:1006, 1952.
18. Brik, M., and Athayde, A.: Bilateral Duane's syndrome, paroxysmal lacrimation and Klippel-Feil anomaly. Ophthalmologica, 167:1, 1973.
19. Brown, M. W., Templeton, A. W., and Hodges, F. J.: The incidence of acquired and congenital fusions in the cervical spine. A. J. R., 92:1255, 1964.
20. Brzezinska, H., Dabkowska, M., Janiszewska-Fronczak, M., Krawczynski, M., and Zgliczynska-Bartoszewicz, M.: Klippel-Feil syndrome coexisting with Sprengel's disease in a 3-year-old child. Pneumonol. Pol., 45:569, 1977.
21. Bucy, P. C., and Ritchey, H.: Klippel-Feil's syndrome associated with compression of the spinal cord by an extradural hemangiolipoma. J. Neurosurg., 4:477, 1947.
22. Burgess, G. H., Ferguson, K. S., and Meyer, W. J.: Recurrent pneumonia in Klippel-Feil syndrome. Tex. Med., 77:56, 1981.
23. Chaurasia, B. D., and Singh, M. P.: Ectopic lungs in a human with Klippel-Feil syndrome. Anat. Anz., 142:205, 1977.
24. Chiari, K.: Doppelseitiger Schiefhals. Z. Orthop., 83:151, 1952.
25. Clarke, J. J.: Congenital deformity of the cervical spine. Lancet, 2:1350, 1906.
26. Clemmesen, V.: Congenital cervical synostosis. Acta Radiol. (Stockh.), 17:480, 1936.
27. Cordier, J., Duprez, A., and Raspiller, A.: Uvéite chronique et syndrome de Klippel-Feil. Bull. Soc. Ophtal. Fr., 70:929, 1970.
28. Creighton, R. E., Relton, J. E., and Meridy, H. W.: Anaesthesia for occipital encephalocoele. Can. Anaesth. Soc. J., 21:403, 1974.
29. Cremers, C. W., Hoagland, G. A., and Kuypers, W.:

Hearing loss in the cervical-oculo-acoustic (Wildervanck syndrome). Arch. Otolaryngol., *110*:54, 1984.

30. DaSilva, E. O.: Autosomal recessive Klippel-Feil syndrome. J. Med. Genet., *19*:130, 1982.
31. Dihlmann, W., and Friedmann, G.: The radiological criteria of juvenile rheumatic cervical synostosis in adults. Fortschr. Geb. Röntgenstr. Nuklearmed., *126*:536, 1977.
32. Dinakar, I., and Rao, S. B.: Spinal tumours associated with Klippel-Feil syndrome. Neurol. India, *20*:60, 1972.
33. Dolan, K. D.: Developmental abnormalities of the cervical spine below the axis. Radiol. Clin. North Am., *15*:167, 1977.
34. Donaldson, J.: The Neck. 3rd Ed. Baltimore, Williams & Wilkins, 1968, pp. 273–291.
35. Duncan, P. A.: Embryologic pathogenesis of renal agenesis associated with cervical vertebral anomalies (Klippel-Feil phenotype). Birth Defects, *13*:91, 1977.
36. Dussault, R. G., and Kaye, J. J.: Intervertebral disk calcification associated with spine fusion. Radiology, *125*:57, 1977.
37. Ehrenhaft, J. L.: Development of the vertebral column as related to certain congenital and pathological changes. Surg. Gynecol. Obstet., *76*:282, 1943.
38. Elowson, S.: Ein Fall mitt Klippel-Feil Syndrome. Acta Chir. Scand., *67*:326, 1939.
39. Erskine, C. A.: Analysis of Klippel-Feil syndrome. Arch. Pathol., *41*:269, 1946.
40. Falk, R. H., and Mackinnon, J.: Klippel-Feil syndrome associated with aortic coarctation. Br. Heart J., *38*:1220, 1976.
41. Feil, A.: L'absence et la diminution des vertèbres cervicales (étude clinique et pathogénique); le syndrome de réduction numérique cervicale. Thèses de Paris, 1919.
42. Feil, A., Roland, J., and Vanbockstael: Les hommes sans cou. Considérations sur la réduction numérique et le tassement des vertèbres cervicales. Rev. Orthop., *11*:281, 1924.
43. Fickentscher, H.: Klippel-Feilsches Syndrom und Schwerhörigkeit. Arch. Ohr. Heilkd., *164*:297, 1954.
44. Fietti, V. G., Jr., and Fielding, J. W.: The Klippel-Feil syndrome: Early roentgenographic appearance and progression of the deformity. A report of two cases. J. Bone Joint Surg., *58-A*:891, 1976.
45. Foggie, W. E.: Clinical record—a case of congenital short neck showing the Klippel-Feil syndrome. Edinburgh Med. J., *42*:421, 1935.
46. Forney, W. R., Robinson, S. J., and Pascoe, D. J.: Congenital heart disease, deafness, and skeletal malformations: A new syndrome? J. Pediatr., *68*:14, 1966.
47. Fragoso, R., Cid-Garcia, A., Hernandez, A., Nazara, Z., and Cantu, J. M.: Frontal nasal dysplasia in the Klippel-Feil syndrome: A new associated malformation. Clin. Genet., *22*:270, 1982.
48. Fraser, W. I., and MacGillivray, R. C.: Cervico-oculo-acoustic dysplasia. Br. Med. J., *1*:283, 1970.
49. Gajic, S. I.: Gallbladder agenesis in a patient with Klippel-Feil syndrome. Arch. Pathol. Lab. Med., *105*:682, 1981.
50. Gardner, W. J.: Diastematomyelia and the Klippel-Feil syndrome. Cleve. Clin. Q., *31*:19, 1964.
51. Gardner, W. J., and Collis, J. S.: Klippel-Feil syndrome. Arch. Surg., *83*:638, 1961.
52. Gehring, G. G., and Shenasky, J. H.: Crossed fusion of renal pelves and Klippel-Feil syndrome. J. Urol., *116*:103, 1976.
53. Giroud, M., Verret, S., and Fortin, G.: Le syndrome cervical-oculo-acoustique. Pediatrie, *36*:479, 1981.
54. Giroud, M., Verret, S., and Fortin, G.: Les anomalies radiologiques dans le syndrome de Wildervanck. J. Radiol., *64*:131, 1983.
55. Gray, S. W., Romaine, C. B., and Skandalakis, J. E.: Congenital fusion of the cervical vertebrae. Surg. Gynecol. Obstet., *118*:373, 1964.
56. Groff, R. A., and Pitts, F. W.: Klippel-Feil syndrome (brevicollis). *In* Rubin, A. (ed.): Handbook of Congenital Malformations. Philadelphia, Saunders, 1969, p. 69.
57. Gunderson, C. H., Greenspan, R. H., and Glaser, G. H.: The Klippel-Feil syndrome: Genetic and clinical reevaluation of cervical fusion. Medicine, *46*:491, 1967.
58. Gunderson, C. H., and Solitaire, G. B.: Mirror movements and patients with Klippel-Feil syndrome. Neuropathologic observations. Arch. Neurol., *18*:675, 1968.
59. Gupta, M., and Singh, R. N.: The Klippel Feil syndrome: (a case report). Indian Pediatr., *15*:437, 1978.
60. Hamacher, P., and Parsch, K.: Differential diagnosis of the "shoulder-arm syndrome". Z. Allg. Med., *46*:1168, 1970.
61. Hensinger, R. N.: Orthopedic problems of the shoulder and neck. Pediatr. Clin. North Am., *24*:889, 1977.
62. Hensinger, R. N., Lang, J. E., and MacEwen, G. D.: Klippel-Feil syndrome: A constellation of associated anomalies. J. Bone Joint Surg., *56-A*:1246, 1974.
63. Hita Perez, J., Barreiro Tella, P., Martin Herrera, L., and Vazquez Rodriquez, J. J.: Klippel-Feil's syndrome associated with horseshoe kidney and brown and white spots. Rev. Clin. Esp., *119*:263, 1970.
64. Holliday, P. O., Davis, C., and Angelo, J.: Multiple meningiomas of the cervical spinal cord associated with Klippel-Feil malformation and atlanto-occipital assimilation. Neurosurgery, *14*:353, 1984.
65. Hrivnakova, J., and Fara, M.: Brevicollis (Klippel-Feil syndrome). Rozhl. Chir., *53*:183, 1974.
66. Illingsworth, R. S.: Attacks of unconsciousness in association with fused cervical vertebrae. Arch. Dis. Child., *31*:8, 1956.
67. Ionescu, A., Lavrov, S., and Milicescu, S.: Bilateral congenital elevation of the scapula associated with the Klippel-Feil syndrome. Chirurgia (Bucur.): *21*:241, 1972.
68. Jalladeau, J.: Malformations congénitales associées au syndrome de Klippel-Feil. Thèse de Paris, 1936.
69. Jarcho, S.: Anomaly of the vertebral column (Klippel-Feil syndrome) in American aborigines. J.A.M.A., *193*:843, 1965.
70. Jarvis, J. F., and Sellars, S. L.: Klippel-Feil deformity associated with congenital conductive deafness. J. Laryngol. Otol., *88*:285, 1974.
71. Kazmin, A. I., and Fomicheva, E. U.: Surgical treatment of Klippel-Feil syndrome. Ortop. Travmatol. Protez., *10*:67, 1974.
72. Khandekar, J. D., Singhal, G. C., and Singh, D.: Klippel-Feil syndrome associated with congenital cyanotic heart disease, Marfan's syndrome and other anomalies. J. Assoc. Physicians India, *19*:203, 1971.
73. Klippel, M., and Feil, A.: Anomalies de la colonne vertébrale par absence des vertèbres cervicales; cage thoracique remontant jusqu'à la base du crâne. Bull. Soc. Anat., Paris, *87*:185, 1912.
74. Klippel, M., and Feil, A.: The classic: a case of absence of cervical vertebrae with the thoracic cage rising to the base of the cranium (cervical thoracic cage). Clin. Orthop., *109*:3, 1975.
75. Lato, S. T., and Stanizcek, J.: Case of Klippel-Feil syndrome coexisting with left lung aplasia. Wiad. Lek., *31*:195, 1978.
76. Lowry, R. B.: The Klippel-Feil anomalad as part of the fetal alcohol syndrome. Teratology, *16*:53, 1977.
77. Luftman, I., and Weintraub, S.: Klippel-Feil syn

drome in a full-term stillborn infant. N.Y. J. Med., *51*:2035, 1951.

78. McElfresh, E., and Winter, R.: Klippel-Feil syndrome. Minn. Med., *56*:353, 1973.

79. McLay, K., and Maran, A. G. D.: Deafness and the Klippel-Feil syndrome. J. Laryngol., *83*:175, 1969.

80. Mackenzie, S.: Klippel-Feil syndrome. Proc. R. Soc. Med., *31*:1162, 1938.

81. Mackenzie, S.: Klippel-Feil syndrome. Br. Child. Dis., *40*:10, 1943.

82. Martischnig, E., and Schmuttermeier, E.: Zur Frage der des Klippel-Feilschen Syndroms. Wien. Klin. Wochenschr., *64*:722, 1952.

83. Mecklenburg, R. S., and Krueger, P. M.: Extensive genitourinary anomalies associated with Klippel-Feil syndrome. Am. J. Dis. Child., *128*:92, 1974.

84. Michie, I., and Clark, M.: Neurological syndromes associated with cervical and craniocervical anomalies. Arch. Neurol., *18*:241, 1968.

85. Milner, L. S., Davidge-Pitts, K. J., Rosen, E. U., and Anderson, M. G.: Recurrent meningitis due to round-window fistula in Klippel-Feil syndrome. A case report. S. Afr. Med. J., *64*:413, 1983.

86. Miyamoto, C., Ishii, H., and Hamamoto, Y.: An autopsy case of the Klippel-Feil syndrome. Bull. Osaka Med. Sch., *17*:11, 1971.

87. Miyamoto, R. T., Yune, H. Y., and Rosevear, W. H.: Klippel-Feil syndrome and associated ear deformities. Am. J. Otol., *5*:113, 1983.

88. Moore, W. B., Matthews, T. J., and Rabinowitz, R.: Genitourinary anomalies associated with Klippel-Feil syndrome. J. Bone Joint Surg., *57-A*:355, 1975.

89. Morrison, S. G., and Perry, L. S., and Scott, L. P., III: Congenital brevicollis (Klippel-Feil syndrome). Am. J. Dis. Child., *115*:614, 1968.

90. Neidengard, L., Carter, T. E., and Smith, D. W.: Klippel-Feil malformation complex in fetal alcohol syndrome. Am. J. Dis. Child., *132*:929, 1978.

91. Noble, T. P., and Frawley, J. M.: The Klippel-Feil syndrome—numerical reduction of cervical vertebrae. Ann. Surg., *82*:728, 1925.

92. Nora, J. J., Cohen, M., and Maxwell, G. M.: Klippel-Feil syndrome with congenital heart disease. Am. J. Dis. Child., *102*:858, 1961.

93. Oggero, R., Bertoletti, M. T., Pioli, M., and Giorla, F.: Inquadramento nosografico della sindrome die Klippel-Feil e descrizione di un caso clinico associato ad ipoacusia. Arch. Sci. Med., *139*:261, 1982.

94. Ohwada, T.: Klippel-Feil syndrome. Nippon Rinsho, *35*:522, 1977.

95. Palant, D. I., and Carter, B. L.: Klippel-Feil syndrome and deafness. A study with polytomography. Am. J. Dis. Child., *123*:218, 1972.

96. Park, I. J., and Jones, H. W., Jr.: A new syndrome in two unrelated females: Klippel-Feil deformity, conductive deafness and absent vagina. Birth Defects, *7*:311, 1971.

97. Pfandler, U., and Gloor, R. D.: Une famille avec syndrome de Klippel-Feil et autres malformations de la colonne vertébrale. J. Genet. Hum., *15*:103, 1966.

98. Poznanski, A. K.: Congenital anomalies of the cervical spine. *In* Bailey, R. W. (ed.): The Cervical Spine. Philadelphia, Lea & Febiger, 1974, pp. 63–69.

99. Ramsey, J., and Bliznak, J.: Klippel-Feil syndrome with renal agenesis and other anomalies. A. J. R., *113*:460, 1971.

100. Rechtman, A. M., and Horwitz, M. J.: Congenital synostosis of the cervico-thoracic vertebrae (the Klippel-Feil syndrome). A. J. R., *43*:66, 1940.

101. Rinvik, R.: A case of the Klippel-Feil syndrome (congenital synostosis of the cervical vertebrae). Acta Paediatr. (Upps.), *31*:417, 1944.

102. Rish, B. L.: Klippel-Feil syndrome: Case report. Va. Med., *109*:520, 1982.

103. Roberts, A. P.: A case of intracranial dermoid cyst associated with the Klippel-Feil deformity and recurrent meningitis. Arch. Dis. Child., *33*:222, 1958.

104. Rodriguez Cuartero, A., Morata Garcia, F., and Machado Quintana, F.: A further case of Klippel-Feil syndrome with associated abnormalities. Rev. Clin. Esp., *126*:541, 1972.

105. Sakai, M., Miyake, H., Shinkawa, A., and Komotsu, N.: Klippel-Feil syndrome with conductive deafness and histological findings of removed stapes. Ann. Otol. Rhinol. Laryngol., *92*:202, 1983.

106. Sauvegrain, J., and Mareschal, J. -L.: Malformations de la charnière craniocervicale chez l'enfant. A propos de 35 observations. Ann. Radiol. (Paris), *15*:263, 1972.

107. Schmorl, G.: Klippel-Feil syndrome (short neck). New York, Grune & Stratton, 1971, pp. 96–97.

108. Sensenig, E. C.: The development of the occipital and cervical segments and their associated structures in human embryos. Contrib. Embryol. Carnegie Inst., *36*:141, 1957.

109. Sherk, H. H., Shut, L., and Chung, S.: Iniencephalic deformity of the cervical spine with Klippel-Feil anomalies and congenital elevation of scapula; report of three cases. J. Bone Joint Surg., *56-A*:1254, 1974.

110. Sherk, H. H., and Dawoud, S.: Congenital os odontoidum with Klippel-Feil anomaly and fatal atlanto-axial instability. Report of a case. Spine, *6*:42, 1981.

111. Shoul, M. L., and Ritvo, M.: Clinical and roentgenological manifestations of the Klippel-Feil syndrome (congenital fusion of the cervical vertebrae, brevicollis). A. J. R., *68*:369, 1972.

112. Sicard, A., and Peres: L'association du syndrome de Klippel Feil, de la surélevation de l'omoplate et du pterygium colli. Presse Méd., *66*:2033, 1958.

113. Singhi, S., Verna, I. C., Kalra, V.: Klippel-Feil syndrome with Bell's palsy. Indian J. Pediatr., *47*:257, 1980.

114. Strax, T. E., and Baran, E.: Traumatic quadriplegia associated with Klippel-Feil syndrome: Discussion and case reports. Arch. Phys. Med. Rehabil., *56*:363, 1975.

115. Southwell, R. B., Reynolds, A. F., Badger, V. M., and Sherman, F. C.: Klippel-Feil syndrome with cervical compression resulting from cervical subluxation in association with an omo-vertebral bone. Spine, *5*:480, 1980.

116. Stadnicki, G., and Rassomowski, D.: The association of cleft palate with the Klippel-Feil syndrome. Oral Surg., *33*:335, 1972.

117. Stark, E. W., and Borton, T. E.: Klippel-Feil syndrome and associated hearing loss. Arch. Otolaryngol., *97*:415, 1973.

118. Stark, E. W., and Borton, T. E.: Hearing loss and the Klippel-Feil syndrome. Am. J. Dis. Child., *123*:233, 1972.

119. Truex, R. C., Jr., and Johnson, C. H.: Congenital anomalies of the upper cervical spine. Orthop. Clin. North Am., *9*:891, 1978.

120. Vaquero, J., Herrero, J., Cabezudo, J., and Leunda, G.: Klippel-Feil syndrome with epidural fibroblastoma in the area of vertebral fusion. Arch. Neurol., *39*:318, 1982.

121. Viegas, C. A.: Charcot-Marie-Tooth disease associated with Klippel-Feil malformation. Report of a

case and review of the literature. (Eng. abstr.) Arq. Neuropsiquiatr., 38:193, 1980.

122. Wang, Y. Y.: Klippel-Feil syndrome (author's transl.). Chung Hua I Hsueh Tsa Chih, 61:293, 1981.

123. Whitehouse, G. H., and Harrison, R. J.: Klippel-Feil syndrome. Proc. R. Soc. Med., 63:287, 1970.

124. Whittle, I. R., and Besser, M.: Congenital neural abnormalities presenting with mirror movements in a patient with Klippel-Feil syndrome. Case Report. Neurosurgery, 59:891, 1983.

125. Willemsen, W. N.: Combination of the Mayer-Rokitansky-Kuster and Klippel-Feil syndrome—a case report and literature review. Eur. J. Obstet. Gynecol. Reprod. Biol., 13:229, 1982.

126. Windle-Taylor, P. C., Emery, P. J., and Phelps, P. D.: Ear deformities associated with the Klippel-Feil syndrome. Ann. Otol. Rhinol. Laryngol., 90:210, 1981.

CONGENITAL HIGH SCAPULA (Sprengel's Deformity)

The scapula initially appears as a cervical appendage, descending to the level of the posterior upper thorax by the end of the third fetal month. Occasionally, however, it fails to descend from the neck to its usual location; the result is an abnormally and permanently elevated scapula, known commonly as Sprengel's deformity.

This rare congenital deformity was first described, in 1863, by Eulenberg of Germany, who reported three cases of "hochgradige Dislocation der Scapula."[31, 32] Willet and Walsham of England, in 1880, were the first to describe the omovertebral bone as a broad osseous band connecting the scapula with the spinous process of the sixth cervical vertebra in a case of congenitally high scapula. The affected scapula differed in shape and size from its counterpart. They also found absence of ribs, and a sharp left dorsal scoliosis.[96] In 1883, the same authors reported a second case in which the omovertebral bone was excised and function was improved.[97] Sprengel, in 1891, described four cases of upward displacement of the scapula without rotation.[90] Kölliker reported cases in 1891 and unjustifiably applied Sprengel's name to the condition.[59] Since then *Sprengel's deformity* has become a common eponym for this congenital deformity.

Etiology

Various theories concerning the pathogenesis of the deformity have been suggested. Horwitz presented a comprehensive study of the subject, in which he set forth the following possibilities: first, that it (Sprengel's deformity) is a failure of descent caused by (a) too great intrauterine pressure, due to either an increased or a diminished amount of amniotic fluid; (b) abnormal articulations of the scapula with the vertebral column; (c) a defective musculature, unable to draw the scapula caudally, where neither (a) nor (b) exists; or (d) a normal musculature, unable to draw the scapula caudally where either (a) or (b) exists; and second, that the changes in the shape and size of the scapula are an arrest of development due to improper or defective muscular tension.[48] Horwitz did not believe heredity to be a factor in Sprengel's deformity, but he had difficulty explaining the presence of a high percentage (67 per cent) of concomitant congenital deformities.

Sprengel's deformity almost always occurs sporadically.[29, 30, 68, 72, 92] Neuhof, however, reported three generations of a family in which, out of 20 members, 7 had Sprengel's deformity, 3 of them bilaterally.[68] Gottesleben reported that there were nine patients in three generations.[40] Walker described a family of 40 individuals, spanning three generations, of which four members had bilateral and six members had unilateral involvement.[92] From these reports it is obvious that, at least in some patients, Sprengel's deformity has an apparent autosomal dominant pattern of inheritance.

The "bleb" theory was advanced by Engel to explain the pathogenesis of the undescended scapula and related syndromes.[29, 30] Normally, cerebrospinal fluid escapes through the area membranacea at the roof of the fourth ventricle to form the subarachnoid space.[93] In some pathologic conditions in which there is either excessive production or deficient reabsorption of cerebrospinal fluid, or when there is failure to achieve midline union and the area membranacea remains unduly patent, cerebrospinal fluid escapes into the subcutis of the adjacent neck region. The subcutaneous blebs so formed spread on the body surface and are driven by physical forces toward areas of least resistance. They are arrested and retained by preformed cavities and pockets such as the orbits and limb buds. The subcutaneous blebs cause damage by pressure and by provoking an inflammatory reaction. By irradiating the ovaries in mice, Bagg and his associates showed experimentally that, in the progeny, these blebs are the direct cause of numerous deformities such as clubfoot, clawhand, and polydactylism.[4–6] Although the deformed second and subsequent generations were not subjected to roentgen radiation, they produced progeny with the same malformations in a high percentage of cases, showing the acquired deformities to be inheritable. Blebs similar to those described in Bagg's strain of mice were observed by Bonnevie in human embryos with anomalies of the fingers and toes.[11] Engel proposed that the bleb mechanism is polyvalent and, as it spreads over the upper limb, may cause a great variety of deformities such as the Klippel-Feil syndrome in the neck, Sprengel's deformity in the shoulder, malformations of the humerus and radius and ulna, and syndactylism and other deformities of the digits.[29, 30]

Pathology

The pathologic changes of Sprengel's deformity reflect the embryology and phylogeny of the scapula. In the human embryo, the arm bud appears in the third week as a slight swelling opposite the fifth cervical to the first thoracic segment; the scapula appears in the fifth week. With further development, the scapula gradually migrates caudally until it reaches its final position. In the adult, the normal scapula is situated on the posterior aspect of the thorax, extending vertically from the second to the seventh or eighth vertebra.

The affected scapula in Sprengel's deformity is abnormally high. It is small, with a smaller vertical diameter and an apparently greater width. Its shape is distorted, its supraspinous portion tilted forward to fit the convexity of the upper thorax. There may be a prolongation or broadening of the superior median angle or the upper third of the median border of the scapula to the spinous process, lamina, or transverse process of one of the lower cervical vertebrae (fourth to seventh).

The omovertebral bone may be attached to the vertebral border of the scapula in a number of ways: by bony continuity, by cartilaginous union, or by a fibrous band (Fig. 2–16). On occasion, it may form a true joint with a small osseocartilaginous protuberance projecting from the midvertebral border of the scapula.

The shoulder girdle musculature is usually defective, the trapezius being most often affected. The muscle may be absent or weak, especially in its lower portion. The rhomboids

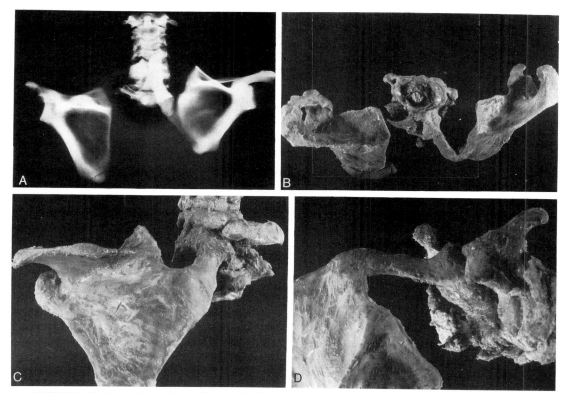

FIGURE 2–16. *Anatomic specimen of Sprengel's deformity on the right with associated Klippel-Feil syndrome.*

A. Radiogram of anatomic specimen with the left scapula in its normal position and the right in its high position. Note the whole right scapula is hypoplastic as compared with the left; the infraspinous portion of the right scapula appears to be wide with decrease in the height-width ratio. **B to D.** Superior, anterior, and oblique views of the anatomic specimen. Note the omovertebral bone connecting the scapula to the lower cervical vertebrae. (Courtesy of J. A. Ogden.)

and levator scapulae are usually hypoplastic and partially fibrosed. The serratus anterior may be weak. The pectoralis major, pectoralis minor, latissimus dorsi, and sternocleidomastoid muscles may be affected.

Histologic findings have indicated interruption of the normal differentiation of the involved muscle fibers at the myoblastic stage. The affected muscles undergo degeneration, necrosis, fibrosis, and secondary contracture.

Other associated congenital deformities are absence or fusion of ribs, cervical ribs, the Klippel-Feil syndrome, congenital scoliosis with hemivertebrae, and spina bifida in the cervical region, syringomyelia, paraplegia, platybasia, situs inversus, and mandibulofacial dysostosis.[12, 21, 27, 37, 46, 51, 55, 88] The humerus may be shortened on the affected side. The clavicle may be malformed or hypoplastic, or it may fail to articulate with the acromion. Congenital shortening of the femur, incomplete intercalary tibial hemimelia, radial hemimelia, and ray defects of the hand and foot are other rare associated congenital anomalies. Kidney malformations, such as ectopia, hypoplasia, or absence of a kidney are infrequent but do occur.[14] It is advisable to perform ultrasonography or intravenous pyelography to rule out renal anomalies. The kidneys, like bone and muscle, are of mesodermal origin and may be similarly affected. Cardiac anomalies such as atrial septal defect may be found.

Clinical Features

The asymmetry of the shoulder caused by the upward and forward displacement of the scapula is the salient physical finding (Fig. 2–17). The deformity is usually noticed at birth; it progresses with growth. It is more preponderant in girls, with female to male sex ratio of about three to one in the series of Ross and Cruess, and four to one in that of Cavendish.[15, 79] The left side is more often affected than the right. The deformity may be bilateral. The level of the scapula in relation to the vertebral column varies with the severity of the condition; it may be situated 1 to 12 cm. higher than its normal opposite, 3 to 5 cm. being the average. The superior angle of the scapula may be found as high as the fourth cervical vertebra with its inferior angle at the second thoracic vertebra. On the affected side, the neck is fuller and shorter, and the cervicoscapular line is diminished. The supraspinous portion of the scapula may be palpable in the supraclavicular area. The affected clavicle is often tilted obliquely upward and laterally at an angle of 25 degrees from the horizontal (Fig. 2–18). On inspection and palpation, its smaller size is evident. It is frequently rotated upon the sagittal axis, bringing the upper medial angle away from the spinal column and the lower angle close to it. The omovertebral bone may be palpable. When the arm is elevated, the lateral motion and rotation of the scapula is diminished. Combined abduction of the affected shoulder is limited (see Fig. 2–17 C). Passive motion of the glenohumeral joint is usually within normal range, however; it is scapulocostal motion that is restricted owing to loss or marked decrease of mobility of the scapula over the thorax secondary to omovertebral bone or fibrous adhesions binding the scapula to the ribs. Other factors are depression of the lateral border of the scapula and motor weakness of the muscles about the affected shoulder resulting from fibrosis or hypoplasia.

A muscle examination is imperative to determine the degree of motor weakness of the defective musculature.

Scoliosis and kyphosis due to congenital deformities of the vertebrae are not uncommon. Torticollis may be present because of contracture of the sternocleidomastoid muscle. Deformities of the rib cage, such as absence of ribs, may be clinically palpable. Other associated congenital deformities such as the Klippel-Feil syndrome may be obvious (Fig. 2–19).

When the condition is bilateral, the neck appears very short and thick. Abduction is limited in both shoulders, and the cervical lordosis may be increased.[10, 82, 83]

Radiographic Findings

Radiograms will demonstrate the elevation of the scapula and its associated bony deformities (see Fig. 2–18). They are best visualized by taking the following views: *anteroposterior views* of both shoulders with the arms at the sides and with the shoulders in both maximal active and passive abduction to show the abnormally high position of the scapula and its limited motion; a *lateral view* of the cervical and dorsal spine; and *oblique and lateral views* of the scapula to demonstrate the omovertebral bone. Computed tomography has been utilized to visualize the omovertebral bone.[8]

Treatment

The goals of treatment are to correct the deformity and improve function. In infants and young children, passive stretching and active

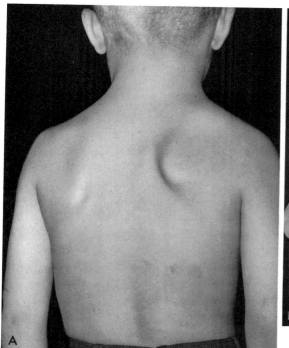

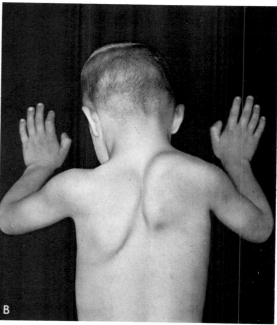

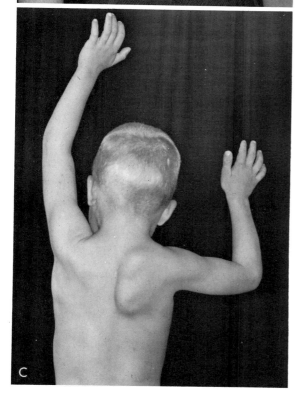

FIGURE 2–17. Sprengel's deformity
of the right shoulder.

A and **B.** The scapula is elevated and hypoplastic, its horizontal diameter being greater than the vertical. **C.** Abduction of the right shoulder is limited.

Illustration continued on following page

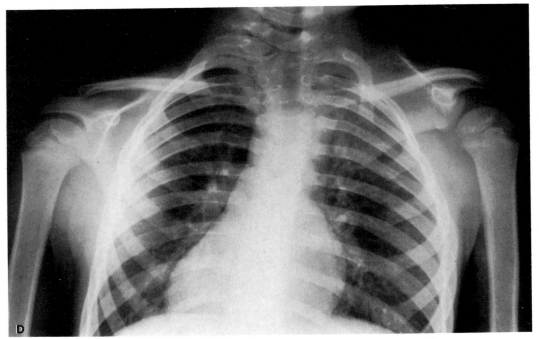

FIGURE 2–17 Continued. Sprengel's deformity of the right shoulder.

D. Preoperative radiogram.

exercises are performed daily in order *to maintain* the maximal degree of range of motion of the involved shoulder and to increase the motor strength of the defective musculature. One should particularly emphasize passive and active abduction of the shoulder, scapular depression and adduction, dorsal hyperextension, trapeze-hanging, and push-ups. It is doubtful, however, whether such conservative treatment will achieve any significant improvement in appearance or function.

If the deformity is especially disfiguring and the function of the shoulder is impaired to a significant degree, operative intervention should be considered. Historically, several operative approaches to correct the deformity have been employed. Putti described a technique in which the scapular insertions of the rhomboids and trapezius (lower and middle fibers) were detached, the omovertebral bone (when present) was resected, and the scapula was displaced to a lower level and fixed at its inferior angle to a rib.[76] Schrock reported an operative procedure that varied from Putti's in that the supraspinous portion of the scapula was resected and the scapula released subperiosteally prior to its transplantation to a lower level.[84, 85] Scaglietti evaluated the end results in

four cases operated on by Putti and advised early intervention to obtain the best results.[83] Smith reviewed the results of various operative procedures performed on 13 patients, and stressed the disadvantages of extensive subperiosteal release. In very young patients, Smith recommended the removal of the omovertebral bone or fibrous band without any attempt to lower the scapula.[89]

Ober's operation differs from Schrock's in that there is less subperiosteal stripping of the scapula and the deformity is gradually corrected by skeletal traction on the scapula. The operation is performed in two stages. With the scapula pulled distally at the desired level, a thick flap of soft tissue and deep fascia is dissected from the adjacent erector spinae and anchored to the inferior angle of the scapula, holding it in the lowered position.[50] The principal drawback of Ober's operation (and Inclan's modification of it) is that it requires two separate stages.

Koenig divides the scapula longitudinally 1.25 cm. lateral to its medial margin, leaving the muscles attached in its vertebral border intact. The lateral part of the scapula is displaced caudally, and the inferior end of the relocated part is inserted into a pocket in the latissimus dorsi muscle. The subscapularis and

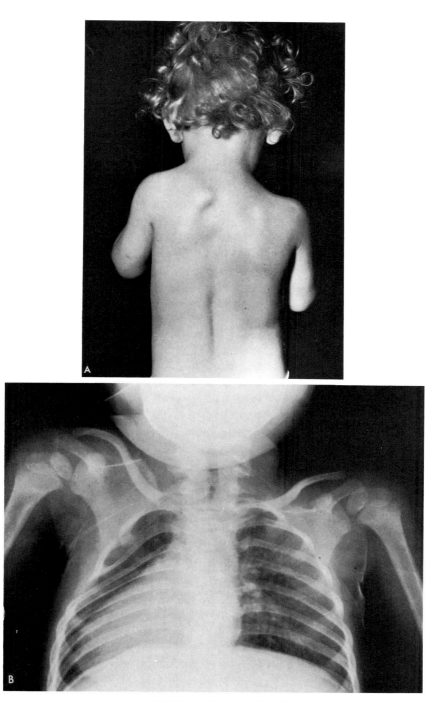

FIGURE 2–18. Sprengel's deformity on the left.

A. Clinical appearance. **B.** Anteroposterior radiogram showing the high position of the left scapula.

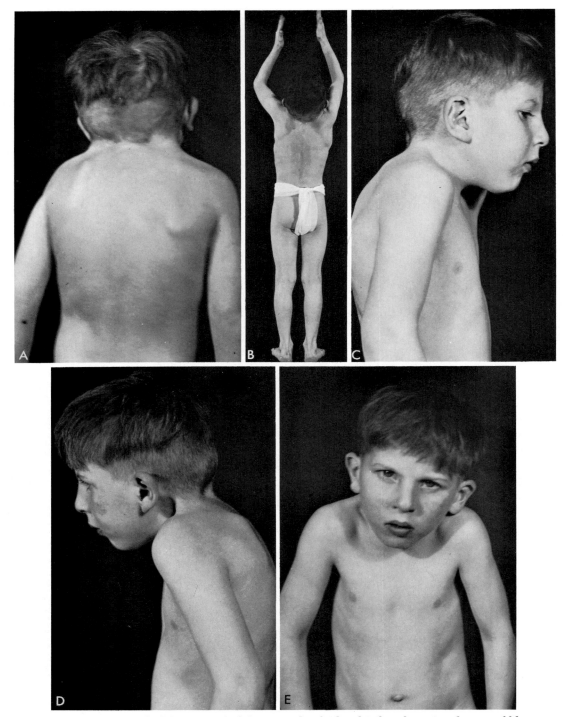

FIGURE 2–19. *Sprengel's deformity on the left associated with Klippel-Feil syndrome in a five-year-old boy.*

A to **E.** Clinical appearance before surgery, showing the high position of the left scapula, limitation of range of abduction of the left shoulder, exaggerated cervical lordosis, and webbing of the neck ("pterygium colli").

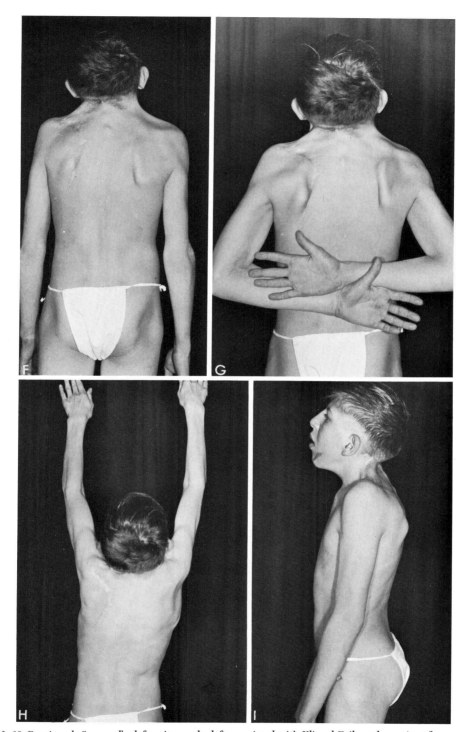

FIGURE 2–19 Continued. Sprengel's deformity on the left associated with Klippel-Feil syndrome in a five-year-old boy.

F to I. Postoperative photographs of same patient nine years after lowering of scapula on the left and soft-tissue release and Z-lengthening of "pterygium colli." Note the normal range of abduction of left shoulder and improvement in clinical appearance.

infraspinatus muscles are sutured to the divided parts of the scapula. The prominent superomedial part of the scapula is excised.[58]

McFarland recommended excision of most of the scapula, leaving only the glenoid cavity and the coracoid process.[64] Subtotal subperiosteal excision of the scapula has also been reported by Chigot and by Cabanac.[13, 17, 18] This author does not recommend subtotal scapulectomy because of its serious disadvantages—namely, further impairment of function as a result of the operation, an unsightly scar, the imperfect cosmetic result, excessive bleeding, and the magnitude of the surgery.

Jeannopoulos reviewed the operative results of 20 cases of Sprengel's deformity from files of the New York Orthopedic Hospital. The Schrock procedure was performed in 16 of them, with results rated as "satisfactory" in only half, "fair" in about one fourth, and "no improvement" in about one fourth. In 9 of the 16 patients, there was regeneration of the bone sufficient to cause an objectionable bulge at the base of the neck. Undesirable cosmetic sequelae of the operation were unsightly, wide, or keloid scars; winging of the inferior angle of the scapula; flaring of the vertebral border of the scapula; and a knoblike prominence of the sternoclavicular joint that simulated a subluxation. The bone regenerated at the site of osteotomy in two patients, and there was no appreciable improvement in their appearance. The abnormal position of the scapula was not corrected in four cases; surgery consisted of extensive subperiosteal stripping of the bone, resection of the supraspinous portion as well as a large part of the body of the scapula, and excision of the omovertebral bone (in three of the four patients). In two patients, the cosmetic result was good. Abduction of the shoulder was increased in two cases.[52]

Green described a procedure in which the muscles connecting the scapula to the trunk are divided at their scapular insertion, the omovertebral bone is removed (if present), and the supraspinous portion of the scapula is excised along with its periosteum. The scapula is displaced distally to a level comparable to the opposite normal side and held in position by wire traction, muscles are again attached to the scapula in its new position so as to hold and control it at the new level, and the traction wire is removed after three weeks.[41] The correction obtained by the Green operation is satisfactory, and there is definite improvement in the range of active and passive abduction of the shoulder. Firm reattachment of the muscles provides better dynamic control to the caudally transferred scapula. Its disadvantages are that it is somewhat difficult, the resulting parascapular scar is unsightly, and prolonged hospitalization is required because of skeletal traction (Fig. 2–20). One of the twenty-six patients reported by Green developed transient brachial plexus paralysis.

Woodward described an operation in which he obtained correction by detaching the origins of the trapezius and rhomboid muscles from the spinous processes and moving them downward after resection of omovertebral bone or any other fibrous bands binding the scapula. Muscles were not stripped from the scapula, and the procedure was combined with extraperiosteal resection of the supraspinous portion of the

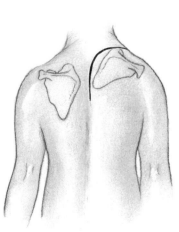

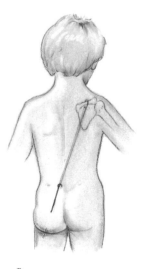

FIGURE 2–20. *Skin incision originally described by Green for distal transfer of scapula.*

A. Skin incision. **B.** Skeletal traction used in the Green technique to maintain the scapula in its lowered position.

A   B

scapula. He reported nine patients with a good to excellent amount of lowering of the scapula, fair to good cosmetic improvement, and satisfactory functional results. In one patient, transient brachial plexus paralysis developed. There was no regeneration of bone.[99]

Robinson and associates, in 1967, noted that in Sprengel's deformity the entire shoulder girdle, of which the clavicle is a major component, is high. In addition, in congenital high scapula the clavicle is shortened and does not have the normal convexity in the frontal plane. They recommended removal of the middle portion of the clavicle, morcellating the removed segment and replacing it in its carefully preserved periosteal sheath as a graft. This morcellation method of softening the clavicle markedly reduced the incidence of neural and vascular complications. In three previous cases neurovascular complications had developed (two patients with partial brachial plexus palsy and one with compression of the subclavian artery). Upon exploration of the subclavicular region they found these neurovascular structures compressed between the deformed clavicle and the first rib, which is also often deformed in this condition. These complications were successfully treated by surgical decompression of the brachial plexus and subclavian artery. In six subsequent shoulders with Sprengel's deformity the clavicles were softened by the morcellation method; in none of these six cases was there any neurovascular complication, and the clavicle re-formed to accommodate to its new position. In addition, the procedure provided greater mobility of the scapula and more ease in its caudal relocation.[78] Chung and Nissenbaum employed the morcellation method of softening the clavicle in six shoulders in five patients. The procedure was combined with the Woodward operation for Sprengel's deformity. In four of the cases (four shoulders) the cosmetic result was excellent; in one patient with bilateral involvement the result was good rather than excellent because his original problem of anencephaly made his final appearance less than normal. Neurovascular complications did not occur in any of the cases. The clavicle healed in all six cases.[20]

Cabanac, in 1954, had previously emphasized the importance of the clavicle as a major deforming force in Sprengel's deformity. He recommended resection of the medial part of the clavicle in conjunction with subtotal subperiosteal scapulectomy.[13]

Sectioning of the base of the coracoid process through a separate anterior incision in conjunction with distal transfer of the scapula (Green type) is advocated by Petrie.[73] This procedure releases the pectoralis minor muscle, providing greater mobility and more distal transplantation of the scapula. It also relieves pressure on the brachial plexus and subclavian vessels. In addition, it allows the scapula to rotate about the acromioclavicular joint as the tethering effect of the coracoclavicular ligaments is released. This author recommends dividing the coracoid process at its base in severe cases of Sprengel's deformity.

This author also recommends osteotomy of the clavicle at two or more levels prior to distal transfer of the scapula. It is not necessary to soften the clavicle by morcellation. After two or three greenstick osteotomies the clavicle heals rapidly in four to six weeks, and the postoperative course is simpler and more benign (see Plate 2).

Ross and Cruess reviewed the results of 77 cases of surgically treated congenital high scapula from 19 Shriners Hospitals throughout North America, Mexico, and Hawaii. Thirty-six of the patients underwent simple excision of the omovertebral bar and the superomedial portion of the scapula along with its periosteum. Functionally this simple procedure gave the best result, producing virtually normal shoulder abduction in a large number of the patients. Structurally and cosmetically, however, proximal scapular and omovertebral resection had no effect on the position of the scapula; the mean elevation observed in the preoperative and postoperative radiograms remained unchanged at 1.8 inches. The scapula did not drift inferiorly following omovertebral release.[79]

Cavendish reviewed 100 cases of congenital elevation of the scapula of which 34 were treated by operation. Eighteen of the patients had excision of the superomedial part of the scapula and omovertebral bone when present. He recommended it as the procedure of choice in grades 2 and 3 of Sprengel's deformity (described later) because of its safety and simplicity, its minimal risk of loss of function, and the simple course of postoperative care. The resultant operative scar is more acceptable than that of the parascapular incision. Cavendish mentions that with division of the structures holding the scapula in the elevated position some degree of "spontaneous" descent of the scapula may occur.[15] In the experience of this author, simple excision of the superomedial part of the scapula and omovertebral bone does not affect the position of the scapula; on the contrary, during a period of rapid growth of the neck, the appearance may deteriorate.

Ross and Cruess studied the results of 41

cases of distal relocation of the scapula—17 had had Woodward's procedure, 14 Schrock's, 4 Green's, and 6 Petrie's modification of the Green procedure. They observed the best functional and cosmetic results when caudal relocation of the scapula was added to simple proximal excision-release surgery. They could not give a valid statistical analysis of the relative effectiveness of one form of scapular transplantation over another. In general the Green and Woodward procedures provided the best functional and cosmetic results. Three of the cases had scapular winging, all following the Woodward procedure. The meticulous reattachment of the muscles to the lowered scapula in the Green procedure provides better scapular stability. Parascapular scars spread and are extremely unsightly; the midline incision provides a more attractive scar. Ross and Cruess observed that the addition of Petrie's coracoid section to the Green operation allowed the scapula to be displaced more distally without neurovascular complications.[79]

This author recommends that the following factors be considered in selecting patients for surgical correction of congenital high scapula: *first, the severity of the deformity*. Cavendish suggested a method of grading appearance. In *Grade I* the deformity is *very mild*; the shoulder joints are level with the deformity, and it is almost invisible when the patient is clothed. Obviously, in such cases surgery is not indicated because it does not offer worthwhile benefit. In *Grade 2*, the deformity is *mild* and the shoulder joints almost level, but when the patient is undressed the superomedial part of the high scapula is visible as a lump in the web of the neck. In such cases, simple excision of the supraspinous portion of the scapula may be indicated. The pros and cons of disfigurement caused by the scar versus the lump in the web of the neck should be weighed and discussed with the family. In *Grade 3, moderate*, the shoulder joint on the affected side is elevated 2 to 5 cm. and the deformity easily visible. In such an instance, the scapula should be lowered. With skeletal growth, the deformity will increase in the adolescent and become unsightly. In *Grade 4, severe*, the position of the scapula is very high, with its superior angle near the occiput, and there is webbing of the neck with brevicollis.[15] Obviously, such a cosmetic classification is difficult when the deformity is bilateral.

The *second factor* to consider in making a decision is *functional impairment*. Limitation of shoulder abduction may be due to fixation of the scapula either by an omovertebral bar or by fibrous adhesion of the scapula to the thoracic cage, or it may be due to motor weakness caused by fibrosis, hypoplasia, or aplasia of the muscles. Shoulder function can be greatly improved by resection of the omovertebral bar and release of scapulocostal adhesions if there is marked winging of the scapula. With motor weakness of shoulder abduction, function and appearance may be improved by fasciodesis of the lowered scapula in a more laterally rotated position.

The *third factor* to consider is the *association with anomalies* such as the Klippel-Feil syndrome or severe congenital scoliosis or kyphosis, which may overshadow the scapular deformity or render prospects of significant cosmetic improvement unlikely.

The *fourth factor* in the decision is the *age of the patient*. Surgical correction of Sprengel's deformity is quite an extensive procedure. In the past the recommended age for surgical correction was between three and seven years. Before the age of three the operation was considered to be extensive and difficult to perform, and after the age of eight there was greater danger of nerve injury to the brachial plexus from stretching. At present this author recommends surgery for severe Sprengel's deformity at six to nine months of age; with modern anesthesia and surgical technique the procedure is relatively simple and not dangerous. With early correction of deformity, function and cosmetic results are much better.

Finally in deciding and in discussing the benefits with the parents, caution must be exercised. Expectations should be realistic. It should be made clear that normal anatomic appearance cannot be provided in such a major malformation, especially if it is associated with other congenital anomalies. The scars are often extensive. These drawbacks should not, however, deter one from offering distal transplantation of the scapula, as it will significantly improve the function of the shoulder and its cosmetic appearance.

The procedure recommended by this author is a modification of Green's scapuloplasty (Plate 2). It has the following advantages: first, the clavicular osteotomy facilitates lowering of the scapula and prevents neurovascular injury. Second, a midline posterior incision is more cosmetically appealing and allows correction of bilateral cases and simultaneous spinal fusion if indicated because of hemivertebrae. Third, it eliminates the need for traction and prolonged hospitalization. The operative technique of the Woodward operation is described in Plate 3 because it is still quite popular with many orthopedic surgeons.[13, 34, 45, 74] This author sees no advantage of the Woodward procedure over the Green operation. Winging of the scapula may be as cosmetically objectionable as the asymmetry of the shoulders due to the high position of the scapula. The cause of winging is hypoplasia or aplasia of the rhomboids or serratus anterior muscles. In such an instance, this author recommends fasciodesis of the scapula on the rib cage with the scapula lowered to its normal position but rotated laterally (see Plate 2, Step Q). In his experience, the laterally rotated fixed position of the scapula will compensate for the lost scapulocostal motion, and the patient will be able to abduct the shoulder fully by motion at the glenohumeral joint. The correction achieved by the modification of Green's scapuloplasty is better and cosmetically more appealing, and most important, motor control of the scapula is re-established (Fig. 2–21).

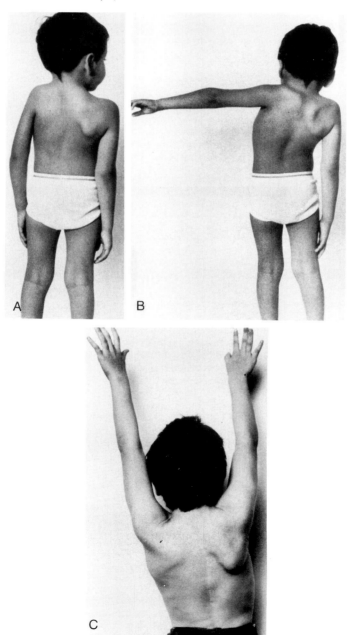

FIGURE 2–21. Clinical results of a modified Green's scapuloplasty in congenital high scapula on the left.

A. Note the asymmetry of the shoulders because of the high scapula on the left. **B.** Limitation of abduction of the left shoulder. **C.** Postoperative result three years later showing full abduction of the left shoulder.

Modified Green's Scapuloplasty for Congenital High Scapula (Sprengel's Deformity)

First, an osteotomy of the clavicle is performed. The patient is placed in the lateral decubitus position, and the upper half of the chest, the entire neck, the entire upper limb, and the posterior aspect of the neck are fully prepared and draped. It is vital that the level of the contralateral normal scapula be visible during surgery. An alternative method is to place the patient in supine position and prepare the neck and the upper half of the chest, perform the osteotomy of the clavicle, and then turn the patient to prone position and reprepare and redrape. This author finds it expedient to use the former method.

OPERATIVE TECHNIQUE

A. A supraclavicular curvilinear incision is made 2 cm. above the clavicle in line with the skin creases of the neck and centered over the midportion of the clavicle. It is best to make the skin incision with the neck in slight flexion (not hyperextension). The subcutaneous tissue is divided in line with the skin incision, and the wound is pulled down directly over the clavicle.

B. The deep fascia is incised; any superficial veins are clamped and coagulated. The periosteum of the clavicle is divided longitudinally on its anterior aspect and, with a periosteal elevator, is gently elevated circumferentially around the clavicle. Two small Chandler elevators are placed deep to the clavicle, protecting the subclavicular vessels and the brachial plexus.

C. With a bone cutter or an oscillating electric saw, the clavicle is sectioned at one or two sites, leaving its posteroinferior cortex intact (if two sites are used they should be 3 cm. apart). Then by gentle force, a greenstick fracture of the clavicle is produced. The periosteum is closed. Skin closure is with subcuticular running sutures. Morcellation of the clavicle is not recommended.

In the older patient the incision may be extended laterally so that the tip of the coracoid process and the origins of the short head of the biceps brachii and the coracobrachialis muscle are exposed. The cartilaginous tip of the coracoid process is sectioned, and then the wound is closed as already described. The purpose of this step in the child over ten years of age is to prevent compression of the neurovascular bundle against the rib.

Plate 2. Modified Green's Scapuloplasty for Congenital High Scapula (Sprengel's Deformity)

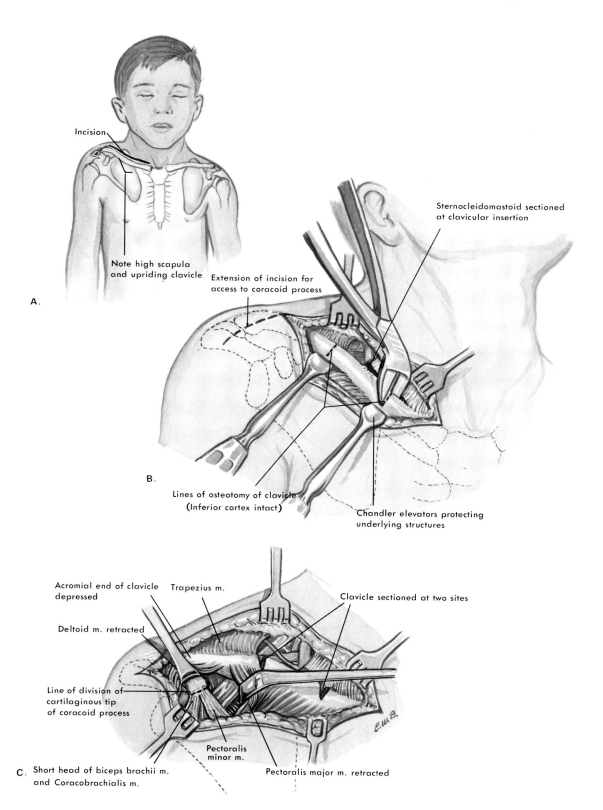

Incision

Note high scapula and upriding clavicle

A.

Sternocleidomastoid sectioned at clavicular insertion

Extension of incision for access to coracoid process

B.

Lines of osteotomy of clavicle (Inferior cortex intact)

Chandler elevators protecting underlying structures

Acromial end of clavicle depressed

Trapezius m.

Clavicle sectioned at two sites

Deltoid m. retracted

Line of division of cartilaginous tip of coracoid process

Pectoralis minor m.

Pectoralis major m. retracted

C. Short head of biceps brachii m. and Coracobrachialis m.

E.W.B.

Modified Green's Scapuloplasty for Congenital High Scapula (Sprengel's Deformity) (Continued)

D. The patient is turned to prone position with the head and neck extending beyond the operating table and supported on a headrest. The chin piece of the headrest should be well padded, and during the procedure, the anesthesiologist should frequently check the chin for pressure areas. Anchoring the patient's buttocks to the operating table with 2- or 3-inch-wide adhesive tape will prevent him from slipping caudally. Care should be taken to guard the sterility of the operating field. First, the vertebral border, the level of the inferior angle and the spine of the elevated scapula, and those of the opposite normal scapula are palpated and marked with indelible ink. A midline skin incision is made that begins at the spinous process of the fourth cervical vertebra and extends distally to terminate at the spinous process of the tenth dorsal vertebra (C-4 to T-10).

E. The skin and the subcutaneous tissue are divided in line with the skin incision, and a plane between the subcutaneous tissue and fascia underlying the trapezius muscle is developed. Dissection is extended laterally to expose the spine of the scapula. Next, the inferior margin of the trapezius muscle, which runs obliquely upward and laterally to the scapular spine, is isolated. Its free lateral border is mobilized and retracted proximally and medially. The insertion of the entire trapezius muscle (superior, middle, and inferior parts) on the scapular spine is sectioned, elevated extraperiosteally, and marked with 2-0 Mersilene sutures. Inferiorly, the lower fibers of the trapezius muscle are separated from the subjacent latissimus dorsi muscle with Metzenbaum scissors.

F. The detached trapezius muscle is reflected medially, exposing underlying muscles and the scapula. The spinal accessory nerve, which is the motor nerve of the trapezius, should not be injured.

Plate 2. Modified Green's Scapuloplasty for Congenital High Scapula (Sprengel's Deformity)

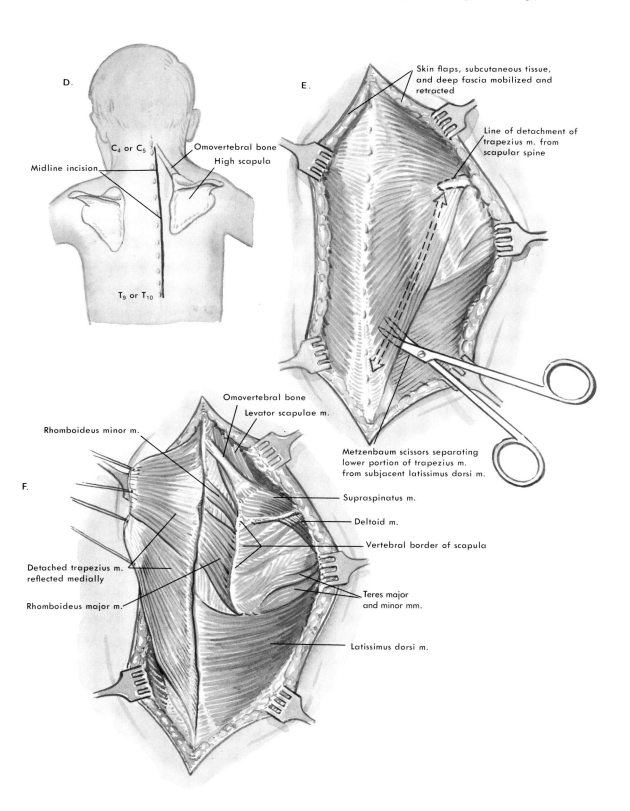

D.

Midline incision

C_4 or C_5

Omovertebral bone

High scapula

T_9 or T_{10}

E.

Skin flaps, subcutaneous tissue, and deep fascia mobilized and retracted

Line of detachment of trapezius m. from scapular spine

Metzenbaum scissors separating lower portion of trapezius m. from subjacent latissimus dorsi m.

F.

Rhomboideus minor m.

Detached trapezius m. reflected medially

Rhomboideus major m.

Omovertebral bone

Levator scapulae m.

Supraspinatus m.

Deltoid m.

Vertebral border of scapula

Teres major and minor mm.

Latissimus dorsi m.

Modified Green's Scapuloplasty for Congenital High Scapula (Sprengel's Deformity) (Continued)

G and **H.** The supraspinatus muscle is then detached from the scapula extraperiosteally to the greater scapular notch. The transverse scapular artery and suprascapular vessels and nerve must be identified and protected in the lateral portion of the wound as they enter the infraspinatus fossa, passing through the greater scapular notch.

I. The omovertebral bar (bony, cartilaginous, or fibrous) is excised by first sectioning it at the scapular end with a bone cutter and then gently detaching its attachment to the cervical vertebra. At the cervical level it may be attached to the spinous process, lamina, or transverse process of one of the lower cervical vertebra (fourth to seventh).

Plate 2. Modified Green's Scapuloplasty for Congenital High Scapula (Sprengel's Deformity)

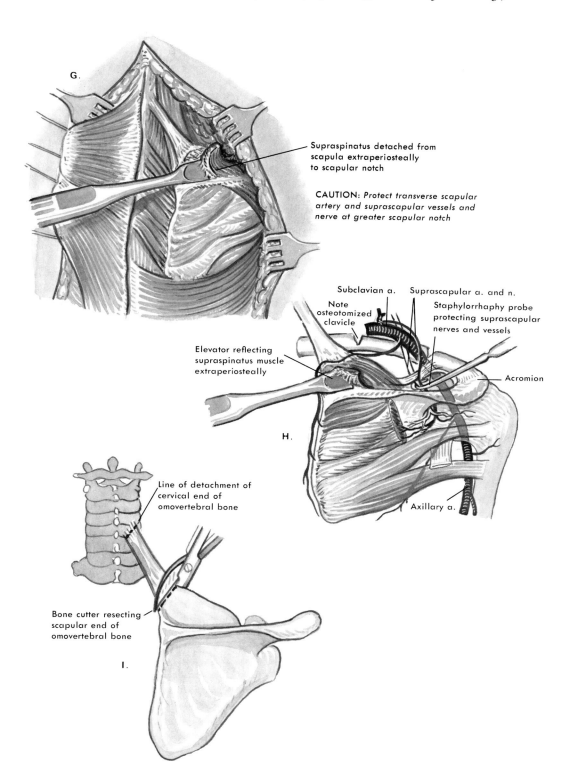

G.

Supraspinatus detached from scapula extraperiosteally to scapular notch

CAUTION: *Protect transverse scapular artery and suprascapular vessels and nerve at greater scapular notch*

Subclavian a.

Note osteotomized clavicle

Suprascapular a. and n.

Staphylorrhaphy probe protecting suprascapular nerves and vessels

Elevator reflecting supraspinatus muscle extraperiosteally

Acromion

H.

Axillary a.

Line of detachment of cervical end of omovertebral bone

Bone cutter resecting scapular end of omovertebral bone

I.

Modified Green's Scapuloplasty for Congenital High Scapula (Sprengel's Deformity) (Continued)

J. The insertions of the levator scapulae muscles on the superior angle of the scapula and of the rhomboideus muscles, major and minor, on the medial border of the scapula are extraperiosteally dissected, divided, and retracted, and their free ends marked with 2-0 Mersilene sutures.

K. The superior margin of the scapula is then retracted posteriorly, and starting medially, the supraspinous portion of the subscapularis muscle is elevated extraperiosteally from the anterior surface of the scapula.

L. Next, a staphylorrhaphy probe is placed in the scapular notch to protect the suprascapular nerves and vessels, and with bone-cutting forceps or an osteotome, the supraspinous part of the scapula along with its periosteum is excised. (Currently this author preserves the normal anatomy of the scapula because often its supraspinous portion is tilted anteriorly toward the rib cage, in which case a greenstick fracture is produced and the tilted portion elevated).

Plate 2. Modified Green's Scapuloplasty for Congenital High Scapula (Sprengel's Deformity)

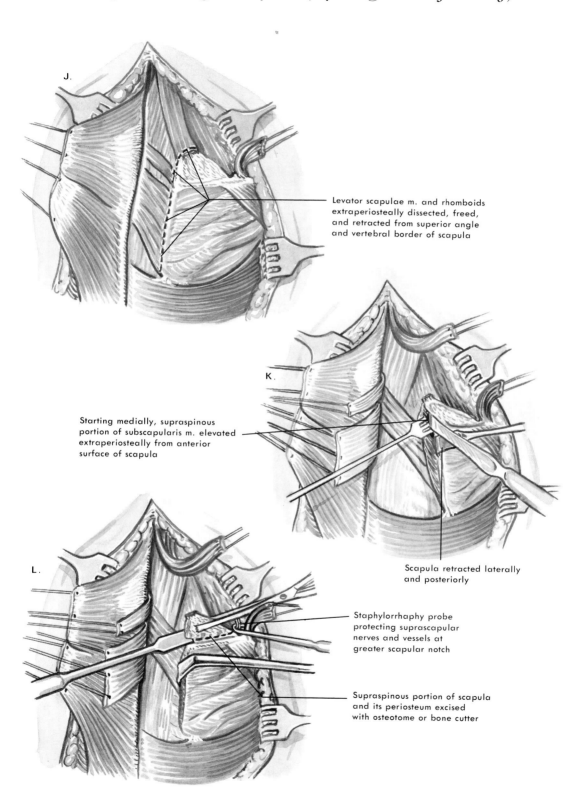

Levator scapulae m. and rhomboids extraperiosteally dissected, freed, and retracted from superior angle and vertebral border of scapula

Starting medially, supraspinous portion of subscapularis m. elevated extraperiosteally from anterior surface of scapula

Scapula retracted laterally and posteriorly

Staphylorrhaphy probe protecting suprascapular nerves and vessels at greater scapular notch

Supraspinous portion of scapula and its periosteum excised with osteotome or bone cutter

155

Modified Green's Scapuloplasty for Congenital High Scapula (Sprengel's Deformity) (Continued)

M. Then attachments of the latissimus dorsi muscle to the scapula are extraperiosteally divided, and by blunt dissection a large pocket is created deep to the superior part of the latissimus dorsi muscle.

N. The medial border of the scapula is everted by retracting it posteriorly and laterally, and the insertions of the serratus anterior muscle to the vertebral margin and to the angle of the scapula are freed extraperiosteally and marked with 2-0 Mersilene sutures.

O. Thick fibrous bands may connect the scapula to the chest wall. They should be divided to mobilize the scapula so that it can be displaced distally enough.

Plate 2. Modified Green's Scapuloplasty for Congenital High Scapula (Sprengel's Deformity)

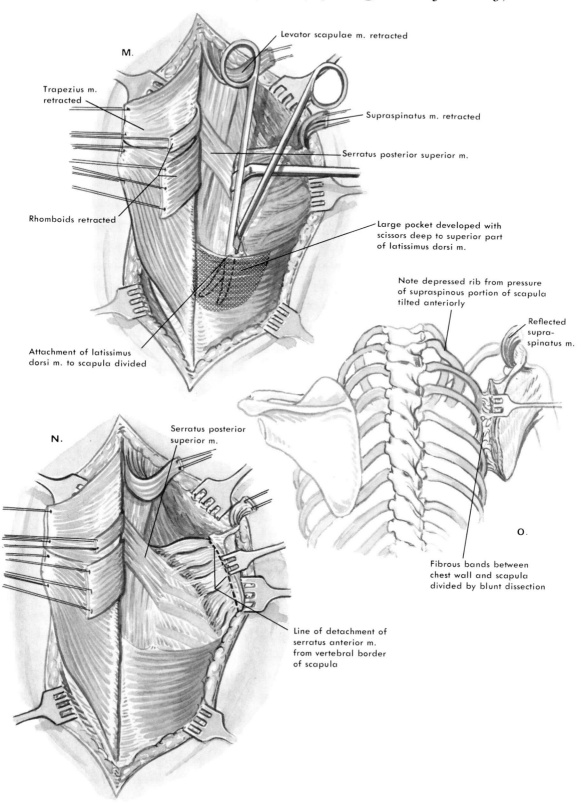

M.

Levator scapulae m. retracted

Trapezius m. retracted

Supraspinatus m. retracted

Serratus posterior superior m.

Rhomboids retracted

Large pocket developed with scissors deep to superior part of latissimus dorsi m.

Attachment of latissimus dorsi m. to scapula divided

Note depressed rib from pressure of supraspinous portion of scapula tilted anteriorly

Reflected supra-spinatus m.

N.

Serratus posterior superior m.

Line of detachment of serratus anterior m. from vertebral border of scapula

O.

Fibrous bands between chest wall and scapula divided by blunt dissection

Modified Green's Scapuloplasty for Congenital High Scapula (Sprengel's Deformity) (Continued)

P. Then, by direct pressure and without traction on the arm, the scapula is gently displaced distally to the desired position. The possibility of stretching of and damage to the brachial plexus must always be kept in mind, and vigorous manipulations should be avoided. The inferior angle and distal quarter of the scapula should be in the large pocket deep to the superior part of the latissimus dorsi muscle.

Q. If there is winging of the scapula, the inferior pole of the scapula is attached to the adjacent rib with two or three absorbable sutures. If the rhomboid muscles and other scapulocostal muscles are hypoplastic or fibrotic and there is marked winging of the scapula, this author recommends fixing the scapula on the rib cage in a lowered and more laterally rotated position. The winging will be corrected, and the laterally rotated fixed position of the scapula will enable the patient to abduct his shoulder fully at the glenohumeral joint.

R. Next, while the assistant holds the scapula in its lowered position, the divided and marked muscles are reattached in the following order. (1) The supraspinatus to the base of the scapular spine. (2) The subscapularis to the vertebral border. (3) The Serratus anterior to the vertebral border at a level more proximal than its original position.

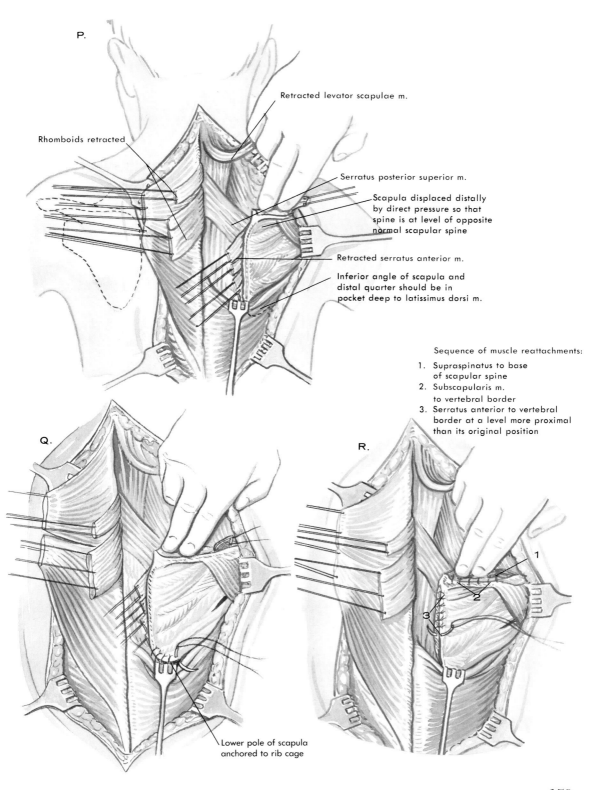

P.

Retracted levator scapulae m.

Rhomboids retracted

Serratus posterior superior m.

Scapula displaced distally by direct pressure so that spine is at level of opposite normal scapular spine

Retracted serratus anterior m.

Inferior angle of scapula and distal quarter should be in pocket deep to latissimus dorsi m.

Sequence of muscle reattachments:
1. Supraspinatus to base of scapular spine
2. Subscapularis m. to vertebral border
3. Serratus anterior to vertebral border at a level more proximal than its original position

Q.

R.

Lower pole of scapula anchored to rib cage

1
2
3

Modified Green's Scapuloplasty for Congenital High Scapula (Sprengel's Deformity) (Continued)

S. (4) The levator scapulae muscle, lengthened if necessary, is attached to the superior border of the scapula. (5) The rhomboids are attached to the medial border of the scapula at a more proximal site than the original position.

T. (6) The superior part of the trapezius is reattached to the scapular spine about 1½ inches medial to its original position. (7) The inferior part of the trapezius is attached to the spine of the scapula more laterally and proximally than before. (8) The superior edge of the latissimus dorsi is attached to the inferolateral edge of the laterally advanced lower part of the trapezius. In the distal part of the incision, the origin of the lower part of the trapezius is followed, the excess tissue is excised, and the free muscle edges are overlapped and sutured. The increased tension in this part of the muscle will serve as an added measure to hold the scapula in its lowered position. The wound is closed in layers. Closure of the skin should be subcuticular. If there is an associated pterygium colli, a Z-plasty repair may be performed.

POSTOPERATIVE CARE

The shoulder is immobilized in a Velpeau cast. Make sure that the elbow is not elevated. The patient is discharged from the hospital in three or four days. About four to six weeks postoperatively, the cast is removed and active shoulder abduction and scapular depression exercises are performed to increase muscle strength. Passive exercises of the glenohumeral and scapulocostal joints are carried out to increase range of joint motion.

Plate 2. Modified Green's Scapuloplasty for Congenital High Scapula (Sprengel's Deformity)

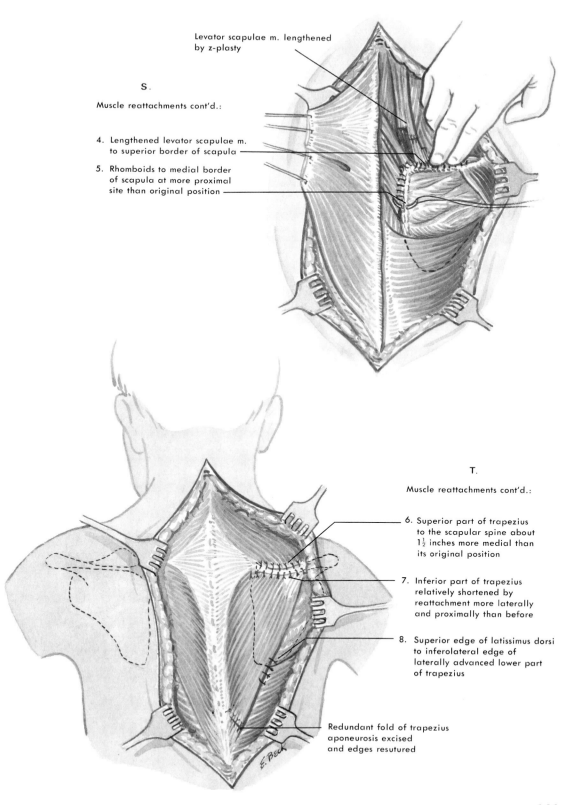

Levator scapulae m. lengthened by z-plasty

S.

Muscle reattachments cont'd.:

4. Lengthened levator scapulae m. to superior border of scapula

5. Rhomboids to medial border of scapula at more proximal site than original position

T.

Muscle reattachments cont'd.:

6. Superior part of trapezius to the scapular spine about $1\frac{1}{2}$ inches more medial than its original position

7. Inferior part of trapezius relatively shortened by reattachment more laterally and proximally than before

8. Superior edge of latissimus dorsi to inferolateral edge of laterally advanced lower part of trapezius

Redundant fold of trapezius aponeurosis excised and edges resutured

E. Beck

161

Woodward Operation for Congenital High Scapula

The operation is performed with the patient in prone position with the head supported on a craniotomy headrest and the neck in slight flexion. The sides and back of the neck, both shoulders, the trunk down to the iliac crests, and the upper limb on the involved side are prepared and draped. One should be able to manipulate the shoulder girdle and arms during the operation without contaminating the surgical field.

OPERATIVE TECHNIQUE

A. A midline longitudinal incision is made, extending from the spinous process of the first cervical vertebra to that of the ninth thoracic vertebra.

B. The subcutaneous tissue is divided in line with the skin incision. The wound margins are undermined laterally to the medial border of the scapula. The muscle arrangement should be clearly visualized.

C. Next, the lateral border of the trapezius muscle is identified at the distal part of the wound. By blunt dissection, the lower portion of the trapezius is separated from the subjacent latissimus dorsi muscle.

D. With a sharp scalpel, the tough and tendinous origin of the trapezius muscle is detached from the spinous process. Numerous sutures are passed at the entire origin of the muscle for marking it and for use at later reattachment.

Plate 3. Woodward Operation for Congenital High Scapula

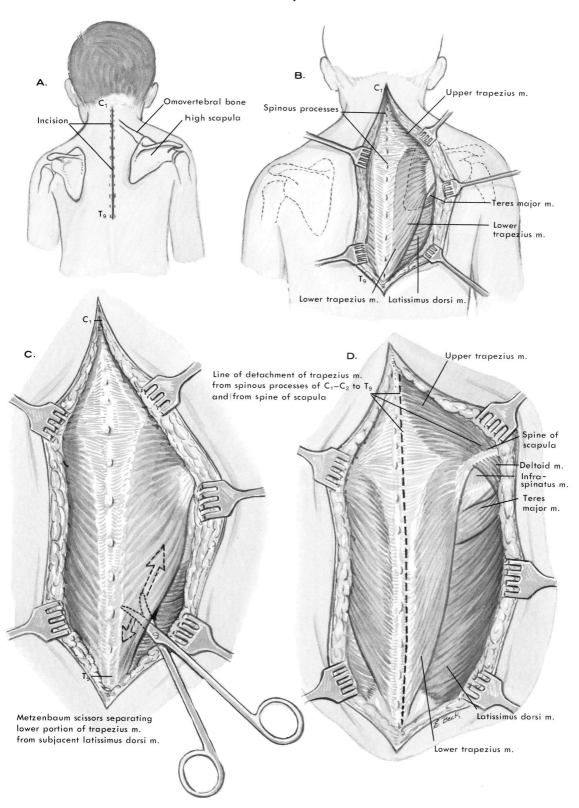

A.
Incision
C_1
Omovertebral bone
high scapula
T_9

B.
Spinous processes
C_1
Upper trapezius m.
Teres major m.
Lower trapezius m.
T_9
Lower trapezius m. Latissimus dorsi m.

C.
C_1
T_9
Metzenbaum scissors separating lower portion of trapezius m. from subjacent latissimus dorsi m.

D.
Line of detachment of trapezius m. from spinous processes of C_1–C_2 to T_9 and from spine of scapula
Upper trapezius m.
Spine of scapula
Deltoid m.
Infra-spinatus m.
Teres major m.
Latissimus dorsi m.
Lower trapezius m.

E. Beck

Woodward Operation for Congenital High Scapula
(Continued)

E. In the upper part of the incision, the origins of the rhomboideus major and minor muscles are sharply divided and tagged with sutures. A well-defined deep layer of fascia separates the rhomboids and the upper part of the trapezius from the serratus posterior superior and erector spinae muscles. It is vital to maintain a proper tissue plane. Preserve the aponeurosis and muscle sheet intact for secure fixation of the scapula at its lowered level.

Next, the entire muscle sheet is retracted laterally, exposing the omovertebral bone or fibrous band, if present. The omovertebral bar is excised *extraperiosteally;* it usually extends from the superior angle of the scapula to the lower cervical vertebrae. It is best to use a bone cutter for resection. Avoid injury to the spinal accessory nerve, the nerves to the rhomboids, and the descending scapular artery. The contracted levator scapulae muscle is sectioned at its attachment to the scapula. Fibrous bands attached to the anterior surface of the scapula usually restrict its downward displacement; if present, they are sectioned. Next, the scapula is everted, and the serratus anterior muscle is detached from its insertion on the vertebral border of the scapula. A periosteal elevator is used to elevate the supraspinatus muscle extraperiosteally from the supraspinous portion of the scapula, and the subscapularis muscle from the deep surface of the scapula midway between the superior and inferior angles. The supraspinous portion of the scapula is resected with its periosteum. Suprascapular vessels and nerves and the transverse scapular artery should be protected from injury. These steps are illustrated in Plate 2, Steps **K** and **L** of the modified Green's scapuloplasty.

F. Next, the scapula is lowered to its normal level and held in the corrected position by an assistant. The subscapularis muscle is reattached to the vertebral border of the scapula, and the supraspinatus muscle is resutured to the scapular spine. The serratus anterior muscle is reattached to the vertebral border of the scapula at a more proximal level. The latissimus dorsi muscle is reattached to the scapula. Proceeding cephalocaudally, the thick aponeurosis of the trapezius and rhomboid muscles is sutured to the spinous processes at a more distal level. It is essential that an assistant maintain the corrected level of the scapula.

G. Since the origin of the trapezius muscle distal to the ninth thoracic vertebra is not disturbed, a redundant fold of aponeurotic tissue is created in the distal end of the trapezius muscle. This fold of soft tissue is excised and resutured.

The wound is closed in the usual fashion. The skin closure is subcuticular.

POSTOPERATIVE CARE

A Velpeau bandage is applied and is worn for three to four weeks. The patient is allowed to be up and around the day after the operation. After removal of the Velpeau bandage, postoperative exercises similar to those described for the modified Green's scapuloplasty are carried out.

Plate 3. Woodward Operation for Congenital High Scapula

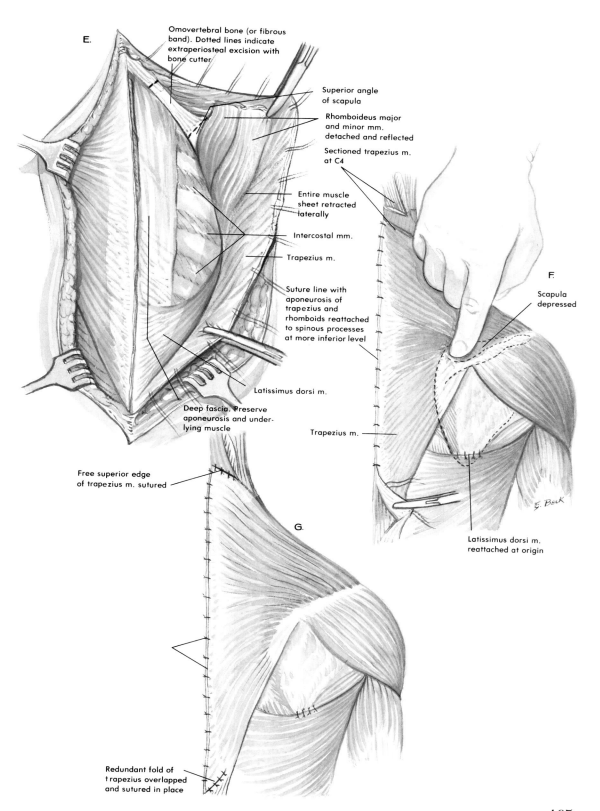

E.

Omovertebral bone (or fibrous band). Dotted lines indicate extraperiosteal excision with bone cutter

Superior angle of scapula

Rhomboideus major and minor mm. detached and reflected

Sectioned trapezius m. at C4

Entire muscle sheet retracted laterally

Intercostal mm.

Trapezius m.

Suture line with aponeurosis of trapezius and rhomboids reattached to spinous processes at more inferior level

Latissimus dorsi m.

Deep fascia. Preserve aponeurosis and under-lying muscle

F.

Scapula depressed

Trapezius m.

Latissimus dorsi m. reattached at origin

E. Beck

Free superior edge of trapezius m. sutured

G.

Redundant fold of trapezius overlapped and sutured in place

References

1. Allan, F. G.: The surgical treatment of Sprengel's shoulder. J. Bone Joint Surg., *46-B*:162, 1964.
2. Arens, W.: Eine seltene angeborene Missbildung des Schultergelenkes. Fortschr. Geb. Röntgenstr., 75:365, 1951.
3. Aubert, L., and Arroyo, H.: Maladie de Sprengel familiale. Marseille Med., *104*:289, 1967.
4. Bagg, H. J.: Hereditary abnormalities of the limbs, their origin and transmission. II. A morphological study with special reference to the etiology of club feet, syndactylism, hypodactylism, and congenital amputation in the descendants of x-rayed mice. Am. J. Anat., *43*:167, 1929.
5. Bagg, H. J., and Halter, C. R.: Further studies on the inheritance of structural defects in the descendants of mice exposed to roentgen-ray irradiation. (Abstract.) Anat. Rec., 37:183, 1927.
6. Bagg, H. J., and Little, C. C.: Hereditary structural defects in the descendants of mice exposed to roentgen ray irradiation. Am. J. Anat., *33*:119, 1924.
7. Bazan, U. B. von: The association between congenital elevation of the scapula and diastematomyelia. J. Bone Joint Surg., *61-B*:59, 1979.
8. Bazan, U. B. von, Redlich, H., Puhl, W., and Best, S.: The omovertebral bone—new possibility of preoperative examination by computed axial tomography. Z. Orthop., *116*:795, 1978.
9. Binnie, J. F.: Congenital elevation of the scapula (Sprengel's deformity). Ann. Surg., 65:488, 1917.
10. Blair, J. D., and Wells, P. O.: Bilateral undescended scapula associated with omovertebral bone. J. Bone Joint Surg., *39-A*:201, 1957.
11. Bonnevie, K.: Embryological analysis of gene manifestation in Little and Bagg's abnormal mouse tribe. J. Exp. Zool., *67*:443, 1934.
12. Brzezinska, H., Dabkowska, M., Janiszewska-Fronczak, M., Krawczynski, M., and Zgliczynska-Bartoszewicz, M.: Klippel-Feil syndrome coexisting with Sprengel's disease in a 3-year-old child. Pneumonol. Pol., *45*:569, 1977.
13. Cabanac, J.: Sur élévation congénitale de l'omoplate. Med. Acad. Chir. (Paris), *80*:474, 1954.
14. Carson, W. G., Lovell, W. W., and Whitesides, T. E., Jr.: Congenital elevation of the scapula. Surgical correction by the Woodward procedure. J. Bone Joint Surg., *63-A*:1199, 1981.
15. Cavendish, M. E.: Congenital elevation of the scapula. J. Bone Joint Surg., *54-B*:395, 1972.
16. Cervenensky, J., and Kalman, E.: Unsere Erfahrungen mit der chirurgischen Therapie der Sprengelschen Deformität. Beitr. Orthop. Traumatol., *15*:545, 1968.
17. Chigot, P. L.: Sur élévation congénitale de l'omoplate. Rev. Chir. Orthop. (Paris), 38:154, 1952.
18. Chigot, P. L., and Ingelrans, R.: Sur élévation congénitale de l'omoplate. Mem. Acad. Chir. (Paris), 89:812, 1963.
19. Chung, S. M. K., and Farahvar, H.: Surgery of the clavicle in Sprengel's deformity. Clin. Orthop., *116*:138, 1976.
20. Chung, S. M. K., and Nissenbaum, M. M.: Congenital and developmental defects of the shoulder. Orthop. Clin. North Am., 6:381, 1975.
21. Collier, M.: Dysostose mandibulo-faciale avec difformité de Sprengel, naevus verruqueux de la face et anomalies du fond de l'oeil. Ophthalmologica, *164*:97, 1972.
22. Creyssel, J., and Cornet, J.: Sur le traitement de la surélévation congénitale de l'omoplate. Lyon Chir., 58:789, 1962.
23. Critchley, M.: Sprengel's deformity with paraplegia. Br. J. Surg., *14*:243, 1926.
24. Currie, A. R., Bird, C. C., Crawford, A. M., and Sims, P.: Embryopathic effects of 7, 12-dimethylbenz(a)anthracene and its hydroxymethyl derivatives in the Sprague-Dawley rat. Nature, 226:911, 1970.
25. DeBastiani, G., Boscaro, C., and Coletti, N.: Green's operation in treatment of elevated scapula. Chir. Organi Mov., *64*:1, 1978.
26. Delchef, J.: L'élévation congénitale de l'omoplate. Bulletin de l'Académie Royale de Médecine de Belgique. 5th Series 2:216, 1922.
27. DuToit, F.: A case of congenital elevation of the scapula (Sprengel's deformity) with defect of the cervical spine associated with syringomyelia. Brain, 54:421, 1931.
28. Ely, L. W.: Sprengel's deformity. Arch. Surg., *11*:598, 1925.
29. Engel, D.: Etiology of multiple deformities. Am. J. Dis. Child., *60*:562, 1940.
30. Engel, D.: The etiology of the undescended scapula and related syndromes. J. Bone Joint Surg., *25*:613, 1943.
31. Eulenberg, M.: Beitrag zur Dislocation der Scapula. Amtliche Berichte über die Versammlungen deutscher Naturforscher und Aerzte fur die Jahre, 37:291, 1863.
32. Eulenberg, M.: Casuistische Mittheilungen aus dem Begiete der Orthopädie. Arch. Klin. Chir., *4*:301, 1863.
33. Fairbank, H. A. T.: Congenital elevation of the scapula: A series of eighteen cases with a detailed description of dissected specimen. Br. J. Surg., *1*:553, 1913–1914.
34. Ferro, R., Perquis, P., Gourul, J. C., Piquard, B., and Auphan, D.: Three cases of congenital elevation of the scapula treated with Woodward's technic. Bull. Soc. Med. Afr. Noire Lang. Fr., *17*:611, 1972.
35. Fetterolf, G., and Arnett, J. H.: A case of Sprengel's deformity. Am. J. Med. Sci., *148*:521, 1914.
36. Fourrier, P., and Cochet: Un cas de surélévation congénitale de l'omoplate. Lyon Chir., 56:603, 1960.
37. Furst, W., and Ostrum, H. W.: Platybasia, Klippel-Feil syndrome and Sprengel's deformity. A. J. R., 47:588, 1942.
38. Gandin, J.: Surgical treatment of congenital elevation of the scapula. 4 cases. Chirurgie, 98:674, 1972.
39. Gill, A. B.: Sprengel's deformity (congenital elevation of the scapula). Trans. Phila. Acad. Surg., Nov., 1919. Abstract in Ann. Surg., 71:229, 1920.
40. Gottesleben, A.: Über der doppelseitigen und einseitigen Schulterblatthochstand. Langenbecks Arch. Klin. Chir., *144*:723, 1927.
41. Green, W. T.: The surgical correction of congenital elevation of the scapula (Sprengel's deformity). Proceedings of the American Orthopedic Association. J. Bone Joint Surg., *39-A*:1439, 1957.
42. Greenberg, L. M.: Sprengel's deformity. Ann. Paediatr., *198*:89, 1962.
43. Greig, D. M.: On congenital high scapula. Edinburgh Med. J. N.S., 6:242, 1911.
44. Greig, D. M.: Congenital high scapula. Edinburgh Med. J. N. S., *31*:22, 1924.
45. Grogan, D. P., Stanley, E. A., and Bobechko, W. P.: The congenital undescended scapula. Surgical correction by the Woodward procedure. J. Bone Joint Surg., *65-B*:598, 1983.
46. Hensinger, R. N.: Orthopedic problems of the shoulder and neck. Pediatr. Clin. North Am., 24:889, 1977.
47. Hensinger, R. N., Lang, J. E., and MacEwen, G. D.:

Klippel-Feil syndrome: A constellation of associated anomalies. J. Bone Joint Surg., 56-A:1246, 1974.

48. Horwitz, A. E.: Congenital elevation of the scapula—Sprengel's deformity. Am. J. Orthop. Surg., 6:260, 1908.
49. Hutchinson, J.: Deformity of shoulder girdle. Br. Med. J., 1:634, 1894.
50. Inclan, A.: Congenital elevation of the scapula or Sprengel's deformity: Two clinical cases treated with Ober's operation. Cir. Ortop. Trauma, Habana, 15:1, 1949.
51. Ionescu, A., Lavrov, S., and Milicescu, S.: Bilateral congenital elevation of the scapula associated with the Klippel-Feil syndrome. Chirurgia (Bucur.), 21:241, 1972.
52. Jeannopoulos, C. L.: Congenital elevation of the scapula. J. Bone Joint Surg., 34-A:883, 1952.
53. Jeannopoulos, C. L.: Observations on congenital elevation of the scapula. Clin. Orthop., 20:132, 1961.
54. Jenkinson, S. G.: Undescended scapula associated with omovertebral bone: Sprengel's deformity. J. La. State Med. Soc., 129:13, 1977.
55. Keats, T. E.: Ocular hypertelorism (Greig's syndrome) associated with Sprengel's deformity. A. J. R., 110:119, 1970.
56. Kieffer, D., Kuntz, J. L., Heitz, A., and Asch, L.: Unusual malformation complex in Sprengel's deformity. (Congenital elevation of the shoulder blade). Rev. Rhum. Mal. Osteoartic., 48:371, 1981.
57. Klisic, P., Filipovic, M., Uzelac, O., and Milinkovic, Z.: Relocation of congenitally elevated scapula. J. Pediatr. Orthop., 1:43, 1981.
58. Koenig, F.: Eine neue Operation des angeborenen Schulterblatthochstandes. Beitr. Klin. Chir., 94: 1914 (cited in Lange, M.: Orthopädisch-Chirurgische Operationslehre. Munchen, Bergmann, 1941, p. 240.)
59. Kölliker, T.: Mittheilungen aus der chirurgischen Casuistik und Kleinere Mittheilungen. Bemerkungen zum Aufsatze von Dr. Sprengel. "Die angeborene Verschiebung des Schulterblattes nach oben." Arch. Klin. Chir., 42:925, 1891.
60. Lance, P., and Maudhuit, J.: L'os omo-cervical dans la surélévation congénitale de l'omoplate. Considerations pathogeniques (à propos de deux observations). Ann. Chir., Infant., 3:243, 1962.
61. Lanier, M., and Lexlercq, L.: Un cas de surélévation de l'omoplate gauche avec malformation vertébrale. Lyon Chir., 55:598, 1959.
62. Lind, T.: Ein Fall von angeborenen linksseitigem Schulterblatthochstand. Fortschr. Röntgenstrahl., 75:754, 1951.
63. McClure, J. G., and Raney, R. B.: Anomalies of the scapula. Clin. Orthop., 110:22, 1975.
64. McFarland, B. I.: Congenital deformities of the spine and limbs. *In* Platt, H. (ed.): Modern Trends in Orthopaedics. London, Butterworth, 1950, Chapter 6, p. 117.
65. Mayfield, J. K.: Use of the Milwaukee brace in the surgical treatment of Sprengel's deformity. J. Pediatr. Orthop., 1:137, 1981.
66. Mensi, E., and Siliquini, P. L.: Aplasia of the greater pectoral muscle associated with congenital elevated scapula. Minerva Ortop., 18:77, 1967.
67. Miura, T., Iwata, H., Kino, Y., and Nakamura, R.: Treatment of congenitally high-positioned scapula. Orthop. Surg. (Tokyo), 22:222, 1971.
68. Neuhof, H.: Angeborenen Schulterhochstand (Sprengel's Deformität). Familiärer Type. Z. Orthop. Chir., 31:519, 1913.
69. Ogden, J. A., Conlogue, G. J., Phillips, M. S., and Bronson, M. L.: Sprengel's deformity. Radiology of

the pathologic deformation. Skeletal Radiol., 4:204, 1979.

70. Ombredanne, I.: Précis Clinique et Opératoire de Chirurgie Infantile. 4th Ed. Paris, Masson, 1944, pp. 701–709.
71. Otter, G. den: Bilateral Sprengel's syndrome with situs inversus totalis. Acta Orthop. Scand., 41:402, 1970.
72. Perls, W.: Beitrag zur familiären Form des angeborenen Schulterhochstandes. Z. Orthop. Chir., 41:428, 1921.
73. Petrie, J. G.: Congenital elevation of the scapula. J. Bone Joint Surg., 55-B:441, 1973.
74. Picault, Ch., and Murat, J.: A propos de troix cas de surélévation congénitale de l'omoplate traités par la technique de Woodward. Ann. Chir., 19:627, 1965.
75. Pinsky, H. A., Pizzutillo, P. D., and MacEwen, G. D.: Congenital elevation of the scapula. Orthop. Trans., 4:288, 1980.
76. Putti, V.: Beitrag zur Ätiologie, Pathogenese und Behandlung des angeborenen Hochstandes des Schulterblattes. Fortschr. Rontgenstrahl., 12:328, 1908.
77. Rigault, P., Pouliquen, J. C., Guyonvarch, G., and Zujovic, J.: Congenital elevation of the scapula in children. Anatomopathological and therapeutic study apropos of 27 cases. Rev. Chir. Orthop., 62:5, 1976.
78. Robinson, A. R., Braun, R. M., Mack, P., and Zadek, R.: The surgical importance of the clavicular component of Sprengel's deformity. J. Bone Joint Surg., 49-A:1481, 1967.
79. Ross, D. M., and Cruess, R. L.: The surgical correction of congenital elevation of the scapula. Clin. Orthop., 125:17, 1977.
80. Roux, H., Acquaviva, P., Allignol, J. -M., and Serratrice, G.: Le syndrome de Sprengel. Rhumatologie, 18:361, 1966.
81. Ruhomally, H.: Letter: Ketamine anaesthesia for a patient with severe bilateral Sprengel's deformity. Br. J. Anaesth., 48:2393, 1976.
82. Salmon, M.: Surélévation congénitale bilatérale de l'omoplate résection sub-totale extra-periostée du scapulum. Marseille Chir., 9:594, 1957.
83. Scaglietti, O.: Indirizzi odierni nel trattamento chirurgico della scapola alta congenita. Chir. Organi Mov., 21:287, 1935.
84. Schrock, R. D.: Congenital elevation of the scapula. J. Bone Joint Surg., 8:207, 1926.
85. Schrock, R. D.: Congenital abnormalities at the cervicothoracic level. A.A.O.S. Instruct. Course Lect., 6, 1949.
86. Schwarzweller, F.: Der angeborene Schulterblatthochstand. Z. Mensch. Vererb. Konstit. Lehre, 20:350, 1937.
87. Serafin, J., and Sotirow, B.: Elévation congénitale de l'omoplate. Rev. Chir., 52:477, 1966.
88. Sherk, H. H., Shut, L., and Chung, S.: Iniencephalic deformity of the cervical spine with Klippel-Feil anomalies and congenital elevation of the scapula; report of three cases. J. Bone Joint Surg., 56-A:1254, 1974.
89. Smith, A. de F.: Congenital elevation of the scapula. Arch. Surg., 42:529, 1941.
90. Sprengel, O.: Die angeborene Verschiebung des Schulterblattes nach oben. Arch. Klin. Chir., 42:545, 1891.
91. Steindler, A.: Congenital elevation of the scapula. Pediatrics, 5:367, 1924.
92. Walker, N.: Familiares Vorkommen des Schulterblatthochstandes. Z. Orthop., 110:203, 1972.
93. Weed, L. H.: The Development of the Cerebrospinal Spaces. (Contribution to Embryology No. 14.) Publication 225, Carnegie Institute of Washington, 1916.

94. Weyers, H.: Anatomy and therapy of congenital high scapula. Dtsch. Krankenpflegez, 27:673, 1974.
95. Wilkinson, J. A., and Campbell, D.: Scapular osteotomy for Sprengel's shoulder. J. Bone Joint Surg., 62-B:486, 1980.
96. Willet, A., and Walsham, W. J.: An account of the dissection of the parts removed after death from the body of a woman the subject of congenital malformation of the spinal column, bony thorax, and left scapular arch; with remarks on the probable nature of the defects in development producing the deformities. Med. Chir. Trans., London, 63:256, 1880.
97. Willet, A., and Walsham, W. J.: A second case of malformation of the left shoulder girdle, with remarks on the probable nature of the deformity. Br. Med. J., 1:513, 1883.
98. Wilson, M. G., Mikity, V. G., and Shinno, N. W.: Dominant inheritance of Sprengel's deformity. J. Pediatr., 79:818, 1971.
99. Woodward, J. W.: Congenital elevation of the scapula. Correction by release and transplantation of muscle origins. J. Bone Joint Surg., 43-A:219, 1961.
100. Zeskov, P., Gvozdanovic, V., and Skarica, R.: Sprengel's syndrome. Neuropsihijatrija, 20:341, 1972.

PSEUDARTHROSIS OF THE CLAVICLE

This rare anomaly was first described by Fitzwilliams as an entity distinct from birth fracture, neurofibromatosis, and cleidocranial dysostosis, and Saint-Pierre reported an additional case in 1930.[15, 34] Since then a number of reports have appeared in the English and European literature.[1-43]

Etiology

The cause of this curious defect remains obscure. The pseudarthrosis is fully present at birth. The clavicle is the first bony mass to form in the embryo, appearing at the fourth week (11 mm. stage) as a mesenchymal bar below the precoracoid area in the neck. It develops in enchondral centers of ossification. There is some controversy as to whether it ossifies from one primary center or two.[2, 14, 18, 23] Recent evidence supports ossification from two centers.[17, 30] At the seventh week the precartilaginous masses with their bony nuclei fuse.[30] Failure of normal ossification of the precartilaginous bridge connecting the acromial and sternal ossific centers of the clavicle or failure of amalgamation of the two clavicular parts may be the cause of congenital pseudarthrosis. Familial incidence is reported in some patients, particularly in bilateral cases.[18, 21, 31] There is no genetic pattern.

The right clavicle has been affected in almost all the reported cases. Lloyd-Roberts, Apley, and Owen have proposed that the pseudarthrosis may be due to exaggerated arterial pulsation and pressure on the clavicle by the subclavian artery, which is normally at a higher level on the right side. Other contributing causative factors are cervical ribs or abnormally elevated first ribs, both of which have been observed in congenital pseudarthrosis of the clavicle. In the occasional left-sided congenital pseudarthrosis of the clavicle, the heart is on the right side (dextrocardia, in which the relative high position of the subclavian artery is reversed). The bilateral cases are attributed to the abnormally high subclavian artery on both sides caused by cervical ribs or high vertically oriented upper ribs.[26]

The defect is *not* due to nonunion of a birth fracture of normal bone. All neonatal clavicular fractures unite rapidly with massive callus. Remodeling takes place within a few months, leaving no trace of deformity. Clinically, in a fracture of the clavicle there is a history of trauma, pseudoparalysis of the arm with lack of voluntary limb motion, and pain on passive movement.

Clinical Findings

A nontender swelling just lateral to the middle of the clavicle is discovered at birth or soon afterward. There is no history of birth injury or other trauma. At the site of pseudarthrosis, the adjacent ends of the clavicular fragments are enlarged, and there is a variable degree of painless mobility between them. The larger sternal fragment is tilted upward and lies in front of and sightly above the medial end of the smaller acromial portion.

In the newborn or young infant, congenital pseudarthrosis of the clavicle should not be misdiagnosed as a fracture of the clavicle. The history of trauma, pseudoparalysis of the arm with lack of voluntary limb motion, pain on passive movement, and massive callus with the characteristic radiographic appearance of fracture union of the latter entity are lacking in congenital pseudarthrosis of the clavicle.

Because of the weight of the upper limb, the lateral segment of the clavicle is tilted inferiorly, and the shoulder droops, is rotated forward, and is nearer to the midline than the opposite normal side (Fig. 2–22). There are no café-au-lait or other stigmata of the skin to suggest neurofibromatosis.

The deformity usually increases and becomes unsightly with further growth, more so when

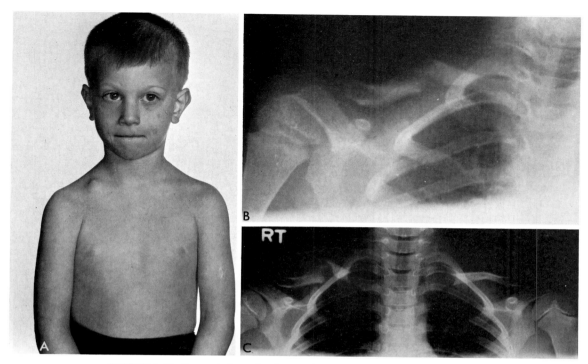

FIGURE 2–22. Congenital pseudarthrosis of right clavicle in a six-year-old boy.

A. Clinical appearance, showing the local swelling. **B.** Anteroposterior radiogram of the right clavicle showing pseudarthrosis. **C.** X-rays two years later, showing persistence of the pseudarthrosis. There was no pain or functional disability.

there is marked mobility at the site of the pseudarthrosis. The overlying skin becomes thin and atrophic. Cosmetically the deformity may be a source of embarrassment to the child (Fig. 2–23). There is some drooping of the affected shoulder with asymmetry and prominence of the vertical border of the scapula. Mild pain around the shoulder girdle and upper arm may be present. There is little or no functional disability. A few children complain of weakness of the arm and limitation of shoulder abduction.

Radiographic Findings

In the radiograph the pseudarthrosis of the clavicle immediately lateral to its middle is evident. In congenital pseudarthrosis the bone ends are enlarged at the pseudarthrosis site—a feature that distinguishes it from both the attenuated bone ends seen in nonunited fractures and the massive callus uniting birth fractures.

In congenital pseudarthrosis of the clavicle there are no other skeletal abnormalities pres-

ent, a feature that distinguishes it from cleidocranial dysostosis. In the latter, a part or whole of the clavicle is simply absent and there is no lump of the pseudarthrosis; in addition there are skull deformities (i.e., bossing), smallness of the facial bones, scoliosis, abnormal epiphyses in the hands and feet, and deficiencies of the pelvis.

Treatment

Treatment consists of excision of the pseudarthrosis mass, curettage of the bone ends, internal fixation with a threaded Steinmann pin, and grafting with cancellous onlay autogenous bone graft from the ilium. The operative technique is illustrated in Plate 4.

In the literature, Owen and Gibson and Carroll consider between three and four years of age the ideal time for operation.[18, 31] This author sees no advantage in postponing surgery and recommends repair of pseudarthrosis at one year of age.

Text continued on page 174

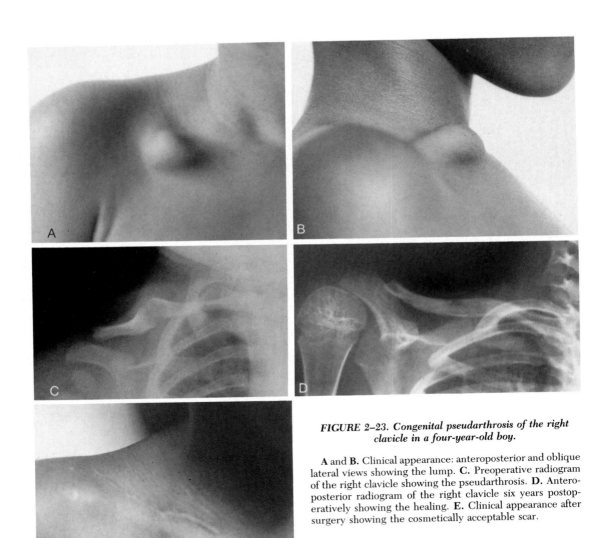

FIGURE 2–23. Congenital pseudarthrosis of the right clavicle in a four-year-old boy.

A and **B.** Clinical appearance: anteroposterior and oblique lateral views showing the lump. **C.** Preoperative radiogram of the right clavicle showing the pseudarthrosis. **D.** Anteroposterior radiogram of the right clavicle six years postoperatively showing the healing. **E.** Clinical appearance after surgery showing the cosmetically acceptable scar.

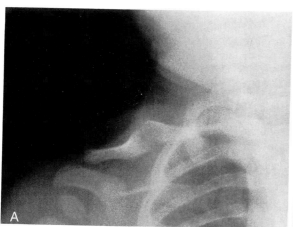
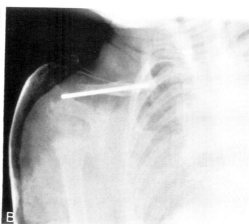
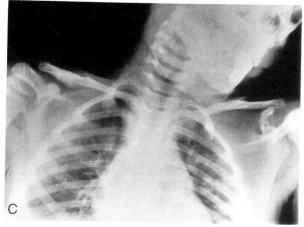

FIGURE 2–24. Congenital pseudarthrosis of the right clavicle.

A. Anteroposterior radiogram at six months of age. Note the enlarged ends of the sternal and acromial fragments. There is no callus formation. **B.** Immediate postoperative radiogram. The pseudarthrosis has been resected, and the bone grafted and internally fixed with a threaded Steinmann pin. **C.** Result showing union two years postoperatively.

Repair of Congenital Pseudarthrosis of the Clavicle

OPERATIVE TECHNIQUE

A. A horizontal incision 4 to 6 cm. long is made in line with the skin creases of the neck about 2 cm. above the clavicle. (It is best to mark the site of the skin incision when the patient is upright and not in supine position because the skin creases will move upward when the neck is hyperextended.) A direct incision over the clavicle is absolutely not recommended. The resultant scar and keloid will be very disfiguring. An arcuate skin incision low down over the second rib (recommended by Owen) avoids supraclavicular nerves, and any keloid can be hidden by clothing, but it makes exposure of the pseudarthrosis difficult.[31] The subcutaneous tissue is divided in line with the skin incision, and the wound is pulled down directly over the clavicle.

B. The fascia is divided. Any superficial veins are clamped and coagulated. The periosteum is divided over the anterior aspect of the sternal and clavicular segments of the clavicle. With a curved elevator, normal bone is exposed subperiosteally before getting to the pseudarthrosis site.

The periosteum is gently elevated circumferentially around the clavicle; small Chandler periosteal elevators are placed behind the clavicle to protect the subclavicular vessels and brachial plexus. The pseudarthrosis site is excised with an oscillating electric saw or bone cutter. Sclerotic bone is removed until healthy osseous tissue is exposed.

C. With a small curet the sternal and acromial ends of the clavicle are cleaned of all sclerotic osseous tissue. Avoid bone splintering. A threaded Steinmann pin of appropriate size is gently drilled, preferably by electric drill, into the acromial segment of the clavicle until it protrudes from the skin lateral to the shoulder; then the two segments are approximated snugly, and the pin is drilled retrograde into the sternal segment of the clavicle.

D. Cancellous autogenous bone for grafting is obtained from the ilium and packed around the pseudarthrosis site, and the periosteum is closed. The wound is closed in the usual fashion—skin closure should be subcuticular. The shoulder is immobilized in a Velpeau bandage reinforced with a second layer of cast.

POSTOPERATIVE CARE

The Velpeau cast is changed as necessary every three weeks. The union is usually solid in eight to ten weeks. At this time the pin across the clavicle is removed under appropriate sedation or, preferably, general anesthesia, and the child is gradually allowed to use the shoulder normally.

Plate 4. Repair of Congenital Pseudarthrosis of the Clavicle

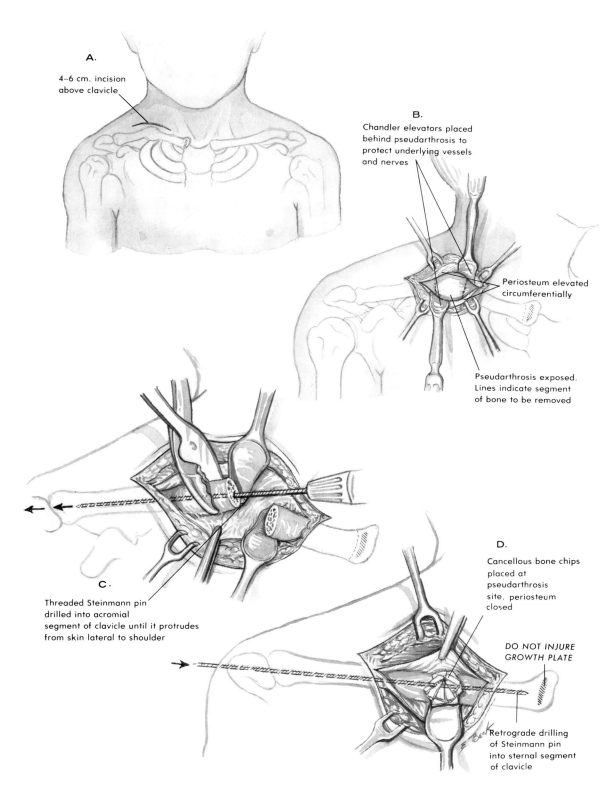

A.

4–6 cm. incision above clavicle

B.

Chandler elevators placed behind pseudarthrosis to protect underlying vessels and nerves

Periosteum elevated circumferentially

Pseudarthrosis exposed. Lines indicate segment of bone to be removed

C.

Threaded Steinmann pin drilled into acromial segment of clavicle until it protrudes from skin lateral to shoulder

D.

Cancellous bone chips placed at pseudarthrosis site, periosteum closed

DO NOT INJURE GROWTH PLATE

Retrograde drilling of Steinmann pin into sternal segment of clavicle

173

Results of surgical repair of pseudarthrosis of the clavicle are very satisfactory (Fig. 2–24). In 12 cases personally operated on by this author, union occurred in every case, and four of them did not require bone grafting. He does not recommend compression plating and bone grafting to maintain the length of the clavicle. Neurovascular injury can occur as a complication.[39] In order to prevent pin migration the intramedullary pin should be threaded and not smooth.

Long-term results show the involved clavicle to be short, causing a drooping-forward of the shoulder; this stunted growth of the clavicle is similar to that of the short leg in congenital pseudarthrosis of the tibia. In the experience of this author, the shortening of the clavicle has been less in the patients operated on in infancy as compared with those operated on later in childhood.

References

1. Ahmadi, B., and Steel, H. H.: Congenital pseudarthrosis of the clavicle. Clin. Orthop., *126*:129, 1977.
2. Alldred, A. J.: Congenital pseudarthrosis of the clavicle. J. Bone Joint Surg., *45-B*:312, 1963.
3. Bauer, U.: Clavicular pseudarthroses in childhood. Munch. Med. Wochenschr., *117*:981, 1975.
4. Behringer, B. R., and Wilson, F. C.: Congenital pseudarthrosis of the clavicle. Am. J. Dis. Child., *123*:511, 1972.
5. Bell, J. F., Kuhlmann, R. F., and Molloy, M. K.: Congenital defects of shoulder girdle, sternum, spine and pelvis. Pediatr. Clin. North Am., *14*:397, 1967.
6. Brunner, C., and Morger, R.: Congenital non-union of the clavicle. Paediatr. Radiol., *16*:137, 1981.
7. Carpenter, E. B., and Garrett, R. G.: Congenital pseudarthrosis of the clavicle. Report of a case with resection and bone-grafting. J. Bone Joint Surg., *42-A*:337, 1960.
8. Cesarani, F.: Pseudo-artrosi della clavicola da pregressa lesione traumatica. Ann. Radiol. Diagn., *19*:160, 1947.
9. Chung, S. M. K., and Nissenbaum, M. M.: Congenital and developmental defects of the shoulder. Orthop. Clin. North Am., *6*:381, 1975.
10. Colavita, N., La Vecchia, G., Book, E., and Vincenzoni, M.: Congenital pseudarthrosis of the clavicle: Roentgenographic appearance and discussion of the aetiological and pathogenetical theories. Radiol. Med. (Torino), *66*:923, 1980.
11. Cotta, H.: Die kindliche Clavicula-Pseudarthrose. Monatsschr. Unfallheilkd., *62*:291, 1959.
12. Deramond, J.: Pseudarthrose de la clavicule. Ann. Chir. Infant., *6*:71, 1965.
13. Engert, J., Klumpp, H., and Simon, G.: Clavicular pseudarthroses in childhood. Chirurgie, *60*:631, 1979.
14. Fawcett, J.: The development and ossification of the human clavicle. J. Anat. Physiol., *47*:225, 1913.
15. Fitzwilliams, D. C. L.: Hereditary cranio-cleido-dysostosis. Lancet, *2*:1466, 1910.
16. Foco, G.: Pseudo-artrosi clavicolare. Ann. Radiol. Diagn., *18*:93, 1946.
17. Gardner, E.: The embryology of the clavicle. Clin. Orthop., *58*:9, 1968.
18. Gibson, D. A., and Carroll, N.: Congenital pseudarthrosis of the clavicle. J. Bone Joint Surg., *52-B*:629, 1970.
19. Gulino, G., and Ragazzi, P. G.: Congenital pseudarthrosis of the clavicle. Considerations of surgical treatment. Chir. Organi. Mov., *65*:701, 1979.
20. Harnapp, O.: Angeborene Klavicula-Pseudarthrose. Beitr. Orthop. Traumatol., *12*:672, 1965.
21. Herman, S.: Congenital bilateral pseudarthrosis of the clavicles. Clin. Orthop., *91*:162, 1973.
22. Kite, J. H.: Congenital pseudarthrosis of the clavicle. South. Med. J., *61*:703, 1968.
23. Koch, A. R.: Die Frühentwicklung der Clavicula beim Menschen. Acta Anat. (Basel), *42*:177, 1960.
24. Koch, F., Papadimitriou, G., and Groher, W.: Clavicular pseudarthrosis, its development and treatment. Monatsschr. Unfallheilkd., *74*:330, 1971.
25. Lilienberg, H.: Ein Beitrag zum Problem der Claviculapseudarthrosen. Beitr. Orthop. Traumatol., *14*:425, 1967.
26. Lloyd-Roberts, G. C., Apley, A. G., and Owen, R.: Reflections upon the aetiology of congenital pseudarthrosis of the clavicle. J. Bone Joint Surg., *57-B*:24, 1975.
27. Manshil, G., and Laufer, S.: Congenital pseudarthrosis of the clavicle: Report of three cases. A. J. R., *132*:678, 1979.
28. Marmor, L.: Repair of congenital pseudarthrosis of the clavicle. Clin. Orthop., *46*:111, 1966.
29. Nawara, J., Januszko, J., and Hryniewicki, T.: Congenital unilateral partial absence of the clavicle. Chir. Narzadow Ruchu Orthop. Pol., *39*:667, 1974.
30. O'Rahilly, R.: *In* Frantz, C. H. (ed.): Normal and Abnormal Embryological Development. National Research Pub. 1497, Washington, D.C., U.S. Govt. Printing Office, 1967, p. 10.
31. Owen, R.: Congenital pseudarthrosis of the clavicle. J. Bone Joint Surg., *52-B*:644, 1970.
32. Pessagno, A.: Sulla pseudoartrosi della clavicola. Radiol. Med., *40*:885, 1954.
33. Quinlan, W. R., Brady, P. G., and Regan, B. F.: Congenital pseudarthrosis of the clavicle. Acta Orthop. Scand., *51*:489, 1980.
34. Saint-Pierre, L.: Pseudarthrose congénitale de la clavicule droite. Ann. Anat. Pathol., *7*:625, 1930.
35. Sakellarides, H.: Pseudarthrosis of the clavicle. J. Bone Joint Surg., *43-A*:130, 1961.
36. Specchiulli, F.: Case of congenital pseudarthrosis of the clavicle with brachial plexus pain. Chir. Organi Mov., *64*:343, 1978.
37. Støren, H.: Old clavicular pseudarthrosis with late appearing neuralgias and vasomotoric disturbances cured by operation. Acta Chir. Scand., *94*:187, 1946.
38. Taylor, S.: Clavicular dysostosis. A case report. J. Bone Joint Surg., *27*:710, 1945.
39. Toledo, C., and MacEwen, G. D.: Severe complication of surgical treatment of congenital pseudarthrosis of the clavicle. Clin. Orthop., *139*:64, 1979.
40. Tuggle, A., and Mitton, K. L.: Clavicular dysostosis. A. J. R., *45*:728, 1941.
41. Veselovski, I.: Pseudarthroses of the clavicle in children and adolescents and their treatment. Ortop. Travmatol. Protez., *10*:44, 1980.
42. Wall, J. J.: Congenital pseudarthrosis of the clavicle. J. Bone Joint Surg., *52-A*:1003, 1970.
43. Zawisch, C.: Die frühe Histogenese der menschlichen Clavicula. Z. Mikrosk. Anat. Forsch., *59*:187, 1952.

CONGENITAL DISLOCATION OF THE SHOULDER

This is a rare abnormality, with few cases recorded.[3, 4] If discovered at birth, it may be

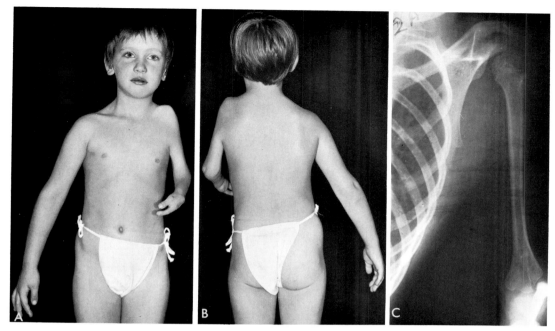

FIGURE 2–25. *Congenital dislocation of the shoulder.*

Congenital dislocation of left shoulder associated with hypoplasia of the glenoid of the scapula and proximal radioulnar synostosis as well as absence of the three ulnar digits. **A** and **B**. Clinical appearance of the patient. **C**. Anteroposterior radiogram of the shoulder.

congenital, i.e., developed in utero. Often the dislocation is paralytic and not congenital, in which case there is associated paralysis of the musculature of the shoulder such as that seen in obstetrical brachial plexus paralysis. Traumatic dislocation of the shoulder in the newborn probably never occurs; experimental work in stillborn infants has disclosed that it could not be produced.[1, 4]

Functional disability varies according to the severity of the condition and the extent of associated abnormalities. Absence or hypoplasia of the glenoid cavity of the scapula or of the humeral head aggravates the deformity and the instability of the shoulder (Fig. 2–25).

Treatment

When functional impairment is minimal no treatment is indicated because there is a possibility of further decreasing functional use of the limb. Manipulative reduction has been advocated by Whitman.[6]

Operative procedures employed depend on the individual case and may consist of reefing of the capsule, tendon transpositions to reinforce the joint, fusion of the shoulder in functional position, and excision of bony blocks (such as a deformed acromion) that may inhibit mo-

tion. In severe aplastic malformations, surgical measures are often futile because function cannot be improved.

References

1. Adreasen, A. T.: Congenital absence of the humeral head. Report of two cases. J. Bone Joint Surg., 30-B:333, 1948.
2. Chari, P. R., Rao, Y. V., and Rao, B. K.: Congenital abduction contracture with dislocation of the shoulder in children: Report of two cases. Aust. N.Z. J. Surg., 49:105, 1979.
3. Cozen, L.: Congenital dislocation of the shoulder and other anomalies. Arch. Surg., 35:956, 1937.
4. Grieg, D. M.: True congenital dislocation of the shoulder. Edinburgh Med. J., 30:157, 1923.
5. Kirmisson and Broca. Quoted by Cozen, L.: Congenital dislocation of the shoulder and other anomalies. Arch. Surg., 35:956, 1937.
6. Whitman, R.: The treatment of congenital and acquired luxations at the shoulder in childhood. Ann. Surg., 42:110, 1905.

RARE CONGENITAL AND DEVELOPMENTAL ANOMALIES OF SHOULDER GIRDLE

Congenital Glenoid Hypoplasia

This rare malformation is due usually to failure of formation of the lower and less often of

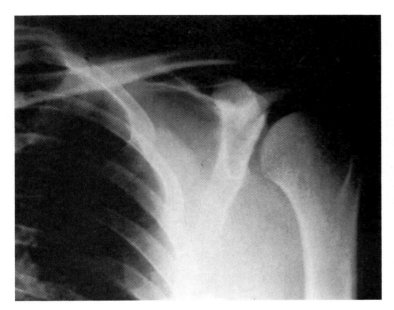

FIGURE 2–26. *Congenital glenoid hypoplasia (dysplasia).*

Note the glenoid cavity is flattened, shallow, and dentate. (From Samilson, R. L.: Congenital and developmental anomalies of the shoulder girdle. Orthop. Clin. North Am., *11*:219, 1980. Reprinted by permission.)

the upper glenoid epiphysis. It is characterized in the radiogram by flattening, shallowness, and a dentate appearance of the glenoid cavity. The lower aspect of the clavicle may be hypertrophied into a bony prominence, and there may be spina bifida in the cervical region (Fig. 2–26). Often, the abnormality is bilateral and is encountered as an isolated malformation. It may be hereditary. Samilson reported congenital glenoid hypoplasia in three successive generations of the same family.[3] Occasionally, it is seen in association with other congenital malformations such as Apert's syndrome, Hurler's syndrome, aglossia-adactylia, oculodento-osseous dysplasia, Holt-Oram syndrome, and Cornelia De Lange's syndrome.

Clinically, in the young child the anomaly is usually asymptomatic and may be found incidentally in the radiogram. In the older patient, however, the glenohumeral joint may be unstable and may become dislocated posteriorly. The range of abduction of the shoulder will be restricted, and occasionally it may cause neurovascular embarrassment.

In the differential diagnosis, one should consider glenoid hypoplasia secondary to obstetrical brachial plexus palsy or multiple epiphyseal dysplasia.

Management should be individualized. Often no treatment is indicated. In symptomatic posterior dislocation of the shoulder, glenoidplasty with a bone graft will improve the glenoid contour and provide stability to the glenohumeral joint.

Aplasia of Scapula

Congenital absence of the scapula is extremely rare and is usually associated with ipsilateral amelia. Treatment consists of fitting with an upper limb prosthesis.

Retrotorsion or Antetorsion of Glenoid Cavity

This deformity will cause posterior or anterior dislocation of the shoulder and can be demonstrated on an axillary radiogram or a computed tomographic torsion study of the glenoid cavity. Treatment consists of osteotomy of the neck of the scapula and insertion of a wedge bone graft to correct the abnormal glenoid torsion.

Nonunion of Ossific Centers of Scapula

Failure of union of the tip of the coracoid process, the lower epiphysis of the glenoid cavity, or the apophysis of the acromion is one of the most common anomalies involving the scapula (Fig. 2–27).

Congenital Varus Deformity of Proximal Humerus

This malformation may be developmental or secondary to neurofibromatosis or rachitic syndromes.

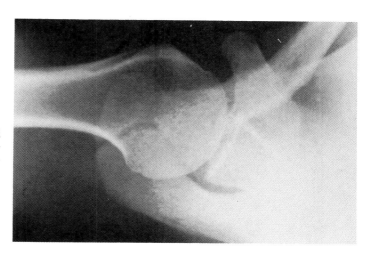

FIGURE 2–27. Nonunion of ossific centers of the scapula. Failure of union of the apophysis of the acromion.

(From Samilson, R. L.: Congenital and developmental anomalies of the shoulder girdle. Orthop. Clin. North Am., *11*:219, 1980. Reprinted by permission.)

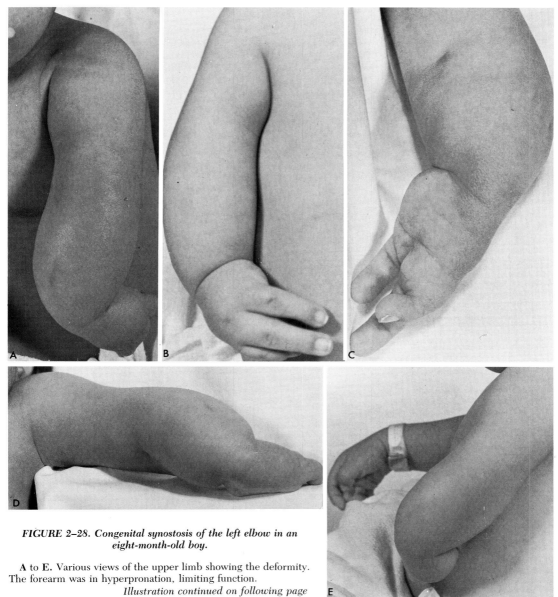

FIGURE 2–28. Congenital synostosis of the left elbow in an eight-month-old boy.

A to **E.** Various views of the upper limb showing the deformity. The forearm was in hyperpronation, limiting function.

Illustration continued on following page

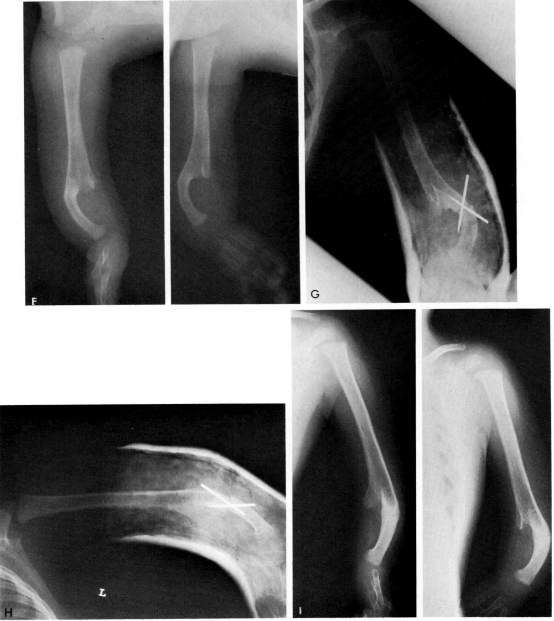

FIGURE 2–28 Continued. Congenital synostosis of the left elbow in an eight-month-old boy.

F. Preoperative radiograms. Note the bony ankylosis of the humeroradial joint, the absence of the ulna and two ulnar rays. G and H. Postoperative radiograms. The patient had a derotation osteotomy of the proximal radius that placed it in neutral position. I. Postoperative radiograms showing the healed osteotomy.

Excessive Retroversion or Anteversion of Humeral Neck

Excessive retroversion will cause posterior dislocation of the glenohumeral joint, and excessive anteversion will cause anterior dislocation. Computed axial tomography will show the degree of humeral torsion. When torsion deformity is severe and is causing shoulder joint instability, it is treated by derotation osteotomy.

References

1. Chung, S. M. K., and Nissenbaum, M. M.: Congenital and developmental defects of the shoulder. Orthop. Clin. North Am., 6:381, 1975.
2. Owen, R.: Bilateral glenoid hypoplasia—report of five cases. J. Bone Joint Surg., 35-B:262, 1953.
3. Samilson, R. L.: Congenital and developmental anomalies of the shoulder girdle. Orthop. Clin. North Am., 11:219, 1980.
4. Sutro, C. J.: Dentated articular surface of the glenoid—an anomaly. Bull. Hosp. Joint Dis., 28:104, 1967.

CONGENITAL SYNOSTOSIS OF ELBOW

This very rare abnormality may occur either as an isolated deformity or in association with other anomalies such as absence of the ulna or fusion or absence of the carpals, metacarpals, or phalanges. In the isolated form, involvement is usually bilateral, whereas in the associated form, it may be unilateral or bilateral. There is no sex predilection.

The ankylosis may occur at the humeroradial, humeroradioulnar, or humeroulnar joints. In humeroulnar or humeroradial synostosis, the radius or ulna is usually absent (Figs. 2–28 and 2–29). In infancy and early childhood the synostosis may be cartilaginous and not visible in the radiogram. With growth and ossification, synostosis of all three joints becomes evident.

Functional disability depends on the position in which the elbow is fixed. In unilateral ankylosis, it is best to perform an osteotomy to achieve a functional position. In cases of bilateral involvement, one may attempt arthroplasty, provided growth centers are not disturbed and there is sufficient motor strength to move the joint. In cases in which there are no epiphyses at the elbow, surgical correction in late childhood can prevent disuse atrophy of the musculature.

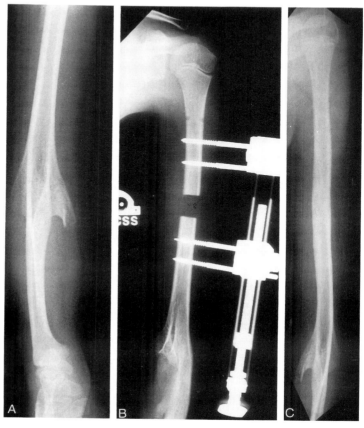

FIGURE 2–29. Radiograms of congenital synostosis of left elbow.

A. Preoperative radiogram. **B.** Following Wagner diaphyseal lengthening of the humerus. **C.** Postoperative radiogram.

References

1. Bagnasco, F. M.: Congenital symmetrical humeroradial synostosis. N.Y. State J. Med., 74:549, 1974.
2. Camera, R.: Congenital ankylosis of elbow. Chir. Organi. Mov., 41:385, 1955.
3. Card, R. Y., and Strachman, J.: Congenital ankylosis of the elbow. J. Pediatr., 46:81, 1955.
4. Frantz, C. H., and O'Rahilly, R.: Ulnar hemimelia. Artif. Limbs, 15:25, 1971.
5. Gherlinzoni, G.: Congenital ankylosis of elbow. Chir. Organi. Mov., 26:162, 1960.
6. Hunter, A. G., Cox, D. W., and Rudd, N. L.: The genetics of and associated clinical findings in humeroradial synostosis. Clin. Genet., 9:470, 1976.
7. Lambert, L. A.: Congenital humeroradial synostosis with other synostotic anomalies. J. Pediatr., 31:573, 1947.
8. Leisti, J., Lachman, R. S., and Rimoin, D. L.: Humeroradial ankylosis associated with other congenital defects. (The "boomerang arm" sign.) Birth Defects, 11:306, 1975.
9. Mnaymneh, W. A.: Congenital radio-humeral synostosis. A case report. Clin. Orthop., 131:183, 1978.
10. Murphy, H. S., and Hanson, C. G.: Congenital humeroradial synostosis. J. Bone Joint Surg., 27:712, 1945.
11. Ogden, J. A., Watson, H. K., and Bohne, W.: Ulnar dysmelia. J. Bone Joint Surg., 58-A:467, 1976.
12. Patriarca, P. L., and Caproni, M.: Congenital humeroradial synostosis. Observations in two siblings. Minerva Pediatr., 30:71, 1978.
13. Say, B., Balci, S., and Atsu, M.: Humeroradial synostosis. A case report. Humangenetik, 19:341, 1973.
14. Sinistrero, G., and Toscano, G.: Radiological and clinical considerations on congenital ankylosis of the elbow. Min. Radiol., 8:529, 1963.
15. Solyom, L.: Two cases of congenital humero-radial synostosis. Magy. Traumatol. Orthop., 21:60, 1978.
16. Surana, R. B., and Sinkford, S. M.: Humero-radial synostosis. Clin. Genet., 13:169, 1978.

CONGENITAL RADIOULNAR SYNOSTOSIS

In this uncommon condition there is congenital fusion of the proximal ends of the radius and ulna, fixing the forearm in varying degrees of pronation. The patient may be affected unilaterally or bilaterally; in about 60 per cent of cases, involvement is bilateral. Male and female incidence is approximately equal.

There are three types of radioulnar synostosis. In *true congenital radioulnar synostosis*, the ulna and the upper end of the radius are closely fused together, with no interjacent cortical bone between their spongiosae (Fig. 2–30). The radial head may be fused to the ulna, or it may be completely absent (the so-called "headless" type). The radial shaft is bowed to a greater degree than normal and is longer and thicker than the ulna. Although, in several cases, the distal ends have been observed to be fused, they are almost always separate. In the headless type, involvement is usually bilateral. The *second type* is that in which the radial head is malformed and posteriorly dislocated (Fig. 2–31). The proximal end of the radius is fused with the upper shaft of the ulna. In the *third type*, the rarest, the ulna and radius may be attached, at a point just distal to their upper ends, by a short, thick, interosseous ligament that prevents any pronation or supination, just as if the bones were fused together. This is not a true synostosis; however, it is so classified because of loss of rotation of the forearm.

Etiology

Congenital radioulnar synostosis is hereditary in some cases, appearing to be a dominant trait with varying degrees of expression. It is caused by a developmental arrest of longitudinal segmentation. Both bones originate as rods of cartilage derived from the same mesodermal tissue. At approximately the fifth week of fetal life, the lower part of the upper limb rests against the trunk, the rods that later mature into the radius and ulna lying in a position halfway between pronation and supination. Synostosis occurs when the rods fail to separate or when the space between their upper ends, which is filled with mesodermal tissue, ossifies. The second type of synostosis, found in conjunction with dislocation of the radial head, is believed to take place at a later stage of fetal life.

It has been theorized that this condition in man is an atavistic process, as fusion of the radius and ulna is normal in lower vertebrates such as the camel and the deer.

Clinical Findings

There is no motion of the radius or the ulna, and the forearm is usually fixed in a position of mid- or hyperpronation (Fig. 2–32). The lack of supination of the forearm is compensated for somewhat by rotation at the glenohumeral joint, though it is impossible for the palm to be fully supinated. The elbow joint and the wrist are able to move freely, though extension of the elbow may be somewhat limited.

The degree of functional disability varies according to the position in which the forearm is fixed. It may be minimal if the condition is unilateral. The child may have difficulty with such activities as turning a doorknob, buttoning shirts, and handling eating utensils.

The involved forearm is thinner than normal and somewhat twisted in appearance. A depression may be found at the normal location of the radial head, caused by its anterior or posterior displacement or its imperfect development.

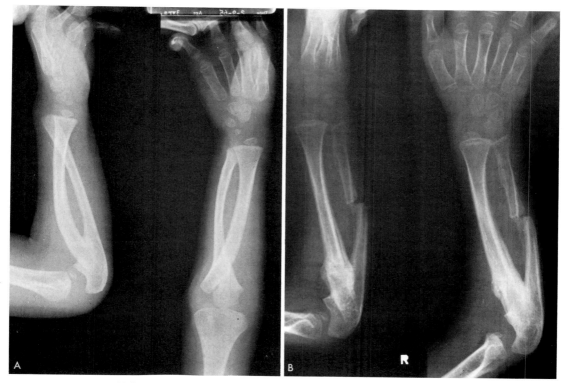

FIGURE 2–30. Congenital radioulnar synostosis of the "headless" type.

A. Preoperative radiograms. The ulna and the upper end of the radius are closely fused together. There is no interjacent cortical bone between their spongiosae. The radial head is almost completely absent, and the radial shaft is bowed anteriorly and somewhat laterally. **B.** Postoperative radiograms of the forearm. Osteotomy of the radius and ulna was performed to turn the forearm from 110 degrees of hyperpronation to functional neutral position.

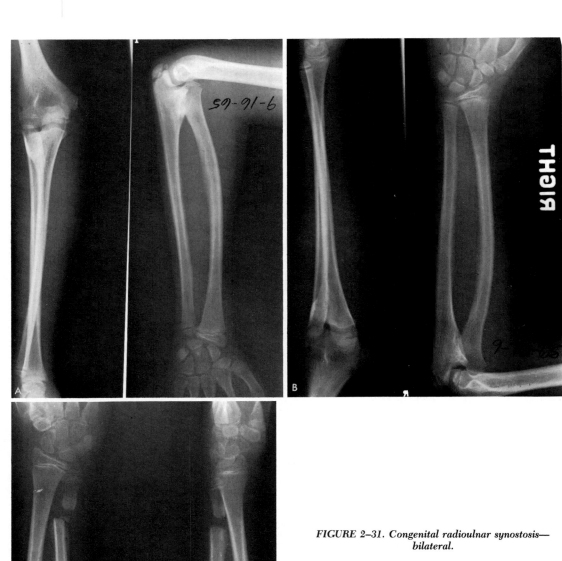

***FIGURE 2–31. Congenital radioulnar synostosis—
bilateral.***

This is the second type, in which the radial head is
malformed and dislocated. Note the fusion of the proximal
radius with the upper shaft of the ulna. **A** and **B.** Preoperative radiograms of both forearms. **C.** Postoperative radiograms. Kelikian's swivel operation was performed to give
active motion of the forearm.

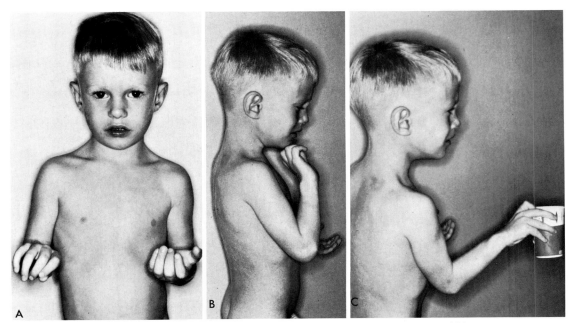

FIGURE 2–32. Congenital radioulnar synostosis on the right in a four-year-old boy.

A. Note the fixed hyperpronation of the right forearm. **B** and **C.** Functional disability is great. He can get only the dorsum of his hand to his mouth. Note the difficulty in handling a paper cup.

Treatment

Each patient should be individually evaluated to determine the treatment required. Surgical separation of the synostosis is not advised, as results have been poor. In cases of extreme pronation, an osteotomy in the proximal thirds of the radius and ulna may be performed to place the forearm in functional position.

Kelikian's swivel operation was designed to provide range of motion in the forearm.[32] It should be combined with resection of the distal shaft of the ulna and transplantation of the flexor carpi ulnaris tendon to restore active supination. The author's experience with this procedure has been disappointing, as associated soft-tissue contractures inhibit motion of the forearm. Kelikian, however, reports gratifying results in seven cases.[31]

References

1. Beck, W.: Beitrag zur radio-ulnaren Synostose. Fortschr. Rontgenstr., 83:734, 1955.
2. Brady, L. P., and Jewett, E. L.: A new treatment of radio-ulnar synostosis. South. Med. J., 53:507, 1960.
3. Cenani, A., and Lenz, W.: Totale Syndactylie und totale radioulnar Synostose bei zwei Brudern. Z. Kinderheilkd., 101:181, 1967.
4. Cohn, B. N. E.: Congenital bilateral radio-ulnar synostosis. J. Bone Joint Surg., 14:404, 1932.
5. Crasselt, C.: Zur operativen Behandlung der radioulnaren Synostose. Z. Orthop., 96:478, 1962.
6. Creyssel, J., Fischer, L., Ray, A., and Machenaud, A.: Congenital upper radiocubital synostosis. Three cases. Lyon Chir., 66:175, 1970.
7. Davenport, C. B., Taylor, H. L., and Nelson, L. A.: Radio-ulnar synostosis. Arch. Surg., 8:705, 1924.
8. Dawson, H. G. W.: A congenital deformity of the forearm and its operative treatment. Br. Med. J., 2:833, 1912.
9. Denischi, A., and Gorun, N.: Therapeutic aspects of proximal radio-ulnar congenital synostosis. Chirurgia (Bucur.), 22:19, 1973.
10. Dubois, H. J.: Nievergelt-Pearlman syndrome. Synostosis in feet and hands with dysplasia of elbows. Report of a case. J. Bone Joint Surg., 52-B:325, 1970.
11. Fahlstrom, S.: Radio-ulnar synostosis: Historical review and case report. J. Bone Joint Surg., 14:395, 1932.
12. Finidori, G., Rigault, P., Barthel, F., Mouterde, P., and Padovani, J. P.: Congenital radio-ulnar synostosis of children. Chir. Pediatr., 19:211, 1978.
13. Fixsen, J.: Congenital abnormalities of the limbs. Br. J. Hosp. Med., 26:194, 1981.
14. Fujita, K., Kamiishi, H., Shioya, N., Anz, E. M., and Iwaizumi, K.: Cleft lip and palate associated with congenital radio-ulnar synostosis: report of a case. Nippon Kyobu Geka Gakkai Zasshi, 21:217, 1975.
15. Gibson, A.: A critical consideration of congenital radio-ulnar synostosis, with special reference to treatment. J. Bone Joint Surg., 5:299, 1923.
16. Gille, P., Sava, P., Mourot, M., and Aubert, D.: Case report of congenital luxation of radial head associated with superior radio-ulnar synostosis. Rev. Chir. Orthop., 62:635, 1976.
17. Grebe, H.: Synostosis radiolunaris congenita. In Becker, P. E. (ed.): Humangenetik. Stuttgart, Thieme, 1964. Vol. 2, pp. 217–218.
18. Green, W. T., and Mital, M. A.: Congenital radio-ulnar synostosis: surgical treatment. J. Bone Joint Surg., 61-A:738, 1979.
19. Hansen, O. H., and Andersen, N. O.: Congenital radio-

ulnar synostosis: Report of 37 cases. Acta Orthop. Scand., *41*:225, 1970.

20. Jancu, J.: Radioulnar synostosis. A common occurrence in sex chromosomal abnormalities. Am. J. Dis. Child, *122*:10, 1971.
21. Keel, A.: Radial-ulnar synostosis. Praxis, *60*:791, 1971.
22. Kelikian, H.: Congenital Deformities of the Hand and Forearm. Philadelphia, Saunders, 1974, pp. 310–407, 714–752, 939–975.
23. Kelikian, H., and Doumanian, A.: Swivel for proximal radio-ulnar synostosis. J. Bone Joint Surg., *39*:945, 1957.
24. Kusswetter, W., and Heisel, A.: Radioulnar synostosis as characteristic feature of chromosome aberrations. Z. Orthop., *119*:10, 1981.
25. Luna, E., and Mannini, G.: Clinico-radiological study of congenital radioulnar synostosis. Chir. Ital., *33*:626, 1981.
26. McCredie, J.: Congenital fusion of bones: Radiology, embrology, and pathogenesis. Clin. Radiol., *26*:47, 1975.
27. Mital, M. A.: Congenital radioulnar synostosis and congenital dislocation of the radial head. Orthop. Clin. North Am., *76*:375, 1976.
28. Mnaymneh, W. A.: Congenital radio-humeral synostosis. A case report. Clin. Orthop., *131*:183, 1978.
29. Rodriguez, A. P., and Bejarno, E. B.: Congenital radioulnar synostosis. Rev. Clin. Esp., *61*:44, 1956.
30. Spiegel, P. G., Pekman, W. M., Rich, B. H., Versteeg, C. N., Nelson, V., and Dudnikov, M.: The orthopedic aspects of the fetal alcohol syndrome. Clin. Orthop., *139*:58, 1979.
31. Wilkie, D. P. D.: Congenital radio-ulnar synostosis. Br. J. Surg., *1*:366, 1913–1914.
32. Wolle, C.: Synostosis of the radius and scaphoid bone in hypoplasia of the thumb. Handchirurgie, *3*:117, 1971.

CONGENITAL DISLOCATION OF THE RADIAL HEAD

Congenital dislocation of the radial head unaccompanied by other congenital abnormalities of the elbow or forearm is very rare. McFarland described 11 cases in 1936; White, in 1943, added one more and mentioned 21 cases in the literature.[18, 22] The total number of cases described in the literature is less than one hundred.[1-22] Some of the reported cases, especially those of anterior dislocation, are of traumatic origin.

The direction of the displacement of the radial head may be anterior, as shown in Figure 2–33, or posterior or lateral, as shown in Figure 2–34. Involvement is often unilateral. Cockshott and Omololu reported bilateral posterior congenital dislocation of the radial heads in a father and daughter; they could not find any report of such familial cases in the literature.[9]

Good and Wicks have described a developmental form of dislocation of the radial head; it is nontraumatic, posterior, and associated with posterior bowing of the upper end of the ulna. The deformity is progressive, similar to Madelung's deformity, but the abnormality of growth involves the proximal growth plate of the radius.[13]

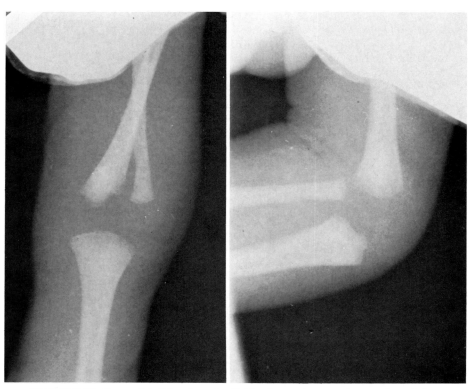

FIGURE 2–33. *Congenital dislocation of radial head, anterior type, in a newborn infant.*

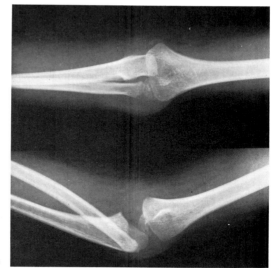

FIGURE 2–34. *Congenital dislocation of radial head.*

A. Posterior type. **B.** Posterolateral type.

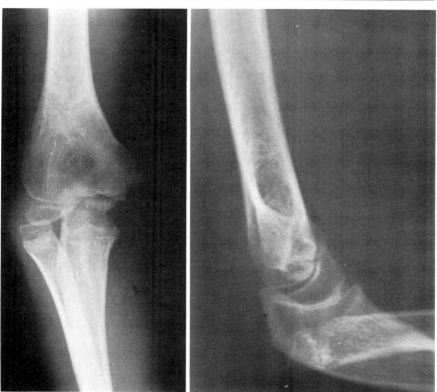

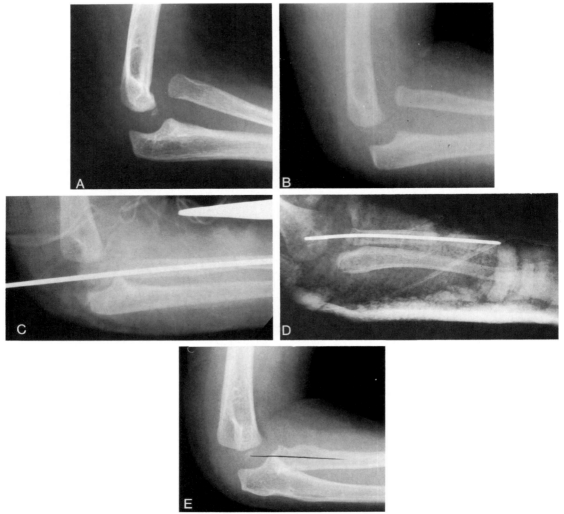

FIGURE 2–35. Bilateral anterior dislocation of the radial heads.

A and **B.** Lateral radiograms of right and left elbows showing the anterior dislocations of the radial heads. **C** and **D.** Intraoperative and immediately postoperative radiograms of the left elbow with the cast on, showing reduction of the dislocated radial head. **E.** Lateral view of the left elbow showing maintenance of reduction.

Diagnosis

The pathologic and clinical findings depend on the age of the patient and the type of dislocation. The abnormality is usually not detected at birth, but is diagnosed later on in childhood when the elbow is examined following some minor injury. Usually the elbows are asymptomatic. Sometimes the presenting complaint is a click or "stiffness" of the elbow with limitation of flexion or extension.

The ulna is bowed, the direction of convexity depending on the type of dislocation; in anterior dislocation of the radial head the convexity of the ulnar bow is forward, in posterior dislocations it is backward, and in lateral dislocations the ulna will bend laterally. In anterior dislocations the range of elbow flexion is limited and the radial head may be palpated in the cubital fossa; in posterior dislocations the elbow will not extend fully and the prominent radial head may be palpated posteriorly.

Radiograms disclose the following findings: a line drawn through the longitudinal axis of the radial shaft does not bisect the capitellum of the humerus, the head of the radius is dome-shaped on its superior surface, and the radial neck articulates with the capitellum and may have a depression at its point of contact.

It is important to distinguish traumatic from congenital dislocations. The types of injury that cause traumatic dislocation of the radial head are missed Monteggia fracture-dislocations, fracture of the radial neck, pulled elbow, and occasionally a primary traumatic dislocation of the radial head with other associated injury. Bowing of the ulna is not pathognomonic of congenital dislocation; it occurs also in unreduced traumatic dislocation. Reliable signs of congenital dislocation are gross underdevelopment of the capitellum of the humerus and the ovoid shape of the radial head. Probably the primary defect is failure of normal growth of the capitellum with alteration in shape of the radial head as a secondary adaptive deformation.[8] The shaft of the radius is relatively long in both congenital and traumatic dislocations. Ossification of soft tissues about the radial head suggests unreduced traumatic dislocation.

In the newborn and infant, arthrography of the elbow is helpful in the definitive diagnosis of radial head dislocation.

Treatment

When the diagnosis is made in the newborn or young infant, closed reduction may be attempted. The posteriorly dislocated radial head is reduced by supination of the forearm and extension of the elbow, whereas the anteriorly dislocated radial head is reduced by flexion of the elbow. Reduction is maintained in an above-elbow cast for four to six weeks.

Closed reduction is often unsuccessful. This author recommends open reduction with shortening of the radius in children up to three years of age. The radius is shortened at its midshaft at the insertion of the pronator teres (shortening it proximally near its neck may disturb growth and result in radioulnar synostosis). The surgical approach at the elbow for open reduction is anterior for anterior dislocations and posterolateral for posterior dislocations. In anterior dislocations the biceps brachii tendon (if contracted and a deforming force) may have to be lengthened by Z or fractional lengthening at its musculotendinous junction. Sometimes the annular ligament is fibrosed and irreparable, acting as an obstacle to reduction; in such an instance the annular ligament is excised and a new annular ligament is constructed with a longitudinal strip of triceps brachii fascia. The reduction is maintained by a smooth Steinmann pin introduced retrograde via the shortened radius at its midshaft, up the radial head, across the elbow joint, into and out of the capitellum, and then reinserted into the distal segment of the radial shaft (Fig. 2–35). The capsule of the elbow is repaired. The operative technique is

described and illustrated in Chapter 8 in the section on Monteggia fracture dislocation. An above-elbow cast is applied for six weeks. The pin and cast are removed, and range-of-motion exercises are performed to mobilize the elbow joint. The elbow is splinted part time for an additional three months.

In the older child it will be impossible to reduce the radial head. The dislocation is left alone until late adolescence, when if symptoms warrant, the radial head is excised.

References

1. Abbott, F. C.: Congenital dislocations of radius. Lancet, *1*:800, 1892.
2. Almquist, E. E., Gordon, L. H., and Blue, A. I.: Congenital dislocation of the head of the radius. J. Bone Joint Surg., *51-A*:1118, 1969.
3. Aritamur, A.: Congenital luxation of the head of the radius. Turk. Tip. Cemiy, Mecm., *36*:106, 1970.
4. Bindman, E.: Congenital dislocation of head of radius. Br. Med. J., *2*:354, 1945.
5. Bozdech, Z., and Muller-Stephann, H.: A contribution to the congenital dislocation of the head of radius. Beitr. Orthop. Traumatol., *15*:547, 1968.
6. Brennan, J. J., Krause, M. E. H., and Harvey, D. M.: Annular ligament construction for congenital anterior dislocation of both radial heads. Clin. Orthop. 29:205, 1963.
7. Bucknill, T. M.: Anterior dislocation of the radial head in children. Proc. R. Soc. Med., *70*:620, 1977.
8. Caravias, D. E.: Some observations on congenital dislocation of the head of the radius. J. Bone Joint Surg., *39-B*:86, 1957.
9. Cockshott, W. P., and Omololu, A.: Familial congenital posterior dislocation of both radial heads. J. Bone Joint Surg., *40-B*:483, 1958.
10. Danielisz, L.: Congenital dislocation of the head of the radius and elbow injury. Arch. Chir. Neerl., *23*:163, 1971.
11. England, J. P. S.: Congenital dislocation of the head of the radius. J. Bone Joint Surg., *47-B*:187, 1965.
12. Exarhou, E. I., and Antoniou, N. K.: Congenital dislocation of the head of the radius. Acta Orthop. Scand., *41*:551, 1970.
13. Good, C. J., and Wicks, M. H.: Developmental posterior dislocation of the radial head. J. Bone Joint Surg., *65-B*:64, 1983.
14. Keats, S.: Congenital bilateral dislocation of the head of the radius in a seven year old child. Orthop. Rev., *3*:33, 1974.
15. Lloyd-Roberts, G. C., and Bucknill, T. M.: Anterior dislocation of the radial head in children: Aetiology, natural history and management. J. Bone Joint Surg., *59-B*:402, 1977.
16. Mardam-Bey, T., and Ger, E.: Congenital radial head dislocation. J. Hand Surg., *4*:316, 1979.
17. Magee, R. K.: Bilateral congenital dislocation of radial head. Lancet, *1*:519, 1947.
18. McFarland, B.: Congenital dislocation of the head of the radius. Br. J. Surg., *24*:41, 1936.
19. Roles, N. C.: Congenital dislocation of the head of the radius. Br. Med. J., *2*:712, 1971.
20. Schubert, J. J.: Dislocation of the radial head in the newborn infant. J. Bone Joint Surg., *47-A*:1019, 1965.
21. Smith, R. W.: Congenital luxations of the radius. Dublin Q. J. Med. Sci., *13*:208, 1852.
22. White, J. R. A.: Congenital dislocation of the head of the radius. Br. J. Surg., *30*:377, 1943.

CONGENITAL LONGITUDINAL DEFICIENCIES OF THE RADIUS

Congenital longitudinal radial deficiencies comprise a spectrum of anomalies that extend from simple hypoplasia of the radius to its complete absence. In the literature, many different names are given to this unsightly defect. The term *radial club hand* is descriptive and, because of its practicality, is commonly used. One of the earliest reports was given in 1733 by Petit.[42]

Incidence

Radial deficiencies are uncommon. Kato, in 1924, reviewed 250 cases from the literature and described an additional 3 cases.[29] Birch-Jensen reported 73 patients in a population of about four million.[5] The deformity probably occurs in 1 of 100,000 live births. It is bilateral in approximately half the cases; and when involvement is unilateral, the right side is affected twice as frequently as the left. Males are more often affected than females, in a ratio of about 1.5 to 1.

Etiology

The exact cause of the longitudinal defect in the radial elements of the upper limb bud is unknown. According to Gegenbauer, the upper limb consists of a main stem and four accessory rays. The humerus, the ulna, the two carpal bones, the fifth metacarpal, and the three phalanges of the fifth finger make up the main stem. The radius, the navicular and greater multangular carpal bones, the first metacarpal, and the two phalanges of the thumb constitute the first accessory ray; the second, third, and fourth accessory rays consist of the index finger, the long finger, and the ring finger, with their respective metacarpals and carpal bones. It is proposed that congenital absence of the radius is due to the suppression of development of the first accessory ray. The cleavage plane between radial and ulnar paraxial hemimelia lies along the index finger; in defects of the ulna, the three ulnar fingers with their respective metacarpals and carpals are often absent; whereas in defects of the radius, the thumb is often missing.[21]

The upper limb develops in an orderly proximal-to-distal sequence. An intact, healthy apical ectoderm is a prerequisite for differentiation of the underlying mesenchymal tissues. Saunders removed part of the apical ectodermal ridge in the developing wings of chick embryos and produced anomalies similar to radial club hand.[48] In the chick embryo, damage to the mesenchymal portion of the upper limb bud on the preaxial side also produces radial deficiencies.[14] It appears that the most probable cause of radial club hand is damage to the apical ectoderm or the deeper mesenchymal tissues on the anterior aspect of the developing upper limb bud.[33]

Environmental factors known to cause radial deficiences are chemicals (such as thalidomide), irradiation, and viral infections.[33] The upper limb is completely formed by the sixth week; therefore, the teratologic factor must affect the limb bud during the first five weeks of fetal life.

Genetics

The defect is usually sporadic. In the University of Iowa series of 81 radial club hands, Flatt could not find any occurrence of the deformity from one generation to the next.[18] Wynne-Davies reviewed the cases of 35 children with radial club hand and investigated the families—70 parents, 71 siblings, 380 second-degree relatives, and 443 third-degree relatives, all of whom were normal.[62] In conclusion, the defect is not genetically patterned. On occasion, however, the absence of the radius is found in association with the Holt-Oram syndrome (atrial septal defect), which is of dominant inheritance; or with Fanconi pancytopenia, which is of recessive inheritance.[33]

Associated Anomalies

Congenital longitudinal radial deficiencies are frequently associated with other malformations (Table 2–5). This is explained by the fact that many organs develop at the same time as the upper limb buds. It behooves the orthopedic surgeon to be aware of these associations and to be sure that the patient has no serious anomalies that would make surgery hazardous and inadvisable. Clinically the most important are those associated with blood dyscrasias (Fanconi pancytopenia and thrombocytopenia with absence of the radius, or TAR syndrome) and with cardiac anomalies (Holt-Oram syndrome, or atrial septal defect with absence of the radius).

The multitude of syndromes that are involved with congenital longitudinal radial deficiencies, according to Goldberg and Meyn, fall into seven groups: chromosomal abnormalities (6), mental

Table 2–5. *Congenital Malformations Associated with Congenital Longitudinal Radial Deficiency*

Hand
  Thumb
    Absent
    Floating
    Hypoplastic
  Digits
    Syndactyly
    Polydactyly
    Symphalangism
    Triphalangism
  Carpus
    Deficient radial side—absence of scaphoid and
      trapezium
    Carpal coalition
  Metacarpal joints (MP)
    Excessive hyperextension with limited flexion
  Proximal interphalangeal joints (PIP)
    Fixed flexion deformity
Spine
  Congenital scoliosis
    Hemivertebrae
  Klippel-Feil syndrome
  Sacral agenesis
  Idiopathic scoliosis
Skeleton
  Hip dislocation
  Congenital high scapula (Sprengel's deformity)
  Bowed and short ulna
  Radioulnar synostosis (in partial absence of distal radius)
  Club foot
  Sternal anomalies
    Pectus excavatum
    Pectus carinatum
Cardiac Anomalies
  Atrial septal defect (Holt-Oram syndrome)
  Ventricular septal defect
  Coarctation of aorta
  Patent ductus arteriosus
  Dextrocardia
  Tetralogy of Fallot
  Pulmonary stenosis
Genitourinary Anomalies
  Renal agenesis
  Hypoplasia of kidney
  Horseshoe kidney
  Pelvic kidney
  Hydronephrosis
  Urethral valve
  Neurogenic bladder
Gastrointestinal Anomalies
  Esophageal atresia
  Tracheoesophageal fistula
  Rectovaginal fistula
  Imperforate anus
  Inguinal hernia
Pulmonary Anomalies
  Agenesis of upper lobe of lung
Head Anomalies
  Cleft lip and palate
  Craniosynostosis
  Hydrocephalus
  Cataracts
  Coloboma
  Ear anomalies
Chromosomal Abnormalities
  Such as Trisomy 18

deficiency (2), craniofacial defects (12), cardiac anomalies (2), blood dyscrasias (2), vertebral anomalies (3), and teratogenic syndromes (2).[22] This list is by no means complete.

Pathologic Anatomy

The anatomic defect has been described and reviewed by many authors.[27, 38, 40, 50, 52, 55] Congenital longitudinal radial deficiencies may be subdivided into three types. *Type A, hypoplasia of the radius,* is the least defective. The distal radial physis is usually deficient, and ossification of its epiphysis is delayed. The distal radius is shortened. Palpation finds the radial styloid process proximal to that of the ulna, normally the former is distal to the latter. The proximal radial epiphysis and the elbow are normal. The radial shortening is minimal. The wrist joint has greater than normal range of radial deviation but is, however, stable and provides adequate functional stability to the carpus. The scaphoid and trapezium bones are hypoplastic but present. The thumb is underdeveloped.

In the more severely hypoplastic radius, both the distal and proximal radial epiphyses are defective. The radius is moderately short and miniature in appearance. The ulna is thickened and bowed, with its concavity toward the radius. There is radial instability of the wrist joint, the instability being directly proportional to the extent of the radial deficiency. The thumb may be hypoplastic, floating, or absent.

In *Type B* there is partial absence of the radius. Frequently it is the distal and middle portion of the bone that has failed to develop (Figs. 2–36 and 2–37). Presence of the proximal part of the radius provides some degree of stability to the elbow joint. The bone may, however, be hypoplastic and fused to the ulna, forming a type of radioulnar synostosis, or on occasion it may be fused to the humerus. The ulna is short, hypertrophic, and bowed, with its concavity to the radial side. The wrist joint is unstable because of the lack of radial support, and the hand tends to deviate toward the radial side.

In *Type C* there is complete absence of the radius (Fig. 2–38). This is the most common type, constituting 50 per cent of the reported cases. There is total lack of radial skeletal support of the carpus; soft-tissue contracture on the radial side of the forearm is severe. Markedly deviated radially, the hand may form an angle of 90 degrees or more with the forearm, and when the elbow is flexed it may even lie directly against and parallel with the arm, its

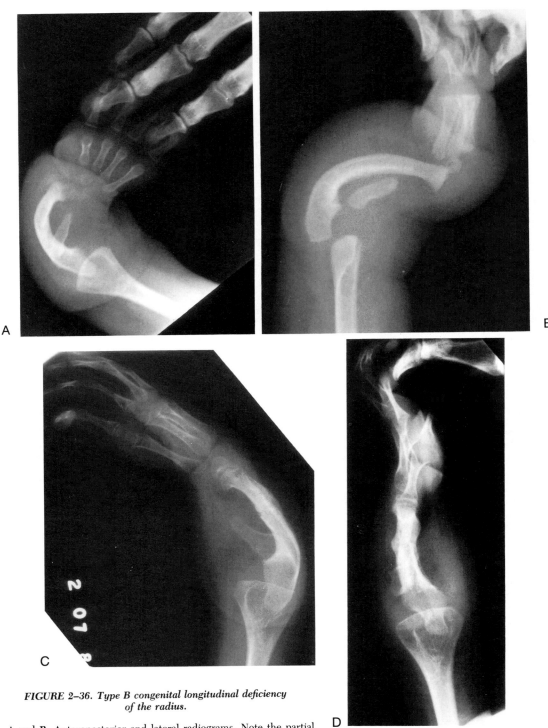

FIGURE 2–36. *Type B congenital longitudinal deficiency of the radius.*

A and **B.** Anteroposterior and lateral radiograms. Note the partial absence of the distal and middle parts of the radius and the deficiency of the proximal radius with abnormality of the elbow. The ulna is markedly bowed. **C** and **D.** Anteroposterior and lateral radiograms of the forearms four years postoperatively following radial lengthening and osteotomy of the ulna to correct its severe bowing.

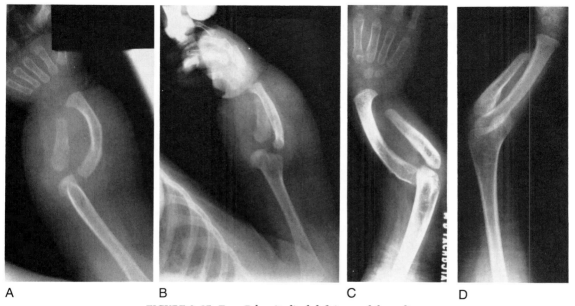

A   B   C   D

FIGURE 2–37. Type B longitudinal deficiency of the radius.

A and **B.** Anteroposterior and lateral radiograms of the radius in a four-month-old child. The ulna is slightly bowed, and the distal third of the radius is absent. **C** and **D.** Anteroposterior and lateral radiograms of the same patient four years later show progressive growth of the radius. Functional use of the right upper limb is quite adequate in this patient.

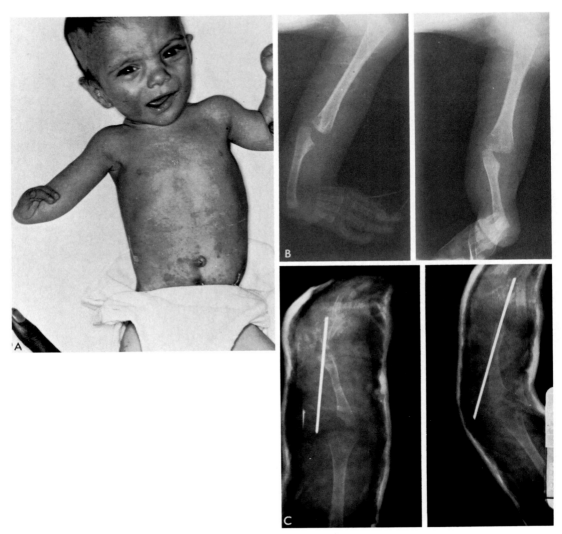

FIGURE 2–38. *Congenital absence of the radius in an infant.*

A. Clinical appearance. **B.** Preoperative radiograms. **C.** Immediate postoperative radiograms through the cast. An arthroplasty was performed implanting the distal end of the ulna into the carpus. A Kirschner bar is used for internal fixation.

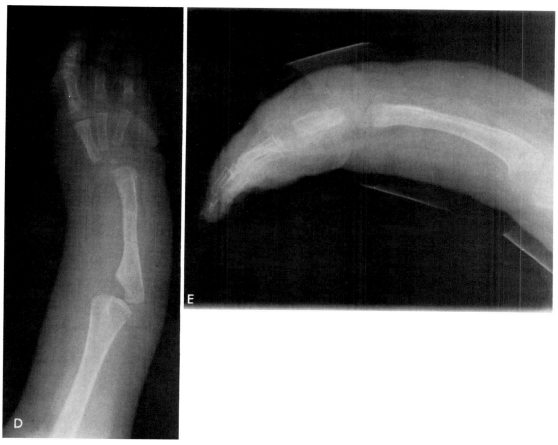

FIGURE 2–38 Continued. Congenital absence of the radius in an infant.

D and E. Postoperative radiograms.

radial border touching the forearm. In complete absence of the radius the bones of the radial ray—the navicular, trapezium, first metacarpal, and phalanges of the thumb—are frequently absent. If the thumb is present it is usually hypoplastic and floating. The humerus is usually short; the capitellum may be hypoplastic or absent. Ossification of the distal humeral epiphysis may be delayed.

The connection between the ulna and carpus is fibrous; the bone ends are not covered with articular cartilage. Occasionally there may be a flat cavity on the radial aspect of the distal ulna that is lined with hyaline cartilage. The carpus is displaced not only radially but also volarly. The radial displacement of the carpus is caused by the taut soft-tissue contracture on the radial side of the forearm. When the deformity is untreated its severity increases with skeletal growth. The volar displacement is caused by the unopposed action of the wrist and finger flexors.

The metacarpophalangeal joints have excessive hyperextension and limited flexion. The proximal interphalangeal joints have fixed flexion deformity, in some cases associated with skin webbing. The radiographic appearance of the metacarpophalangeal and proximal interphalangeal joints is normal. The joint stiffness appears to be related to extra-articular causes such as abnormality of the extensor mechanism. The severity of contracture of the finger joints progressively diminishes from the radial to the ulnar side of the hand.

The elbow joint may be stiff in extension in about one fourth of the cases of radial club hand. Extension contracture of the elbow, if it cannot be corrected, is a definite contraindication to any centralization of the hand over the ulna. It is caused by fibrous contracture of the capsule and soft tissues on the posterior aspect of the elbow joint and by muscle imbalance between weak elbow flexors and strong elbow extensors.[33]

It must be borne in mind that radial club hand is not a simple skeletal deficiency of the preaxial side of the upper limb; there are also abnormalities of muscles and neurovascular structures.

MUSCLES

Muscular involvement in the affected limb is diffuse. In general the muscles arising from the common extensor origin and from the radius are absent, hypoplastic, or fibrotic and fused to each other. Normal muscle and fascial planes are lacking. The pronator quadratus, the extensors carpi radialis longus and brevis, and the brachioradialis and supinator brevis are usually absent; sometimes they are fibrotic and fused with the extensor digitorum communis, which is normal. From the volar surface of the radius arises the flexor digitorum profundus to the index finger; its absence influences the decision about subsequent pollicization of the index finger. If the thumb and first metacarpal are absent, the flexor pollicis longus, extensor pollicis longus, extensor pollicis brevis, abductor pollicis brevis, and muscles of the thenar eminence are usually lacking. The interossei, lumbricales, and hypothenar muscles are usually present.

The flexor muscles of the wrist and fingers are usually normal but occasionally may be fused to each other. The flexor digitorum sublimis shows more variation than the flexor digitorum profundus. The superficial finger flexors may be hypoplastic, fibrotic, or fused to the deep flexors.

The long head of the biceps is almost always absent; the short head of the biceps is always present but usually is abnormal. Insertion of the biceps tendon is usually into either the joint capsule or the radial rudiment, if present; occasionally the tendon inserts into the medial epicondyle of the humerus. The pectoralis major and minor and the deltoid muscles are usually present but may have abnormal insertions or may fuse with the triceps or with the brachialis.

NERVES

The axillary nerve and the ulnar nerve are usually present and normal. The musculocutaneous nerve is often absent. The radial nerve usually terminates at the elbow. Sensory nerve supply to the radial aspect of the hand is provided by the median nerve, which anastomoses with the sensory branch of the ulnar nerve. The ulnar and median nerves are normal. The median nerve is thicker than normal because it contains sensory fibers normally distributed by the radial nerve. It lies consistently on the radial aspect of the forearm immediately beneath the fibers of the deep fascia, a fact that should be remembered at operation (Fig. 2–39). It presents a great challenge when soft-tissue release is performed on the radial aspect of the forearm. In order to prevent inadvertent injury to the median nerve the deep fascia should be split widely up the forearm, the nerve isolated, and its peripheral distribution identified.

VESSELS

The ulnar artery is present and is usually the major arterial supply for the forearm and hand. Therefore, at surgery it is vital to find the ulnar artery and protect it from damage. The interosseous arteries are usually present and well developed. The radial and palmar arterial arches are anomalous, the degree of involvement corresponding closely to the extent of radial dysplasia.[6] The radial aspect of the forearm is supplied by the anterior interosseous artery, which arises from the ulnar artery and accompanies the median nerve through the forearm. Because the radial artery is often rudimentary or absent, damage to the ulnar artery may thus seriously compromise vascular supply to the hand.

Clinical Findings

In total or partial absence of the radius the clinical picture is characteristic—the forearm is short and bowed radially with a prominent knob at its lower end, which represents the ulnar styloid process (Fig. 2–40). The radial styloid process cannot be palpated. The hand is deviated radially owing to loss of skeletal support at the wrist. The diffuse nature of involvement should be realized, and its functional implications thoroughly assessed. The permanent consideration is the function of the upper limb and hand.

Functional disability depends on whether involvement is unilateral or bilateral. The patient with unilateral deficiency uses the opposite normal upper limb as the dominant one and the deficient limb simply as an aid; these children are functionally independent even though the hand on the involved side is clumsy and lacks skill.

In bilateral cases functional disability is great; the child has difficulty performing activities of daily living such as dressing, feeding, and washing himself. Limitation of elbow flexion aggravates the functional impairment.

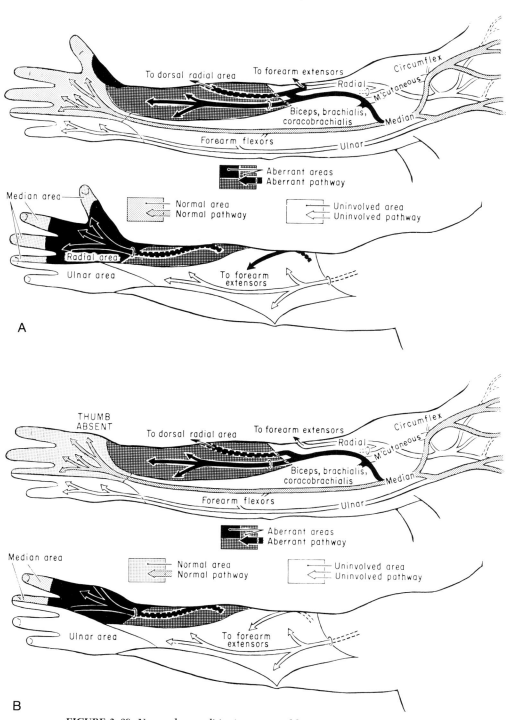

FIGURE 2–39. *Nerve abnormalities in congenital longitudinal radial deficiency.*

A. Thumb present. **B.** Thumb absent. From Skerik, S. K., and Flatt, A. E.: The anatomy of congenital radial dysplasia. Its surgical and functional implications. Clin. Orthop. *66*:125, 1969. Reprinted by permission.

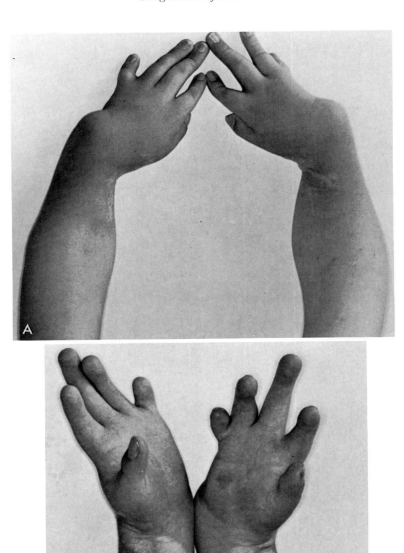

FIGURE 2–40. Bilateral congenital absence of the radius with Fanconi's syndrome in an eight-year-old boy.

Two years earlier, a soft-tissue release was performed. **A** and **B**. Posteroanterior and anteroposterior photographs of the hand and forearm disclosing radial deviation of the carpus and hand and the hypoplastic thumb and little finger. The healed surgical scars are obvious.

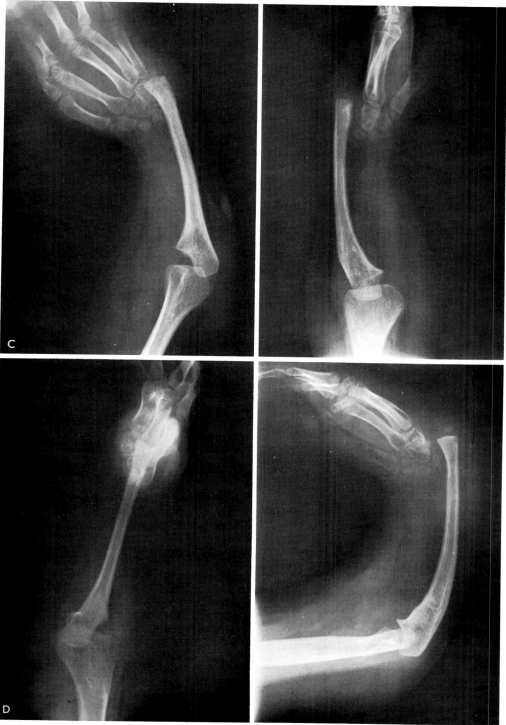

FIGURE 2–40 Continued. Bilateral congenital absence of the radius with Fanconi's syndrome in an eight-year-old boy.

C and **D.** Anteroposterior and lateral radiograms of the right forearm, **C,** and of the left, **D.**

The radial two fingers, especially the index, are abnormal with varying degrees of flexion contracture, weakness of active motion, and hypoplasia. The ulnar two digits are almost always normal and more functional.

In the absence of the thumb, the index finger tends to deviate ulnarward and the little finger radialward. On finger flexion the marginal two digits tend to lie beneath the central two digits. Also there is greater than normal range of abduction-adduction between the index and long fingers; the degree of pronation of the index finger increases in time, enhancing its ability to substitute for the thumb. The grip is usually spherical and sometimes cylindrical. Hook grip is least used because of the lack of full range of finger flexion and the weakness of finger flexors.

Rudimentary thumbs are attached by a soft-tissue pedicle and have no active motion; they are of no functional value. Hypoplastic thumbs have markedly restricted range of motion, especially interphalangeal flexion-extension; the hypoplastic thumb can touch the little and ring fingers, but opposition between the thumb and index and long fingers is greatly impaired. The thumb is weak; when strength is needed the index finger is substituted for the thumb.

Treatment

The type of treatment depends on the degree of longitudinal radial deficiency. For the *hypoplastic radius* it consists of a stretching cast to correct contractural deformity on the radial side of the forearm and the use of night splints and passive stretching exercises to maintain alignment. At age eight to ten years, if progressive shortening of the radius is causing instability of the wrist, one-stage lengthening of the radius can be performed. This, if necessary, can be repeated at 12 to 14 years of age. The technique of radial lengthening is as follows: A longitudinal skin incision is made on the dorsoradial aspect of the forearm, beginning at the radial styloid process and extending proximally to the upper one fourth of the radius. The subcutaneous tissue is divided in line with the skin incision. The interval between the brachioradialis and extensor carpi radialis longus is developed. The pronator teres is detached at its insertion. Avoid injury to the dorsal sensory branch of the radial nerve and the median nerve. Then the deep fasciae on the dorsal, radial, and volar surfaces of the forearm are incised and partially excised. All contracted fibrous soft tissue should be removed. A thorough soft-tissue release is cru-cial. The middle two thirds of the radius is exposed subperiosteally on its dorsal and radial aspects. The outline of Z-lengthening of the radial shaft is marked with multiple small drill holes; there should be enough overlap of the radial bone segments to allow internal fixation with three or four small-fragment cortical screws. Next, two small Schanz screws are inserted distally into the radius (avoid injury to the distal radial physis), and two small Schanz screws are inserted proximally. The Schanz screws are connected to the small Wagner limb lengthening apparatus. The Z-osteotomy is performed. The radius is lengthened the desired amount. Interosseous membrane division is usually not necessary. The tourniquet is released to ensure that circulation is adequate. Range of elbow motion and rotation of the forearm and wrist are checked. The osteotomized segments are fixed either with three or four bicortical small-fragment screws or with an AO plate. The proximal and distal defects in the radius are grafted with autogenous iliac cancellous bone. The Schanz screws and Wagner limb lengthening device are removed. The flexor carpi ulnaris, brachioradialis, and extensors carpi radialis longus and brevis, if taut, are fractionally lengthened at their musculotendinous junctions. A closed-suction Hemovac tube is placed in the wound, which is closed in routine fashion. An above-elbow cast is applied with the elbow in 60 to 70 degrees of flexion, the forearm in full supination, and the wrist in functional position. The cast extends distally to the metacarpal heads. Passive and active exercises are performed to maintain finger and thumb motion. Postoperatively the cast is changed as necessary. The radius usually heals in eight to ten weeks. The screws and plate are removed 6 to 12 months after surgery.

If the *radius is totally or partially absent* the carpus is unstable, the hand rolling over radially around the end of the ulna. Treatment should begin immediately following birth. Every effort should be made to align the radially deviated hand and carpus over the distal end of the ulna to prevent further contracture of soft tissues and muscles. Passive exercises are performed to stretch the shortened muscles on the radial and volar sides, followed by application of a retentive cast. Once full passive correction and alignment are achieved, they are maintained by a light dynamic splint or a plastic mold with Velcro straps (Fig. 2–41). Passive exercises are also performed to develop elbow flexion, volar flexion of metacarpophalangeal joints, and extension of proximal interphalangeal joints.

With progressive radial deviation of the hand and instability of the wrist, the appearance becomes very unsightly, and the function of the hand is interfered with. Correction of the deformity and stabilization of the wrist by centralization of the carpus over the distal ulna are recommended. The procedure is combined with capsular reefing on the ulnar and dorsal sides of the wrist, tendon transfers to balance the hand dynamically over the end of the ulna, release of contracted soft tissues on the radial side, and straightening of the bowed ulna by a wedge osteotomy if necessary. The operative technique used by this author is illustrated in Plate 5.

The procedure is best performed in early infancy, preferably at six months of age. Adequate time is required to assess the functional status of the upper limb and also to evaluate the whole infant for associated malformations and syndromes.

Centralization of the carpus over the distal ulna was originally proposed by Sayre, who sharpened the distal end of the ulna to fit into a notch of the carpus.[49] The technique has been modified by Lidge and by Lamb, and at present is recommended by almost all authors.[33, 34]

Bayne recommends two skin incisions. First, a transverse wedge-shaped incision over the distal end of the ulna allows excision of the excessive ulnar bulge of redundant skin and subcutaneous tissue that is usually present. A separate Z-plasty on the radial side of the forearm and wrist helps to correct the skin webbing

Text continued on page 204

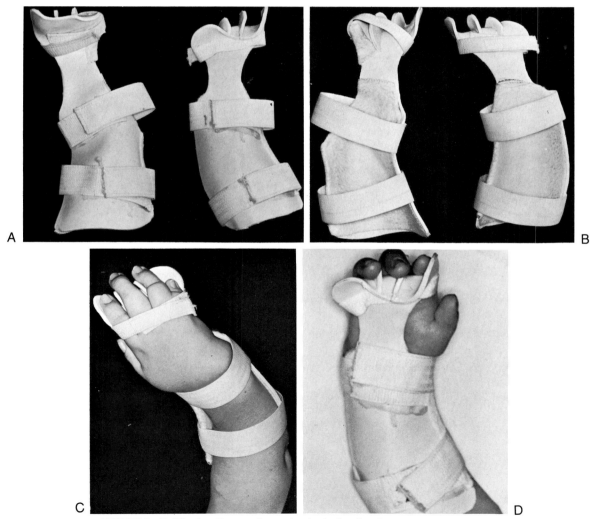

FIGURE 2–41. Plastic splints used to maintain the hand and wrist in neutral position.

Centralization of the Carpus Over the Distal End of the Ulna

OPERATIVE TECHNIQUE

A. The skin incision begins on the dorsum of the hand on the radial border of the distal third of the second metacarpal; it extends proximally and ulnarward toward the prominence of the ulnar head, where it deviates radially and proximally to terminate at the proximal third of the volar surface of the forearm at its radial border. This approach permits an extensive view of the dorsal, radial, and volar aspects of the hand, wrist, and forearm. Subcutaneous tissue is divided in line with the skin incision. Damage to the veins should be avoided.

B. Next, the deep fascia is split widely in the forearm, and the median nerve with its peripheral distribution is identified. The median nerve is thicker than normal and almost invariably aberrant. About 6 to 7 cm. proximal to the wrist, it may divide into two large terminal branches, one passing to the volar surface of the forearm and wrist and through the carpal tunnel, and the second continuing along the radial side of the forearm and wrist, supplying the innervator normally provided by the radial nerve. It is very easy to divide the radial branch inadvertently; it should be isolated and protected.

The median nerve is always preaxial, acting as a bowstring to the radially deviated forearm and wrist. Its course may vary in a number of ways. It may traverse superficially along the radial margin of the brachioradialis muscle until it enters the palm; it may lie beneath the palmaris longus and flexor digitorum sublimus; it may traverse along the radial edge of the flexor digitorum sublimus; or it may emerge superficially beneath the flexors at the middle of the forearm and course distally between the brachioradialis and the extensor digitorum communis. The median nerve can withstand a great deal of stretching and still provide sensory and motor conduction but cannot tolerate external compression by taut fascia and fibrous bands. Therefore it is crucial to relieve it of all constricting bands and perform a thorough release of the deep fascia. Caution! The median nerve is radial in its course and lies immediately beneath the deep fascia.

C and **D.** The incision is developed to the level of the tendons on the dorsal, ulnar, and volar surfaces of the distal ulna. The *dorsal sensory branch of the ulnar nerve* is identified and gently retracted. The extensor carpi ulnaris tendon is identified, detached at its insertion, marked with 2-0 Mersilene suture, and reflected proximally and medially (later to be advanced distally on the fifth metacarpal as tautly as possible). The flexor carpi ulnaris tendon is identified next by blunt dissection. (Avoid injury to the ulnar artery, the major blood supply to the hand; identify, isolate, and protect the ulnar vessels and nerve from injury.) The tendon is detached at its insertion to the pisiform bone; later on, along with the extensor carpi ulnaris, it will be sutured as snugly as possible to the dorsal and radial aspect of the fifth metacarpal.

E. Next, identify the distal end of the ulna and develop the interval between its borders and the carpus. Stay extraperiosteal! *Do not damage growth of the distal ulnar physis!* There will be a thickened false joint capsule covering the distal end of the ulna; carefully and gently section it, dissect it, and elevate it distally, leaving the capsule attached to the dorsoulnar aspect of the carpus. (After implantation of the carpus, the distally based ulnocarpal capsule will be advanced proximally and sutured to the dorsum of the ulna.) The wrist tendons will have aberrant insertions to the capsule.

Plate 5. Centralization of the Carpus Over the Distal End of the Ulna

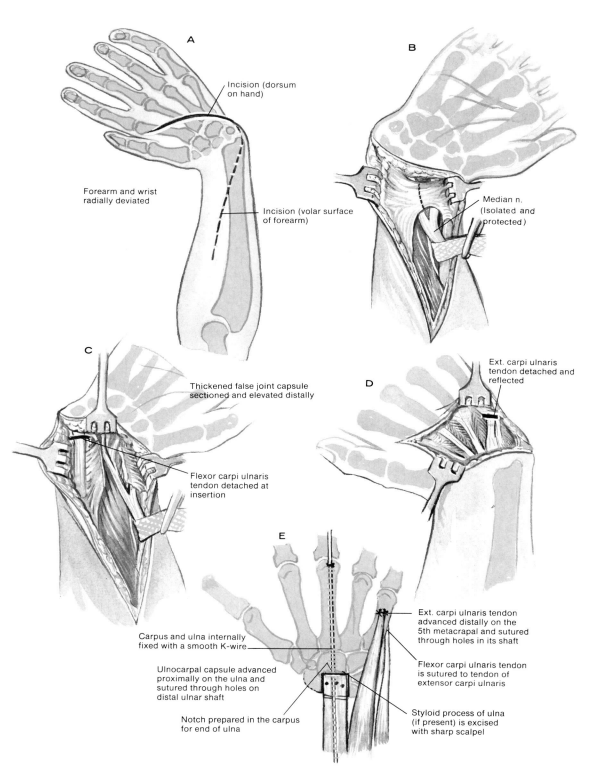

A

Incision (dorsum on hand)

Forearm and wrist radially deviated

Incision (volar surface of forearm)

B

Median n. (Isolated and protected)

C

Thickened false joint capsule sectioned and elevated distally

Flexor carpi ulnaris tendon detached at insertion

D

Ext. carpi ulnaris tendon detached and reflected

E

Carpus and ulna internally fixed with a smooth K-wire

Ulnocarpal capsule advanced proximally on the ulna and sutured through holes on distal ulnar shaft

Notch prepared in the carpus for end of ulna

Ext. carpi ulnaris tendon advanced distally on the 5th metacrapal and sutured through holes in its shaft

Flexor carpi ulnaris tendon is sutured to tendon of extensor carpi ulnaris

Styloid process of ulna (if present) is excised with sharp scalpel

201

The flexor carpi radialis and brachioradialis tendons insert to the radial aspect of the carpus and joint capsule, acting as a strong radial tethering force. When sectioning the constricted fibrotic tendons be sure not to buttonhole and weaken the capsule. To maintain alignment, it must be tautly reefed. It is sectioned on the radial and volar surfaces of the wrist. Caution—any fibrous anlage of the radius is excised. Do not injure the median nerve and anterior interosseous vessels.

Measurements for the notch in the carpus for insertion of the distal end of the ulna are made on the radiograms. The sides of the slot should be as long as the diameter of the end of the ulna, the insertion being mechanically stable only when its depth is at least equal to its diameter—a vital basic biomechanical principle. Specific carpal bones are difficult to identify; the trapezium and navicular are often absent. Often the entire capitate bone is excised to achieve stability. An adequate buttress of carpal wall must be maintained on the radial side.

The styloid process of the ulna is excised and its cartilage slightly shaved with a sharp scalpel. Use no osteotomes, no hammering! Do not impair growth of the distal ulnar physis!

With the elbow flexed, the carpus is reduced over the end of the ulna. Avoid excessive force. The fit must be easy but snug. The shaft of the third metacarpal should be perpendicular to the distal growth plate of the ulna. A single-bone forearm will have no rotation and no radioulnar deviation. With functional range of elbow and shoulder motion it is best to place the distal ulna into the carpus in a position of 30 to 45 degrees of pronation.

Next, the carpus and ulna are internally fixed with a smooth Kirschner wire inserted proximally to distally through the shaft of the third metacarpal and out through its head. Be sure it is not volar. Then the pin is drilled proximally through the center of the distal ulnar epiphysis and up the medullary cavity. If the ulna is markedly bowed, wedge osteotomy of its shaft is performed to correct the curvature.

After internal fixation the tourniquet is deflated and complete hemostasis is obtained. Circulation in the hand is assessed. First, the distally based ulnocarpal capsule is advanced proximally on the ulna and sutured through holes on the distal ulnar shaft. Second, the *extensor carpi ulnaris tendon* is advanced distally on the fifth metacarpal as tautly as possible and sutured through holes in the bone's shaft. It is best to make the holes with an electric drill. Third, the *flexor carpi ulnaris tendon* is sutured to the extensor carpi ulnaris tendon as far dorsally and distally as possible. Thus the hand is balanced dynamically over the distal end of the ulna.

A closed-suction Hemovac drainage tube is inserted in the wound, and the skin incisions are closed in the usual fashion.

An above-elbow cast is applied with the elbow flexed 90 degrees and the hand in neutral position. The metacarpophalangeal and interphalangeal joints are left free for active and passive exercises to correct extension contracture of the metacarpophalangeal joints and flexion contracture of the proximal interphalangeal joints.

Some surgeons (and sometimes this author) prefer to apply a fluffy compression dressing with a dorsal plaster of Paris slab holding the elbow in 90 degrees of flexion. The hand is elevated for several days to minimize postoperative swelling, which will usually subside within a week. Then a new circular plaster of Paris above-elbow cast that extends distally to the metacarpal heads is applied.

POSTOPERATIVE CARE

The cast and sutures are removed in four weeks. A new above-elbow cast is worn for an additional four weeks, by which time a simultaneously performed osteotomy of the ulna should be consolidated. Make radiograms to verify bone healing. There is some controversy about the duration of Kirschner wire fixation. This author recommends its removal in eight weeks when the final cast is taken off. This allows some wrist motion, prevents potential damage to the distal ulnar physis, and obviates breakage of the wire at the wrist or pin extrusion and pin tract infection.

After pin and cast removal a plastic dorsal hand orthosis is made; the splint should extend proximally to just below the elbow for proper lever support and should support the wrist in a few degrees of ulnar deviation and 10 to 20 degrees of dorsiflexion. Leaving the volar aspect relatively free encourages prehension and hand function. Initially the orthosis is worn day and night. Several times a day the splint is removed, and passive and active exercises are performed to develop wrist motion. Day use of the splint is discontinued at two to three years of age, but night use is continued for an additional two years.

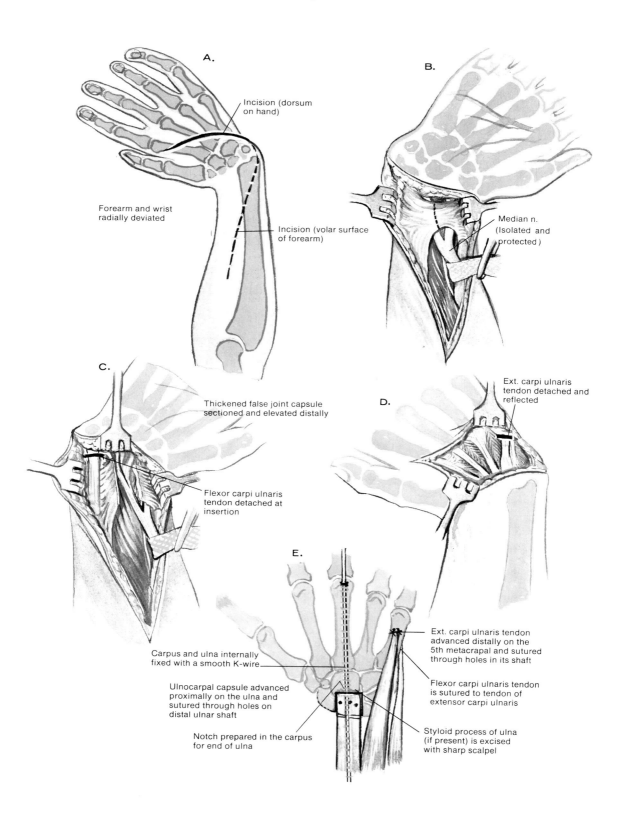

A.

Incision (dorsum on hand)

Forearm and wrist radially deviated

Incision (volar surface of forearm)

B.

Median n. (Isolated and protected)

C.

Thickened false joint capsule sectioned and elevated distally

Flexor carpi ulnaris tendon detached at insertion

D.

Ext. carpi ulnaris tendon detached and reflected

E.

Carpus and ulna internally fixed with a smooth K-wire

Ulnocarpal capsule advanced proximally on the ulna and sutured through holes on distal ulnar shaft

Notch prepared in the carpus for end of ulna

Ext. carpi ulnaris tendon advanced distally on the 5th metacrapal and sutured through holes in its shaft

Flexor carpi ulnaris tendon is sutured to tendon of extensor carpi ulnaris

Styloid process of ulna (if present) is excised with sharp scalpel

203

and at the same time permits release of contracted soft tissues on the radial side of the forearm.[4]

This author prefers the incision used by Lamb because it allows better visualization of the pathologic structures and evaluation of anomalous and normal neurovascular tissues, and permits extensive soft-tissue release and tendon transfers to balance the hand dynamically over the distal ulna. The redundant soft tissue over the ulnar head can be excised later on as a second stage, if indicated.[32]

There is also controversy about the method of internal fixation. An alternative to the method described in Plate 5 is to drill the Kirschner wire from distally to proximally up the center of the ulnar epiphysis and the medullary cavity of its shaft. If the ulna is bowed the wire will extrude from its shaft; if the ulna is straight the wire will curve out of the olecranon. Next, a second wire of similar size is drilled through the notch in the carpus and through the base of the third metacarpal into its shaft. The second Kirschner wire is removed because its purpose is to establish a tract for the ulnar Kirschner wire. The protruded end of the ulnar wire is then fitted into this pin tract in the carpus and drilled into the third metacarpal shaft. The wire should not protrude through the metacarpal head. Passive motion of the metacarpophalangeal joint should be free. The wire is left slightly protruding from the ulnar shaft to facilitate its later removal.

The size of the Kirschner wire should be appropriate for the patient's age. An important point is that both ends of the wire be pointed. A flattened spear end on the wire (often made by cutting it at an angle) will make its top broader than the diameter of the wire. The diameter of the hole made in the bone will be larger than that of the wire; thereby internal fixation will be loose and inadequate. Wires pointed at both ends are commercially available. The use of rods or large Steinmann pins is not recommended because they may damage the distal ulnar physis. Anteroposterior and lateral radiograms are made to ensure correct placement of the pin.

Contraindications to surgical intervention: First is association with severe anomalies (such as Fanconi's pancytopenia) that are not compatible with long life; in such an instance the infant should not be subjected to the unnecessary dangers of operation. Second is persistent extension contracture of the elbow that does not permit the child to bring the straightened hand to the mouth is another contraindication. All

attempts should be made to provide 90-degree elbow flexion. A continuous-motion elbow machine has been successful in the experience of this author. Posterior capsulotomy of the elbow and anterior transfer of the triceps tendon may be indicated in some cases. Third, older patients (adolescents and adults) who have adjusted their functional activities according to their deformity should be left untreated; these patients have marked bowing of the ulna with severe contracture of vital neurovascular structures and soft tissues that precludes surgical correction without further shortening of an already short forearm. They have established their prehension patterns. A straight and stiff wrist will seriously compromise function. Function is of paramount importance in treatment; never sacrifice function for appearance's sake.

There is some controversy about whether centralization of the ulna should be performed in bilateral cases. Goldner advises against performing the procedure bilaterally because he found considerable stiffness of the wrists when he reviewed the results of 32 centralization procedures.[24] In Lamb's experience with four patients who had bilateral centralization he found no postoperative decrease in functional self-care. In fact, one boy became totally independent in toilet and dressing functions postoperatively, which he had not been before surgery.[33] In bilateral cases this author recommends centralizing one side at four to six months of age and assessing the development of function and prehension; if these are satisfactory, the opposite side is operated on at three years of age.

Some surgeons take a negative approach to surgical treatment of both unilateral and bilateral radial club hand; they advise that the deformity be left untreated in order to allow the child to develop the best function possible. They claim that as adults these patients can do almost anything they desire with their hands. These hands are, nevertheless, clumsy and lack skill; they do not possess the required anatomic components for adequate function. Such a nihilistic posture is not recommended by this author.

The results of centralization are satisfactory. Surgery can provide good correction of deformity without loss of function. Cosmetic improvement is considerable. If the operation is performed correctly and the hand is balanced by tendon transfers and supported in splints, the correction can be maintained. Injudicious surgery can disturb growth of the distal ulnar physis; however, if a smooth pin is utilized and removed three to six months postoperatively one can obviate growth arrest and serious shortening of the forearm. Early surgery in the young infant will permit development of an adequate prehension pattern, and one can expect definite improvement of overall function of the upper limb. Function will be further enhanced if the index finger is pollicized, provided its muscle and joint structures are adequate to provide good function as a thumb. (Details of indications, requisites, contraindications, and technique of pollicization are given in Plate 10.)

Complications can occur. Inadvertent division of the median nerve or ulnar vessels should be avoided. Growth of the distal ulnar physis should not be disturbed. Pin tract infection and wound infection are problems that can be adequately treated by appropriate local wound care and antibiotics. Recurrence of deformity is usually due to failure of initial operative reduction, inadequate internal pin fixation, failure to balance the hand dynamically over the distal ulna, and poor postoperative care in respect to wearing of the splint. Progressive bowing of the ulna may be troublesome; it may be due to asymmetrical growth of the distal ulnar physis or response of the ulna to muscle imbalance caused by the stronger pull of muscles on the radial side. Repeat osteotomy of the ulna may be indicated in some cases. One should not hesitate to recentralize a poorly executed and failed centralization.

In the literature, one will find reports of many other methods of surgical correction of radial club hand. The various approaches have included:

Release of contracted soft tissues on the radial side of the forearm to correct existing fixed deformity. The correction provided is temporary. Radial deviation of the forearm inevitably recurs. At present soft-tissue release is performed as a preliminary step or in conjunction with other types of surgery.

Osteotomy of the ulna designed to provide permanent correction was proposed by Hoffa and by Sayre.[28, 49] By itself osteotomy of the ulna does not maintain alignment. At present it is combined with centralization of the carpus over the distal end of the ulna when necessary in severe cases.

Replacement of the absent or dysplastic radius by a bone graft has been another approach. The bones used as sources of the bone graft have been the tibia (by Albee) and the proximal fibula with its epiphysis (by Starr and by Riordan).[1, 45, 53] In reviewing results in 18 patients with fibular transplants with an average post-operative follow-up of nine years, Carroll and Louis found recurrence of deformity in all.[10] All failed to maintain the alignment. At present Riordan has abandoned the fibular transplant and recommends implantation of the distal ulna into the carpus in early infancy.[46] Microsurgical transfer of the fibula with its vascular supply intact is a possibility, but potential for further growth of the transplanted epiphysis has not been demonstrated.

Arthrodesis of the wrist stabilizes the wrist and corrects the ugly deformity. Mobility in the wrist is lost, however, and therefore the procedure is not recommended for the treatment of bilateral deformity. Arthrodesis should not be carried out before growth of the distal ulna has stopped. When performed in the adolescent, it requires a total change of the pattern of prehension that has been used from childhood. Functional results of wrist arthrodesis are not as adequate as those of centralization of the ulna, which can be performed in infancy, allowing the development of a satisfactory pattern of prehension with the deformity corrected and the wrist stabilized.

References

1. Albee, F. H.: Formation of radius congenitally absent; condition seven years after implantation of bone graft. Ann. Surg., 87:105, 1928.
2. Armendares, S., Salamanca, F., and Cortex, R.: A case of trisomy 18 with bilateral absence of thumbs and aplasia of the left radius. Bol. Med. Hosp. Infant. Mex., 32:115, 1975.
3. Barsky, A. J., Kahn, S., and Simon, B. E.: Congenital Anomalies of the Hand, Reconstructive Plastic Surgery. Philadelphia, Saunders, 1964.
4. Bayne, L. G.: Reconstruction of congenital hand deformities. *In* Green, D. P. (ed.): Operative Hand Surgery. New York, Churchill-Livingstone, 1982, pp. 562–568.
5. Birch-Jensen, A.: Congenital Deformities of the Upper Extremities. Copenhagen, Munksgaard, 1949.
6. Blauth, W., and Schmidt, H.: The implication of arteriographic diagnosis in malformation of the radial marginal ray. Z. Orthop., 106:102, 1969.
7. Bora, F. W., Jr., Nicholson, J. T., and Cheema, H. M.: Radial meromelia: The deformity and its treatment. J. Bone Joint Surg., 52-A:966, 1970.
8. Bora, F. W., Osterman, A. L., Kaneda, R. R., and Esterhai, J.: Radial club-hand deformity. Long-term follow-up. J. Bone Joint Surg., 63-A:741, 1981.
9. Butts, D. E., and Goldberg, M. J.: Congenital absence of the radius: the occupational therapist and a new orthosis. Am. J. Occup. Ther., 31:95, 1977.
10. Carroll, R. E., and Louis, D. S.: Anomalies associated with radial dysplasia. J. Pediatr., 84:409, 1974.
11. Davidson, A. J., and Horwitz, M. T.: Congenital clubhand deformity associated with absence of radius, its surgical correction; case report. J. Bone Joint Surg., 21:462, 1939.
12. Define, D.: Treatment of congenital radial club hand. Clin. Orthop., 73:153, 1970.
13. DeLorme, T. L.: Treatment of congenital absence of

the radius by transepiphyseal fixation. J. Bone Joint Surg., 51-A:117, 1969.

14. Duraiswami, P. K.: Experimental causation of congenital skeletal defects and its significance in orthopaedic surgery. J. Bone Joint Surg., 34-B:646, 1952.

15. Eaton, R. G.: Hand problems in children: a timetable for management. Pediatr. Clin. North Am., 14:643, 1967.

16. Edelberg, S. E., Cohn, J., and Brandt, N. J.: Congenital hypomegakaryocytic thrombocytopenia associated with bilateral absence of the radius—the TAR syndrome. Hum. Hered., 27:147, 1977.

17. Faed, M., Stewart, A., and Keay, A. J.: Chromosome abnormalities in two cases with bilateral radial element defects. J. Med. Genet., 6:342, 1969.

18. Flatt, A.: The Care of Congenital Hand Anomalies. St. Louis, Mosby, 1977, pp. 286–327.

19. Forbes, G.: A case of congenital club hand with a review of the etiology of the condition. Anat. Rec., 71:181, 1938.

20. Frias, J. L., and Felman, A. H.: Absence of the pectoralis major, with ipsilateral aplasia of the radius, thumb, hemidiaphragm and lung: An extreme expression of Poland anomaly? Birth Defects, 10:55, 1974.

21. Gegenbauer, C.: Zur Morphologie der Gliedmassen der Wirbelthiere. Morph. Jahrb., 2:396, 1876.

22. Goldberg, M. J., and Meyn, M.: The radial clubhand. Orthop. Clin. North Am., 7:341, 1976.

23. Goldenberg, R. R.: Congenital bilateral complete absence of the radius in identical twins. J. Bone Joint Surg., 30-A:1001, 1948.

24. Goldner, J. L.: Congenital absence of the radius and digital deformities (club hand). Inter-Clinic Information Bulletin, 1965.

25. Hall, J. G., Levin, J., Kuhn, J. P., Ottenheimer, E. J., Van Berkum, K. A. P., and McKusick, V. A.: Thrombocytopenia with absent radius (TAR). Medicine, 48:411, 1969.

26. Harrison, S. H.: Pollicization in cases of radial club hand. Br. J. Plast. Surg., 23:192, 1970.

27. Heikel, H. V. A.: Aplasia and hypoplasia of the radius. Acta Orthop. Scand., 39:1, 1959.

28. Hoffa, A.: Lehrbuch der orthopadischen Chirurgie. Ed. 4. Stuttgart, Enke, 1902, p. 557.

29. Kato, K.: Congenital absence of the radius. J. Bone Joint Surg., 6:589, 1924.

30. Kelikian, H.: Congenital Deformities of the Hand and Forearm. Philadelphia, Saunders, 1974, pp. 780–824.

31. Lamb, D. W.: Club hand: absent radius. In Pulvertaft, R. G. (ed.): Operative Surgery, 2nd Ed. London, Butterworth, 1970, pp. 12–16.

32. Lamb, D. W.: The treatment of radial club hand. Absent radius, aplasia of the radius, hypoplasia of the radius, radial paraxial hemimelia. Hand, 4:22, 1972.

33. Lamb, D. W.: Radial club hand, a continuing study of sixty-eight patients with one hundred and seventeen club hands. J. Bone Joint Surg., 59-A:1, 1977.

34. Lidge, R.: Congenital radial deficient club hand. J. Bone Joint Surg., 51-A:1041, 1969.

35. Lloyd-Roberts, G. S.: Orthopaedics in Infancy and Childhood. London, Butterworth, 1972.

36. MacCon, M. B.: Radial club hand: a review of 106 cases. Thesis. Liverpool, England, 1974.

37. Menelaus, M. B.: Radial club hand with absence of the biceps muscle treated by centralisation of the ulna and triceps transfer. J. Bone Joint Surg., 58-B:488, 1976.

38. O'Rahilly, R.: Radial hemimelia and the functional anatomy of the carpus. J. Anat., 80:181, 1946.

39. O'Rahilly, R.: An analysis of cases of radial hemimelia. Arch. Pathol., 44:28, 1947.

40. O'Rahilly, R.: Morphologic patterns in limb deficiencies and duplications. Am. J. Anat., 89:135, 1956.

41. Pardini, A. G., Jr.: Radial dysplasia. Clin. Orthop., 57:153, 1968.

42. Petit, J. L.: Remarques sur un enfant nouveau-né, dont les bras étaient difformés. Paris, Mem. l'Acad. Roy. Sci., 1733, p. 17.

43. Pulvertaft, R. G.: Twenty-five years of hand surgery. J. Bone Joint Surg., 55-B:32, 1973.

44. Ray, R., Zorn, E., Kelly, T., Hall, J. G., and Sommer, A.: Lower limb anomalies in the thrombocytopenia absent-radius (TAR) syndrome. Am. J. Med. Genet., 7:523, 1980.

45. Riordan, D. C.: Congenital absence of the radius. J. Bone Joint Surg., 37-A:1129, 1955.

46. Riordan, D. C.: Congenital absence of the radius. In Lovell, W. W., and Winter, R. B. (eds.): Pediatric Orthopedics. 1st Ed., Vol II. Philadelphia, Lippincott, 1978, pp. 708–714.

47. Roberts, A., Wickstrom, J., and McKay, D.: Congenital absence of the radius. South. Med. J., 73:702, 1980.

48. Saunders, J. W., Jr.: The proximo-distal sequence of origin of the parts of the chick wing and the role of the ectoderm. J. Exp. Zool., 108:363, 1948.

49. Sayre, R. H.: A contribution to the study of club-hand. Trans. Am. Orthop. Assoc., 6:208, 1893.

50. Schaeffer, J. P., and Nachamopsky, L. H.: Some observations on the anatomy of the upper extremities of an infant with complete bilateral absence of the radius. Anat. Rec., 8:1, 1914.

51. Simcha, A.: Congenital heart disease in radial clubbed hand syndrome. Arch. Dis. Child., 46:345, 1971.

52. Skerik, S. K., and Flatt, A. E.: The anatomy of congenital radial dysplasia: Its surgical and functional implications. Clin. Orthop., 66:125, 1969.

53. Starr, D. E.: Congenital absence of radius. A method of surgical correction. J. Bone Joint Surg., 27:572, 1945.

54. Steindler, A.: Livre jubilaire offert au docteur Albin Lambotte. Brussels, Vromant S.A., 1936.

55. Stoffel, A., and Stempel, E.: Anatomische studien über die klumphand. Z. Orthop. Chir., 23:1, 1909.

56. Sugiura, Y.: Congenital absence of the radius with hemifacial microsomia, ventricular septal defect and crossed renal ectopia. Birth Defects, 7:109, 1971.

57. Sultan, Y., Scrobohaci, M. L., Rendu, F., and Caen, J. P.: Abnormal platelet function, population, and survival-time in a boy with congenital absent radii and thrombocytopenia. Lancet, 2:653, 1972.

58. Taylor, H. L.: Congenital absence of the radius. Trans. Am. Orthop. Assoc., 10:1897.

59. Temtamy, S. A., and McKusick, V. A.: The Genetics of Hand Malformations. Birth Defects, Original Article Series, 14:1, 1978.

60. Warkamy, J., and Schraffenberger, E.: Congenital malformations induced in rats by roentgen rays. A.J.R., 57:455, 1947.

61. Wilson, J. N.: Epiphyseal transplantation. A clinical study. J. Bone Joint Surg., 48-A:245, 1966.

62. Wynne-Davies, R.: Heritable Disorders in Orthopedic Practice. Oxford, Blackwell, 1973, p. 177.

63. Zaricznyj, B.: Centralization of the ulna for congenital radial hemimelia. J. Bone Joint Surg., 59-A:694, 1977.

CONGENITAL LONGITUDINAL DEFICIENCY OF THE ULNA

This is one of the rarest of the upper limb anomalies, ranking second to absence of the humerus.[16] According to Birch-Jensen its incidence is 1 in 100,000 live births.[1] The anomaly was first described by Goller in 1683; just over 100 cases have been reported in the literature.[10] The defect is referred to in the literature by various terms: *ulnar club hand, ulnar dysmelia, para-axial ulnar hemimelia, congenital absence of the ulna,* and *longitudinal arrest of the development of the ulna.** According to the new classification of congenital deformities it should be called congenital longitudinal deficiency of the ulna.

Classification

Ogden described three primary patterns based on radiographic findings: *Type I,* hypoplasia of an otherwise complete ulna that has a distal epiphysis; *Type II,* partial absence with absence of the distal part of the ulna including its epiphysis; and *Type III,* total absence of the ulna. If, with skeletal growth, an ossification center becomes visible in the fibrocartilaginous anlage of the ulna in the older child, the Type III anomaly should be reclassified as Type II.[21]

Swanson classified the anomaly according to the degree of anatomic and functional deficiency. In the *mild* form there is minimal shortening of the ulna (this corresponds to Ogden Type I). In the *moderate* form a substantial portion of the ulna is absent, the radius is bowed, and the radial head is dislocated; the ulnar digits may be absent or present. In the *severe* form the ulna is completely absent, as are the ulnar digits; the radius may be normal, slightly bowed, or fused with the humerus.[38]

Kummel proposed a classification based on the elbow morphology: in *Type A* the radiohumeral joint is normal or nearly normal; in *Type B* the radiohumeral joint is fused; in *Type C* the radial head is dislocated.[15]

There are multiple defects involved in congenital longitudinal deficiency of the ulna; not only the forearm but the whole upper limb should be considered in classification and assessment of the anomaly.

Associated anomalies are less frequent in congenital longitudinal deficiency of the ulna than in radial longitudinal deficiency. Often they involve the musculoskeletal system. They include ipsilateral hypoplasia of the scapula or glenoid cavity, short humerus, absence or hypoplasia of the ulnar rays of the hand, congenital scoliosis, spina bifida, proximal femoral focal deficiency, congenital dislocation of the hip, absence of the patella, longitudinal deficiency of the fibula, and talipes equinovarus. Associated visceral malformations are very rare. Congenital longitudinal deficiency of the ulna may be found in syndromes such as Cornelia de Lange.

Treatment

Treatment depends on the type of ulnar deficiency and the age of the patient. In Type I in which the ulna is short but complete, the hand, wrist, and forearm are splinted to prevent progressive ulnar deviation of the carpus. At about eight years of age the ulna is elongated by one-stage Z-lengthening, grafted with autogenous bone from the ilium, and internally fixed with screws. The one-stage lengthening may be repeated at 12 and 16 years of age if necessary. Experience with lengthening of the short ulna in multiple hereditary exostoses has made this procedure relatively simple. It should be emphasized, however, that it is mandatory to perform a simultaneous release of contracted soft tissues and to excise the fibrous distal ulnar anlage.

In Type II ulnar longitudinal deficiency, in which there is partial absence of the distal ulna (including its epiphysis), the distal fibrocartilaginous anlage of the ulna is resected at 6 to 12 months of age. Any fibrous insertions to the carpus and radius are excised as far distally as possible. This will eliminate any tethering effect of the ulnar anlage on the growth of the radius and will prevent progressive radial bowing. The importance of early treatment to prevent increasing deformity as the child grows cannot be overemphasized.

A one-bone forearm should not be created by proximal radioulnar fusion if there is an adequate proximal ulnar segment that will provide a stable forearm with functional range of pronation and supination. Creation of a one-bone forearm is indicated only when the forearm is unstable and the radial head is dislocated. Unless the radial head is dislocated, the radius should not be swung over and fused to the ulna. Another prerequisite for radioulnar fusion is functional range of flexion-extension of the elbow.

Conversion of the forearm into a one-bone member preserves the growth from the proximal physis of the ulna and the distal physis of the radius. The *operative technique* is as follows: an incision is made that begins on the radial aspect of the lower third of the humerus and extends to terminate on the radial aspect of the middle third of the forearm. The radial nerve is identified and traced distally to its posterior interosseous and superficial branches. The supinator brevis muscle is dissected extra

*See references 8, 14, 16, 21, 26, 29, 36, 37.

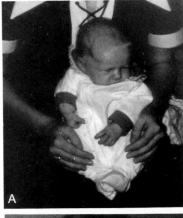

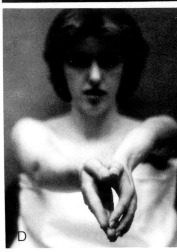

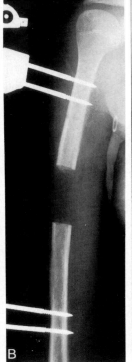

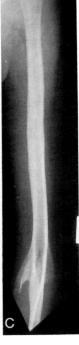

FIGURE 2–42. *Congenital longitudinal deficiency of the ulna with synostosis of the humeroulnar joint.*

A. Clinical appearance: photograph of the child at one month of age in mother's lap. **B.** Anteroposterior radiogram of the humerus showing Wagner diaphyseal lengthening. **C.** Radiogram showing result after third operation for a total of 12 cm. of lengthening. **D.** The patient's upper limbs are nearly equal in length.

periosteally off the proximal radius. Dissection should be meticulous and injury to the radial nerve avoided.

With an electric oscillating saw, the proximal radial shaft including the radial head is removed at the appropriate level, and depending on where the proximal ulnar shaft terminates, the radius and ulna are transfixed by screws or an intramedullary Steinmann pin passed through the olecranon and the distal radial shaft.

In Type III complete absence of the ulna, the cartilaginous anlage of the ulna is excised between 6 and 12 months of age. Often the radius has a marked bow, especially in older children. The radial bow is corrected by wedge osteotomy. When there is radiohumeral synostosis, both the radius and the humerus are lengthened according to the Wagner tibial lengthening technique (Fig. 2–42).

References

1. Birch-Jensen, A.: Congenital Deformities of the Upper Extremities. Odense, Munksgaard, 1949.
2. Birnbacher, G.: Drei Beobachtungen über Verkümmerung der oberen Extremitäten. Konigsberg, 1891.
3. Broudy, A. S., and Smith, R. J.: Deformities of the hand and wrist with ulnar deficiency. J. Hand Surg., 4:304, 1979.
4. Bychowsky, C.: Ein Fall von angeborener Ellbogenankylose eines im Wachstum zuruckgebleibenen und missgebildeten Armes. Z. Orthop. Chir., 31:480, 1913.
5. Carroll, R. E., and Bowers, W. H.: Congenital deficiency of the ulna. J. Hand Surg., 2:169, 1977.
6. Conway, H., and Wagner, K. J.: Congenital anomalies reported on birth certificates in New York City (1952–1962 inclusive). N.Y. State J. Med., 65:1087, 1965.
7. Deville: Absence d'une grande partie du cubitus. Bull. Soc. Anat. Paris, 24:153, 1849.
8. Frantz, C. H., and O'Rahilly, R.: Ulnar hemimelia. Artif. Limbs, 15:25, 1971.
9. Goddu, L. A. O.: Reconstruction of elbow and bone graft of rudimentary ulna. N. Engl. J. Med., 202:1142, 1930.
10. Goller: Cited in Meckel.
11. Grimault, L., and Epitalbra, A.: Un cas d'absence congénitale bilatérale du cubitus. Bull. Soc. Anat. Paris, 93:738, 1923.
12. Jones, H. W., and Roberts, R. E.: A rare type of congenital club hand. J. Anat., 60:146, 1926.
13. Kajon, C.: Angeborener doppelseitiger Ulnadefekt und Pollex bifidus dexter. Z. Orthop. Chir., 41:526, 1921.
14. Klippel, M., François-Dainville, and Feil, A.: L'absence congénitale du cubitus. Un nouveau cas. Paris Med., 55:107, 1925.

15. Kummel, W.: Die Missbildungen der Extremitäten durch Defekt, Verwachsung und Ueberzähl. Hefte 3. Bibliotheca Medica, Kassel, 1895.

16. Laurin, C. A., and Farmer, A. W.: Congenital absence of ulna. Can. J. Surg., 2:204, 1959.

17. Lausecker, H.: Der angeborne Defekt der Ulna. Virchows Arch. Pathol. Anat., 325:211, 1954.

18. Liu, S. H.: A case of congenital partial absence of right ulna and associated deformities. Chin. Med. J., 47:1052, 1933.

19. Meckel, J. F.: Handbuch der pathologischen Anatomie. Leipzig, 1812.

20. Mouchet, A., and Pakowski: Deux cas d'absence du cubitus (une absence totale et une absence partielle). Rev. Orthop., 10:147, 1923.

21. Ogden, J. A.: Ulnar dysmelia. J. Bone Joint Surg., 58-A:467, 1976.

22. Pardini, A. G., Jr.: Congenital absence of the ulna. J. Iowa Med. Soc., 57:1106, 1967.

23. Pircard: Hemimelie cubitale. Absence presque complète du cubitus droit. Rev. Orthop., 12:269, 1925.

24. Piulachs, M.: Absence congénitale partielle du cubitus fracture de l'extrémité inférieure du radius. Rev. Orthop., 26:672, 1939–1940.

25. Pringle, J. H.: Notes of a case of congenital absence of both ulnae. J. Anat. Physiol., 27:239, 1993.

26. Rabaud, E., and Hovelacque, A.: Absence congénitale du cubitus, du radius, du tibia et du péroné. Rev. Orthop., 11:21, 1924.

27. Reimann-Hunziker, G.: Ueber den angeborenen Ulnadefekt. Z. Orthop., 73:160, 1942.

28. Reinhardt, K., and Pfeiffer, R. A.: Ulna-fibulare Dysplasie. Eine autosomal-dominant verebte. Mikromesomelie ahnlich dem Nievergeltsyndrom. Fortschr. Geb. Röntgen., 107:379, 1967.

29. Riordan, D. C.: Congenital absence of the radius or ulna. (Abstract). J. Bone Joint Surg., 54-B:381, 1972.

30. Riordan, D. C.: Congenital absence of the ulna. *In* Lovell, W. W., and Winter, R. B. (eds.): Pediatric Orthopaedics. Philadelphia-Toronto, Lippincott, 1978, pp. 714–719.

31. Riordan, D. C., Mills, E. H., and Aldredge, R. H.: Congenital absence of the ulna. J. Bone Joint Surg., 43-A:614, 1961.

32. Roberts, A. S.: A case of deformity of the fore-arm and hands, with an unusual history of hereditary congenital deficiency. Ann. Surg., 3:135, 1886.

33. Romanus, R.: Ein Fall von Angeborener Ankylose im Ellbogengelenk. Acta Orthop. Scand., 4:291, 1933.

34. Roth, P. B.: A case of congenital defect of the ulna. Lancet, 1:1457, 1914.

35. Southwood, A. R.: Partial absence of the ulna and associated structures. J. Anat., 61:346, 1926–1927.

36. Spinner, M., Freundlich, B. D., and Abeles, E. D.: Management of moderate longitudinal arrest of development of the ulna. Clin. Orthop., 69:199, 1970.

37. Straub, L. R.: Congenital absence of ulna. Am. J. Surg., 109:300, 1965.

38. Swanson, A. B.: Classification of limb malformation on the basis of embryologic failures. Inter-clin. Info. Bull. N.Y.U. Postgrad. Med. Sch., 6:3, 1966.

39. Vitale, C. C.: Reconstructive surgery for defects in shaft of ulna in children. J. Bone Joint Surg., 34-A:804, 1952.

40. Watson, H. K., and Bohne, W. H.: The role of the fibrous band in ulnar deficient neonates. J. Bone Joint Surg., 53-A:816, 1971.

41. Watt, J. C.: Anatomy of seven months' foetus exhibiting bilateral absence of ulna accompanied by monodactyly (and also diaphragmatic hernia). Am. J. Anat., 22:385, 1917.

42. Wierzejewski, I.: Über den kongenitalen Ulnadefekt. Z. Orthop. Chir., 27:101, 1910.

ULNAR DIMELIA

In ulnar dimelia the radial ray, i.e., the radius, scaphoid, trapezium, first metacarpal, and the phalanges of the thumb are absent. The ulna is duplicated, and there are seven or eight fingers in the hand. At the elbow the olecranon fossae face each other (Fig. 2–43). This malformation is extremely rare; about 60 cases have been reported in the literature. The abnormality may be associated with duplication of the fibula, absence of the tibia, or duplication of the feet.[6, 11] Ulnar dimelia is usually not hereditary.

Clinical Picture

Involvement is usually unilateral. The multidigited hand is palmar-flexed at the wrist and radially deviated. The wrist and elbow are broad. Forearm rotation and elbow motion are restricted. The fingers are held in flexion because of absence or hypoplasia of the extensor digitorum longus muscles. Intrinsic muscles are weak. As a rule the ulnar (postaxial) fingers tend to be more normal and functional than the radial (preaxial) digits. Syndactyly of some of the digits may be present. Metacarpals diverge, and there is a cleft in the palm.

Treatment

The objective of treatment is to improve function and provide a cosmetically more attractive hand. The most normal preaxial digit is chosen for pollicization. The intervening supernumerary one or two digits are ablated by filleting. The excess skin is utilized to create a thumb web. The remaining divergent metacarpals may be osteotomized to close the palmar cleft. A free tendon graft is used to hold the metacarpals together. Appropriate tendon transfers are performed to increase the strength of finger extensors.

Flexion–radial deviation contracture of the wrist is corrected by soft-tissue release and splinting in neutral position. In the adolescent, arthrodesis of the wrist is performed if the wrist joint is unstable and soft-tissue repair is unable to correct and maintain correction of flexion deformity of the wrist. Range of elbow motion and rotation of the forearm are increased by excision of the olecranon process of the preaxial ulna. If the forearm is fixed in marked pronation, rotation osteotomy of one or both ulnae is performed, and the forearm is placed in neutral

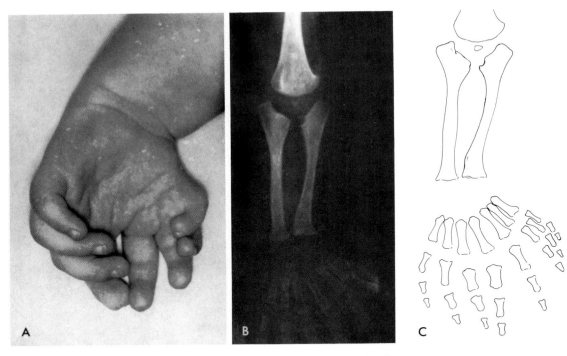

FIGURE 2–43. *Ulnar dimelia (mirror hand).*

Note that the thumbs are absent. There are eight digits. The wrist is flexed and radially deviated. There are two ulnae, no radius. The olecranon fossae face each other. (From Kelikian, H. A.: Congenital Deformities of the Hand and Forearm. Philadelphia, W. B. Saunders, 1974. Reprinted by permission.)

position. Surgical reconstruction of the mirror hand is very difficult; it requires the expertise of a capable hand surgeon.

References

1. Buck-Gramcko, D.: Operative Behandlung einer Spiegelbild-Deformität der hand (mirror hand-doppelte ulna mit polydaktylie). Traitement opératoire d'une difformité en miroir de l'avant bras (dedoublement du cubitus et des doigts cubitaux). Ann. Chir. Plast., 9:180, 1964.
2. Burman, M.: An historical perspective of double hands and double feet. The survey of cases reported in the 16th and 17th centuries. Bull. Hosp. Joint Dis., 29:241, 1968.
3. Davis, R. G., and Farmer, A. W.: Mirror hand anomaly: A case presentation. Plast. Reconstr. Surg., 21:80, 1958.
4. Harrison, R. G., Pearson, M. A., and Roaf, R.: Ulnar dimelia. J. Bone Joint Surg., 42-B:549, 1960.
5. Kelley, J. W.: Mirror hand. Plast Reconstr. Surg., 30:374, 1962.
6. Laurin, C. A., Fevreau, J. C., and Labelle, P.: Bilateral absence of the radius and tibia with bilateral duplication of the ulna and fibula. J. Bone Joint Surg., 46-A:137, 1964.
7. Manaresi, C.: La dimelia ulnare e il sui trattamento. Chir. Organi Mov., 51:76, 1962.
8. Mukerji, M.: Congenital anomaly of hand: "Mirror hand." Br. J. Plast. Surg., 9:222, 1957.
9. Perini, G.: Dimelia ulnare e suo trattamento chirurgico. Arch. Putti. Chir. Organi Mov., 6:363, 1965.
10. Pintilie, D., Hatmanu, D., Olaru, I., and Panoza, G.: Double ulna with symmetrical polydactyly. J. Bone Joint Surg., 46-B:89, 1964.
11. Sandrow, R. E., Sullivan, P. D., and Steel, H. H.: Hereditary ulnar and fibular dimelia with peculiar facies. J. Bone Joint Surg., 52-A:367, 1970.
12. Santero, N.: Dichiria con duplicita dell ulna e assenza del radio. Arch. Ital. Chir., 43:173, 1936.

MADELUNG'S DEFORMITY

Madelung's deformity is a congenital abnormality of the wrist caused by a growth disturbance that retards development of the ulnar and volar portions of the distal radial physis.

The eponym gives credit to Madelung, who published a paper entitled "Die spontane Subluxation der Hand" in 1879.[7, 28] Various other terms have been used to describe the condition, such as *carpus curvus, radius curvus, progressive subluxation of the wrist, manus valgus,* and *manus furca.*

The primary deformity is bowing of the distal end of the radius, which in the most typical form curves in a volar direction while the ulna continues to grow in a straight line. The distal ends of the radius and ulna are at different levels in the lateral plane; that of the ulna has maintained its original normal position, while that of the radius has curved down to a volar level. It is the distal end of the radius that is displaced. Because of its curvature and growth disturbance, the radius has become short while the ulna has continued to grow normally and has become relatively longer.

Etiology

The exact nature of the pathologic process that causes the disturbance in the growth of the distal radial physis is unknown. This partial growth arrest has also been referred to as "dyschondroplasia," "osteochondrodystrophy," and "hemiatrophy of the distal radial epiphysis." The asymmetrical growth disturbance is similar to that seen in Blount's disease or tibia vara. Madelung's deformity is a hereditary disorder, transmitted as an autosomal dominant trait with incomplete penetrance. Sporadic forms do occur. It is more common in the female; involvement is frequently bilateral.

Pathologic Anatomy

Normally, the ossification center of the distal radial epiphysis appears around the age of two years as a small rounded seed, lying closer to the radial than to the ulnar aspect of the bone. The ossific nucleus begins to flatten at the age of six years, extending radially to form the radial styloid process, but at this time there is no evidence of the ulnar third of the distal epiphysis. The styloid process of the radius is ossified around the age of ten years, when the ulnar portion of the epiphysis is still very small. From this age on until its closure at 19 years, the distal radial epiphysis maintains its wedge-shaped appearance, having a broad radial base and a tapered ulnar point. In Madelung's deformity, this wedge configuration of the distal radial epiphysis is greatly accentuated. In some cases, the ulnar half of the epiphysis is not ossified.

Normally, the distal articular surface of the radius is tilted 5 degrees toward its volar surface and 25 degrees toward the ulna, with its dorsal surface and radial margin convex and its volar surface and ulnar border concave.

There are two types of Madelung's deformity—typical, or regular, and atypical, or reverse.

In the *typical form*, the distal articular surface of the radius may tilt toward its palmar surface as much as 80 degrees and ulnarward as much as 90 degrees. In the normal wrist, the proximal row of the carpal bones is arranged in an arc,

with its proximal surface forming a convex dome. In Madelung's deformity, this dome becomes peaked, its apex resting on the lunate bone. The radius and ulna are separated, with the peak of the carpal bones wedged into the interosseous space. The entire carpus is shifted toward the ulnar and volar side of the wrist. Coalition of carpal bones may be present.[12]

In *reverse, or atypical, Madelung's deformity* (which is rare), the distal end of the radius is tilted dorsally, reversing the plane of the distal end of the articular surface with a shift of the carpus toward the dorsal side. The distal end of the ulna then appears to be displaced volarly instead of dorsally.

Clinical Features

Deformity of the wrist is the initial presenting complaint; it usually becomes obvious in late childhood or early adolescence, between the ages of 8 and 12 years. Occasionally it may be noted much earlier.

In *typical Madelung's deformity* the distal end of the ulna remains in its normal anatomic position and grows distally, causing a visible prominence on the dorsal and ulnar aspects of the wrist (Fig. 2–44). Normally, the radial styloid process is long and is located 1 cm distal to the ulnar styloid. In Madelung's deformity, the radius is shortened at the wrist; the radial styloid process may be on the same horizontal line as the ulnar styloid or may reach a point proximal to it. The range of motion of the wrist is limited, especially in dorsal extension and ulnar deviation. Because of the diasthesis between the distal radius and ulna and the displacement of the carpus between the two separated bones of the forearm, pronation and supination of the forearm are also limited; as a rule, supination is definitely decreased, and pronation is impaired to a slight degree.

In *reverse Madelung's deformity* palmar flexion of the wrist is decreased, while dorsiflexion is increased. Range of rotation of the forearm, especially pronation, is decreased. When it is minimal, Madelung's deformity may be asymptomatic. In moderate or severe deformity, however, pain develops insidiously at the wrist. Initially it is minimal, disappearing on rest. With progression of the deformity and impingement of the displaced carpus on the distal ulna, the pain increases. Volar displacement of the carpus may cause discomfort in the region of the median nerve and flexor tendons. Weakness of the wrist may result from progressive instability of the joint.

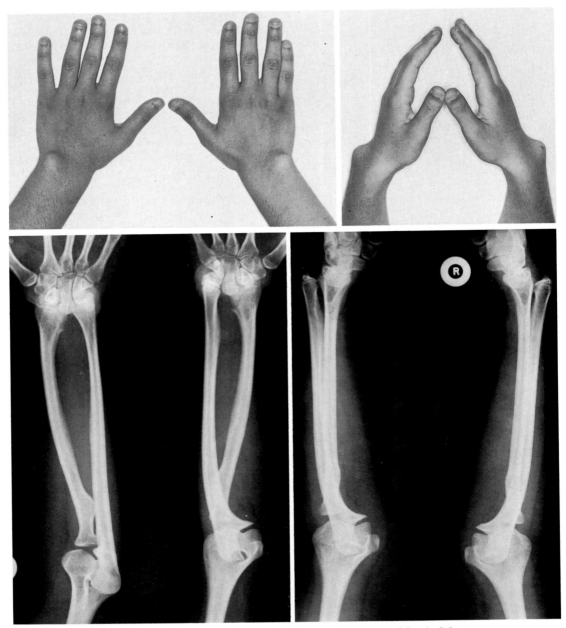

FIGURE 2–44. *Clinical appearance and radiograms of typical Madelung's deformity.*

Note the marked prominence on the dorsoulnar aspect of the wrist. It is due to the normal ulnar styloid process, which is longer than the radial styloid process, which is shortened and tilted volar.

Diagnosis

Characteristic radiographic findings include dorsal and radial curvature of the distal radius; exaggerated palmar and ulnar tilt of the distal articular surface of the radius; pyramiding of the carpal bones; greater length of the ulna as compared with the radius; wide interosseous space; and assumption of a relatively dorsal position by the ulnar head, which appears to be enlarged (see Fig. 2–44). In the differential diagnosis, one should consider the possibility of trauma (dislocation of the distal radioulnar joint), rickets, inflammatory conditions of the wrist such as rheumatoid arthritis, and infection involving the ulnar half of the distal radial physis. These are acquired deformities, are usually unilateral, and have other distinguishing features.

Differential Diagnosis

A skeletal radiographic survey should be performed to rule out bone dysplasia involving other bones. In Léri-Weill syndrome, a dyschondro-osteosis, the deformity of the wrist is similar to Madelung's deformity with the ulnar part of the distal radial physis closing early and the carpal angle decreased, but the radius is involved proximally as well as distally and there is associated deformity of the tibiae and fibulae. The phalanges of the hand may be short. Léri-Weill syndrome is an autosomal dominant condition, occurring mostly in females. The affected individuals average less than 5 feet in height. It is a part of the spectrum of mesomelic dwarfism.[25]

Other bone dysplasias that present with Madelung-like deformity include multiple hereditary exostoses, multiple epiphyseal dysplasia, enchondromatosis (Ollier), and Turner, or XO, syndrome (gonadal dysgenesis) (Fig. 2–45).[21]

Early fusion of the ulnar half of the distal radial physis may also be acquired and due to trauma or infection.

Treatment

Treatment is primarily directed toward the relief of pain and the restoration of function, with cosmetic improvement as a secondary consideration. The majority of patients with Madelung's deformity do not require surgical treatment. Conservative measures consist of curtailing physical activities that may cause

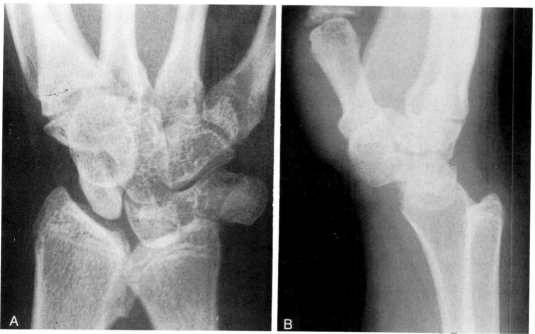

FIGURE 2–45. *Madelung's deformity in Turner's syndrome.*

A. Anteroposterior radiogram showing that the normal gentle arch of the proximal carpal bones has become a sharp V-shape. **B.** Lateral view showing the dorsal prominence of the distal end of the ulna. (A from Poznanski, A. K.: The Hand in Radiologic Diagnosis. Philadelphia, W. B. Saunders Co., 1984. B from Poznanski, A. K., and Holt, J. F.: The carpals in congenital malformation syndromes. Am. J. Roentgenol. *112:*443, 1971. Reprinted by permission.)

forced dorsiflexion of the wrist and wearing a plastic wrist splint to provide support and relieve symptoms. Surgical treatment is directed toward shortening the ulna, correcting the bowing deformity of the distal radius by wedge osteotomy, stabilizing the carpus, and preventing recurrence of deformity by controlling the asymmetrical growth of the distal radius. Realignment procedures are not performed in childhood because pain is usually not a symptom and because recurrence of the deformity will require repeat operations. As a rule surgical correction is delayed until 11 to 13 years of age.

Shortening of the Ulna. The ulna can be

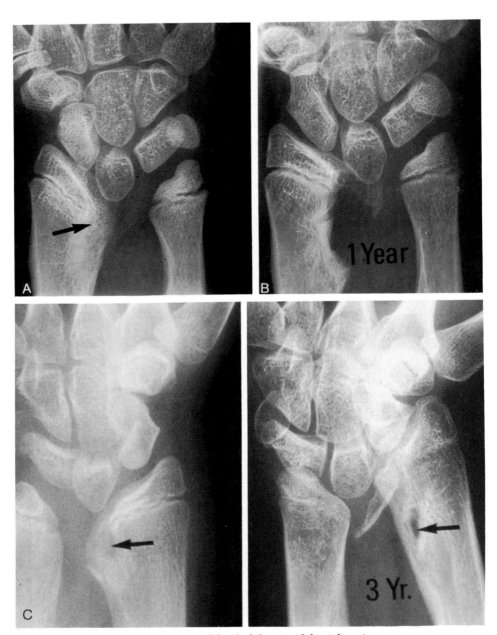

FIGURE 2–46. *Madelung's deformity of the right wrist.*

A. Preoperative radiogram. Note the premature fusion of the ulnar part of the distal radial physis. **B.** Radiogram of same wrist one year postoperatively shows excision of the fusion across the ulnar part of the distal radial physis. Note the improvement in the orientation and tilting of the distal radial physis. **C.** Radiogram of the wrist. The right (**D**) is three years postoperative. The arrow marks the metaphysis for comparison. Note the marked improvement of the deformity with growth of the distal radius.

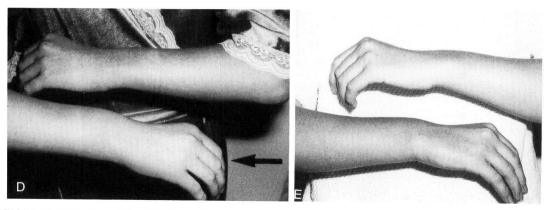

FIGURE 2–46 Continued **D** and **E.** Pre- and postoperative photographs of both wrists. Madelung's deformity is bilateral. The right wrist has been operated on. Note the deformity of the left wrist has increased, whereas that of the right wrist has become less. Clinically function in the wrist has improved and it is pain free. (Courtesy of D. W. Vickers, M.D., B.S., F.R.A.C.S., Watkins Medical Centre, Brisbane, Australia.)

shortened by Milch's cuff resection in children or Darrach's resection of the distal ulna in the adult.[9, 32] In early adolescence epiphyseodesis of the distal ulnar physis will stop growth and result in shortening. Burrows shortened the ulna by resecting a bone segment from the distal ulnar metaphyseal-diaphyseal junction and creating a gap between the lower end of the ulnar shaft and the radial head, the objective being to prevent interference with rotation of the forearm.[6] The procedure aggravates the ulnar shift of the carpus, requiring fusion of the distal ulnar segment (head) to the adjacent radius. This operation of gapping the ulna and bone-blocking is meddlesome and not recommended by this author.

Correction of Bowing of the Distal Radius.
This is achieved by either a closing wedge or an opening wedge osteotomy of the distal radius at its metaphyseal-diaphyseal junction. The objective is to restore the inclination of the articular surface of the distal radius to normal. This author prefers the opening wedge osteotomy because it simultaneously elongates the radius and corrects the angular deformity.

Control of Asymmetrical Growth of the Distal Radius.
Fusion of the radial half of the distal radial physis will prevent recurrence of deformity. Soft-tissue bands tethering the ulnar half of the distal radial physis, if present, should be released. Excision of the prematurely fused ulnar half of the distal radial physis and interposition of fat (Langenskiöld procedure) may restore normal growth of the distal radius (Fig. 2–46). This is advocated by Vickers.[47] The *operative technique* according to Vickers is as follows:

A volar approach through a transverse incision gives adequate access to the pathologic zone of the radius and is cosmetically better than a dorsal approach. The dissection passes to the radial side of the flexor carpi radialis tendon. The median nerve and radial artery are identified and protected. A longitudinal osteotomy is made from proximal to distal in the radius approximately one third of the width of the bone across from the radioulnar joint. A triangle of bone and cartilage is elevated carefully to preserve what remains of the distal radioulnar joint and the articular cartilage on the distal radius. A wavy growth plate will be seen just proximal to a narrowed bony epiphysis. Bone is removed with a fine rongeur until a healthy cartilaginous physis is seen across the bone. Magnification is recommended. A ball burr is then used to excise a little more bone on the metaphyseal side of the physis so that the cartilage stands up well clear of the bone. After the cavity has been washed out with saline, a small amount of bone wax may be applied to the trough on both sides of the physis. A generous free fat graft is then inserted into the space between the reflected triangular ulnar segment of the radius and the physis. Sutures are placed to secure these tissues over the fat graft.

The supplementary procedure of shortening the ulna by resection of the physis and internal fixation may be indicated at the time the physis of the radius is lysed or at a subsequent stage closer to skeletal maturity. This procedure is cosmetically good, and any growth remaining in the radius further improves function and appearance.

Text continued on page 221

Correction of Madelung's Deformity by Resection of Ulnar Head and Open-Wedge Osteotomy of Distal Radius

OPERATIVE TECHNIQUE

A. Two longitudinal incisions are made. The first, on the dorsoulnar aspect of the wrist and forearm, begins on the dorsum of the base of the fourth metacarpal and extends proximally to the wrist where, at the dorsal crease, it traverses ulnarward immediately above the prominent distal ulnar head, and then extends proximally for a distance of 5 to 7 cm. The second longitudinal incision is 7 cm. long on the radial margin of the volar surface of the wrist, beginning at the radial styloid process. The subcutaneous tissues are divided in line with the skin incisions. Injury to dorsal veins and branches of sensory nerves should be avoided.

B. The extensor retinaculum is divided and reflected ulnarward. The extensor carpi ulnaris is retracted radially. With an oscillating saw, an oblique resection of the distal ulna is performed. The dorsal and radial part of the ulnar head, including its epiphysis, is removed. The osteotomy begins 3 cm. proximal to the distal articular surface of the ulna on its dorsoradial aspect and slants ulnarward. The resected ulnar head is kept sterile for bone graft.

C. Next, the extensor carpi ulnaris tendon is split into halves. A tunnel is made with an electric drill through the lower end of the ulnar shaft, and the free split half of the extensor carpi ulnaris tendon is passed through it and sutured to the continuous other half of the tendon.

Plate 6. *Correction of Madelung's Deformity by Resection of Ulnar Head and Open-Wedge Osteotomy of Distal Radius*

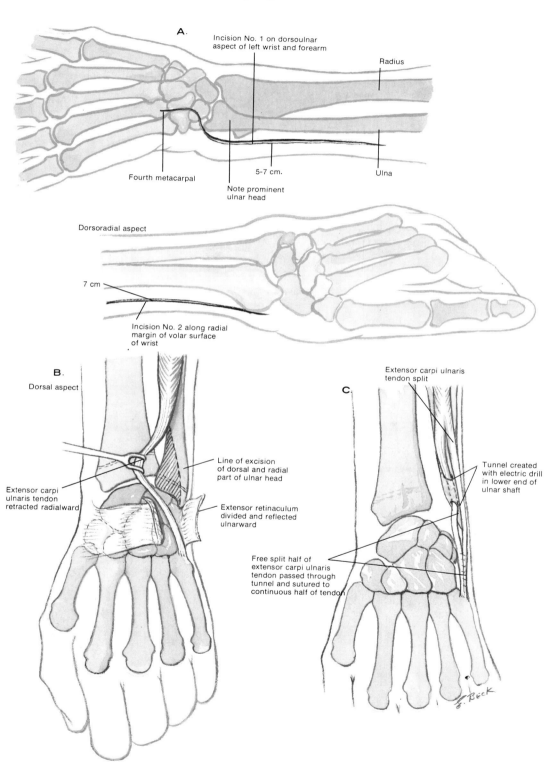

A.

Incision No. 1 on dorsoulnar aspect of left wrist and forearm

Radius

Fourth metacarpal

5-7 cm.

Note prominent ulnar head

Ulna

Dorsoradial aspect

7 cm

Incision No. 2 along radial margin of volar surface of wrist

B.

Dorsal aspect

Extensor carpi ulnaris tendon retracted radialward

Line of excision of dorsal and radial part of ulnar head

Extensor retinaculum divided and reflected ulnarward

C.

Extensor carpi ulnaris tendon split

Tunnel created with electric drill in lower end of ulnar shaft

Free split half of extensor carpi ulnaris tendon passed through tunnel and sutured to continuous half of tendon

E. Beck

Correction of Madelung's Deformity by Resection of Ulnar Head and Open-Wedge Osteotomy of Distal Radius
(Continued)

D. Next an open-up wedge osteotomy of the radius is performed through the volar incision to correct the marked bowing of the distal radius. The subcutaneous tissue is divided in line with the skin incision. The flexor carpi radialis along with the radial artery is retracted ulnarward. The distal shaft of the radius is exposed; injury to the distal radial physis should be avoided. With an oscillating saw, osteotomy of the distal radial shaft is performed on its volar and ulnar aspects. The dorsoradial cortex is left intact.

E. With a periosteal elevator and small laminar bone spreader, the distal radial segment is elevated dorsally and radially. A triangular piece of bone fashioned from the resected distal end of the ulna is inserted on the volar and ulnar aspect of the radius. The osteotomy and bone graft are transfixed with two crisscrossed, threaded Kirschner wires inserted with an electric drill. Anteroposterior and lateral roentgenograms are made to ensure adequacy of correction and internal fixation with the Kirschner wires. The tourniquet is released, and after complete hemostasis, a Hemovac suction tube is inserted, and the wound is closed in the usual fashion. An above-elbow cast is applied.

F and G. Some surgeons prefer to perform the osteotomy of the distal radius through the dorsal incision. In such an instance the skin incision begins dorsally at the base of the second metacarpal and extends proximally to the dorsal crease of the wrist, where it swings ulnarward immediately above the ulnar head and then continues longitudinally upward for a distance of 5 to 7 cm. The distal radial shaft is exposed by developing a plane between the extensor carpi radialis and the extensor digitorum longus. The pronator quadratus is elevated and retracted distally. The osteotomy of the radius is performed from its ulnar side.

A close-up biplane osteotomy of the distal radial shaft is preferred by some surgeons. The base of the wedge to be resected is dorsal and radial. The osteotomized segments are apposed and anteromedially fixed internally with two crisscrossed, threaded wires.

POSTOPERATIVE CARE

The osteotomy usually heals in six to eight weeks. The cast is changed as necessary. The two pins are removed, and passive exercises to restore range of motion of the wrist and active and progressive resistive exercises to increase motor strength of the wrist and hand are begun.

Plate 6. Correction of Madelung's Deformity by Resection of Ulnar Head and Open-Wedge Osteotomy of Distal Radius

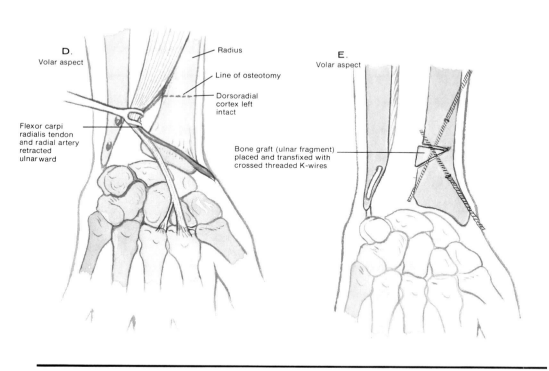

D.
Volar aspect

Radius

Line of osteotomy

Dorsoradial cortex left intact

Flexor carpi radialis tendon and radial artery retracted ulnarward

E.
Volar aspect

Bone graft (ulnar fragment) placed and transfixed with crossed threaded K-wires

Alternate procedure

Correction with closing wedge bi-plane osteotomy and distal ulnar resection (shaded areas)

F.
Dorsal aspect

Bone to be resected

G.
Dorsal aspect

Postoperative fixation with crossed, threaded K-wires

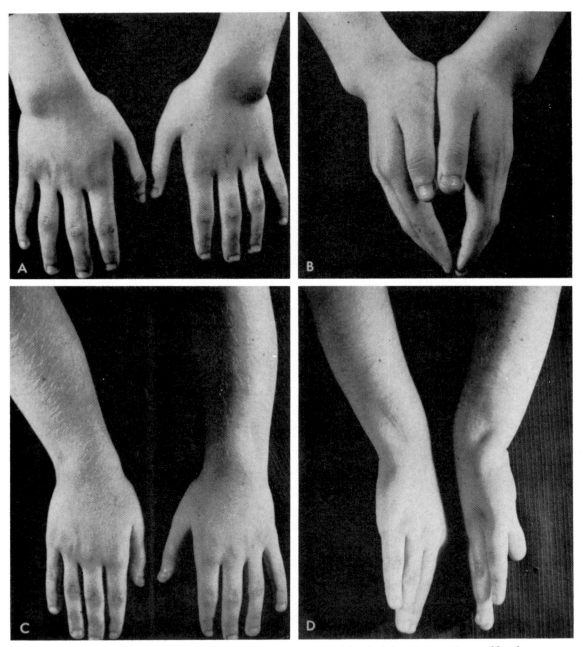

FIGURE 2–47. *Clinical result of operative treatment of Madelung's deformity in a 12-year-old girl.*

A. Preoperative dorsal view. **B.** Preoperative radial view. **C.** Postoperative dorsal view. **D.** Postoperative ulnar view. (From Kelikian, H.: Congenital Deformities of the Hand and Forearm. Philadelphia, W. B. Saunders Co., 1974. Reprinted by permission.)

A well-padded above-elbow cast should be applied, and some compression of the radius toward the ulna is usually possible. After three weeks the cast can be shortened to below the elbow for a further four weeks.

Experience with the Langenskiöld procedure is limited; the number of cases in which it has been performed is small and follow-up short.

Stabilization of the Carpus. Stabilization is indicated if the wrist joint is unstable and if there is ulnar shift of the carpus after resection of the ulnar head. Kelikian recommends passing the split half of the extensor carpi ulnaris tendon through a tunnel in the lower part of the ulnar shaft and suturing it to the other half of the tendon.[20] In the adult with painful arthritis, fusion of the radiocarpal joint is the best way to relieve symptoms and provide stability of the wrist joint.

Choice of Procedure. Factors determining the type of operative procedure depend on the age of the patient, the severity of the deformity, the degree of instability of the wrist, and the intensity of pain. The operation recommended by this author in the adolescent patient near skeletal maturity with severe deformity is Milch's cuff resection of the ulna with an open-up osteotomy of the distal radius to correct its angular deformity, as described in Plate 6 (Fig. 2–47). In the younger patient the Lengenskiöld procedure is performed as described by Vickers. The distal ulna is not resected. An open-up osteotomy of the distal radius (at its diaphyseal-metaphyseal junction) is performed to correct the angular deformity.

References

1. Argenta, L. C., McClatchey, K. D., Ferrell, W. J., and Newman, M. H.: Benign symmetrical lipomatosis (Madelung's disease). Head Neck Surg., 3:240, 1981.
2. Bazy, L., and Galtier, M.: Traitement sanglant de la luxation isolée de l'extrémité inférieure du cubitus en avant. J. Chir., 45:868, 1935.
3. Beals, R. K. and Lovrien, E. W.: Dyschondrostéosis and Madelung's deformity. Report of three kindreds and review of the literature. Clin. Orthop., 116:24, 1976.
4. Berdon, W. E., Grossman, H., and Baker, D. H.: Dyschondrostéose (Léri-Weill syndrome). Congenital short forearms, Madelung-type of wrist deformities and moderate dwarfism. Radiology, 85:678, 1965.
5. Bielecka, A.: Surgical treatment of Madelung's deformity. Wiad. Lek., 25:1787, 1972.
6. Burrows, H. J.: An operation for the correction of Madelung's deformity and similar conditions. Proc. R. Soc. Med., 30:565, 1937.
7. Christ, F.: Ulno-volar bayonet hand: its differential diagnosis from Madelung's deformity. R.O.F.O., 134:426, 1981.
8. Dannenberg, M., Anton, J. I., and Spiegel, M. B.: Madelung's deformity: Consideration of its roentgenological diagnostic criteria. A. J. R., 42:671, 1939.
9. Darrach, W.: Habitual forward dislocation of the head of the ulna. Ann. Surg., 57:928, 1913.
10. Dorogan, C. A., and Borodulia, L. V.: Case of Madelung's syndrome. Klin. Khir., 1:59, 1980.
11. Duplay, S.: Un cas de rachitisme tardif des poignets. Gaz. Hôp., 64:1397, 1891.
12. Felman, A. H., and Kirkpatrick, J. A.: Madelung's deformity: Observation on 17 patients. Radiology, 93:1037, 1969.
13. Felman, A. H., and Kirkpatrick, J. A., Jr.: Dyschondrostéose: Mesomelic dwarfism of Leri and Weill. Am. J. Dis. Child., 120:329, 1970.
14. Gelberman, R. H., and Bauman, T.: Madelung's deformity and dyschondrosteosis. J. Hand Surg., 5:338, 1980.
15. Golding, J. S. R., and Blackburne, J. S.: Madelung's disease of the wrist and dyschondrosteosis. J. Bone Joint Surg., 58-B:350, 1976.
16. Goncalves, D.: Correction of disorders of the distal radioulnar joint by artificial pseudarthrosis of the ulna. J. Bone Joint Surg., 56-B:462, 1974.
17. Goodwin, D. R., Michels, C. H., and Weissman, S. L.: Spontaneous rupture of extensor tendons in Madelung's deformity. Hand, 11:72, 1979.
18. Henry, A., and Thorburn, M. J.: Madelung's deformity—a clinical and cytogenetic study. J. Bone Joint Surg., 49-B:66, 1967.
19. Ismael, A., Elmanouar, M., Jirari, M., Ismael, M. A., and Hermas, M.: The Madelung syndrome. Maroc. Med., 1:229, 1979.
20. Kelikian, H.: Congenital Deformities of the Hand and Forearm. Philadelphia, Saunders, 1974, pp. 753–779.
21. Kosowicz, J.: The radi appearance of the hand and wrist in gonadal dysgenesis. A. J. R., 93:354, 1965.
22. Kozlowski, K., and Zychowicz, C.: Dyschondrostosis. Acta Radiol., 11:459, 1971.
23. Kovalenko, V. S., and Koval, N. S.: A rare case of Madelung's disease. Stomatologiia (Mosk.), 57:94, 1978.
24. Leone, G.: Stenosis of the lumbar spinal canal and dolichophalangy in a case of dyschondrostéosis. Radiol. Med., 65:905, 1979.
25. Léri, A., and Weill, J.: Une affection congénitale et symétrique du développement osseux: La dyschondrostéose. Bull. Mem. Soc. Med. Hôp. Paris, 53:1491, 1929.
26. Levin, B.: Gonadal dysgenesis. Clinical and roentgenographic manifestations. A. J. R., 87:11, 1962.
27. Linscheid, R. L.: Madelung's deformity. Correspondence Newsletter. No. 24. Correspondence Club. American Society for Surgery of the Hand, 1979.
28. Madelung, V.: Die spontane Subluxation der Hand nach vorne. Verh. Dtsch. Ges. Chir., 7:259, 1878; Arch. Klin. Chir., 23:395, 1979.
29. Malowiejski, J.: Madelung's disease. Chir. Narzadow Ruchu Ortop. Pol., 36:263, 1971.
30. Mansat, M., Lebarbier, P., Cahuzac, J. P., Gay, R., and Pasquie, M.: Madelung's disease. A study of nine wrists operated on. Ann. Chir., 33:669, 1979.
31. Matev, I., and Karagancheva, S.: The Madelung deformity. Hand, 7:152, 1975.
32. Milch, H.: Cuff resection of the ulna for malunited Colles' fracture. J. Bone Joint Surg., 23:311, 1941.
33. Nagura, S.: Madelung's deformity. Z. Orthop., 109:813, 1971.
34. Naljdihin, G., Bajec, D., Cvetanovi, C. S., Tomi, C. M., and Luki, C. B.: Therapeutic possibilities in the treatment of Madelung's deformity in children. Acta Chir. Iugosl., 22:313, 1975.
35. Nielsen, J. B.: Madelung's deformity: A follow-up study of 26 cases and a review of the literature. Acta Orthop. Scand., 48:379, 1977.
36. Phemister, D. B.: Operative arrestment of longitudinal growth of bones in the treatment of deformities. J. Bone Joint Surg., 15:1, 1933.

37. Poznanski, A. K., Garn, S. M., and Shaw, H. A.: The carpal angle in congenital malformation syndromes. Ann. Radiol., *19*:141, 1976.
38. Poznanski, A. K., and Holt, J. F.: The carpals in congenital malformation syndromes. A. J. R., *112*:443, 1971.
39. Ranawat, C. S., DeFiore, J., and Straub, L. R.: Madelung's deformity: An end-result study of surgical treatment. J. Bone Joint Surg., 57-A:772, 1975.
40. Rigault, P., Kipfer, M., and Beneux, J.: Treatment of so-called Madelung's deformity of the forearm. Rev. Chir. Orthop., *58*:341, 1972.
41. Schnek, F.: Federnde Dorsalluxation der Elle. Konsolenradius-Madelungsche Deformität. Z. Orthop. Chir., *53*:101, 1930.
42. Schuler, F. A., III, Graham, J. K., and Horton, C. E.: Benign symmetrical lipomatosis (Madelung's disease). Case report. Plast. Reconstr. Surg., *57*:662, 1976.
43. Schulstad, I.: Madelung's deformity with extensor tendon rupture. Case report. Scand. J. Plast. Reconstr. Surg., *5*:153, 1971.
44. Stypa, Z.: Post-traumatic Madelung's deformity of the hand. Acta Chir. Orthop. Traumatol. Cech., *40*:436, 1973.
45. Thompson, C. F., and Kalayjian, B.: Madelung's deformity and associated deformity at the elbow. Surg. Gynecol. Obstet., *69*:221, 1939.
46. Vickers, D. W.: Premature incomplete fusion of the growth plate: Causes and treatment by resection (physolysis) in fifteen cases. Aust. N.Z. J. Surg., *50*:393, 1980.
47. Vickers, D. W.: Personal communication, 1982.

SYNDACTYLY

Syndactyly is webbing or fusion of two digits. At the sixth week of intrauterine life the hand plate develops five ridges; these digital buds rapidly grow distally and separate. Failure of differentiation between adjacent digits results in syndactyly. It takes place between the sixth and eighth weeks of intrauterine life.

Incidence

Syndactyly is the most common congenital anomaly of the hand, occurring once in every 2250 births.[40] Involvement is bilateral and symmetrical in about 50 per cent of cases. Syndactyly is most common between the long and ring fingers (57 per cent); next, in decreasing order of frequency, between the little and ring fingers (27 per cent), between the long and index fingers (14 per cent), and least frequently between thumb and index fingers (3 per cent) because the thumb develops earlier than the fingers.[46] Males are affected twice as often as females.

Inheritance

Syndactyly is sporadic, occurring spontaneously in about 80 per cent of cases. In the literature, however, reports of a family history vary from 10 to 40 per cent.[40, 46] In the familial cases, especially with fusion between the long

and ring fingers, the trait appears to be autosomal dominant with reduced penetrance and variable expressivity. Genetic counseling is difficult, however, because all known types of genetic transmission have been observed.

Classification

Syndactyly is classified according to the degree of webbing and the presence or absence of bony fusion. In the normal hand the commissure area of a web between two fingers slopes from dorsal and proximal to distal and palmar; the distal edge of the web is about two fifths of the way between the metacarpal head and the distal end of the proximal phalanx. In *complete* syndactyly the skin interconnection extends to the tips of the involved digits, as shown in Figure 2–48 A; the fingernail may be common to both. In *incomplete* syndactyly the web does not reach the fingertip, stopping at any point between the normal commissure and the finger ends (Fig. 2–48 B). Syndactyly may be simple or complex. In *simple* syndactyly the web contains only skin and soft tissue; there is no bony fusion. In *complex* syndactyly there is osseous connection between the digits to a varying degree (Fig. 2–48 C). In complex syndactyly there may be abnormalities of nerves, vessels, and tendons. Accessory phalanges may be interposed between the webbed fingers (Fig. 2–48 D). Syndactyly may be associated with a multitude of other malformations and syndromes (Table 2–6). The webbed fingers may be associated with polydactyly or brachydactyly. In almost every case of Apert's syndrome and Poland's syndrome the fingers are webbed, and the incidence of syndactyly is very high in congenital constriction band syndrome.

Treatment

The objective of surgery is to separate the webbed fingers so that they can be spread normally and to improve function and appearance. The *timing of surgery* is important and depends on the fingers involved and the degree of completeness and complexity of syndactyly. Fingers of unequal length, such as thumb and index fingers or little and ring fingers, should be separated early in life because the longer finger will develop lateral deviation and flexion contracture (Figs. 2–49 and 2–50). Early separation of the digits permits unimpeded growth. As a rule, thumb–index finger syndactyly should be separated by six months of age, and ring–little finger syndactyly before one year of age. In index–long finger syndactyly the inter-

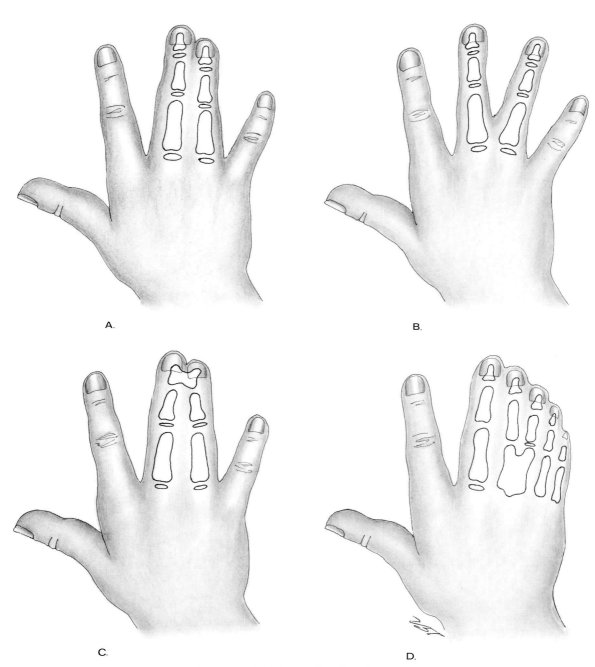

A.   B.   C.   D.

FIGURE 2–48. *Classification of syndactyly.*

A and **B.** *Simple syndactyly.* The interconnection is only by skin and soft tissue. There is no bony fusion. **A.** Complete—the web extends to the tips of the fingers. **B.** Incomplete—the web does not reach the ends of the fingers, stopping at any point between the normal commissure and the fingertip. **C** and **D.** *Complex syndactyly.* There is bony fusion between the phalanges of adjacent digits. **C.** Note the osseous synostosis between the distal phalanges. **D.** Complex syndactyly complicated by duplication of digits.

Table 2–6. *Syndromes Associated with Syndactyly*

Chromosomal Disorders
  5p−
  13q−, right D+
  Trisomy 13
  Triploidy
Craniofacial Syndromes
  Acrocephalosyndactyly
    Apert*
    Others
  Acrocephalopolysyndactyly
    Carpenter*
  Aglossia-adactyly
  Ankyloglossia superior
  Cohen
  Cryptophthalmos
  Greig*
  Lacrimoauriculodentodigital
  Lenz microphthalmos
  Möbius*
  Oculodentodigital*
  Orofaciodigital I
  Pierre-Robin
Other Syndromes
  Aarskog*
  Bloom
  Brachydactyly A-2*
    B*
    C
  Camptobrachydactyly
  Chondrodysplasia punctata (Conradi)
  De Lange
  F
  Goltz focal dermal hypoplasia
  Incontinentia pigmenti
  Laurence-Moon-Biedl
  Meckel
  McKusick-Kaufman*†
  Pancytopenia-dysmelia
  Pectoral aplasia–dysdactyly*
  Popliteal pterygium
  Pseudothalidomide*†
  Robert *†
  Rothmund-Thomson†
  Scalp defect
  Sclerosteosis*†
  Short-rib polydactyly (Saldino-Noonan)†
  Smith-Lemli-Opitz
  Spondylothoracic dysplasia
  Thrombocytopenia–absence of radius
  WT

*Common
†Osseous syndactyly
From Poznanski, A. K.: The Hand in Radiologic Diagnosis. Philadelphia, W. B. Saunders Co., 1984, p. 295. Reprinted by permission.

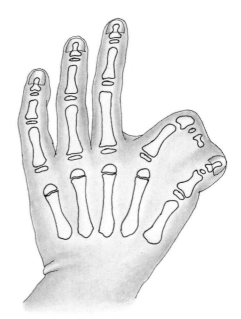

FIGURE 2–49. *Syndactyly of index finger and thumb.*

Note the radial subluxation of the distal interphalangeal joint. Separation of syndactyly should be performed before six months of age.

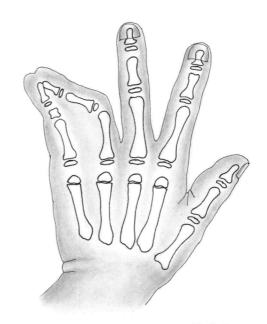

FIGURE 2–50. *Syndactyly of ring and little fingers.*

The digits are of unequal length and the longer finger will develop lateral deviation and flexion contracture because its growth is impaired. Separate before one year of age.

phalangeal joints, especially the distal ones, are not at the same level, and flexion contracture will develop if separation of syndactyly is delayed; it is best to separate the index and long fingers at about one year of age (Fig. 2–51). The long and ring fingers are almost even in length, and there is no urgency to separate them; one can wait until the child is two or three years of age (Fig. 2–52). While awaiting the appropriate age for surgery, parents are

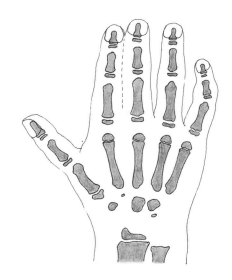

FIGURE 2–51. Syndactyly of index with long finger.

Note that the interphalangeal joints, especially the distal ones, are not at the same level. Joint contracture will develop if surgery is delayed; separate at about one year of age.

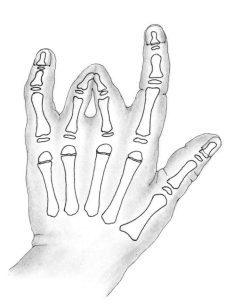

FIGURE 2–52. Syndactyly of long and ring fingers.

The digits are almost of equal length. One can delay surgery until the child is two or three years of age; there is no urgency.

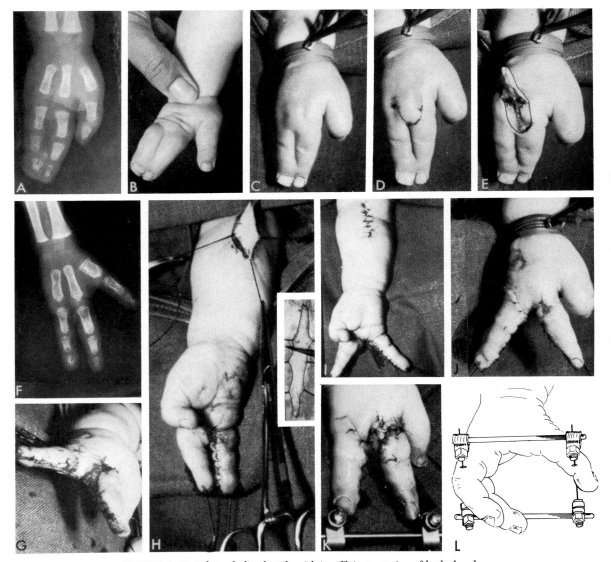

FIGURE 2–53. Bilateral oligodactyly with insufficient rotation of both thumbs.

Note that there are only two ulnar digits in each hand. The index and middle fingers are syndactylized in the right hand.
A and **B.** Radiogram and dorsal photograph of the right hand. **C** and **D.** Intraoperative views showing the incisions for the dorsal commissural skin flap. **E.** Dissection and elevation of the skin flap. **F.** Radiogram of the hand after surgical separation of the webbed fingers. **G.** Surfacing of the deepened interdigital commissure with a dorsal flap. **H.** Full-thickness skin graft is removed from the forearm. The insert shows the "raw" side of the graft scraped free of fat and areolar tissue. **I.** Closure of the incision on the forearm by Z-plasty. **J.** Surfacing of the raw areas on the sides of the separated digits. **K.** and **L.** Photograph and sketch showing the use of percutaneous wires and a spreader bar to maintain the fingers apart. Rotation osteotomy of the first metatarsal has been performed.

instructed to perform massage and stretching exercises to widen the skin web between the digits and maintain range of motion of the interphalangeal joints. When there is syndactyly of three digits, one should stage the operations and separate the webbed fingers at different sessions, preferably at intervals of three months. Circulatory embarrassment of the central digit is a definite hazard. Oligosyndactyly is webbing of a diminished number of digits (Fig. 2–53). An arteriogram will depict the digital vessels (Fig. 2–54). A preoperative Doppler examination is also helpful. When two joined fingers have a single blood supply they should not be separated.

Operative technique of complete separation of syndactyly is shown in Plate 7.

Broader syndactyly such as between the thumb and index finger may be deepened by the four-flap Z-plasty shown in Figure 2–55 or the V-Y release with lateral Z's shown in Figure 2–56.

Text continued on page 235

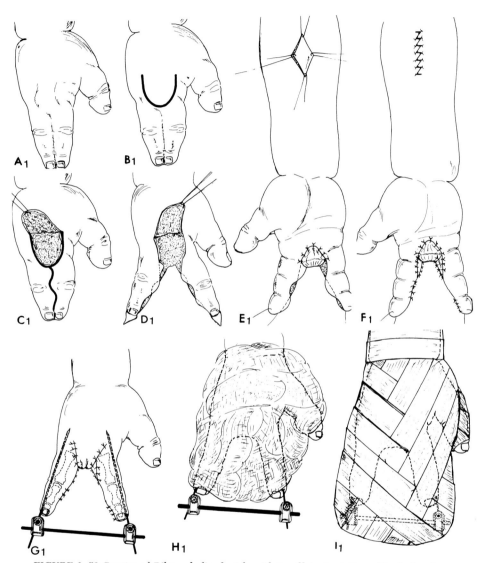

FIGURE 2–53 *Continued Bilateral oligodactyly with insufficient rotation of both thumbs.*

A_1 to I_1. The surgical steps for separation of the webbed digits of the right hand.

A_1. Sketch of the hand. B_1. Dorsal horseshoe-shaped incision. C_1. Elevation of the dorsal flap. D_1. Separation of the digits by undulating incision. E_1. Suturing the dorsal flap to the skin of the palm and lifting a free graft from the volar aspect of the forearm. F_1. Closure of the donor site with Z-plasty and surfacing the raw areas on the sides of the separated digits. G_1. Digits held apart with the aid of percutaneous K-wire and spreader bar. H_1. Packing the interdigital spaces and surrounding the hand with fluffy fine-meshed gauze. I_1. Pressure dressing.

(From Kelikian, H.: Congenital Deformities of the Hand and Forearm. Philadelphia, W. B. Saunders Co., 1974. Reprinted by permission.)

Separation of Simple Complete Syndactyly Between Ring and Long Fingers

The operation is performed with the aid of tourniquet ischemia. To save tourniquet time, the incisions are planned and outlined before it is applied. It is crucial to release the tourniquet before skin closure to obtain hemostasis and also at the end of the operation before a compression dressing is applied. If a finger is blue and congested or palish the sutures at its base are removed.

OPERATIVE TECHNIQUE

A. The first step is to raise a commissural flap. An incision shaped like a broad horseshoe is made on the dorsum of the hand between the webbed digits. It is based proximally, beginning from the distal one fourth of the metacarpals and extending distally at least two thirds of the way from the metacarpal heads to the proximal interphalangeal joints. This dorsal flap should be broad in order to provide adequate width to the commissure; its proximal base is somewhat wider than its distal end. Flatt recommends sloping the end of the dorsal flap so that the first dorsal interdigital flap has a wider base.[16] Because the skin of the dorsum of the hand is mobile and thin, the dorsal flap is made thicker as it is elevated proximally toward its base in order to provide it with adequate circulation. This maneuver also gives the newly constructed commissure a dorsopalmar slope similar to that of the normal interdigital web, increasing the length of the palm as compared with the dorsum of the hand. The proximal placement of the dorsal flap and the resultant deeper commissure is in anticipation of the distal advancement of the interdigital web consequent to the child's growth. Utilization of two triangular flaps, one dorsal and the other palmar, is not recommended because the reconstructed interdigital commissure will be narrow and V-shaped.

B. Next, a palmar transverse incision is made, which will mark the palmar margin of the web space. As children grow the interdigital web advances distally; therefore, make the commissure deeper by placing the palmar incision 5 to 6 mm. proximal to the normal level of that web. In the palm the normal interdigital webs between the long and ring fingers and between the ring and little fingers incline from distal-radial to proximal-ulnar. In placing the incisions, the surgeon should pay attention to this detail.

C to E. The syndactylized fingers are separated by two interdigital undulating or zigzag longitudinal incisions. There is always insufficient skin, and it is difficult to cover the two digits totally with flaps. It is best not to favor one finger by providing greater flap size. Because the interdigital groove in the web is usually present on the dorsum but not on the palmar aspect of the conjoined fingers, the dorsal interdigital incision is made first, the apices of its flaps corresponding to the midpoint of the base of the palmar interdigital flap. From these apices, straight needles are inserted to emerge on the palmar aspect to serve as guideposts for the bases of the palmar interdigital flaps. If the base of the flap release incision on the dorsum includes the crease of the proximal interphalangeal joint, the crease on the palmar aspect should be at the apex of the palmar flap. The bases and apices of the flaps should extend approximately to the midlines of the digits. The palmar incisions should not cross the interphalangeal flexion creases.

Plate 7. Separation of Simple Complete Syndactyly Between Ring and Long Fingers

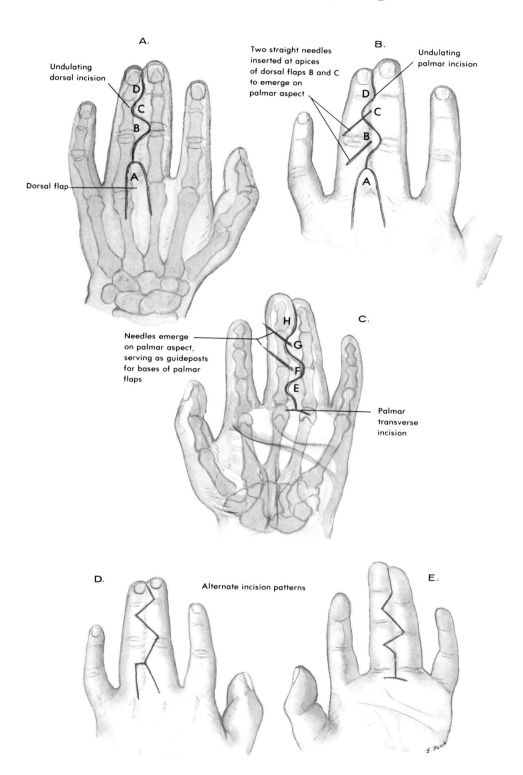

A.

Undulating dorsal incision

Dorsal flap

B.

Two straight needles inserted at apices of dorsal flaps B and C to emerge on palmar aspect

Undulating palmar incision

C.

Needles emerge on palmar aspect, serving as guideposts for bases of palmar flaps

Palmar transverse incision

D.

Alternate incision patterns

E.

E. Beck

Separation of Simple Complete Syndactyly Between Ring and Long Fingers *(Continued)*

F. Next, the neurovascular bundle of each finger is identified; this is simpler from the palmar side. The digital vessels and nerves are traced proximally by sharp and blunt dissection with tiny scissors and fine probe to the bifurcation of the common digital artery. The configuration, branching pattern, and size of the digital vessels are determined. In simple syndactyly there is usually no crossing of vessels or nerves between the fingers.

The fascial interconnections are released next. If there is any bony union between the digits it is sectioned with a very sharp scalpel. The adjacent flaps of the digits are defatted, especially if they are abnormally contoured. Take care not to injure digital vessels and nerves. Next, check the span of the palm.

G. Often the deep transverse metacarpal ligament has to be sectioned to provide adequate spread between the fingers. The bifurcation of the common digital vessels is retracted palmarly, and the deep transverse metacarpal ligament, lying immediately behind the vessels, is divided. Should one ligate an arterial branch to one of the conjoined fingers to allow a more proximal commissure? This author recommends it in simple syndactyly and in complex syndactyly provided preoperative studies by Doppler examination and arteriography show that the opposite side of the webbed finger has another feeder artery.

H and I. At this stage, the tourniquet is released, and complete hemostasis is obtained by coagulating the bleeders. The commissural dorsal flap is pulled toward the palm and sutured into the palmar incision with unabsorbable sutures such as 3-0 or 4-0 nylon. Kelikian prefers No. 34 stainless steel suture; in his procedure the threads of the steel are not tied but are twisted together until the skin edges are brought together. The unabsorbable nylon or wire sutures are supplemented by 5-0 absorbable sutures (such as Dexon or polyglycoline).

J. Next, a pattern exactly the size and shape of the defect is cut and with a sharp scalpel, an elliptical full-thickness skin graft of appropriate size is obtained from the hairless area of the groin. It is not necessary to use a dermatome and very thick split-thickness graft. The hairless area of the inguinal region is preferable to either the medial aspect of the upper arm, the volar surface of the upper forearm immediately distal to the cubital crease, or the inner aspect of the upper thigh. The donor site at the groin heals well and cosmetically is hidden, and the scar is much more pleasing. The skin graft removed is turned with its raw side up and is spread by tying it to a tongue depressor. All areolar tissue and fat are scraped off, and the skin is serrated like a piecrust. Two such skin grafts are prepared; one for each digit. By undermining and immobilizing the margins of the donor site, the groin wound is closed as a linear incision.

Plate 7. Separation of Simple Complete Syndactyly Between Ring and Long Fingers

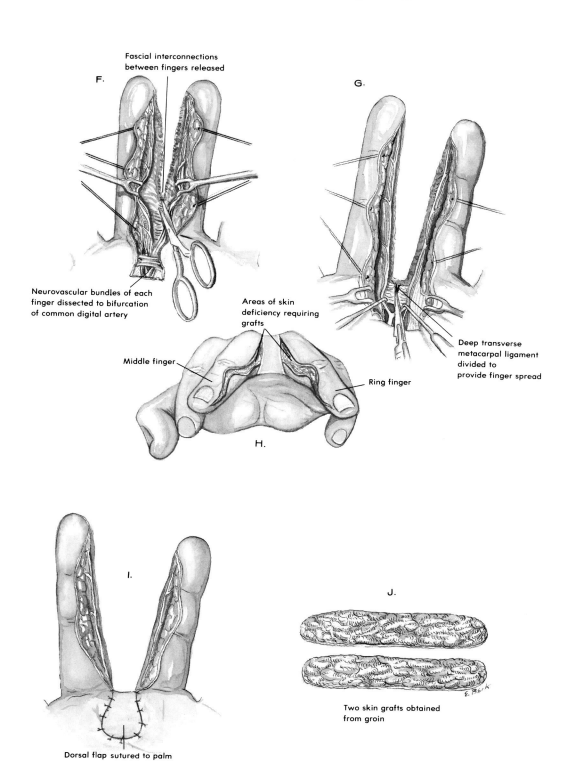

F.

Fascial interconnections between fingers released

Neurovascular bundles of each finger dissected to bifurcation of common digital artery

G.

Deep transverse metacarpal ligament divided to provide finger spread

Areas of skin deficiency requiring grafts

Middle finger

Ring finger

H.

I.

Dorsal flap sutured to palm

J.

Two skin grafts obtained from groin

E. Beck

Separation of Simple Complete Syndactyly Between Ring and Long Fingers (Continued)

K. The temptation is to close the skin flaps primarily, but often this will result in tension and cause deformity of the growing fingers. *There should be no lines of tension* on the reconstructed sides of the separated fingers. It is best to graft skin on the adjacent sides of *both* fingers. It is time consuming, but results justify the extra time spent. The skin grafts are carefully sutured into place. The sutures are tied on the finger skin, not on the graft. The use of 5-0 plain catgut or Dexon sutures obviates the trauma of later suture removal. Sometimes the interdigital webs are loose and broad; in such an instance the interdigital flaps of one finger may be closed loosely, without tension. Select the "dominant" finger, i.e., the one that will carry the flap. As a rule the "dominant" digit is the ring finger in ring–long finger syndactyly, the little finger in ring–little finger syndactyly, the thumb in thumb–index finger syndactyly, and the index finger in index–long finger syndactyly.

L. The digits may be kept apart by introducing fine Kirschner wires subcutaneously and holding the wires apart with a spreader bar as recommended by Kelikian.[23] This author does not recommend that method.

M. *Postoperative bandaging* should be simple but effective in immobilizing the upper limb. The separated fingers are spread apart widely, and sterile wet cotton dressings are placed in the space between them (wet dressings can be molded to the web configuration). Fluff dressings are placed over the wet dressing with sufficient pressure to maintain them snugly in place in the interdigital space. Fluff dressings are placed between the other fingers, sheet-wadding is rolled over them, and a very light above-elbow plaster of Paris cast is applied with the wrist in neutral extension and the elbow flexed to 90 degrees. The small child is active and uncooperative; adequate immobilization is vital.

Other methods used are Xeroform gauze or fine mesh gauze.

N and **O.** If the nails are conjoined in syndactyly, a sufficient amount of the nail and nail bed are excised to provide lateral-wall closure. The subjacent fibrofatty tissue of the digital pad may have to be partially excised. This management of adjacent nail borders is an important detail. Any osseous connections distal to the metacarpal phalangeal joint are sharply divided.

POSTOPERATIVE CARE

The initial dressing is not disturbed for three weeks; at that time there is usually adequate healing. Unabsorbable sutures over the dorsal commissural flap are removed. Crustings over the incision and grafts are left alone. Another glovelike soft dressing is applied for an additional five to seven days. Following this, all dressings are removed, the wound is exposed to air, and the child is allowed to use the hand fully.

Separation of Incomplete Simple Syndactyly

Incomplete webbing of the fingers that extends beyond the proximal interphalangeal joint is treated by the same surgical technique as for complete syndactyly. In incomplete syndactyly that stops short of the proximal interphalangeal joint, the commissure is deepened by an interdigital butterfly flap that utilizes two opposing Z-plasties. The two dorsal halves of each Z-plasty provide a common broad dorsal flap, which is turned palmarward and proximally to create a deep commissure. There are two possibilities for the palmar halves of each Z-plasty. The first choice is to create a wide-angle V. The second choice is an inverted Y—this is utilized when the web is abundant. It provides skin to be transferred on each side of the separated fingers. Thumb–index finger web contracture can be widened and deepened by four-flap Z-plasty, as illustrated in Figure 2–55, or by the central V-Y with lateral Z-plasties shown in Figure 2–56.

Plate 7. Separation of Simple Complete Syndactyly Between Ring and Long Fingers

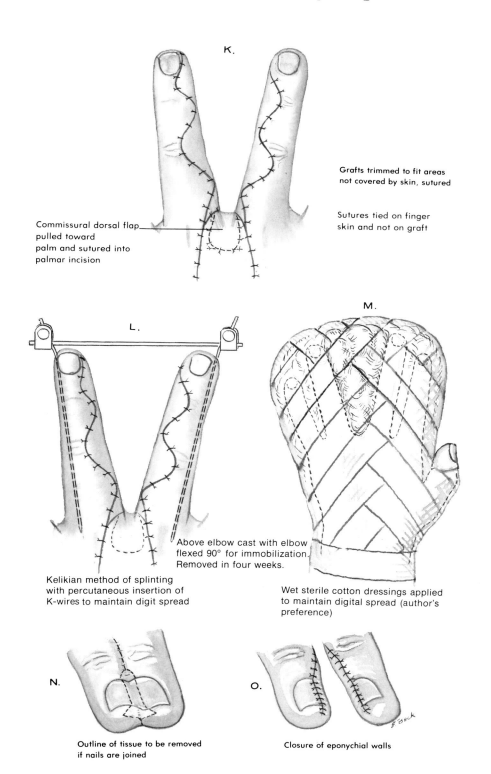

K.

Commissural dorsal flap pulled toward palm and sutured into palmar incision

Grafts trimmed to fit areas not covered by skin, sutured

Sutures tied on finger skin and not on graft

L.

Kelikian method of splinting with percutaneous insertion of K-wires to maintain digit spread

Above elbow cast with elbow flexed 90° for immobilization. Removed in four weeks.

M.

Wet sterile cotton dressings applied to maintain digital spread (author's preference)

N.

Outline of tissue to be removed if nails are joined

O.

Closure of eponychial walls

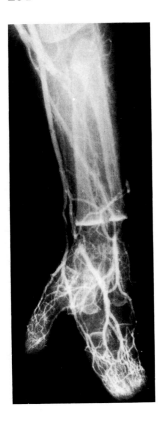

FIGURE 2–54. Arteriogram in syndactyly showing one central digital artery supplying both fingers.

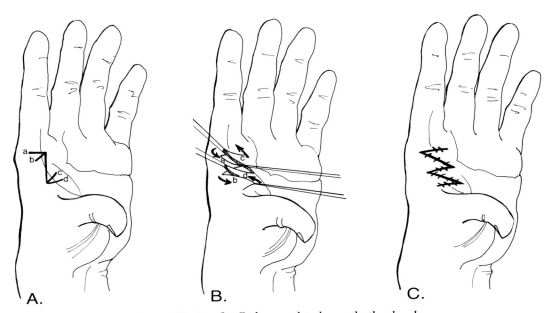

FIGURE 2–55. Four-flap Z-plasty used to deepen the thumb web.

A. Skin incision. **B.** Raising of skin flaps. **C.** Skin closure with interrupted sutures.

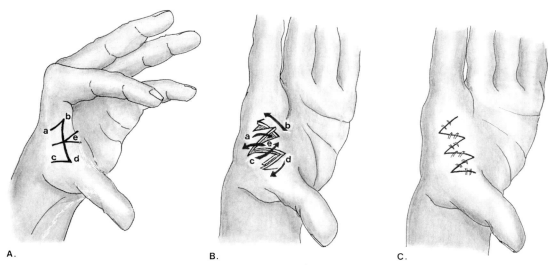

FIGURE 2–56. *The V-Y release with lateral Z's to deepen the thumb web.*

A. Skin incisions—V-Y. **B.** Raising of skin flaps. **C.** Skin closure with interrupted sutures.

References

1. Apert, E.: De l'acrocephalosyndactylie. Bull. Mem. Soc. Med. Hôp. Paris, 23:1310, 1906.
2. Bauer, T. B., Tondra, J. M., and Trusler, H. M.: Technical modification in repair of syndactylism. Plast. Reconstr. Surg., 17:385, 1956.
3. Beals, R. K., and Crawford, S.: Congenital absence of the pectoral muscles. Clin. Orthop., 119:166, 1976.
4. Bell, J.: On syndactyly and its association with polydactyly. In Penrose, L. S. (ed.): The Treasury of Human Inheritance. Cambridge, Cambridge University Press, 1953, Vol. 5, Part II, pp. 33–43.
5. Bing, R.: Weber angeborene muskeldefekta. Virchows Arch. Pathol., 170:175, 1902.
6. Blank, C. E.: Apert's syndrome (a case of acrocephalosyndactyly)–observations on a British series of thirty-nine cases. Ann. Hum. Genet., 24:151, 1960.
7. Brooksaler, F. S.: Poland's syndrome. Am. J. Dis. Child., 121:263, 1971.
8. Brown, J. B., and McDowell, F.: Syndactylism with absence of the pectoralis major. Surgery, 7:599, 1940.
9. Carpenter, G.: Two sisters showing malformations of the skull and other congenital abnormalities. Rep. Soc. Study Dis. Child., 1:110, 1900–1901.
10. Carpenter, G.: A case of acrocephaly, with other congenital malformations. Proc. R. Soc. Med., 2:45, 1909.
11. Christopher, F.: Congenital absence of the pectoral muscles. J. Bone Joint Surg., 10:350, 1928.
12. Clarkson, P.: Poland's syndactyly. Guys Hosp. Rep., 111:335, 1962.
13. Conway, H., and Bowe, J.: Congenital deformities of the hand. Plast. Reconstr. Surg., 18:460, 1956.
14. Cross, H. E., Lerberg, D. B., and McKusick, V. A.: Type II syndactyly. Am. J. Hum. Genet., 20:368, 1968.
15. Ebskov, B., and Zachariae, L.: Surgical methods in syndactylism. Acta Chir. Scand., 131:258, 1966.
16. Flatt, A. E.: Practical factors in the treatment of syndactyly. In Littler, J. W., Cramer, L. M., and Smith, J. W. (eds.): Symposium on Reconstructive Hand Surgery. St. Louis, Mosby, 1974, pp. 144–156.
17. Gellis, S., and Feingold, M.: Poland's syndactyly. Am. J. Dis. Child., 110:85, 1965.
18. Goodman, R. M.: A family with polysyndactyly and other anomalies. J. Hered., 56:37, 1965.
19. Holmes, L. B., Wolf, E., and Miettinen, O. S.: Metacarpal 4–5 fusion with X-linked recessive inheritance. Am. J. Hum. Genet., 24:562, 1972.
20. Hoover, G. H., Flatt, A. E., and Weiss, M. W.: The hand and Apert's syndrome. J. Bone Joint Surg., 52-A:878, 1970.
21. Ireland, D. C. R., Takayama, N., and Flatt, A. E.: Poland's syndrome: A review of forty-three cases. J. Bone Joint Surg., 58-A:52, 1976.
22. Iselin, F.: Traitement chirurgical des syndactylies congenitales. Résultats d'après 42 observations. Rev. Prat., 10:2611, 1960.
23. Kelikian, H.: Congenital Deformities of the Hand and Forearm. Philadelphia, Saunders, 1974, p. 331–407.
24. Kettelkamp, D. B., and Flatt, A.: An evaluation of syndactylia repair. Surg. Gynecol. Obstet., 133:471, 1961.
25. Lewandowski, R. C., and Yunis, J. J.: New chromosomal syndromes. Am. J. Dis. Child., 129:515, 1975.
26. Losch, G. M., and Duncker, H. R.: Acrosyndactylism, Transactions of the International Society of Plastic and Reconstructive Surgery, 5th Congress, Australia, 1971. Butterworth, 1971, pp. 671–676.
27. MacCollum, D. W.: Webbed fingers. Surg. Gynecol. Obstet., 71:782, 1940.
28. McKusick, V. A.: Mendelian Inheritance in Man: Catalogs of Autosomal Dominant, Autosomal Recessive, and X-Linked Phenotypes. Ed. 3. Baltimore, Johns Hopkins University Press, 1971.
29. Maisels, D. O.: Acrosyndactyly. Br. J. Plast. Surg., 15:166, 1962.
30. Miller, P. R.: Syndactyly. N. Engl. J. Med., 269:112, 1963.
31. Ombrédanne, L.: Technique Chirurgicale Infantile. Paris, Masson, 1912, pp. 271–274.
32. Ombrédanne, L., and Fevre, M.: Précis Clinique et Operatoire de Chirurgie Infantile. 5th Ed. Paris, Masson, 1949, pp. 708–713.
33. Pers, M.: Aplasia of the anterior thoracic wall, the pectoral muscle and the breast. Scand. J. Plast. Reconstr. Surg., 2:125, 1968.
34. Poland, A.: Deficiency of the pectoralis muscle. Guys Hosp. Rep., 6:191, 1841.
35. Poznanski, A. K.: The Hand in Radiologic Diagnosis. Philadelphia, Saunders, 1974, p. 278–283.

36. Robinow, M., Johnson, G. F., and Broock, G. J.: Syndactyly type V. Am. J. Med. Genet., *11*:475, 1982.
37. Saldino, R. M., Steinbach, H. L., and Epstein, C. J.: Familial acrocephalosyndactyly (Pfeiffer syndrome). J. Roentgenol., *116*:609, 1972.
38. Suguira, Y.: Poland's syndrome. Clinico-roentgenographic study on 45 cases. Cong. Anom., *16*:17, 1976.
39. Temtamy, S. A.: Carpenter's syndrome: Acrocephalopolysyndactyly, an autosomal recessive syndrome. J. Pediatr., *69*:111, 1966.
40. Temtamy, S. A.: Genetic Factors in Hand Malformations. Thesis. Baltimore, Johns Hopkins University, 1966.
41. Walker, J. D., Jr., Meijer, R., and Aranda, D.: Syndactylism with deformity of the pectoralis muscle: Poland's syndrome. J. Pediatr. Surg., *4*:569, 1969.
42. Walsh, R. J.: Acrosyndactyly: a study of 27 patients. Clin. Orthop., *71*:99, 1970.
43. Warkany, J.: The Upper Extremities. Chicago, Year Book, 1971, pp. 258–261.
44. Warkany, J.: Congenital Malformations. Notes and Comments. Chicago, Year Book, 1971.
45. Woolf, C. M., and Myrianthopoulos, N. C.: Polydactyly in American Negroes and whites. Am. J. Hum. Genet., *25*:397, 1973.
46. Woolf, C. M., and Woolf, R. M.: A genetic study of syndactyly in Utah. Soc. Biol., *20*:335, 1973.

ACROCEPHALO-SYNDACTYLISM
(Apert's Syndrome)

Acrocephalosyndactylism was first described as a syndrome by Apert in 1906.[1] Primarily affecting the head, hands, and feet, it is characterized by synostosis of the cranial sutures and varying degrees of complex syndactyly of the hands and feet. It appears to be a primary germ plasm defect that causes primary synostosis. The growth disturbance results in failure of the nonosteogenic mesenchymal tissue to isolate the various ossification centers. The condition is very rare, probably occurring in one in 200,000 births. Its etiology is not known. It is, however, a genetic disturbance with a strong dominant inheritance; sporadic cases due to mutation do occur.

Clinical Features

Appearance of the patient is characteristic (Figs. 2–57 and 2–58). The head is peaked and vertically elongated in its anteroposterior diameter, with the planes of the face and the back of the skull being parallel. The enlarging brain causes increased intracranial pressure. The protuberant eyes are wide-spaced, with divergence of the transverse axis. Strabismus and progressive impairment of vision are common. Often the posterior palate is high-arched, and there are fusion defects of the maxilla and mandible. Convolutional atrophy of the brain and mental retardation are not uncommon. Some patients with normal mentation, however, have been placed in institutions for the mentally retarded because of their grotesque appearance.

In true Apert's syndrome the hand looks like a mitten, with complete complex syndactyly of the index, long, and ring fingers. The three central digits are fused with interdigital osseous union and a common nail. The little finger often shows a soft-tissue syndactyly with the ring finger but with an independent nail. The thumb is short and deviated radially at the metacarpophalangeal joint; it is often separate, but sometimes may be webbed with the fingers. The palm is spoon-shaped and functions like a paddle for gross movements. The deformity is bilateral. The feet show complete syndactyly of all toes and coalition of carpal and tarsal bones, and usually both bones of the forearm are shortened, the elbows are stiff, and shoulder abduction is limited.

Treatment

Treatment is a multidisciplinary neurosurgical and plastic surgical reconstruction. An osteotomy of the cranial bones is performed to prevent an increase in intracranial pressure, and the facial bones are reconstructed. With modern techniques of surgery, the success rate is very high. At 6 to 12 months of age the hands are treated according to the same surgical principles as those for treatment of syndactyly. In severe complex syndactyly it is best to strive to provide three fingers instead of four. Liberation of adhering fingertips permits normal longitudinal growth of the fingers and prevents progressive deformation of the interphalangeal joints. The skin coverage of the separated fingers is provided by local flaps and skin grafting; full-thickness skin grafts are better than split-thickness skin grafts. Range-of-motion exercises are performed to increase the arcs of flexion of the proximal interphalangeal and distal interphalangeal joints. Long-term follow-up studies show marked improvement in function.

References

1. Apert, E.: De l'acrocephalosyndactylie. Bull. Mem. Soc. Med. Hôp. Paris, *23*:1210, 1906.
2. Blank, C. E.: Apert's syndrome (a type of acrocephalosyndactyly)—observations on a British series of thirty-nine cases. Ann. Hum. Genet., *24*:151, 1960.
3. Book, J. A., and Hesselvik, L.: Acrocephalosyndactyly. Acta Paediatr., *42*:359, 1953.
4. Buckley, R. W., and Yakovlev, P. I.: Dysostosis of skull, face and extremities (acrocephalosyndactyly). Am. J. Dis. Child., *75*:688, 1948.
5. Carter, C. O.: The skeletal system. Localized abnormalities of the skeleton. Acrocephalosyndactyly (Apert's

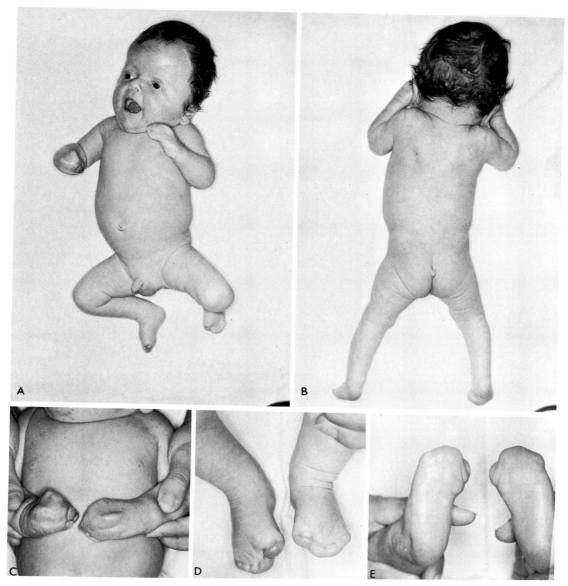

FIGURE 2–57. *Apert's syndrome (acrocephalosyndactylism) in a newborn infant.*

A and **B.** Anteroposterior and posteroanterior photographs of patient, depicting the typical deformities. (See text for description.) **C** to **E.** Views of the feet and hands showing complete syndactylism.

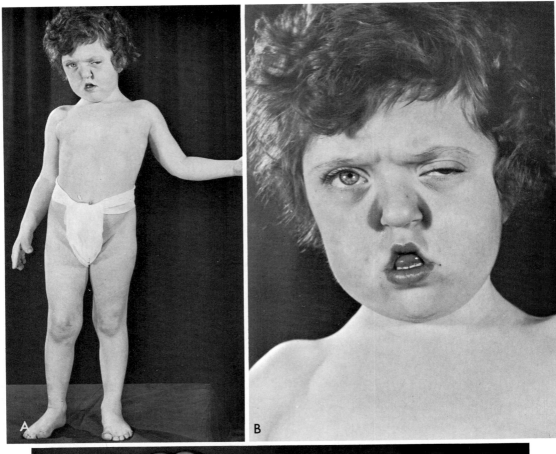

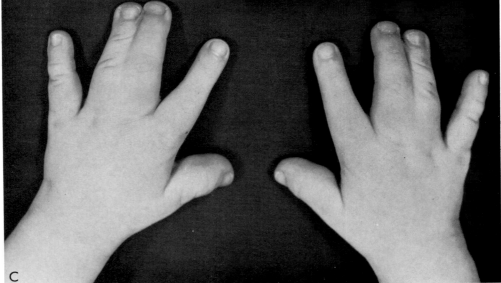

FIGURE 2–58. Apert's syndrome in an eight-year-old girl.

(See text for description.)

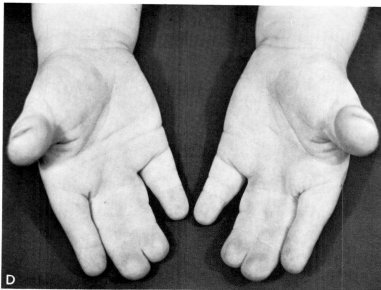

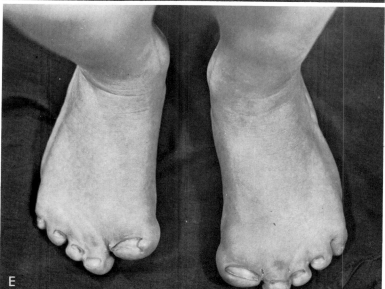

FIGURE 2–58 Continued. Apert's syndrome in an eight-year-old girl.

(See text for description.)

syndrome). *In* Sorsby, A. (ed.): Clinical Genetics. 2nd Ed. London, Butterworth, 1973, p. 193.

6. Dell, P. C., and Sheppard, J. E.: Deformities of the great toe in Apert's syndrome. Clin. Orthop., *157*:113, 1981.

7. Dunn, F. H.: Apert's acrocephalosyndactylism. Radiology, 78:738, 1962.

8. Gray, H., and Dickey, L. B.: Acrocephalosyndactyly. Am. J. Dis. Child., 74:213, 1947.

9. Hogan, G. R., and Bauman, M. L.: Hydrocephalus in Apert's syndrome. J. Pediatr., 79:782, 1971.

10. Hoover, G. H., Flatt, A. E., and Weiss, M. W.: Hand and Apert's syndrome. J. Bone Joint Surg., 52-A:878, 1970.

11. Kahn, A., Jr., and Fulmer, J.: Acrocephalo-syndactylism. N. Engl. J. Med., 252:379, 1955.

12. Kelikian, H.: Craniosynostosis. *In* Congenital Deformities of the Hand and Forearm. Philadelphia, Saunders, 1974, pp. 345–351.

13. Martsolf, J. T., Cracco, J. B., Carpenter, G. G., and O'Hara, A. E.: Pfeiffer syndrome: Unusual type of acrocephalosyndactyly with broad thumbs and great toes. Am. J. Dis. Child., *121*:257, 1971.

14. Meyer, J. L.: Apert's syndrome (acrocephalosyndactylism). J. Foot Surg., 20:210, 1981.

15. Owens, R. H.: Acrocephalosyndactyly. A case with congenital cardiac abnormalities. Br. J. Radiol., 25:103, 1952.

16. Pfeiffer, R. A., Tunte, W., and Reinken, M.: Das Kniepterygium-Syndrom. Z. Kinderheilkd., *108*:102, 1970.

17. Pillay, V. K.: Acrocephalosyndactyly in Singapore. A study of five Chinese males. J. Bone Joint Surg., *46*:94, 1964.

18. Rubin, M. B., Pirozzi, D. J., and Heaton, C. L.: Acrocephalosyndactyly. Report of a case with review of the literature. Am. J. Med., 53:127, 1972.

19. Sakati, N., Nyhan, W. L., and Tisdale, W. K.: A new syndrome with acrocephalopolysyndactyly, cardiac disease and distinctive defects of the ear, skin, and lower limbs. J. Pediatr., 79:194, 1971.

20. Saldino, R. M., Steinbach, H. L., and Epstein, C. J.: Familial acrocephalosyndactyly (Pfeiffer syndrome). A. J. R., *116*:609, 1972.

21. Spranger, J. W., Langer, L. O., Jr., and Weideman, H. R.: Acrocephalosyndactyly, Type I. *In* Bone Dysplasias. Philadelphia, Saunders, 1974, pp. 261–263.

22. Walsh, R. J.: Acrosyndactyly: Study of twenty-seven patients. Clin. Orthop., 71:99, 1970.

23. Woolf, R. M.: Acrocephalosyndactyly—Apert's syndrome. Acrocephaly with syndactylism. Plast. Reconstr. Surg., 24:201, 1959.

24. Wynne-Davies, R.: Acrocephalosyndactyly (Apert's syndrome). *In* Heritable Disorders in Orthopaedic Practice. London, Blackwell, 1973, pp. 107–108.

25. Yonenobu, K., Tada, K., and Tsuyuguchi, Y.: Apert's syndrome—a report of five cases. Hand, *14*:317, 1982.

POLYDACTYLY

Digits in excess of five in the human are anomalous, and *polydactyly* is the term used to denote duplication of digits. In polydactyly there are usually six digits per hand; occasionally, however, there may be more, such as seven or eight.[51]

In the literature it has been proposed that polydactylism is an expression of atavism, a reversion to our phylogenetic ancestors, to the multi-rayed manus of earlier animals.[12, 19, 105]

Are five fingers on the human hand the result of reduction from a greater number of digits existing in lower species of animals in the evolutionary scale? This theory has been contested.[33, 34] When an infant is born with two heads does that represent derivation of the single head of the human from a phylogenetic ancestry of polycephaly? At present polydactylism is ascribed to twinning or duplication of a single embryologic bud. Polydactyly may be caused by maternal ingestion of thalidomide in the embryonic period of limb bud formation.

Incidence

Polydactyly is the second most common congenital deformity of the hand, the first being syndactyly. It has been reported in all countries of the world. No race is immune; there is, however, definite racial preference. In the black, the incidence is about 1 in 300, and in the white it is 1 in 3000, i.e., polydactyly is ten times as frequent in the black as in the white race. In the black, duplication of the little finger is ten times as common as of the thumb, whereas in the white and the Oriental, duplication of the thumb is the most frequent polydactyly. The incidence of thumb polydactyly is about 0.08 per 1000 live births in both blacks and whites (Table 2–7). It is slightly more common in the American Indian.[113] Supernumerary digits are more common in the male.

*Table 2–7. Incidence of Polydactyly in American Black and American White Populations**

Polydactyly	Incidence per 1,000	
	American Black (N = 25,126 infants)	American White (N = 24,153 infants)
Preaxial	0.08	0.08
Postaxial	13.53	1.24

*Adapted from Woolf, C. M., and Myrianthopoulos, N. C.: Polydactyly in American Negroes and whites. Am. J. Hum. Genet., 25:397, 1973.

The extra digit may be *postaxial*, i.e., lying on the side of the little finger, or it may be *preaxial*, lying on the side of the thumb. Very occasionally the surplus digit may be *central* or *axial*, i.e., the ring, long, or index finger is duplicated. These various morphologic types are discussed separately.

Postaxial Polydactyly

Although any one of the five digits of the hand may be duplicated, the little finger is the most commonly duplicated one.

TYPES

The spectrum of duplication of the little finger varies from a skin tag to a completely developed extra little finger with its own phalanges and metacarpal. Duplication of the fingers, according to Stelling and Turek, may be classified into three main types: In *Type I* there is an extra soft-tissue mass that has no bony attachment to the skeleton of the hand, often does not have bones or joints or tendons, and is connected to the hand by a narrow pedicle (Fig. 2–59 A). In *Type II*, a part or all of the finger is duplicated with normal bony, cartilaginous, or tendinous components; it articulates with an enlarged or bifid metacarpal or phalanx (Fig. 2–59 B). In *Type III*, the entire finger with its own metacarpal and all soft-tissue components is duplicated; Type III is rare (Fig. 2–59 C).[107, 119]

INHERITANCE

Postaxial polydactyly, when it occurs as an isolated anomaly, is a dominant trait with marked penetrance in some families and variable penetrance in others. Temtamy and McKusick subdivided duplication of the little finger into two types. In Type A the extra digit is fully developed; in Type B it is rudimentary and pedunculated. Persons with Type A polydactyly can produce progeny with either Type A or Type B extra digits, whereas persons with Type B polydactyly can produce only children with Type B extra digits. The genetic pattern of Type B is complicated, involving one or two dominant genes and variable penetrance.[112, 113]

ASSOCIATED ANOMALIES AND SYNDROMES

In the *black*, duplication of the little finger often occurs as an isolated deformity without any associated abnormalities; it is often bilateral. In some individuals both feet and both hands are polydactylous, whereas in others only two or three limbs are involved.

In the *white*, postaxial polydactyly is often associated with a variety of anomalies and syndromes; when it occurs as part of a syndrome it is not uncommon for it to be transmitted as an autosomal recessive trait. In contrast, duplication of the thumb is rarely part of a syndrome. Thumb polydactyly is seen in the two types of acrocephalopolysyndactyly—the Noack type,

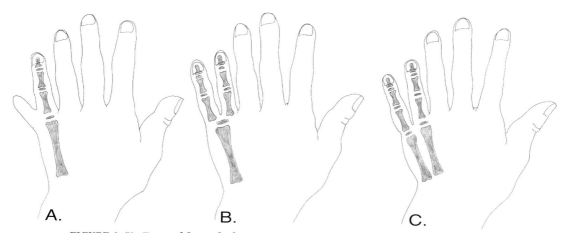

FIGURE 2–59. *Types of finger duplication according to classifications of Stelling and Turek.*

A. *Type I* polydactyly consists of an extra soft-tissue mass that is connected to bone. Often it does not contain bone, cartilage, or tendon. Treatment consists of simple ablation of the accessory soft-tissue mass. **B.** *Type II* polydactyly consists of duplication of a digit. Note it articulates with an enlarged metacarpal head. Treatment of this type of polydactyly is complex. **C.** *Type III* polydactyly. The extra digit is complete with its own metacarpal and all its soft-tissue components. Treatment is simple ablation of the entire digit and metacarpal.

Table 2–8. *Some Abnormalities Associated with Postaxial Polydactyly*

Hand—Syndactyly, triphalangeal thumb, absence of thumb, fingernail dystrophy, mirror hand, accessory carpal bones, coalition of carpal bones, radioulnar synostosis
Foot-Leg—Polydactyly of toes, hypoplasia or aplasia of tibiae and fibulae
Skeleton—Hemivertebrae, dwarfism, bowed femur
Head—Hydrocephalus, cleft lip, eye defects, cataracts, deafness, mental deficiency
Genitourinary—Hypogonadism, chronic nephritis, horseshoe kidney, bladder obstruction, micropenis
Other—Imperforate anus, Hirschsprung's disease, tooth anomalies

transmitted by dominant inheritance, and the Carpenter type, which is recessive. Thumb polydactyly occurs in syndromes such as Fanconi's and Holt-Oram.

The most common regional anomaly associated with polydactyly is syndactylism. Other accompaniments in the hand are nail dystrophy, brachydactyly, absence of thumb, triphalangeal thumb of the contralateral hand, and mirror hand. Over 40 abnormalities have been reported in association with postaxial polydactyly (Table 2–8). Postaxial polydactyly is also part of a variety of syndromes and chromosomal abnormalities (Table 2–9). When a white infant presents with duplication of the little finger, the whole child should be thoroughly examined, and if necessary genetic consultation should be obtained to rule out the presence of associated syndromes, chromosomal aberrations, or other serious abnormalities. A thorough diagnostic work-up will prevent embarrassment later on.

Preaxial Polydactyly (Duplication of the Thumb)

Extra thumbs are the most common type of polydactyly in the white. In both blacks and whites the incidence of the deformity is 0.08 per 1000.

It manifests itself in many forms, ranging from a small fleshy webbing on the radial border of the hand to triplication. On the basis of the degree of bony union, Wassel classified thumb polydactyly into seven types (Fig. 2–60). In Type I the distal phalanx is bifid (most rare, 2 per cent); in Type II the distal phalanx is duplicated (15 per cent); in Type III the proximal phalanx is bifid but the distal phalanx is duplicated (6 per cent); in Type IV, the most common (43 per cent), both the proximal and distal phalanges of the thumb are duplicated; in Type V (10 per cent), the metacarpal of the thumb is bifid, and both its proximal and distal phalanges are duplicated; in Type VI (4 per cent), the thumb metacarpal and both proximal and distal phalanges are duplicated; in Type VII (20 per cent), the thumb is triphalangeal.[122]

Preaxial polydactyly may be associated with syndactyly, as shown in Figure 2–61; it is inherited as an autosomal dominant trait. Temtamy refers to this form of polydactyly as polysyndactyly.[111, 112]

In thumb duplication, circulation may be anomalous, being supplied by one artery instead of two (Fig. 2–62). Often one of the thumbs is dominant while the other is underdeveloped; sometimes, however, both thumbs are of equal size, posing a problem as to which one to ablate.

Table 2–9. *Some Syndromes Associated with Postaxial Polydactyly*

Syndrome	Inheritance
Ellis–Van Creveld (chondroectodermal) dysplasia	Autosomal recessive
Jeune's (infantile thoracic dystrophy)	Autosomal recessive
Biemond II (coloboma of iris, mental retardation, obesity, and hypogonadism)	Autosomal dominant (irregular)
Laurence-Moon-Bardet-Biedl (LMBB)	Autosomal recessive
Meckel (plus syndactyly, encephalocele, polycystic kidney, cleft lip and palate)	Autosomal recessive
Goltz (focal dermal hypoplasia)	X-linked dominant
Orofaciodigital Type I	X-linked dominant
Orofaciodigital Type II (Mohr)	Autosomal recessive
Patau (trisomy 13)	Sporadic

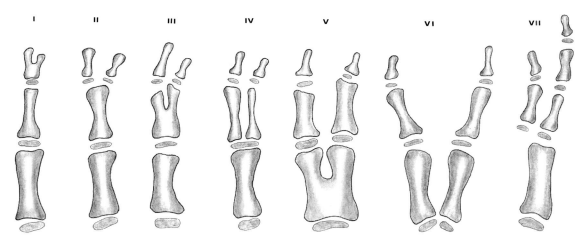

FIGURE 2–60. Wassel's classification of thumb duplication.

The most common type is Type IV, in which both the proximal and distal phalanges are duplicated (43 per cent). In Type I the distal phalanx is bifid. It is the least common, constituting 2 per cent. In Type II (15 per cent) the distal phalanx is duplicated. In Type III (6 per cent) the distal phalanx is duplicated and the proximal phalanx is bifid. In Type V (10 per cent) the metacarpal of the thumb is bifid and both phalanges are duplicated. In Type VI (4 per cent) the thumb metacarpal and both proximal and distal phalanges are duplicated. In Type VII the thumb is triphalangeal.

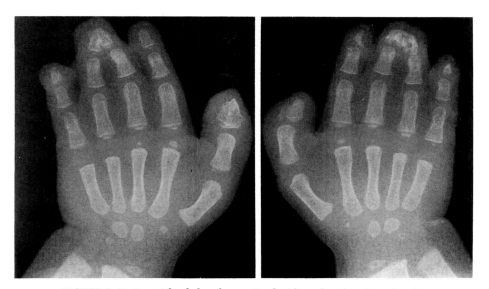

FIGURE 2–61. Preaxial polydactyly associated with syndactyly-polysyndactyly.

The deformity is inherited as an autosomal dominant trait. (From Poznanski, A.: The Hand in Radiologic Diagnosis. Philadelphia, W. B. Saunders Co., 1984. Reprinted by permission.)

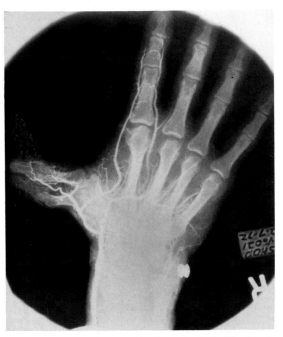

FIGURE 2–62. Anomalous blood supply in double thumb.

Instead of two arteries a single artery supplies both thumbs. (From Poznanski, A.: The Hand in Radiologic Diagnosis. Philadelphia, W. B. Saunders Co., 1984. Reprinted by permission.)

Involvement is usually unilateral. In the University of Iowa series (reported by Wassel) bilateral involvement was found in 7 of the 70 patients with thumb duplication; in the series of Barsky 1 of the 25 cases was bilateral, and in that of Handforth, 11 of 13 cases were unilateral.[2, 40, 122]

Thumb polydactyly is usually sporadic, though if associated with triphalangeal thumb it may be familial.[111]

Preaxial polydactyly may be associated with vertebral anomalies, absence of the tibia, cleft palate, and imperforate anus.[46, 87, 95] It may also be seen in a number of syndromes; of special clinical importance are Down's syndrome, Fanconi pancytopenia, and acrocephalosyndactyly (Table 2–10).

Central Polydactyly

Duplication of the index, long, and ring fingers is referred to as axial or central polydactyly. Often the extra digit of a long or ring finger is concealed in a web between adjoining normal digits (Fig. 2–63). The tendons, nerves and vessels of the supernumerary digits are usually abnormal, as are the epiphyses of the extra digit. The epiphysis of the extra digit usually does not lie in the normal line of growth; as a result its phalanges diverge from the longitudinal axis into ulnar or radial deviation and distort adjacent digits.

Duplication of the index finger is very rare, representing about 3.5 per cent of all cases of polydactyly.[127] This anomaly should not be confused with triphalangeal thumb. The extra index finger may consist of a pedunculated soft-tissue mass or it may have normal bony and soft-tissue components. It may be associated with congenital radioulnar synostosis, and occasionally the duplicated index finger may be fused to the long finger.

Treatment

Treatment of postaxial polydactyly is relatively simple. If the duplicated small finger is hypoplastic, rudimentary, and attached to the hand by a narrow pedicle it can be removed in the newborn nursery; simple tying off of the pedicle, however, can cause serious bleeding problems. It is best to ablate by division of the pedicle with a scalpel and coagulation of the stump by electrocautery.

The fully developed and complete extra little finger is excised as described and illustrated in Plate 8.

Operative treatment for preaxial polydactyly is more complicated and surgically more challenging. The important considerations are to maintain size and stability, to provide adequate motor control and strength, and to establish anatomic alignment. The type of treatment varies according to the type of thumb duplication. If one of the two thumbs is significantly smaller

Text continued on page 254

***Table 2–10.** Some Syndromes Associated with Preaxial Polydactyly*

Syndrome	Inheritance
Acrocephalopolysyndactyly—Noack type	Autosomal dominant
Acrocephalopolysyndactyly—Carpenter type	Autosomal recessive
Bloom (chromosomal break)	Autosomal recessive
Holt-Oram	Autosomal dominant
Fanconi (pancytopenia-dysmelia)	Autosomal recessive

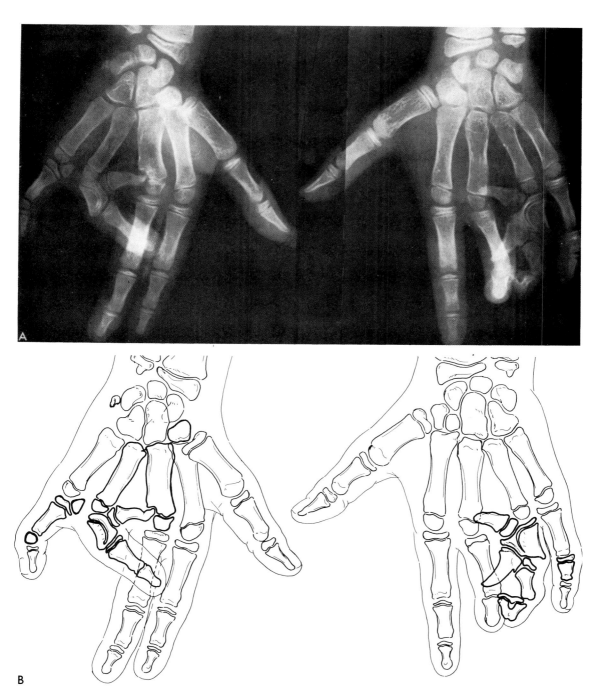

FIGURE 2–63. Central polydactyly.

Note the polyphalangy of the ring finger of both hands. **A** and **B.** Radiograms and sketches of both hands. (From Kelikian, H.: Congenital Deformities of the Hand and Forearm. Philadelphia, W. B. Saunders Co., 1974. Reprinted by permission.)

Ablation of Duplicated Little Finger (Postaxial Polydactyly)

OPERATIVE TECHNIQUE

A. A racquet incision is made. The solid lines are on the dorsal surface and the dotted lines are on the volar surface. Avoid longitudinal straight scars. Be generous and err on the safe side. Excess skin can always be trimmed later. Preserve volar skin as much as possible because it is thicker and more durable and has better two-point discrimination than the thin dorsal skin. Subcutaneous tissue is divided in line with the skin incision. Next, a midline incision is made on the radial aspect of the extra little finger for exposure of the long flexor and extensor tendons of the little finger.

B. The digital nerves and vessels are carefully isolated and protected. Next, the hypothenar muscles are dissected off their insertions to the extra digit and the long flexor and extensor tendons are identified, divided at their insertions, and dissected and reflected proximally.

C. The collateral ligaments are dissected; leaving their insertions to the metacarpal intact. Next, the extra digit is excised by division of the capsule at the metacarpophalangeal joint.

Plate 8. Ablation of Duplicated Little Finger
(Postaxial Polydactyly)

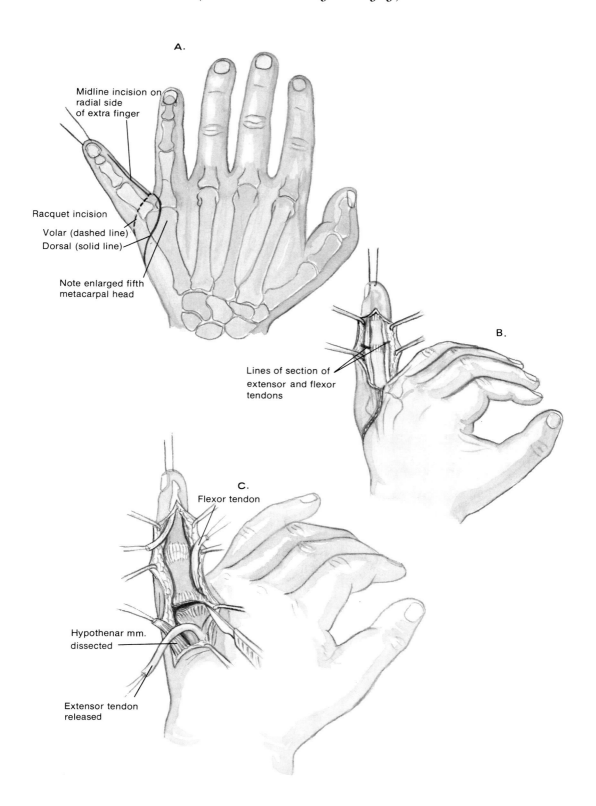

A.

Midline incision on radial side of extra finger

Racquet incision

Volar (dashed line)

Dorsal (solid line)

Note enlarged fifth metacarpal head

Lines of section of extensor and flexor tendons

B.

C.

Flexor tendon

Hypothenar mm. dissected

Extensor tendon released

Ablation of Duplicated Little Finger (Postaxial Polydactyly)
(Continued)

D. The fifth metacarpal head is usually enlarged, with a ridge separating the individual articular surfaces of the duplicated little fingers. The portion of the metacarpal head for the extra digit with a part of the subjacent thickened metacarpal shaft is removed with a thin sharp osteotome or a small oscillating saw. The cut is made parallel to the ridge on the articular surface of the metacarpal head. If the fifth metacarpal is angulated ulnarward it may be necessary to perform an osteotomy of the metacarpal shaft for proper anatomic alignment.

E. The long flexor and extensor tendons of the ablated digit are transferred to the adjoining remaining little finger. The collateral ligament and hypothenar muscles are reattached to the base of the remaining proximal phalanx on its ulnar aspect. Avoid injury to the growth plate. The capsule of the metacarpophalangeal joint is repaired with interrupted sutures.

F. A smooth Kirschner wire is used for internal fixation; it extends from the tip of the little finger to the base of the fifth metacarpal. It will protect the repair of the collateral ligament and hold the metacarpophalangeal joint and the osteotomized metacarpal shaft in proper alignment. The tourniquet is removed, and after complete hemostasis, the wound is closed in routine fashion. An above-elbow cast or splint is applied.

POSTOPERATIVE CARE

In four weeks the cast and Kirschner wire are removed, and the infant is allowed to use the hand.

Plate 8. Ablation of Duplicated Little Finger (Postaxial Polydactyly)

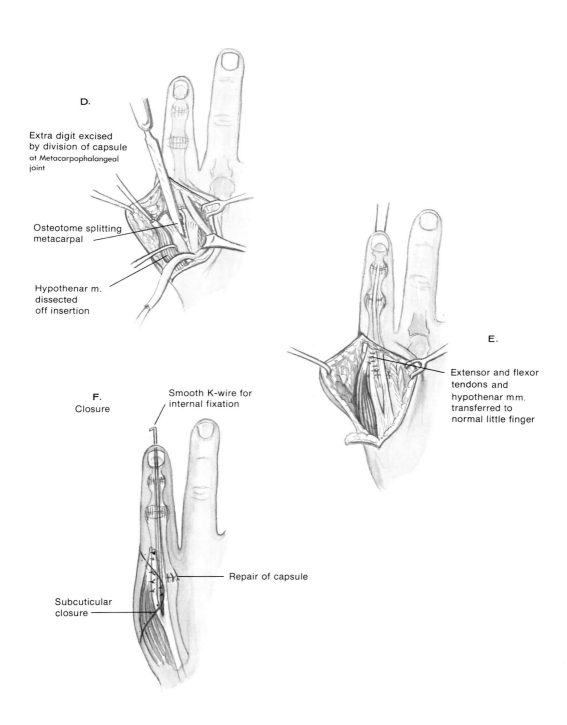

D.

Extra digit excised
by division of capsule
at Metacarpophalangeal
joint

Osteotome splitting
metacarpal

Hypothenar m.
dissected
off insertion

E.

Extensor and flexor
tendons and
hypothenar mm.
transferred to
normal little finger

F.
Closure

Smooth K-wire for
internal fixation

Repair of capsule

Subcuticular
closure

Ablation of Duplicated Radial Accessory Thumb (Preaxial Polydactyly)

OPERATIVE TECHNIQUE

A and **B.** A racquet incision is made over the base of the radial thumb to be ablated as illustrated. The dorsal incision is shown by a solid line and the volar incision by a dashed line. A midline incision is made on the radial aspect of the accessory thumb to facilitate exposure of tendons and nerves.

C. The subcutaneous tissue is divided in line with the skin incision. Care is taken not to injure digital vessels and nerves. The extensor pollicis longus tendon is identified and sectioned over the middle of the proximal phalanx of the accessory thumb. The flexor pollicis longus tendon of the accessory thumb is identified and sectioned near its insertion. The long flexor and extensor tendons are reflected proximally. The thenar muscles are transected at their insertions. The capsule of the metacarpophalangeal joint is identified and divided by a transverse incision. The nerves and vessels of the ulnar thumb are identified, and if they are present and adequate, the digital vessels of the radial thumb are divided and ligated, and the digital nerve of the radial thumb is divided with a sharp scalpel and allowed to retract (formation of a neuroma is ordinarily not a problem).

Plate 9. Ablation of Duplicated Radial Accessory Thumb (Preaxial Polydactyly)

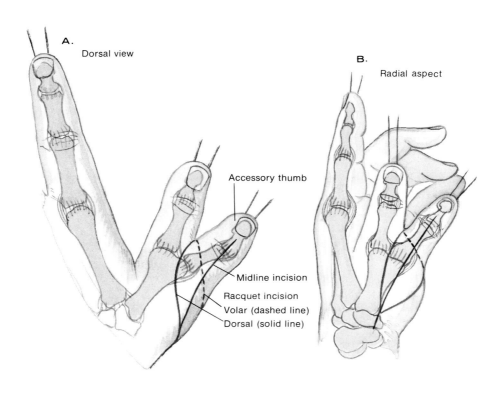

A. Dorsal view

B. Radial aspect

Accessory thumb

Midline incision

Racquet incision
Volar (dashed line)
Dorsal (solid line)

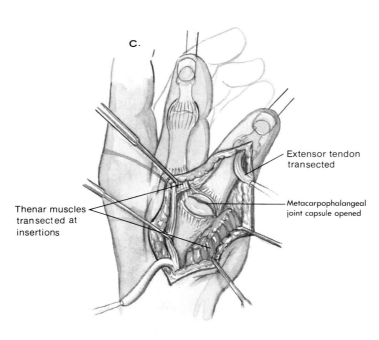

C.

Thenar muscles transected at insertions

Extensor tendon transected

Metacarpophalangeal joint capsule opened

Ablation of Duplicated Radial Accessory Thumb (Preaxial Polydactyly) (Continued)

D. The radial thumb is ablated, and the first metacarpal head is exposed. With a sharp osteotome or a small oscillating saw the enlarged metacarpal head is trimmed (the growth plate of the first metacarpal is proximal).

E. The flexor pollicis longus and extensor pollicis longus are transferred to those of the remaining thumb. The collateral ligament and the capsule are repaired with interrupted sutures. Thenar muscles are reattached to the base of the proximal phalanx of the remaining thumb.

F. A smooth Kirschner wire is used to transfix the metacarpophalangeal joint of the thumb. The tourniquet is released, and after hemostasis is obtained, the wound is closed in the usual fashion. An above-elbow cast is applied, incorporating the thumb. A cap is put over the thumb portion of the cast to protect the pin.

POSTOPERATIVE CARE

The cast and pin are removed in four to six weeks. Exercises are begun to restore function.

Plate 9. Ablation of Duplicated Radial Accessory Thumb (Preaxial Polydactyly)

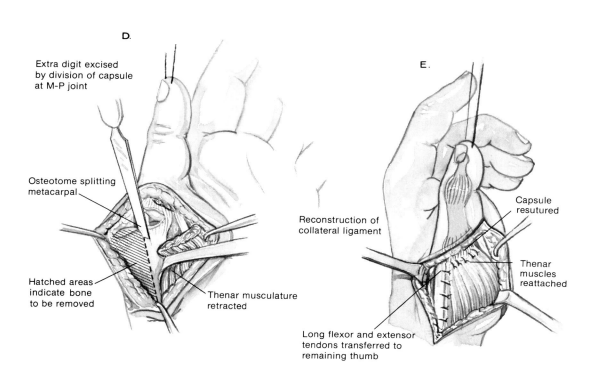

D.

Extra digit excised by division of capsule at M-P joint

Osteotome splitting metacarpal

Hatched areas indicate bone to be removed

Thenar musculature retracted

E.

Reconstruction of collateral ligament

Capsule resutured

Thenar muscles reattached

Long flexor and extensor tendons transferred to remaining thumb

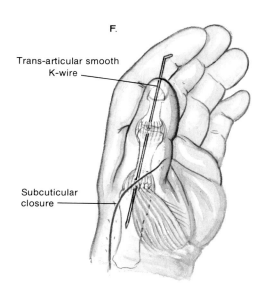

F.

Trans-articular smooth K-wire

Subcuticular closure

or if only one deviates from the anatomic axis, the smaller accessory thumb is ablated. It is vital to forewarn the parents that at skeletal maturity the thumb will be smaller than the contralateral normal thumb. The surgical technique follows the same details and principles as those for ablation of the extra little finger. Linear incisions result in contracted scars that cause or aggravate an angular deformity at the interphalangeal or metacarpophalangeal joint, pulling the distal part to the side of the scar. If a linear incision is inevitable, Z-flaps are made to break it up. If a Z-plasty is inadequate, a dorsally based triangular skin flap is rotated from the dorsum and transferred to the side of the interphalangeal joint. The dorsal skin defect is covered with split-thickness skin grafts.[76] Reattachment of the thenar muscles is crucial.

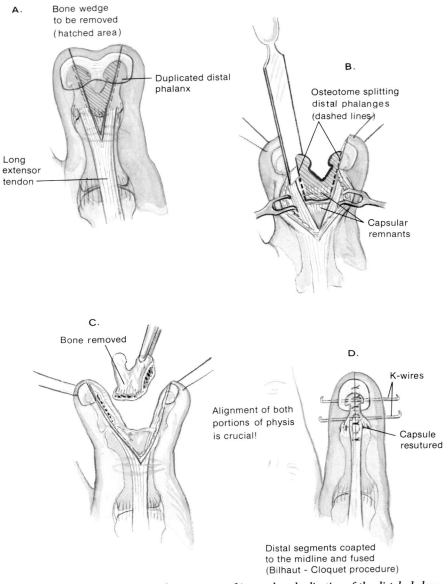

FIGURE 2–64. *The Bilhaut-Cloquet operation for treatment of incomplete duplication of the distal phalanx of the thumb.*

   A. The objective of surgery is to create a normally shaped distal phalanx of the thumb by a central wedge resection and coaptation of the remaining parts. A dorsal and palmar triangular wedge area of the skin is excised. The long extensor tendon is split. **B.** With an osteotome the distal phalanges are split as shown. **C.** The bone is removed. **D.** The retained parts are anatomically coapted to the midline and fixed with two Kirschner wires. It is vital to align the physis. The capsule is repaired, and the extensor tendons are sutured together.

Reconstruction of the collateral ligaments prevents instability of the interphalangeal or metacarpophalangeal joints. The long flexor and extensor tendons of the ablated thumb are transferred to the remaining thumb. The operative technique is described and illustrated in Plate 9.

When only the distal phalanx of the thumb is duplicated and both components diverge equally from the longitudinal axis, a triangular wedge is resected centrally, and the retained parts of the distal segments are coapted in the midline and fused to form one distal phalanx—the Bilhaut-Cloquet procedure (Fig. 2–64). During the excision of the central wedge care is taken not to injure the growth plate at the base of the distal phalanges. Anatomic positioning of the phalanges and their physes is crucial; in the radiogram the growth plate should be continuous and horizontal; there should be no step-ups. Anatomic alignment is maintained by smooth Kirschner wires. A single nail is reconstructed by bringing together the nail beds and matrices in the midline. This procedure is not simple; it presents several technical problems. Accurate approximation of the distal phalanges and the physis is difficult. Often the thumb is not reduced to normal size because of an insufficient central wedge resection of bone and soft tissues. The collateral ligaments of the interphalangeal joint of the thumb are taut owing to abnormal enlargement of the head of the proximal phalanx. A cosmetically objectionable midline fissure in the nail often results, and the scar on the volar surface of the thumb will be bothersome to the patient.

References

1. Aznar, J., and Vaya, A.: Homozygous form of the Pelger-Huet leukocyte anomaly in man. Acta Haemat., *66*:59, 1961.
2. Barsky, A. J.: Congenital anomalies of the hand. J. Bone Joint Surg., 33-A:35, 1951.
3. Barsky, A. J.: Congenital Anomalies of the Hand and Their Surgical Treatment. Springfield, Thomas, 1958, pp. 48–64.
4. Barsky, A. J.: Congenital anomalies of the thumb. Clin. Orthop., *15*:96, 1959.
5. Barsky, A. J., Kahn, S., and Simon, B. E.: Congenital anomalies of the hand. Reconstr. Plast. Surg., *4*:1704, 1964.
6. Baumann, L., and Landauer, W.: Polydactyly and anterior or horn cells in fowl. J. Comp. Neurol., *79*:153, 1943.
7. Beckmann, E., and Widdlund, L.: On inheritance of poly- and syndactyly in man. Acta Genet. Med. Gemellol., *11*:43, 1962.
8. Bienvenue, F.: Un cas de pouce supplementaire à trois phalanges. Rev. Orthop. Chir. Paris, *111*:91, 1912.
9. Bilhaut, M.: Guérison d'un pouce bifide par un nouveau procédé opératoire. Congr. Fr. Chir., *4*:576, 1890.
10. Blankenburg, H.: Die Polydaktylie. Beitr. Orthop. Traumatol., *14*:160, 1967.
11. Blumel, J., and Kniker, W. T.: Laurence-Moon-Bardet-Biedl syndrome. Review of the literature and a report of five cases including a family group with three affected males. Tex. Rep. Biol. Med., *17*:391, 1959.
12. Boinet, E.: Polydactylie et atavisme. Rev. Med., *19*:316, 1898.
13. Bornstein, N. B.: Aniridie bilatérale avec polydactylie. Relations des anomalies oculaires du type colobomateux associées à des malformations sequelettiques avec les formes atypiques du syndrome de Bardet-Biedl. J. Genet. Hum., *1*:211, 1952.
14. Buck-Gramcko, D.: Congenital malformations of the hand: indications, operative treatment and results. Scand. J. Plast. Surg., *9*:192, 1975.
15. Bunge, R. G., and Bradbury, J. T.: Two unilaterally cryptorchid boys with spermatogenic precocity in the descended testis, hypertelorism and polydactyly. J. Clin. Endocrinol., *19*:1103, 1959.
16. Burman, M.: An historical perspective of double hands and double feet. The survey of the cases reported in the 16th and 17th centuries. Bull. Hosp. Joint Dis., *29*:241, 1968.
17. Burman, M.: Note on duplication of the index finger. J. Bone Joint Surg., 54-A:884, 1972.
18. Christiaens, L., Laude, M., and Fontaine, G.: Les polydactylies: à propos d'un case familial. Pediatrie, *18*:709, 1963.
19. Darwin, C.: The Variation of Animals and Plants under Domestication. 2nd ed. New York, Appleton, 1896. Vol. I, pp. 457–460. (The first edition was published in 1868.)
20. DeMarinis, F., and Sobbota, A.: On inheritance and development of preaxial and postaxial types of polydactyly. Acta Genet., *7*:215, 1957.
21. DeMarinis, F., and Wildervanck, L. S.: Pre-axial polydactylia (double thumb and triphalangia). Ned. Tijdschr. Geneeskd., *104*:2169, 1960.
22. Dignan, P. St. J.: Polydactyly in Down's syndrome. Am. J. Ment. Defic., *77*:486, 1973.
23. Dungy, C. I., Aptekar, R. G., and Cann, H. M.: Hereditary hydrometrocolpos with polydactyly in infancy. Pediatrics, *47*:138, 1971.
24. Eaton, G. O., and McKusick, V. A.: A seemingly unique polydactyly-syndactyly syndrome in four persons in three generations. In Bergsma, D. (ed.): Birth Defects. Original Article Series. New York, National Foundation—March of Dimes, Vol. V, No. 3, 1969, pp. 221–225.
25. Ecke, H.: Beitrag zu den Doppelmissbildungen im Bereich der Finger. Beitr. Klin. Chir., *205*:463, 1962.
26. Egawa, T.: Surgical treatment of polydactyly of the thumb. Jpn. J. Plast. Reconstr. Surg., *9*:97, 1966.
27. Entin, M. A.: Reconstruction of congenital abnormalities of the upper extremities. J. Bone Joint Surg., 41-A:681, 1959.
28. Flatt, A. E.: The Care of Congenital Hand Anomalies, St. Louis, Mosby, 1977, pp. 99–117.
29. Flatt, A. E.: The Care of Congenital Hand Anomalies, St. Louis, Mosby, 1977, p. 248.
30. Flatt, A. E.: Problems in polydactyly. In Cramer, L. M., and Chase, R. A. (eds.): Symposium on the Hand, Vol. 3. St. Louis, Mosby, 1971, pp. 150–167.
31. Frazier, T. M.: A note on race-specific congenital malformation rates. Am. J. Obstet. Gynecol., *80*:184, 1960.
32. Fuhrmann, W., Fuhrmann-Rieger, A., and de Sousa, F.: Poly-, syn- and oligodactyly, aplasia or hypoplasia of fibula, hypoplasia of pelvis and bowing of femora in

three sibs—a new autosomal recessive syndrome. Eur. J. Pediatr., *133*:123, 1980.

33. Gegenbaur, C.: Kritische Bemerkungen über Polydactylie als Atavismus. Morph. Jahrb., *6*:584, 1880. See also translation in J. Anat. Physiol. Norm. Pathol., *16*:615, 1882.

34. Gegenbaur, C.: Über polydactylie. Morph. Jahrb., *14*:394, 1888. See also review of this article in Rev. Sci. Med. en France et a L'Etranger, *34*:46, 1889.

35. Gellis, S. S., and Feingold, M.: Picture of the month: Denouement and discussion of Smith-Lemli-Opitz syndrome. Am. J. Dis. Child., *115*:603, 1968.

36. Goodman, R. M.: A family with polysyndactyly and other anomalies. J. Hered., *56*:37, 1965.

37. Grebe, H.: Polydaktylia. *In* Becker, P. E. (ed.): Humangenetik. Stuttgart, Thieme, 1964. Vol. 2, p. 182.

38. Gustavson, K.-H., Kreuger, A., and Petersson, P. O.: Syndrome characterized by lingual malformation, polydactyly, tachypnea, and psychomotor retardation (Mohr syndrome). Clin. Genet., *2*:261, 1971.

39. Halal, F.: Minor manifestations in preaxial polydactyly type I and Poland complex. Am. J. Med. Genet., *8*:221, 1981.

40. Handforth, J. R.: Polydactylism of the hand in southern Chinese. Anat. Rec., *106*:119, 1950.

41. Hanissian, A. S., Riggs, W. W., Jr., and Thomas, D. A.: Infantile thoracic dystrophy—a variant of Ellis-van Creveld syndrome. J. Pediatr., *71*:855, 1967.

42. Hare, P. J.: Rudimentary polydactyly. Br. J. Dermatol., *66*:407, 1954.

43. Harrison, R. G., Pearson, M., and Roaf, R.: Ulnar dimelia. J. Bone Joint Surg., *42-B*:549, 1960.

44. Hartrampf, C. R., Vasconez, L. O., and Mathes, S.: Construction of one good thumb from both parts of a congenitally bifid thumb. Plast. Reconstr. Surg., *54*:148, 1974.

45. Hefner, R. A.: Hereditary polydactyly. J. Hered., *31*:25, 1940.

46. Ho, C. K., Kaufman, R. L., and McAlister, W. H.: Congenital malformations. Cleft palate, congenital heart disease, absent tibiae, and polydactyly. Am. J. Dis. Child., *129*:714, 1975.

47. Hootnick, D., and Holmes, L. B.: Familial polysyndactyly and craniofacial anomalies. Clin. Genet., *3*:128, 1972.

48. James, J. I. P., and Lamb, D. W.: Congenital abnormalities of the limbs. Practitioner, *191*:159, 1963.

49. Jeune, M., Beraud, C., and Carron, R.: Dystrophie thoracique asphyxiante de caractère familial. Arch. Fr. Pediatr., *12*:886, 1955.

50. Johnston, O., and Davis, R. W.: On the inheritance of hand and foot anomalies in six families (2. Polydactyly). Am. J. Hum. Genet., *5*:356, 1953.

51. Kanavel, A. B.: Congenital malformations of the hands. Trans. Sect. Surg. Gen. Abdom. Am. Med. Assoc., *17*:121, 1931.

52. Kanavel, A. B.: Congenital malformations of the hands. Arch. Surg., *25*:282, 1932.

53. Kanavel, A. B.: Congenital malformations of the hands. Arch. Surg., *25*:308, 1932.

54. Karchinov, K.: The treatment of polydactyly of the hand. Br. J. Plast. Surg., *15*:362, 1962.

55. Kelikian, H.: Congenital Deformities of the Hand and Forearm. Philadelphia, Saunders, 1974, pp. 408–456.

56. Kelikian, H., and Doumanian, A.: Congenital anomalies of the hand. J. Bone Joint Surg., *39-A*:1002, 1974.

57. Kelikian, H., and Doumanian, A.: Congenital anomalies of the hand. J. Bone Joint Surg., *39-A*:1002, 1957.

58. Khoo, C. T. K., and Saaol, M. N.: Median cleft of upper lip in association with bilateral hexadactyly and accessory toes. Br. J. Plast. Surg., *33*:407, 1980.

59. Kleinert, H. E., Grundberg, A. B., and Kutz, J. E.: Treatment of the reduplicated thumb. (Abstract.) J. Bone Joint Surg., *55-A*:874, 1973.

60. Komai, T., Ozaki, Y., and Inokuma, W.: A Japanese kindred of hyperphalangism of thumbs and duplication of thumbs and big toes. Folia Hered. Pathol., *2*:307, 1953.

61. Laurence, K. M., Prosser, R., Rocker, I., Pearson, J. F., and Richards, C.: Hirschsprung's disease associated with congenital heart malformation, broad big toes, and ulnar polydactyly in sibs: A case for fetoscopy. J. Med. Genet., *12*:334, 1975.

62. Le Marec, B., and Coutel, Y.: La polydactylie. Maladie ou symptome? Pediatrie, *25*:735, 1970.

63. Lucas, R. C.: On a remarkable instance of hereditary tendency to the production of supernumerary digits. Guy's Hosp. Rep., *25*:417, 1881.

64. Lyonnet, R.: Cinq polydactyles dans la même fraterie grandpère maternel lui-même polydactyle et originaire de lzeaux. Bull. Feder. Soc. Gynecol. Obstet. Langue Fr., *13*:298, 1961.

65. MacCarthy, W. C., Jr., and Russell, D. G.: Tuberous sclerosis: Report of a case with ependymoma. Radiology, *71*:833, 1958.

66. McClintic, B. S.: Five generations of polydactylism. J. Hered., *26*:141, 1935.

67. McKusick, V. A.: Mendelian Inheritance in Man. Baltimore, Johns Hopkins University Press, 1971, pp. 237–239.

68. McKusick, V. A., Egeland, J. A., Eldridge, R., and Krusen, D. E.: Dwarfism in the Amish. I. The Ellis-van Creveld syndrome. Bull. Johns Hopkins Hosp., *115*:306, 1964.

69. Manoiloff, E. O.: A rare case of hereditary hexodactylism. Am. J. Phys. Anthrop., *15*:503, 1931.

70. Marks, T. W., and Bayne, L. G.: Polydactyly of the thumb: Abnormal anatomy and treatment. J. Hand Surg., *3*:107, 1978.

71. Maroteaux, P., and Savart, P.: La dystrophie thoracique asphyxiante. Etude radiologique et rapports avec le syndrome d'Ellis et van Creveld. Ann. Radiol., *7*:332, 1964.

72. Maurizio, E.: Primus digitus varus, triphalangism of the thumb and radial polydactylia. Arch. Putti Chir. Organi Mov., *19*:449, 1964.

73. Mecke, S., and Passarge, E.: Encephalocele, polycystic kidneys, and polydactyly as an autosomal recessive trait simulating certain other disorders: The Meckel syndrome. Ann. Genet., *14*:97, 1971.

74. Mellin, G. W.: The Frequency of Birth Defects. *In* Fishein, M.: Birth Defects. Philadelphia, Lippincott, 1963, Chapter 1.

75. Millesi, H.: Deformations of the fingers following operations for polydactylia. Klin. Med. (Wien), *22*:266, 1967.

76. Miura, T.: An appropriate treatment for postoperative Z-formed deformity of the duplicated thumb. J. Hand Surg., *2*:380, 1977.

77. Mohan, J.: Postaxial polydactyly in three Indian families. J. Med. Genet., *6*:196, 1969.

78. Muller, W.: Die angeborenen Fehlbeldunger der menschlicher Hand. Leipzig, Thieme, 1937.

79. Nathan, P. A., and Keniston, R. C.: Crossed polydactyly. J. Bone Joint Surg., *57-A*:847, 1975.

80. Nylander, E. S.: Pre-axiale Polydaktylie in funf Generationen einer schwedischen Sippe. Upsala lak. Foren. Forh., *36*:275, 1931.

81. Odiorne, J. M.: Polydactylism in related New England families. J. Hered., *34*:45, 1943.

82. Ohkura, K.: Clinical genetics of polydactylism. Jpn. J. Hum. Genet., *1*:11, 1956.

83. Palmieri, T. J.: Polydactyly of the thumb: Incidence, etiology, classifications and treatment. Bull. Hosp. Joint Dis., *34*:200, 1973.

84. Pfeiffer, R. A.: Associated deformities of the head and hands. Birth Defects, Original Article Series, 5:18, 1969.

85. Pintilie, D., Hatmanu, D., Olaur, I., and Panoza, G.: Double ulna with symmetrical polydactyly. Case report. J. Bone Joint Surg., 46-B:89, 1964.

86. Prakash, C., and Singh, S.: Coarctation of the aorta with hypertelorism, pilonidal sinus and polydactyly. J. Indian Med. Assoc., 35:267, 1960.

87. Reber, M.: Un syndrome osseous peu commun associant une heptadactylie et une aplasie des tibias. J. Genet. Hum., 16:15, 1967–1968.

88. Refior, H. J.: Beitrage zur postaxialen familiaren Polydaktylie. Arch. Orthop. Unfallchir., 63:293, 1968.

89. Ricciardi, L.: La polidattilia transitoria. Clin. Orthop., 6:441, 1954.

90. Rimoin, D. L., and Edgerton, M. T.: Genetical and clinical heterogeneity in the oral-facial-digital syndromes. J. Pediatr., 71:94, 1967.

91. Rogers, J. G., Levin, L. S., Dorst, J. P., and Temtamy, S. A.: A postaxial polydactyly-dental vertebral syndrome. J. Pediatr., 90:230, 1977.

92. Rosenverg, T., Palombini, B. C., and Peterson, N.: Simultaneous occurrence of spherocytosis and polydactyly in a Brazilian family. Acta Genet. Med. Gemellol., 11:55, 1962.

93. Ruby, L., and Goldberg, M. J.: Syndactyly and polydactyly. Orthop. Clin. North Am., 7:361, 1976.

94. Say, B., Balci, S., Pirnar, T., and Tuncbilek, E.: A new syndrome of dysmorphogenesis: Imperforate anus associated with polyoligodactyly and skeletal (mainly vertebral) anomalies. Acta Paediatr. Scand., 60:197, 1971.

95. Say, B., and Gerald, P. S.: A new polydactyly/imperforate anus/vertebral anomalies syndrome? Lancet, 2:688, 1968.

96. Schoolfield, B.: Bilateral polydactylism with multiple syndactylism: Case report. South. Med. J., 49:716, 1956.

97. Segmi, G., Serra, A., Mastrangelo, R., Plidori, G., and Massasso, J.: Sindrome OFD in un Maschio. Rilivi sulla genetica della sindrome OFD dell analisi 33 famiglie. Acta Genet. Med. Gemellol., 19:546, 1970.

98. Sehgal, V. N., and Dube, B.: Polydactyly with ainhum in all the extra digits, hyperkeratosis palmaris et plantaris, and idiopathic eosinophilia. Dermatologica, 138:39, 1969.

99. Sergeant, P. W.: The Life of Anne Boleyn. New York, Appleton, 1924.

100. Shapiro, R. N., Eddy, W., Fitzgibbon, J., and O'Brien, G.: The incidence of congenital anomalies discovered in the neonatal period. Am. J. Surg., 96:396, 1958.

101. Sharma, N. L., Singh, R. N., and Anand, J. S.: Polydactylosyndactylism with unusual skeletal anomalies in mother and her six children. Indian J. Pediatr., 32:233, 1965.

102. Simopoulos, A. P., Brennan, G. G., Alwan, A., and Fidis, N.: Polycystic kidneys, internal hydrocephalus and polydactylism in newborn siblings. Pediatrics, 39:931, 1967.

103. Simpkiss, M., and Lowe, A.: Congenital abnormalities in the African newborn. Arch. Dis. Child., 36:404, 1961.

104. Smith, D. W., Lemli, L., and Opitz, J. M.: A newly recognized syndrome of multiple congenital anomalies. J. Pediatr., 64:210, 1964.

105. Smith, S., and Boulgakoff, B.: A case of polydactylia showing certain atavistic characters. J. Anat., 58:350, 1924.

106. Sobbota, A., and DeMarinis, F.: On the inheritance and development of preaxial and postaxial types of polydactylism. Acta Genet. Med. Gemellol., 6:85, 1957.

107. Stelling, F.: The upper extremity. In Ferguson, A. B. (ed.): Orthopedic Surgery in Infancy and Childhood. 3rd Ed. Baltimore, Williams & Wilkins, 1967, pp. 292–334.

108. Stevenson, A. C., Johnston, H. A., Stewart, M. I. P., and Golding, D. R.: Congenital malformations. A report of a study of series of consecutive births in 24 centres. Bull. W.H.O., 34:Suppl., 1966.

109. Strickland, A.: Lives of the Queens of England, Vol. II. London, Colburn, 1840–1848, pp. 589–590.

110. Sverdrup, A.: Postaxial polydactylism in six generations of a Norwegian family. J. Genet., 12:217, 1922.

111. Temtamy, S. A.: Genetic factors in hand malformations. Thesis. Johns Hopkins University, Baltimore, Maryland, 1966.

112. Temtamy, S., and McKusick, V. A.: Synopsis of hand malformations with particular emphasis on genetic factors. Birth Defects, 5:125, 1969.

113. Temtamy, S. A., and McKusick, V. A.: Polydactyly. Birth Defects, 14:364, 1978.

114. Tessari, L.: Sulla polidattilia. Arch. Ortop., 74:1186, 1961.

115. Thuline, H. C.: Current status of a family previously reported with the oral-facial-digital syndrome. In Bergsma, D. (ed.): Birth Defects: Original Article Series. New York, National Foundation-March of Dimes, Vol. V, No. 2:102, 1969.

116. Tollner, U., Horst, J., Manzke, E., Schmid, M., Nestler-Wocher, H., and Weckler, C.: Heptacarpo-octatarso-dactyly combined with multiple malformations. Eur. J. Pediatr., 136:207, 1981.

117. Townes, P. L., and Brocks, E. R.: Hereditary syndrome of imperforate anus with hand, foot, and ear anomalies. J. Pediatr., 81:321, 1972.

118. Tuch, B. A., Lipp, E. B., Larsen, I. J., and Gordon, L. H.: A review of supernumerary thumb and its surgical management. Clin. Orthop., 125:159, 1977.

119. Turek, S. L.: Orthopaedic Principles and Their Application. Philadelphia, Lippincott, 1967, p. 123.

120. Vardi, V., Szabo, L., and Papp, Z.: Syndrome of polydactyly, cleft lip/palate, or lingual lump and psychomotor retardation in endogamic gypsies. J. Med. Genet., 17:119, 1980.

121. Walker, J. T.: A pedigree of extra-digit V polydactyly in a Batutsi family. Ann. Hum. Genet., 25:65, 1961.

122. Wassel, H. D.: The results of surgery for polydactyly of the thumb: A review. Clin. Orthop., 64:175, 1969.

123. Weyers, H.: Über eine korrelierte Missbildung der Kiefer und Extremitätenakren (Dysostosis acrofacialis). Fortschr. Röntgenstr., 77:562, 1952.

124. Weyers, H.: Hexadactylie, Unterkieferspalt und Oligodontie ein neuer Symptom Komplex. Dysostosis acrofacialis. Ann. Paediatr., 181:45, 1953.

125. Wood, V. E.: Duplication of the index finger. J. Bone Joint Surg., 52-A:569, 1970.

126. Wood, V. E.: Treatment of central polydactyly. Clin. Orthop., 74:196, 1971.

127. Wood, V. E.: Polydactyly and the triphalangeal thumb. J. Hand Surg., 3:436, 1978.

128. Woolf, C. M., and Myrianthopoulos, N. C.: Polydactyly in American Negroes and Whites. Am. J. Hum. Genet., 25:397, 1973.

129. Woolf, C. M., and Woolf, R. M.: A genetic study of polydactyly in Utah. Am. J. Hum. Genet., 22:75, 1970.

130. Woolf, R. M., and Broadbent, T. R.: The four-flap Z-plasty. Plast. Reconstr. Surg., 49:48, 1972.

131. Yano, M., and Soma, H.: A kindred of polydactyly. Jpn. J. Hum. Genet., 6:124, 1961.

132. Zabolotikov, P. V.: On the problem of polydactylia (Russian). Arkh. Anat., 50:91, 1966.

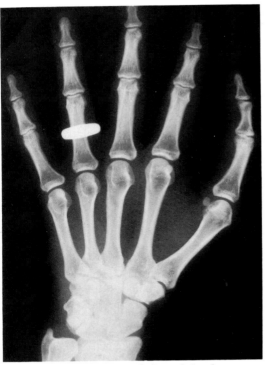

FIGURE 2–65. Triphalangeal thumb.

(From Poznanski, A.: The Hand in Radiologic Diagnosis. Philadelphia, W. B. Saunders Co., 1984. Reprinted by permission.)

TRIPHALANGEAL THUMB

In the normal human hand the thumb has two phalanges; the triphalangeal thumb contains three phalanges instead of the normal two (Fig. 2–65). Dubois is credited with being the first, in 1826, to describe a thumb with three instead of two phalanges.[14] The triphalangeal thumb may be an isolated anomaly without duplication. It occurs in about one per 25,000 births, constituting the second most common type of thumb duplication (20 per cent in the series reported by Wassel).[80] It is inherited as an autosomal dominant trait.[14] Its occurrence in a large family of 30 persons spanning four generations was reported by Swanson and Brown.[73] There is no sex predilection. In about 87 per cent of the cases involvement is bilateral. The thumb of the contralateral hand may be normal, absent, or duplicated.

Triphalangeal thumb may be part of a generalized syndrome such as Holt-Oram, Blackfan-Diamond anemia, or Fanconi's anemia.[1, 13, 16, 27, 28, 46, 56] It may be associated with other anomalies such as duplication of the hallux or the little toe; lobster feet and hands; or absence of the tibia, of carpal bones, or of pectoral muscles.[52, 54, 63] Other associated findings may be hypoplasia of nails, tooth anomalies, deafness, and mental retardation.[59] The anomaly may occur in diastrophic dwarfism.[4]

Phylogenetically, in all forms of life from the amphibians and up, the preaxial (or first) digit is composed of three phalanges. In the thalidomide-caused birth defects, triphalangeal thumb occurred when thalidomide was ingested between the forty-fifth and fiftieth days of gestation. The triphalangeal thumb with full-length normal second phalanx and without duplication resembles a finger; when it does not oppose because the thenar muscles are absent, the hand is referred to as a "thumbless" five-finger hand. In the adult, the triphalangeal thumb is

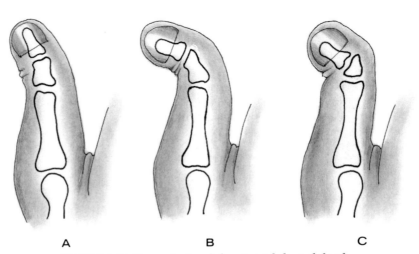

A   B   C

FIGURE 2–66. Types of extra phalanx in triphalangeal thumb.

A. Full. **B.** Rectangular. **C.** Delta.

extra long, cosmetically unattractive, and not normal. Functionally, fine motor activities such as precision handling are defective. The extra phalanx may be delta-shaped, rectangular, or normal (Fig. 2–66). A small trapezoid second phalanx will cause ulnar angulation.[19]

Treatment

In thumb duplication, when a triphalangeal thumb accompanies a normal thumb, the three-phalanxed thumb is ablated. When the accompanying two-phalanx thumb is hypoplastic but functional, again it is best to ablate the triphalangeal thumb. When both thumbs are triphalanxed and hypoplastic, the more functional of the duplicated thumbs is retained.

Excision of the accessory phalanx of a triphalangeal thumb results in instability at the site of excision. Surgery should be performed early in life, preferably prior to one year of age. The whole accessory phalanx is excised. The first and third phalanges are fused and internally fixed with a Kirschner wire. Providing stability of the interphalangeal joint of the thumb is of vital importance. The long extensor and flexor tendons are shortened. If the web space of the thumb is contracted it is widened by Z-plasty or a larger rotation flap from the dorsum of the hand. The Kirschner wire is removed in six weeks. Splinting is continued for an additional two months.

References

1. Aase, J. M., and Smith, D. W.: Congenital anemia and triphalangeal thumbs. J. Pediatr., 74:471, 1969.
2. Abramowitz, I.: Triphalangeal thumb in a Bantu family. J. Bone Joint Surg., 41-B:766, 1959.
3. Abramowitz, I.: Triphalangeal thumb—a case report and evaluation of its importance in the morphology and function of the thumb. S. Afr. Med. J., 41:104, 1967.
4. Amuso, S. J.: Diastrophic dwarfism. J. Bone Joint Surg., 50-A:113, 1968.
5. Barsky, A. J.: Congenital anomalies of the hand. J. Bone Joint Surg., 33-A:35, 1951.
6. Barsky, A. J.: Congenital Anomalies of the Hand and Their Surgical Treatment. Springfield, Thomas, 1958.
7. Barsky, A. J.: Congenital anomalies of the thumb. Clin. Orthop., 15:96, 1959.
8. Bienvenue, F.: Un cas de pouce supplémentaire à trois phalanges. Rev. Orthop., 111:91, 1912.
9. Buck-Gramcko, D.: Pollicization of the index finger. J. Bone Joint Surg., 53-A:1605, 1971.
10. Carstam, N., and Theander, G.: Surgical treatment of clinodactyly caused by longitudinal bracketed diaphysis (delta phalanx). Scand. J. Plast. Reconstr. Surg., 9:199, 1975.
11. Converse, J. M.: Plastic and Reconstructive Surgery. Philadelphia, Saunders, 1964, p. 1720.
12. Cotta, H., and Jager, M.: Die familiäre Triphalangie des Daumens und ihre operative Behandlung. Arch. Orthop. Unfallchir., 58:282, 1965.
13. Diamond, L. R., Allen, D. M., and Magill, F. B.:

14. Dubois, P.: Le pouce à de plus 3 phalanges. Arch. Gen. Med., 7:148, 1826.
15. Dubreuil-Chambardel, L.: Un cas d'hyperphalangie du pouce. Gaz. de Centre, Tours., 15:26, 1910.
16. Ferber, C.: A contribution to the three-phalangia of the thumb. Z. Orthop., 83:55, 1952.
17. Flatt, A.: The Care of Congenital Hand Anomalies. St. Louis, Mosby, 1977, pp. 109–117.
18. Francesconi, G.: Clinical considerations on a thumb malformation of a familial nature. Minerva Chir., 21:618, 1966.
19. Frere, J. M.: A case having thumbs with three phalanges simulating fingers. South. Med. J., 23:536, 1930.
20. Fuerst: Ein Fall von verkverzten und zweigliedrigen Fingern begleitet von Brustmuskeldefekten usw. Z. Morphol. Anthropol., 2:1900.
21. Girjia, A.: The occurence of an additional phalanx in the thumb. Indian J. Pediatr., 25:374, 1958.
22. Grobelnik, S.: Triphalangeal thumb. Z. Orthop., 80:294, 1951.
23. Haas, S. L.: Three-phalangeal thumb. A. J. R., 42:677, 1939.
24. Hersch, A. H., DeMarinis, F., and Stecher, R. M.: On the inheritance and development of clinodactyly. Am. J. Hum. Genet., 5:257, 1953.
25. Hilgenfelt, O.: Operativer Daumenersatz und Beseitigung von Griefstörungen bie Fingerverlusten. Stuttgart, Enke, 1950.
26. Hilgenreiner, H.: Ueber Hyperphalangie des Daumens. Beitr. Klin. Chir., 54:585, 1907.
27. Holmes, L. B.: Congenital heart disease and upper extremity deformities. A report of two families. N. Engl. J. Med., 272:437, 1965.
28. Holt, M., and Oram, S.: Familial heart disease with skeletal malformations. Br. Heart J., 22:236, 1960.
29. Holthusen, W.: The Pierre Robin syndrome: Unusual associated developmental defects. Ann. Radiol., 15:253, 1972.
30. Hoover, G. H., Flatt, A. E., and Weiss, M. W.: The hand and Apert's syndrome. J. Bone Joint Surg., 52-A:878, 1970.
31. Jaeger, M., and Refior, H. J.: The congenital triangular deformity of the tubular bones of the hand and foot. Clin. Orthop., 81:139, 1971.
32. Joachimsthal, G.: Ueber brachydaktylie und Hyperphalangie. Virchows Arch., 151:429, 1898.
33. Jones, G. B.: Delta phalanx. J. Bone Joint Surg., 46-B:226, 1964.
34. Juberg, R. C., and Hayward, J. R.: A new familial syndrome of oral, cranial, and digital anomalies. J. Pediatr., 74:755, 1969.
35. Kirmission, E.: Pouces à trois phalanges. Rev. Orthop., 10:249, 1909.
36. Komai, T., Ozaki, Y., and Inokuma, W.: A Japanese kindred of hyperphalangism of thumbs and duplication of thumbs and big toes. Folia Hered. Pathol., 2:307, 1953.
37. Krisjansen, A.: Supernumerary phalanx in the thumbs, "hyperphalangeal pollicis." Hospitalstid, 69:109, 1926.
38. Lapidus, P. W., and Guidotti, F. P.: Triphalangeal bifid thumb. Arch. Surg., 49:228, 1944.
39. Lapidus, P. W., Guidotti, F. P., and Coletti, C. J.: Triphalangeal thumb—report of six cases. Surg. Gynecol. Obstet., 77:178, 1943.
40. Lenz, W.: Zur Diagnose und Aetiologie der Akrocephalosyndaktylie. Z. Mund. Kieferheilkd., 79:546, 1957.
41. Lenz, W., Theopold, W., and Thomas, J.: Thiphalangie des daumens als folge von thalidomidschadgung. Munch. Med. Wochenschr., 106:2033, 1964.
42. Malek, R., and Oger, P.: Les pouces à trois phalanges. Ann. Chir., 30:849, 1976.

Congenital (erythroid) hypoplasia anemia. A 25 year study. Am. J. Dis. Child., 102:403, 1961.

43. Manzke, H.: Symmetrische Hyperphalangie des zweiten Fingers durch ein akzessorisches Metacarpale. Fortschr. Geb. Rontgenstr. Nuklearmed., *105*:425, 1966.

44. Maurizio, E.: Primus digitus varus, triphalangism of the thumb and radial polydactylia. Arch. Putti Chir. Organi Mov., *19*:449, 1964.

45. Milch, H.: Triphalangeal thumb. J. Bone Joint Surg., *33-A*:692, 1951.

46. Minagi, H., and Steinbach, H. L.: Roentgen appearance of anomalies associated with hypoplastic anemias of childhood. A. J. R., *97*:100, 1966.

47. Miura, T.: Triphalangeal thumb. Plast. Reconstr. Surg., *58*:587, 1976.

48. Mueller, W.: Contributions to knowledge of the triphalangeal thumb. Arch. Klin. Chir., *185*:377, 1936.

49. Murphy, S., and Lubin, B.: Triphalangeal thumbs and congenital erythroid hypoplasia: Report of a case with unusual features. J. Pediatr., *81*:987, 1972.

50. Palmieri, T. J.: Polydactyly of the thumb: incidence, etiology, classification and treatment. Bull. Hosp. Joint Dis., *34*:200, 1973.

51. Pashayan, H., Fraser, F. C., McIntyre, J. M., and Dunbar, J. S.: Bilateral aplasia of the tibia, polydactyly and absent thumb in father and daughter. J. Bone Joint Surg., *53-B*:495, 1971.

52. Phillips, R. S.: Congenital split foot (lobster claw) and triphalangeal thumb. J. Bone Joint Surg., *53-B*:247, 1971.

53. Pol, R.: Brachydaktylie—Klinodaktylie—Hyperphalangie und ihre Grundlogen. Virchows Arch., *229*: 388, 1921.

54. Polinelli, U.: A case of familial hyperphalangia of the thumbs. Minerva Nefrol., *12*:373, 1962.

55. Poznanski, A. K.: Rubeinstein Taybi syndrome (broad thumb syndrome). *In* Poznanski, A. K. (ed.): The Hand in Radiologic Diagnosis. Philadelphia, Saunders, 1974, pp. 369–370.

56. Poznanski, A. K., Gall, J. C., Jr., and Stern, A. M.: Skeletal manifestations of the Holt-Oram syndrome. Radiology, *94*:45, 1970.

57. Poznanski, A. K., Garn, S. M., and Holt, J. F.: The thumb in the congenital malformation syndromes. Radiology, *100*:115, 1971.

58. Poznanski, A. K., Pratt, G. B., Manson, G., et al.: Clinodactyly, camptodactyly, Kirner's deformity and other crooked fingers. Radiology, *93*:573, 1969.

59. Qazi, Q. H., and Smithwick, E. M.: Triphalangy of thumbs and great toes. Am. J. Dis. Child., *120*:255, 1970.

60. Rath, F.: Triphalangia of the thumb as a manifestation of thalidomide embryopathy. Arch. Orthop. Unfallchir., *62*:339, 1967.

61. Rubinstein, J. H.: The broad thumb syndrome—progress report 1968. Birth Defects, *5*:25, 1969.

62. Sallam, A. M.: Triphalangeal thumb. Arch. Surg., *71*:257, 1955.

63. Salzer, M.: Über den kongenitales Tibiadefekt. Zbl. Chir., *85*:673, 1960.

64. Scharizer-Mannheim, E.: On the surgical treatment of the 3-joint thumb. Langenbecks Arch. Chir., *309*:47, 1965.

65. Schatzki, P.: Ueber verdeckte Syndaktyle Polydaktylie und euber "Triangelbildung" in der menschlichen Hand. Arch. Orthop. Unfallchir., *34*:637, 1934.

66. Schrader, E.: Three-jointed thumbs, case. Fortschr. Geb. Roentgenstr., *40*:693, 1929.

67. Schonenberg, H.: Missbildungen der Gliedmassen-extremitaetenfehlbildungen. *In* Opitz, H., and Schmid, F. (eds.): Handbuch der Kinderheilkunde. Berlin, Springer, 1967.

68. Sella, E. J.: Delta phalanx. Conn. Med., *36*:437, 1972.

69. Smith, R. J.: Osteotomy for "delta-phalanx" deformity. Clin. Orthop., *123*:91, 1977.

70. Stieve, H.: Ueber Hyperphalangie des Daumens. Anat. Anz., 565, 1915.

71. Stover, C. N., Hayes, J. T., and Holt, J. F.: Diastrophic dwarfism. A. J. R., *89*:914, 1963.

72. Strauch, B., and Spinner, M.: Congenital anomaly of the thumb: Absent intrinsics and flexor pollicis longus. J. Bone Joint Surg., *58-A*:115, 1976.

73. Swanson, A. B., and Brown, K. S.: Hereditary triphalangeal thumb. J. Hered., *53*:259, 1962.

74. Taybi, H.: Diastrophic dwarfism. Radiology, *80*:1, 1963.

75. Temtamy, S., and McKusick, V. A.: Synopsis of hand malformations with particular emphasis on genetic factors. Birth Defects, *3*:125, 1969.

76. Theander, G., and Carstam, N.: Longitudinally bracketed diaphysis. Ann. Radiol., *17*:355, 1974.

77. Theander, G., and Carstam, N.: Triphalangism and pseudotriphalangism of the thumb in children. Acta Radiol. [Diagn.] (Stockh.), *20*:223, 1979.

78. Townes, P. L., and Brocks, E. R.: Hereditary syndrome of imperforate anus with hand, foot, and ear anomalies. J. Pediatr., *81*:321, 1972.

79. Unger, H.: Missbildungen. *In* Matzen, P. F. (ed.): Lehrbuch der Orthopaedie. Berlin, VEB Bolk und Gesundheit, 1967.

80. Wassel, H. D.: The results of surgery for polydactyly of the thumb. Clin. Orthop., *64*:175, 1969.

81. Watson, H. K., and Boyes, J. H.: Congenital angular deformity of the digits. J. Bone Joint Surg., *49-A*:333, 1967.

82. Wertheman, A.: Die Entwicklungsstoerungen der Extremitaeten. *In* Lubarsch, O., Heinke, F., Roessle, R., et al. (eds.): Handbuch der Speziellen pathologischen Anatomie und Histologie. Berlin, Springer, 1952.

83. Witt, A. M., Cotta, H., and Jaeger, M.: Die angeborenen Fehlbildungen der Hand und ihre operative Behandlung. Stuttgart, Thieme, 1966.

84. Wood, V. E.: The treatment of central polydactyly. Clin. Orthop., *74*:196, 1971.

85. Wood, V. E.: Treatment of the triphalangeal thumb. Clin. Orthop., *120*:188, 1976.

86. Wood, V. E., and Flatt, A. E.: Congenital triangular bones in the hand. J. Hand Surg., *2*:179, 1977.

87. Woolf, R. M., and Broadbent, T. R.: The four-flap Z-plasty. Plast. Reconstr. Surg., *49*:48, 1972.

88. Woolf, R. M., Broadbent, T. R., and Woolf, C. M.: Practical genetics of congenital hand abnormalities. *In* Littler, J. W., Cramer, L. M., and Smith, J. W. (eds.): Symposium on Reconstructive Hand Surgery. St. Louis, Mosby, 1974, pp. 141–143.

89. Zderkiewicz, W.: Familial occurrences of triphalangeal thumbs. Chir. Narzadow Ruchu Ortop. Pol., *22*:551, 1957.

90. Zrubecky, G., and Scharizer, E.: Triphalangia of the thumb. Arch. Orthop. Unfallchir., *57*:45, 1965.

CONGENITAL LONGITUDINAL DEFICIENCY OF THE THUMB

Congenital absence or hypoplasia of the thumb is often associated with congenital longitudinal deficiency of the radius. The spectrum of the defect varies from simple hypoplasia and miniature thumb to total absence of the thumb.

Hypoplastic Thumb

In the normal hand, the tip of the thumb reaches to the middle of the proximal phalanx of the index finger. When the thumb is shorter than this it can be classified as hypoplastic. It is crucial to rule out associated abnormalities because often this malformation is a manifestation of a syndrome. One should rule out abnormalities of the heart, spine, and gastrointestinal tract. A short slender first metacarpal may be a feature of the Fanconi or Holt-Oram syndrome, whereas a short broad first metacarpal may be associated with such disorders as Cornelia de Lange syndrome or diastrophic dwarfism. If the small thumb is associated with a

Text continued on page 268

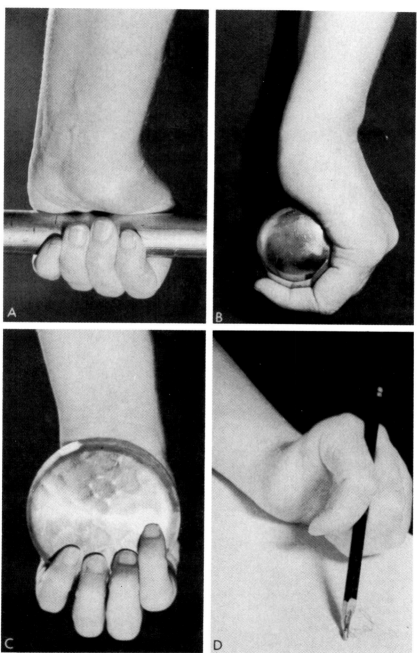

FIGURE 2–67. *Congenital absence of the thumb.*

A and **B.** Grasping a bar against the palm. Note the absence of the thenar eminence. **C.** Curling the four digits on a disc. Effective rotation of a doorknob will be difficult. **D.** Side-to-side pinch. (From Kelikian, H.: Congenital Deformities of the Hand and Forearm. Philadelphia, W. B. Saunders Co., 1974. Reprinted by permission.)

Pollicization of the Index Finger (Buck-Gramcko Technique)

OPERATIVE TECHNIQUE

A and **B.** A lazy S–shaped incision is made on the radial side of the palmar surface of the hand, beginning on the volar aspect of the index finger near its base and terminating at the wrist. Another curvilinear incision is made across the base of the index finger at right angles and connected to the distal end of the first incision. The two ends of the incision are connected on the dorsum of the hand as shown in **B.** The third incision is made on the dorsum of the proximal phalanx of the index finger.

C. The transverse fascicles of the palmar aponeurosis are divided to gain access to the neurovascular bundle between the index and middle fingers.

D. The artery to the radial side of the long finger is ligated. Next, the common digital nerve is carefully separated into its component parts for the index and the long fingers. It is important that there be no tension on the neurovascular structures when the index finger is rotated. If an anomalous neural ring is present, it is sectioned so that there is no angulation of the digital artery. It is crucial that the digital veins be preserved.

Plate 10. Pollicization of the Index Finger
(Buck-Gramcko Technique)

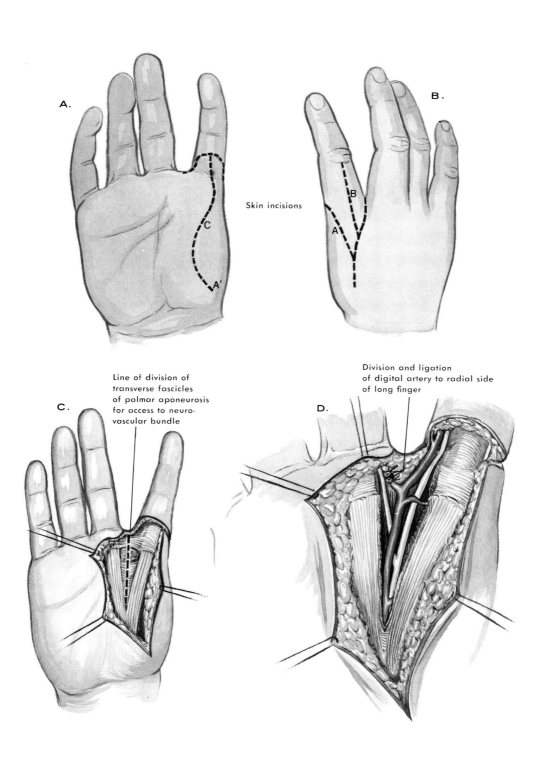

A.

B.

Skin incisions

C.

Line of division of
transverse fascicles
of palmar aponeurosis
for access to neuro-
vascular bundle

D.

Division and ligation
of digital artery to radial side
of long finger

Pollicization of the Index Finger (Buck-Gramcko Technique) (Continued)

E and F. The long extensor tendon of the index finger is sectioned at the level of the metacarpophalangeal joint, and the interosseous muscles of the index finger are detached from the proximal phalanx and lateral bands of the dorsal aponeurosis. A subperiosteal incision is made on the dorsum of the second metacarpal, and the interosseous muscles are stripped subperiosteally. Caution! Do not injure neurovascular structures. The metacarpal of the index finger is excised but its head is preserved. If the phalanges of the index finger are short, the base of the metacarpal is preserved. The index finger is rotated 160 degrees, and the head of the index metacarpal is fixed to its base by two Kirschner wires. At the completion of the operation the 160-degree rotation of the index finger becomes only 120 degrees. It is important to have the proximal phalanx of the index finger in complete hyperextension in relation to the metacarpal head to provide maximal joint stability.

G. The extensor digitorum communis tendon is fixed to the base of the former proximal phalanx, which now acts as the first metacarpal. The extensor digitorum communis functions now as an abductor pollicis longus. The extensor indicis proprius is shortened to the appropriate length and sutured end-to-end to function as an extensor pollicis brevis. The origins of the first dorsal and first volar interosseous muscles are sutured to their respective bases on the shaft of the new metacarpal (former proximal phalanx).

Plate 10. Pollicization of the Index Finger
(Buck-Gramcko Technique)

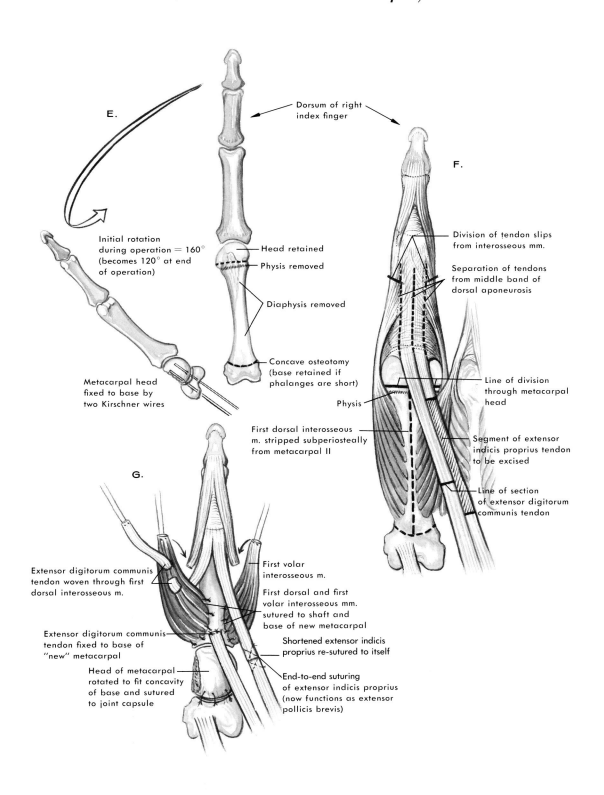

E.

Dorsum of right index finger

Initial rotation during operation = 160° (becomes 120° at end of operation)

Head retained

Physis removed

Diaphysis removed

Metacarpal head fixed to base by two Kirschner wires

Concave osteotomy (base retained if phalanges are short)

Physis

First dorsal interosseous m. stripped subperiosteally from metacarpal II

F.

Division of tendon slips from interosseous mm.

Separation of tendons from middle band of dorsal aponeurosis

Line of division through metacarpal head

Segment of extensor indicis proprius tendon to be excised

Line of section of extensor digitorum communis tendon

G.

First volar interosseous m.

First dorsal and first volar interosseous mm. sutured to shaft and base of new metacarpal

Shortened extensor indicis proprius re-sutured to itself

End-to-end suturing of extensor indicis proprius (now functions as extensor pollicis brevis)

Extensor digitorum communis tendon woven through first dorsal interosseous m.

Extensor digitorum communis tendon fixed to base of "new" metacarpal

Head of metacarpal rotated to fit concavity of base and sutured to joint capsule

Pollicization of the Index Finger (Buck-Gramcko Technique) (Continued)

H. The distal segment of the extensor digitorum communis tendon is woven through the first dorsal interosseous muscle as shown in **G** and sutured to itself and the radial lateral band of the aponeurosis; it will serve as abductor pollicis brevis. The first volar interosseous muscle is sutured to the ulnar lateral band to function as adductor pollicis.

I. View of the volar surface of the hand showing the rotated and shortened index finger that will serve as the thumb.

J. The skin is closed with interrupted sutures, and an above-elbow cast is applied incorporating the pollicized index finger.

POSTOPERATIVE CARE

The cast is removed in four weeks. The pins are removed. Bony fusion is not necessary because fibrous union of the head of the former metacarpal to its base is adequate for satisfactory function.

Plate 10. Pollicization of the Index Finger
(Buck-Gramcko Technique)

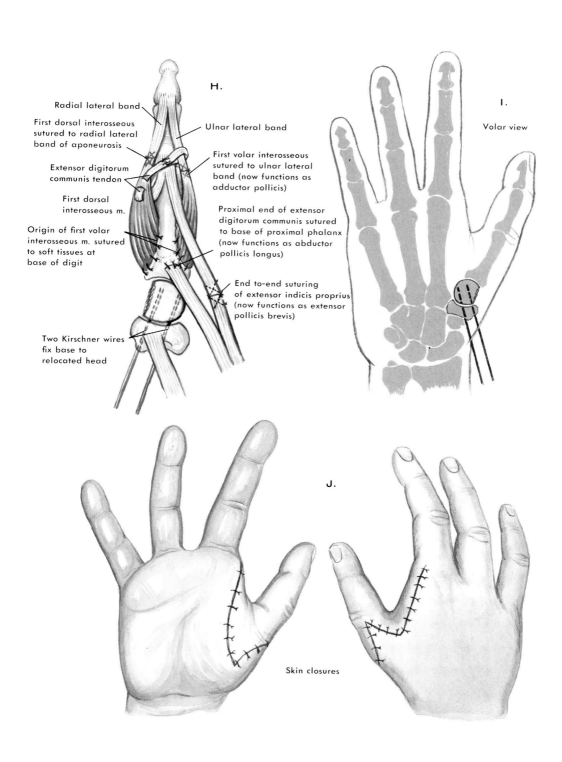

H.

Radial lateral band

First dorsal interosseous sutured to radial lateral band of aponeurosis

Extensor digitorum communis tendon

First dorsal interosseous m.

Origin of first volar interosseous m. sutured to soft tissues at base of digit

Two Kirschner wires fix base to relocated head

Ulnar lateral band

First volar interosseous sutured to ulnar lateral band (now functions as adductor pollicis)

Proximal end of extensor digitorum communis sutured to base of proximal phalanx (now functions as abductor pollicis longus)

End to-end suturing of extensor indicis proprius (now functions as extensor pollicis brevis)

I.

Volar view

J.

Skin closures

short great toe, beware of myositis ossificans progressiva. Brachydactyly of the proximal or the distal phalanx of the thumb may be an isolated finding or a manifestation of such syndromes as Rubinstein-Taybi, Apert's, or Carpenter's.

Grasp and prehension are hampered when the thumb is short. Recessing the web proximally will effectively lengthen the thumb, but stability of the carpometacarpal joint is a prerequisite. Two- or four-flap Z-plasties are the best techniques to deepen the web space between the thumb and index finger.

Floating Thumb (Pouce Flottant)

This anomaly is characterized by a hypoplastic thumb with a nail and two phalanges but the metacarpal partially or entirely absent. Its extrinsic tendons are absent, and functionally the thumb is useless. Treatment consists of ablation of the vestigial thumb and pollicization

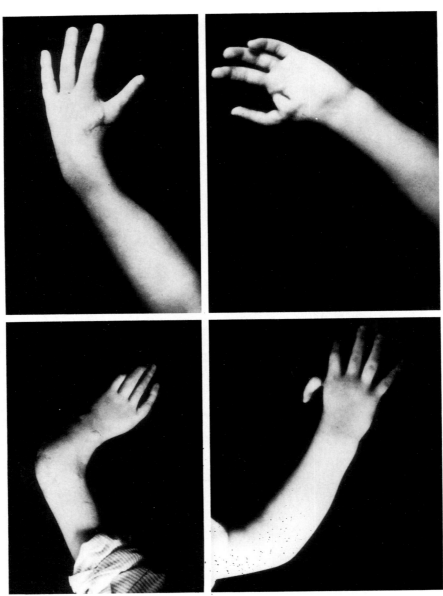

FIGURE 2–68. Bilateral congenital absence of the thumbs.

Left side has been pollicized; the right thumb is absent. In addition, the right forearm has congenital longitudinal deficiency of the radius and ulna.

of the index finger. There may be associated neurovascular anomalies, such as a neural ring encircling the common digital artery.

The severely hypoplastic thumb attached to the hand by a small skin pedicle is ablated, and the index finger is pollicized.

Pollicization of the index finger, described in detail by Littler in 1953 and later refined by Buck-Gramcko, is a safe and successful means of providing a thumb.[4, 26] There is some controversy whether it should be performed in unilateral absence of the thumb, because the deficiency can be compensated for by a strong lateral pinch grip between the ulnar side of the index finger and the pad of the long finger, and there will be considerable rotation of the index finger. This is a poor substitute for a normal tip or pulp pinch produced by transposing the index finger. In bilateral absence of the thumbs there should be no question about pollicizing the index finger in one hand (Figs. 2–67 and 2–68).

Timing of surgery with respect to the age of the patient depends on the skill and experience of the surgeon. Sometime between 6 and 12 months of age is the best time for pollicization, provided it is performed by meticulous surgical technique. The infant then learns normal prehension patterns at an early age. The operative technique of pollicization of the index finger is illustrated in Plate 10.

In recent years development of microsurgical techniques has made it feasible to transplant a toe to the hand.[7, 10–12, 14, 18, 19, 32] At present esthetic and functional results are dubious. Further experience may open new vistas. At the present time, this author does not recommend this procedure.

References

1. Ahstrom, J. P., Jr.: Pollicization in congenital absence of the thumb. Curr. Pract. Orthop. Surg., 5:1, 1973.
2. Bowe, J. J.: Thumb reconstruction by index transpositions. Plast. Reconstr. Surg., 32:414, 1963.
3. Broadbent, T. R., and Woolf, R. M.: Thumb reconstruction with contiguous skin-bone pedicle graft. Plast. Reconstr. Surg., 26:494, 1960.
4. Buck-Gramcko, D.: Pollicization of the index finger: Method and results in aplasia and hypoplasia of the thumb. J. Bone Joint Surg., 53-A:1605, 1971.
5. Bunnell, S.: Physiological reconstruction of a thumb after total loss. Surg. Gynecol. Obstet., 52:245, 1931.
6. Bunnell, S.: Reconstruction of the thumb. Am. J. Surg., 95:168, 1958.
7. Clarkson, P.: Reconstruction of hand digits by toe transfers. J. Bone Joint Surg., 37-A:270, 1955.
8. Clarkson, P.: On making thumbs. Plast. Reconstr. Surg., 29:325, 1962.
9. Clarkson, P.: Erratum (on making thumbs). Plast. Reconstr. Surg., 30:491, 1962.
10. Clarkson, P., and Chandler, R.: A toe to thumb transplant with nerve graft. Am. J. Surg., 95:315, 1958.
11. Clarkson, P., and Furlong, R.: Thumb reconstruction by transfer of big toe. Br. Med. J., 2:1332, 1949.
12. Cobbett, J. R.: Free digital transfer: report of a case of transfer of a great toe to replace an amputated thumb. J. Bone Joint Surg., 51-B:677, 1969.
13. Cuthbert, J. B.: Pollicization of the index finger. Br. J. Plast. Surg., 1:56, 1948–1949.
14. Davis, J. E.: Toe to hand transfer (pedochyrodactyloplasty). Plast. Reconstr. Surg., 33:422, 1964.
15. De Oliveira, J. C.: Some aspects of thumb reconstruction. Br. J. Surg., 57:85, 1970.
16. Dunlop, J.: The use of the index finger for the thumb: Some interesting points in hand surgery. J. Bone Joint Surg., 5:99, 1923.
17. Edgerton, M. T., Snyder, G. B., and Webb, W. L.: Surgical treatment of congenital thumb deformities (including psychological impact of correction). J. Bone Joint Surg., 47-A:1453, 1965.
18. Freeman, B. S.: Reconstruction of thumb by toe transfer. Plast. Reconstr. Surg., 17:393, 1956.
19. Gilbert, A.: Toe transfers for congenital hand defects. J. Hand Surg., 7:118, 1982.
20. Harrison, S. H.: Restoration of muscle balance in pollicization. Plast. Reconstr. Surg., 34:236, 1964.
21. Hung-Yin, C., Ta-Mei, W., Fan-Yu, K., and Chu-Jen, H.: Reconstruction of the thumb. Chin. Med. J., 79:541, 1959. (Abstracted by David E. Hallstrand, Int. Abstr. Surg., 111:177, 1960.)
22. Iselin, M.: Chirurgie de la Main. 10th Ed. Paris, Masson, 1955.
23. Jeffery, C. C.: A case of pollicisation of the index finger. J. Bone Joint Surg., 39-B:120, 1957.
24. Joyce, J. L.: A new operation of the substitution of a thumb. Br. J. Surg., 5:499, 1918.
25. Kaplan, I., and Plaschkes, J.: One stage pollicisation of little finger. Br. J. Plast. Surg., 13:272, 1960–1961.
26. Littler, J. W.: The neurovascular pedicle method of digital transposition for reconstruction of the thumb. Plast. Reconstr. Surg., 12:303, 1953.
27. Littler, J. W.: Digital transposition. In Adams, J. P. (ed.): Current Practice In Orthopaedic Surgery, Vol. 3. St. Louis, Mosby, 1966.
28. Littler, J. W.: On making a thumb: One hundred years of surgical effort. J. Hand Surg., 1:35, 1976.
29. Matthews, D.: Congenital absence of functioning thumb. Plast. Reconstr. Surg., 26:487, 1960.
30. Miura, T.: Thumb reconstruction using radial-innervated cross-finger pedicle graft. J. Bone Joint Surg., 55-A:563, 1973.
31. Moore, F. T.: The technique of pollicisation of the index finger. Br. J. Plast. Surg., 1:60, 1948–1949.
32. O'Brien, B. M., MacLeod, A. M., Sykes, P. J., et al.: Hallux-to-hand transfer. Hand, 7:128, 1975.
33. Reid, D. A. C.: Reconstruction of the thumb. J. Bone Joint Surg., 42-B:444, 1960.
34. Schmauk, B.: On the problem of thumb substitution (Zur Problematik des Daumenersatzes). Med. Welt, 9:482, 1960. (Abstr. by Joseph C. Mulier, Int. Abstr. Surg., 111:178, 1960.)
35. Shaw, M. H., and Wilson, I. S. P.: An early pollicisation. Br. J. Plast. Surg., 3:214, 1950–1951.
36. Tanzer, R. C., and Littler, J. W.: Reconstruction of the thumb. Plast. Reconstr. Surg., 3:533, 1948.
37. Verdan, C.: The reconstruction of the thumb. Surg. Clin. North Am., 48:1033, 1968.
38. White, W. F.: Fundamental priorities in pollicization. J. Bone Joint Surg., 52-B:438, 1970.
39. Zancolli, E.: Transplantation of the index finger in congenital absence of the thumb. J. Bone Joint Surg. 42-A:658, 1960.

CONGENITAL CLASPED THUMB

Congenital clasped thumb, also referred to as thumb-clutched (or clasped) hand, is characterized by marked flexion of the metacarpophalangeal joint and adduction into the palm. It is a syndrome and not a specific entity because the flexion-extension imbalance of the thumb is the result of several causes, not a single cause.

Classification

Weckesser, Reed, and Heiple suggested subdivision of the syndrome into four groups: Group I—deficient extension only; Group II—deficient extension combined with flexion contracture; Group III—hypoplasia of the thumb associated with deficiencies of muscles and tendons; and Group IV—the few cases not falling in the first three groups.[21]

Incidence

Congenital clasped thumb is a rare anomaly. Group I is the most common (about 70 per cent of reported cases). Next in frequency is Group II (about 23 per cent). Groups III and IV are very rare (about 3.5 per cent each).[21] Involvement is almost always bilateral. There is definite sex predilection for the male with a male to female ratio of two to one. Familial incidence is observed, with a possible sex-linked inheritance in the Group I syndrome. There are usually no associated abnormalities with the exception, occasionally, of talipes equinovarus.

Anatomic and Clinical Findings

The original description of Zadek, in 1934, depicts the characteristic deformity in the infant—"the thumbs laying helplessly in the palms of the hands" (Fig. 2–69).[24]

In *Group I* cases it is principally the extensor pollicis brevis that is hypoplastic or absent, although sometimes the extensor pollicis longus muscle may also be involved. The tendons of these thumb extensors are not completely absent. They are attenuated into thin thread-like tendinous structures that narrow proximally and terminate into fibrofatty tissue; usually there is no real muscle attached to them. The thumb can be passively extended and abducted—there is no fixed contractural deformity. There are no other finger or hand anomalies.

In *Group II* there is definite flexion contracture of the thumb, but in addition there are

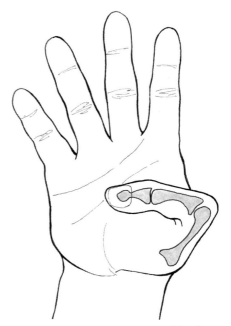

FIGURE 2–69. *Thumb-clasped hand.*

significant flexion contracture of the other digits and, occasionally, mild flexion contracture of elbows and knees. The disorder in this group may represent a form of arthrogryposis multiplex congenita. A thorough physical examination is crucial; Sheldon-Freeman (or whistling face) syndrome should be ruled out.

In *Group III*, the involvement is more severe and diffuse. The thumb is small, the first metacarpal and its phalanges are hypoplastic, and the metacarpophalangeal joint is unstable. There is partial or complete absence of the extensor tendons of the thumb, thenar muscles, and abductor pollicis longus. In addition to the flexion contracture there is marked adduction contracture of the thumb. This group probably represents a mild form of longitudinal deficiency of the radial ray.

Group IV cases usually represent varying degrees of polydactyly with associated musculotendinous weakness rather than aplasia.

In the newborn and during the first three to four months of infancy, grasp reflex is normal—the thumb is flexed across the palm and the fingers are flexed over the clutched thumb. Spontaneously and upon stimulation, the infant will actively extend his fingers and thumb. This normal grasp posture should be distinguished from congenital clasped thumb. In spastic cerebral palsy, hypertonicity of the thumb adductors and flexors will clutch the thumb across the palm. A thorough neurologic examination will establish the degree of cerebral palsy.

Treatment

The treatment depends on the type of clasped thumb. Group I thumbs usually respond to conservative nonsurgical measures. The thumbs are splinted into extension and abduction; splints are preferably manufactured of plastics such as polypropylene or Orthoplast. Some surgeons may prefer to use plaster of Paris casts. The splints should be well molded to keep the metacarpophalangeal and interphalangeal joints of the thumbs in complete extension and the thumb metacarpal in abduction. The splints are changed as needed to accommodate growth of the infant's hand. Splinting should be continuous and not only at night. Immobilization of the thumbs out of flexion-abduction is continued for at least three months, at which time one can determine with a certain degree of accuracy whether the thumb extensors are absent or nonfunctional. If at the end of three months there has been improvement with some active extension, the splinting is continued for another three months. It appears that the weak thumb extensors become stronger with growth if protected early in life against the overpowering pull of the thumb flexors. Long-term results have shown that recovery of strength persists and thumb extension remains functionally good.

If at the end of three months there is no power of active extension of the thumb and the clasped deformity immediately recurs, immobilization of the thumb in extension-abduction is continued for another three months. Occasionally, active extension of the thumb will develop after this extra period of splinting; this is unlikely, however, and a tendon transfer usually is required to provide it. What is the best age for surgery? It is preferable that the child be sufficiently cooperative to train the tendon transfer. Therefore this author recommends delay of the operation until the child is at least three years of age. In the interim waiting period, exercises for passive stretching of the thumb into abduction-extension and splinting at night are utilized to prevent development of fixed contractural deformity.

The most suitable tendon for transfer is the extensor indicis proprius; it is of adequate motor strength and appropriate length, and is in phase. The transfer should be anchored fairly tautly into the base of the distal phalanx of the thumb in order to provide a certain degree of tenodesis effect against the pull of the strong flexor pollicis longus muscle. Injury to the growth plate at the base of the distal phalanx should be avoided. It is best to attach the transferred tendon to the attenuated tendon of the extensor pollicis longus at its insertion. The use of a smooth Kirschner wire of adequate size ensures that the interphalangeal and metacarpophalangeal joints of the thumb are in complete extension and the thumb metacarpal is in abduction. An above-elbow cast is applied for external immobilization for a period of six weeks.

Other possible motors for tendon transfers are the extensor carpi ulnaris (Kelikian), the extensor carpi radialis (Gold and Perlman, Zadek), the brachioradialis (Flatt), and the flexor digitorum sublimis of the ring or long finger (Littler, Crawford and associates).[5, 6, 8, 11, 12, 24] Most of these tendon transfers require extension with a graft taken from the palmaris longus, the plantaris, or one of the long toe extensors (usually the fourth). The long-term results of tendon transfers to provide thumb extension are very satisfactory.

In Group II or in late cases of Group I with contractural deformity of soft tissues, a preliminary soft-tissue release will be required as a first stage. The thumb–index finger skin contracture is widened by Z-plasty. In the severe case a full dorsal rotation flap and a full-thickness skin graft may be required; also one may have to release the adductor pollicis from the third metacarpal through a separate midpalmar incision, lengthen the flexor pollicis longus at the wrist level, and release the flexor pollicis brevis at its insertion and the first dorsal interosseous from the metacarpal. To allow full correction, the joint capsule may have to be sectioned. Such extensive release requires internal splinting of the interphalangeal and metacarpophalangeal joints of the thumb in extension and the thumb in abduction. Tendon transfers to provide active thumb extension are performed three to six months after correction of contractural deformity. Normal range of joint motion is a vital prerequisite for success of tendon transfer.

In Group III cases the metacarpophalangeal joint is unstable; it is treated by arthrodesis in the patient over 12 years of age and chondrodesis in the younger child. Tendon transfers are required to provide thumb extension and abduction, and also, sometimes, opposition.

Most Group IV cases involve the residual clutched thumb after the supernumerary thumb has been excised; the thumb extensors are present but weak. Treatment consists of prolonged retention of the remaining thumb in extension-abduction in a plaster of Paris cast or plastic splint. With such therapy, good active abduction and extension of the thumb can often be restored.

References

1. Barsky, A. J.: Congenital anomalies of the hand. J. Bone Joint Surg., *33-A*:35, 1951.
2. Barsky, A. J.: Congenital Anomalies of the Hand and Their Surgical Treatment. Springfield, Thomas, 1958, p. 112.
3. Broadbent, T. R., and Woolf, R. M.: Flexion adduction deformity of the thumb—congenital clasped thumb. Plast. Reconstr. Surg., *34*:612, 1964.
4. Bunnell, S.: Surgery of the Hand. 3rd Ed. Philadelphia, Lippincott, 1956, p. 26.
5. Crawford, H. H., Horton, C. E., and Adamson, J.: Congenital aplasia or hypoplasia of thumb and finger extensor tendons. J. Bone Joint Surg., *48-A*:82, 1966.
6. Flatt, A. E.: The Care of Congenital Hand Anomalies. St. Louis, Mosby, 1977, pp. 60–63.
7. Gesell, A.: An Atlas of Infant Behavior. Vol. 1. New Haven, Yale University Press, 1934, pp. 243–249.
8. Gold, A. M., and Perlman, R. D.: Congenital clasped thumb deformity. Case report. Bull. Hosp. Joint Dis., *29*:255, 1968.
9. Granberry, W. M.: American Society for Surgery of the Hand Correspondence Newsletter, No. 1975–36, October 30, 1975.
10. Huber, E.: Hifsoperation bei Medianeeslähmung. Dtsch. Z. Chir., *162*:271, 1921.
11. Kelikian, H.: Congenital Deformities of the Hand and Forearm. Philadelphia, Saunders, 1974, pp. 555–565.
12. Littler, J. W.: The prevention and the correction of adduction contracture of the thumb. Clin. Orthop., *13*:182, 1959.
13. Loomis, L. K.: Congenital "clasped thumb." J. La. State Med. Soc., *110*:23, 1958.
14. Miller, J. W.: Pollex varus: A report of two cases. Univ. Hosp. Bull., Ann Arbor, *10*:10, 1944.
15. Miura, T.: Congenital absence of the flexor pollicis longus. A case report. Hand, *9*:272, 1977.
16. Namba, K., Muda, Y., and Hachiguchi, T.: Congenital clasped thumb. Orthop. Surg., *16*:1031, 1965.
17. Neviaser, R. J.: Congenital hypoplasia of the thumb with absence of the extrinsic extensors, abductor pollicis longus, and thenar muscles. J. Hand Surg., *4*:301, 1979.
18. Strauch, B., and Spinner, M.: Congenital anomaly of the thumb: Absent intrinsics and flexor pollicis longus. J. Bone Joint Surg., *58-A*:115, 1976.
19. Su, C. T., Hoopes, J. E., and Daniel, R.: Congenital absence of the thenar muscle innervated by the median nerve. Report of a case. J. Bone Joint Surg., *54-A*:1087, 1972.
20. Weckesser, E. C.: Congenital flexion-adduction deformity of the thumb (congenital "clasped thumb"). J. Bone Joint Surg., *37-A*:977, 1955.
21. Weckesser, E. C., Reed, J. R., and Heiple, K. G.: Congenital clasped thumb (congenital flexion-adduction deformity of the thumb). J. Bone Joint Surg., *50-A*:1417, 1968.
22. White, J. W., and Jensen, W. E.: The infant's persistent thumb clutched hand. J. Bone Joint Surg., *34-A*:680, 1952.
23. Wood, V. E.: Thumb-clutched hand. In Green, D. P. (ed.): Operative Hand Surgery. New York, Churchill-Livingstone, 1982, pp. 335–341.
24. Zadek, I.: Congenital absence of the extensor pollicis longus of both thumbs. Operation and cure. J. Bone Joint Surg., *16*:432, 1934.

TRIGGER THUMB

Trigger thumb, or stenosing tendovaginitis of the flexor pollicis longus, is a relatively rare deformity in which the fibrous tendon sheath is thickened and constricted.[1-20] Characteristically there is a palpable nodule on the volar aspect of the thumb in the region of the metacarpophalangeal joint. The incongruity of the tendon's surface interferes with its normal gliding within its sheath. Snapping or triggering results from the blockage of the tendon prominence against the constricted sheath and the sudden release following application of passive force and passage past the obstruction. In most cases the thumb is locked in flexion, but occasionally it may be locked in extension. The nodule is not painful. The infant or child has no complaints. It is the concern of the parents that brings the patient to the surgeon.

In about 25 per cent of cases, the trigger thumb is noted at birth. This congenital form resolves spontaneously within 12 months in about 30 per cent of cases. Involvement is bilateral in about 50 per cent of the cases noted at birth.[4]

The childhood form develops later on, between 6 and 30 months of age, and has a spontaneous recovery rate of about 12 per cent. In this later form, involvement is bilateral in about one fourth of the cases. Compere reported a 27-year-old woman with bilateral snapping thumbs that had been present since she was three years old.[2] Some patients have several digits involved.

The etiology is unknown. In some cases the deformity is familial but not genetic in origin. It may be present as a feature of trisomy 13 syndrome.[6]

Treatment

Gentle passive stretching exercises can be performed several times a day; they do no harm provided they cause the infant no pain. Part-time splinting of the thumb in extension may be tried. Full-time splinting should not exceed three weeks because of the possibility of locking in the reverse direction. Hydrocortisone injection into the thickened fibrous sheath and nodule has not succeeded; it is not fair to try a painful invasive method of treatment when previous experience has demonstrated lack of success.

Because of the possibility of spontaneous recovery it is wise to postpone operation on the trigger thumbs until the child is two years of age. Fixed deformities do not develop even when the deformity is left alone until the age of three and then corrected.

Operative treatment consists of simple surgical release of the fibrosed tendon sheath through a transverse incision in the flexion crease of the metacarpophalangeal joint of the thumb. The operative technique is described and illustrated in Plate 11. The operation should be performed before the child is four years of age. Problems and complications of surgery are inadvertent division of digital nerves or flexor tendon, adherence of tendon, and infection. If inadvertently sectioned, digital nerves and the flexor pollicis longus tendon should be repaired at the time of surgery.

References

1. Bollinger, J., and Fahey, J.: Snapping thumb in infants and children. J. Pediatr., *41*:445, 1952.
2. Compere, E. L.: Bilateral snapping thumbs. Ann. Surg., 97:773, 1933.
3. Cotton, F. J.: Trigger finger. Am. J. Orthop. Surg., 8423:587, 1910–1911.
4. Dinham, J. M., and Meggitt, B. F.: Trigger thumbs in children. A review of the natural history and indications for treatment in 105 patients. J. Bone Joint Surg., *56-B*:153, 1974.
5. Fahey, J. J., and Bollinger, J. A.: Trigger-finger in adults and children. J. Bone Joint Surg., *36-A*:1200, 1954.
6. Flatt, A. E.: The Care of Congenital Anomalies. St. Louis, Mosby, 1977, pp. 58–60.
7. Gharib, R.: Stenosing tenovaginitis (trigger finger). J. Pediatr., 69:294, 1966.
8. Hart, G. M.: Trigger thumb. Lancet, 80:436, 1960.
9. Hauck, G.: Ueber eine Tendovaginitis stenosans der Beugeschnenschcide mit dem Phanomen des schnellende Finger. Arch. Klin. Chir., *123*:232, 1932.
10. Hodgins, T., and Lipscomb, P.: Bilateral trigger fingers in a child: Report of a case. Proc. Staff Meet. Mayo Clin., 31:279, 1956.
11. Houston, J. P., and Wilson, W. F.: The etiology of the trigger finger. Hand, 4:257, 1972.
12. Hudson, H. W.: Snapping thumb in childhood. N. Engl. J. Med., *210*:854, 1934.
13. Jahss, S. A.: Trigger finger in children. J.A.M.A., *107*:1463, 1936.
14. James, T.: Bilateral trigger thumb in infants. Arch. Dis. Child., 35:302, 1960.
15. Rose, T. F.: Bilateral trigger finger in infants. Med. J. Aust., 1:18, 1946.
16. Sprecher, E. E.: Trigger thumb in infants. J. Bone Joint Surg., *31-A*:672, 1949.
17. Van Neck, M.: Nodules congénitaux des tendons. Etiologie des pouces à ressort. Arch. Franco-Belges Chir., 29:924, 1926.
18. White, J. W., and Jensen, W. E.: Trigger thumb in infants. Am. J. Dis. Child., 85:1412, 1953.
19. Wilks, J.: Trigger thumb. Practitioner, *177*:725, 1956.
20. Zadek, I.: Congenital absence of extensor pollicis longus of both thumbs: Operation and cure. J. Bone Joint Surg., 16:432, 1934.

SYMPHALANGISM

Symphalangism is failure of separation of the digits in which there is fusion of one phalanx to another within the same digit. The term *symphalangism* was first used by Harvey Cushing in 1916.[3] He described clinical stiffness of the proximal interphalangeal joints with normal or near normal length of all the phalanges. The

Table 2–11. *Symphalangism in Syndromes**

Acrocephalosyndactyly, Apert
Acrocephalosyndactyly, other
Brachydactyly B
Brachydactyly C
Cushing symphalangism
Diastrophic dwarfism
Drey symphalangism
Kirmisson symphalangism
Multiple synostosis
WL symphalangism-brachydactyly
Popliteal pterygium

*From Poznanski, A. K.: The Hand in Radiologic Diagnosis. Philadelphia, W. B. Saunders Co., 1984, p. 295. Reprinted by permission.

cases he reported were hereditary. Subsequently the term *symphalangism* has been used by other authors to describe stiffness of any of the interphalangeal joints. This congenital malformation is in the general category of failure of differentiation of parts. It may occur as a simple isolated malformation or it may be associated with other deformities of the hands or feet, and it may also occur in numerous congenital syndromes such as Apert's, Poland's, Möbius', and the like (Table 2–11).

Symphalangism is usually inherited as a Mendelian dominant trait. It is most frequently found in Caucasians, occasionally in Orientals, and hardly ever in blacks. The classification given by Flatt and Wood is the most practical and simple (Table 2–12).[9]

Clinically the disorder is characterized by lack of motion of the affected joint in the finger. The skin overlying the fused articulation is smooth, and the transverse skin creases are absent (Fig. 2–70). At birth it is easy to detect the condition. One cannot, however, make a diagnosis radiographically at birth because of lack of ossification of the phalanges around the affected joint. With growth and maturation, when the bones ossify, there is a decrease in the articular width with eventual fusion. Usually

Text continued on page 276

Table 2–12. *Classification of Symphalangism**

True symphalangism
Single
Multiple
Symbrachydactylism
Short middle phalanges
Absent middle phalanges
Symphalangism and syndactylism
Apert syndrome
Poland syndrome
Hypoplasia

*From Poznanski, A. K.: The Hand in Radiologic Diagnosis. Philadelphia, W. B. Saunders Co., 1984, p. 294. Reprinted by permission.

Release of Congenital Trigger Thumb

The operation is performed under general anesthesia with tourniquet ischemia.

OPERATIVE TECHNIQUE

A. A transverse incision 2 cm. long is made on the volar surface of the thumb at the metacarpophalangeal joint but not in the flexion crease.

B. The subcutaneous tissue is divided in line with the skin crease. Do not cut the digital nerves and vessels, which are close to the undersurface of the very thin skin. By blunt dissection in the longitudinal plane, the neurovascular structures are retracted to either side of the tendon. The flexor sheath and the tendon with its nodule are exposed. On flexion or extension of the thumb, the thickened and constricted sheath blocks gliding of the nodule.

C. A longitudinal incision is made in the flexor sheath in line with the flexor tendon. The thickened sheath is excised; inadvertent division of the flexor pollicis longus tendon must be avoided. Flexion and extension of the thumb should be fully restored. Partial excision of the thickened nodule of the flexor tendon is not necessary. Resist the temptation to reduce the nodule.

D. The tourniquet is released, and after hemostasis is obtained, the wound is closed with 4-0 or 6-0 plain catgut or Dexon absorbable sutures.

POSTOPERATIVE CARE

A simple soft dressing is applied. The child is encouraged to move the thumb freely. Bow-stringing of the tendon is not a problem.

Plate 11. Release of Congenital Trigger Thumb

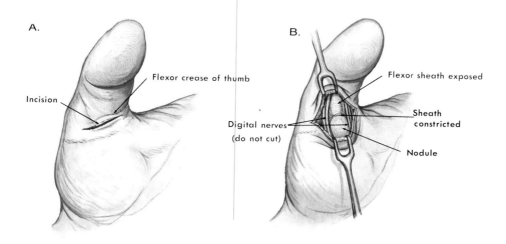

A.

Incision

Flexor crease of thumb

B.

Flexor sheath exposed

Digital nerves
(do not cut)

Sheath
constricted

Nodule

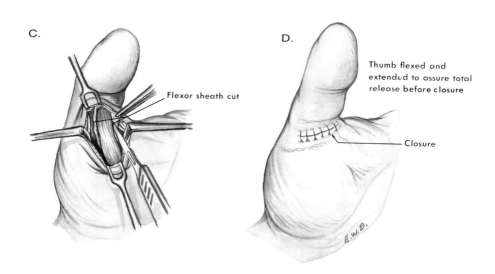

C.

Flexor sheath cut

D.

Thumb flexed and
extended to assure total
release before closure

Closure

E.W.B.

more than one finger is affected. When the proximal interphalangeal joint is affected, the digit is usually fixed in extension. At the level of the fused joint the soft tissues are narrowed. The patient cannot make a fist and has difficulty in picking up small objects.

Treatment

Treatment is individualized. Attempts to provide motion by arthroplasty are usually unsuccessful and not recommended by this author, especially in growing children. Digits that are fixed in extension will be functionally improved by flexion osteotomy. Also, the cosmetic benefits of such surgical intervention are obvious in the extended long finger.

In symbrachydactyly, when there is an associated shortening of the fingers, one may gain relative length by recessing the interdigital webs into the spaces between the metacarpal heads. Also, one may lengthen digits surgically.

The management of symphalangism with associated anomalies is complex. One should individualize the care; often it is difficult to improve function.

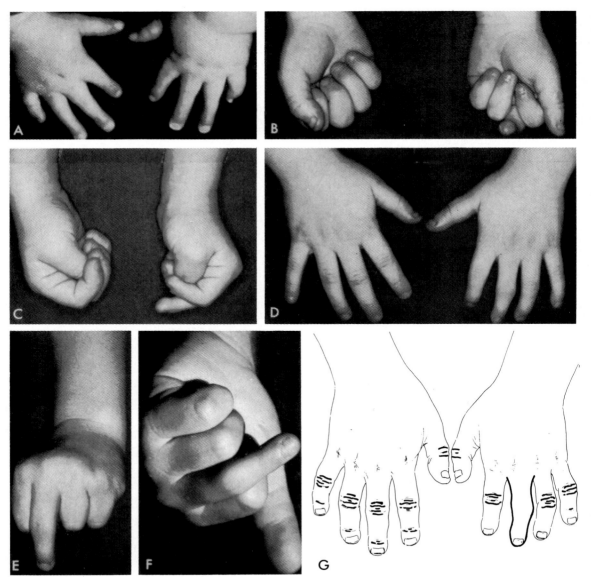

FIGURE 2–70. Symphalangism in a three-month-old infant.

A to **D.** Dorsal, palmar, and lateral views of both hands. **E** and **F.** Dorsal and oblique views of the hand of the same patient at age five and six years. **G.** Sketch illustrating the findings in **D.** (From Kelikian, H.: Congenital Deformities of the Hand and Forearm. Philadelphia, W. B. Saunders Co., 1974. Reprinted by permission.)

References

1. Bell, J.: On brachydactyly and symphalangism. *In* Penrose, L. S. (ed.): The Treasury of Human Inheritance. Vol. 5, Part 1. Cambridge, Cambridge University Press, 1951, pp. 1–31.
2. Comings, D. E.: Symphalangism and fourth digit hypophalangism. Arch. Intern. Med., *115*:580, 1965.
3. Cushing, H.: Hereditary ankylosis of the proximal phalangeal joint (symphalangism). Genetics, *1*:90, 1916.
4. Daniel, G. H.: A case of hereditary anarthrosis of the index finger, with associated abnormalities in the proportions of the fingers. Ann. Eugen., 7:281, 1936.
5. Dellon, A. L., and Gaylor, R.: Bilateral symphalangism of the index finger. J. Bone Joint Surg., *58-A*:270, 1976.
6. Drachman, D. B.: Normal development and congenital malformation of joint. Bull. Rheum. Dis., *19*:536, 1969.
7. Drinkwater, H.: Phalangeal anarthrosis (synostosis, ankylosis) transmitted through 14 generations. Proc. R. Soc. Med., *10*:60, 1917.
8. Elkington, S. G., and Huntsman, R. G.: The Talbot fingers: A study of symphalangism. Br. Med. J., *1*:407, 1967.
9. Flatt, A. E., and Wood, V. E.: Rigid digits or symphalangism. Hand, 7:197, 1975.
10. Geelhoed, G., Neel, J. V., and Davidson, R. G.: Symphalangism and tarsal coalitions: A hereditary syndrome. A report on two families. J. Bone Joint Surg., *51-B*:278, 1969.
11. Gorlin, R. J., Kietzer, G., and Wolfson, J.: Staple fixation and proximal symphalangism. Z. Kinderheilkd., *108*:12, 1970.
12. Harle, T. S., and Stevenson, J. R.: Hereditary symphalangism associated with carpal and tarsal fusions. Radiology, 89:91, 1967.
13. Hermann, J.: Symphalangism and brachydactyly syndrome: Report of the WL symphalangism-brachydactyly syndrome: Review of the literature and classification. Birth Defects, Original Article Series, *10*:23, 1974.
14. Kelikian, H.: Congenital Deformities of the Hand and Forearm. Philadelphia, Saunders, 1974, pp. 310–330.
15. Palmieri, T. J.: The use of silicone rubber implant arthroplasty in treatment of true symphalangism. J. Hand Surg., 5:242, 1980.
16. Savarinathan, G., and Centerwall, W. R.: Symphalangism. A pedigree from South India. J. Med. Genet., *3*:285, 1966.
17. Schwarz, P., and Rivellini, G.: Symphalangism. A. J. R., 89:1256, 1963.
18. Strasburger, A. K., Hawkins, M. R., Eldridge, R., Hargrave, R. L., and McKusick, V. A.: Symphalangism: Genetic and clinical aspects. Johns Hopkins Med. J., *117*:108, 1965.
19. Sugiura, Y., and Inagaki, Y.: Symphalangism associated with carpal and tarsal fusions. Jpn. J. Hum. Genet., 5:117, 1960.
20. Temtamy, S. A., and McKusick, V. A.: Symphalangism as an essentially isolated malformation. Birth Defects, *14*:495, 1978.
21. Vessel, E. S.: Symphalangism, strabismus and hearing loss in mother and daughter. N. Engl. J. Med., 263:839, 1960.
22. Wildervanck, L. S., Goedhard, G., and Meijer, S.: Proximal symphalangism of fingers associated with fusion of os naviculare and talus and occurrence of two accessory bones in the feet (os paranaviculare and os tibiale externum) in a European-Indonesian-Chinese family. Acta Genet., *17*:166, 1967.
23. Wray, J. B., and Herndon, C. N.: Hereditary transmission of congenital coalition of calcaneus and navicular (symphalangism associated with tarsal synostosis). J. Bone Joint Surg., *45-A*:370, 1963.

MACRODACTYLY

Macrodactyly, also referred to in the literature as megalodactyly or digital gigantism, is a rare congenital deformity in which there is hyperplasia of all the elements of the involved digit—soft tissues, subcutaneous fat, bone, and digital nerves. The hypertrophy of the digits is symmetrical, and enlargement of the nerves may extend proximal to the level of local gigantism.[1-42] There is no sensory loss. In childhood the interphalangeal and metacarpophalangeal joints are flexible, with full range of motion; with advancing age in the adult, however, joint stiffness may develop.

There are two forms of macrodactyly—static and progressive. In the *static type* the growth of the enlarged digit is proportional to the growth of the rest of the hand, whereas in the *progressive type* the growth of the enlarged digit is accelerated out of proportion to that of the remainder of the hand (Fig. 2–71). The static form is much more common than the progressive type. There is great variety in the degree and extent of gigantism affecting the digit.

The cause of macrodactyly is unknown. In the differential diagnosis one should consider lymphedema, neurofibromatosis, hemangiomata, arteriovenous fistulae, and skeletal lesions such as aneurysmal bone cyst or fibrous dysplasia.

Treatment varies according to the severity of involvement. In mild megalodactyly, soft-tissue reduction is achieved by a defatting procedure through a midlateral incision, one side of the digit at a time. Ordinarily a three-month interval between operations is desirable. To prevent skin flap necrosis, the skin, subcutaneous tissue, and fat are excised in one piece; then the skin is defatted and resutured as a full-thickness skin graft.

In the moderate and severe form, in addition to the soft-tissue excision, bone reduction is carried out; longitudinal growth is arrested by curetting the growth plate. The transverse diameter of the phalanx is reduced by resecting its middle third. Stripping and incising the small twigs of the digital nerves into the subcutaneous fat will retard or prevent recurrence. Again, one side of a finger is operated on at a time, the operations being performed three months apart. Severe cases in which the likelihood of ending with an acceptable digit is slim may require ablation of the digit or the entire ray.

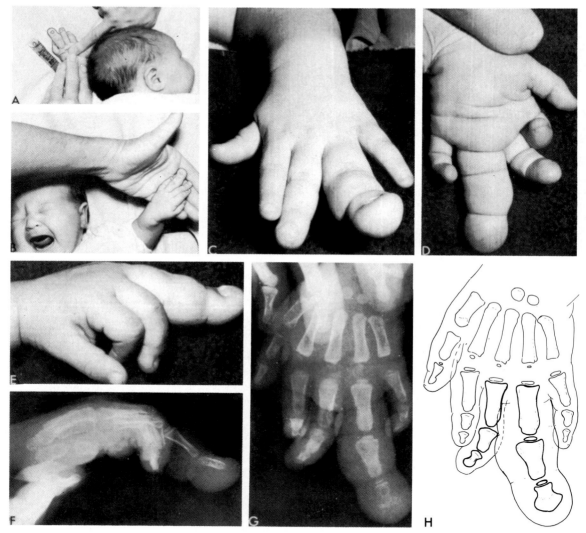

FIGURE 2–71. *Progressive macrodactyly of the ring and middle fingers.*

A and **B.** Dorsal views of the hand at birth. **C** to **E.** Dorsal, palmar, and lateral views of the left hand three months later. Note the fulminant, fast-growing macrodactyly of the long and ring fingers. The ring finger is deviated ulnarward. **F** and **G.** Lateral and dorsopalmar radiograms of the left hand. **H.** Sketch illustrating the macrodactyly of the long and ring fingers. (From Kelikian, H.: Congenital Deformities of the Hand and Forearm. Philadelphia, W. B. Saunders Co., 1974. Reprinted by permission.)

References

1. Allende, B. T.: Macrodactyly with enlarged median nerve associated with carpal tunnel syndrome. J. Plast. Reconstr. Surg., 39:578, 1967.
2. Alosio, S. and Novellino, L.: Due casi di gigantismo parziale congenito. Acta Ortop. Ital., 7:245, 1961.
3. Barsky, A. J.: Macrodactyly. J. Bone Joint Surg., 49-A:1255, 1967.
4. Battelli, L.: Rilievi patogenitici e clinici sulle macrosomie parziali. Chir. Organi Mov., 55:138, 1966.
5. Bean, W. B., and Peterson, P. K.: Note on a monstrous finger. Arch. Intern. Med., 104:433, 1959.
6. Ben-Bassat, M., Casper, J., Kaplan, I., and Laron, Z.: Congenital macrodactyly. A case report with a three-year follow-up. J. Bone Joint Surg., 48-B:359, 1966.
7. Boyes, J. G.: Macrodactylism—a review and proposed management. Hand, 9:172, 1977.
8. Boyes, J. H. (ed.): Bunnell's Surgery of the Hand. 5th Ed. Philadelphia, Lippincott, 1970, p. 95.
9. Brihaye, J., Milaire, J., Dustin, P., and Retif, J.: Local gigantism of the hand associated with a plexiform neurofibroma of the ulnar nerve. J. Neurosurg. Sci., 18:271, 1974.
10. Byrne, J. J.: Megalodactylism. Am. J. Surg., 88:470, 1954.
11. Charters, A. D.: Local gigantism. J. Bone Joint Surg., 39-B:542, 1957.
12. Chung, I. H., Kim, N. H., and Choi, I. Y.: Macrodactylism associated with neurofibroma of the median nerve. Yonsei Med. J., 14:49, 1973.
13. Edgerton, M. T., and Tuerk, D. B.: Macrodactyly (digital gigantism): Its nature and treatment. *In* Littler, J. S., Carmer, L. M., and Smith, J. W. (eds.): Symposium on Reconstructive Hand Surgery, Vol. 9. St. Louis, Mosby, 1974, p. 157.
14. El-Shami, I. N.: Congenital partial gigantism: Case report and review of literature. Surgery, 65:683, 1969.
15. Flatt, A. E.: The Care of Congenital Hand Anomalies. St. Louis, Mosby, 1977, pp. 249–262.
16. Fontana, A. M., Vinay, L., and Verga, G.: La macrodattilia. Ethiopathogenesi e trattamento chirurgico riparatore. Bull. Soc. Piedmont. Chir., 34:447, 1964.
17. Frykman, G. K., and Wood, V. E.: Peripheral nerve hemartomas with macrodactyly in the hand: Report of three cases and review of the literature. J. Hand Surg., 3:307, 1978.
18. Golding, F. C.: Localized gigantism. *In* McLaren, J. E. (ed.): Modern Trends in Diagnostic Radiology. 3rd Ed. New York, Hooker, 1960, pp. 160–163.
19. Goldman, A. B., and Kaye, J.: Macrodystrophia lipomatosa. Radiographic diagnosis. A. J. R., 128:101, 1977.
20. Hellmann, K.: Ueber die Behandlung der Makrodaktylies. Ann. Chir. Plast., 9:184, 1964.
21. Hueston, J. T., and Millroy, P.: Macrodactyly associated with hamartoma of major peripheral nerves. Aust. N.Z. Surg., 37:394, 1968.
22. Inglis, K.: Local gigantism (a manifestation of neurofibromatosis): Its relation to general gigantism and to acromegaly. Am. J. Pathol., 26:1059, 1950.
23. Iselin, M., and Iselin, F.: Traité de Chirurgie de la Main. Paris, Editions Médicales Flammarion, 1967, pp. 295–299.
24. Kaplan, E. B.: Congenital giant thumb. Bull. Hosp. Joint Dis., 8:38, 1947.
25. Kelikian, H.: Congenital Deformities of the Hand and Forearm. Philadelphia, Saunders, 1974, pp. 610–660.
26. Khanna, N., Gupta, S., Khanna, S., and Tripathi, F.: Macrodactyly. Hand, 7:215, 1975.
27. McCarroll, H. R.: Clinical manifestations of congenital neurofibromatosis. J. Bone Joint Surg., 32-A:601, 1950.
28. Millesi, H.: Macrodactyly: A case study. *In* Littler, J. W., Cramer, L. M., and Smith, J. W. (eds.): Symposium on Reconstructive Hand Surgery, Vol. 9. St. Louis, Mosby, 1974, p. 173.
29. Minkowitz, S., and Minkowitz, F.: A morphological study of macrodactylism: A case report. J. Pathol. Bacteriol., 90:323, 1965.
30. Moore, B. H.: Macrodactyly and associated peripheral nerve changes. J. Bone Joint Surg., 24:6, 1942.
31. Mouly, R., and Debeyre, J.: Le gigantisme digital. Etiologie et traitement. A propos d'un cas. Ann. Chir. Plast., 6:187, 1961.
32. Rechnagel, K.: Megalodactylism, report of seven cases. Acta Orthop. Scand., 38:47, 1967.
33. Rousso, M., Katz, S., and Khodadadi, D.: Treatment of a case of macrodactyly of the thumb. Hand, 8:131, 1976.
34. Shima, Y., Kasahara, K., and Nakeseko, T.: Experiences in the treatment of macrodactylia (Japanese). Orthop. Surg. (Tokyo), 18:292, 1967.
35. Tagliabue, D., and Spina, G. M.: Le macrodattilie. Arch. Orthop., 73:792, 1960.
36. Temtamy, S. A., and Rogers, J. G.: Macrodactyly, hemihypertrophy and connective tissue nevi: Report of a new syndrome and review of the literature. J. Pediatr., 89:924, 1976.
37. Thorne, F. L., Posch, J. L., and Mladick, R. A.: Megalodactyly. Plast. Reconstr. Surg., 41:232, 1968.
38. Tsuge, K.: Treatment of macrodactyly. Plast. Reconstr. Surg., 39:590, 1967.
39. Tsuge, K., and Ikuta, Y.: Macrodactyly and fibro-fatty proliferation of the median nerve. Hiroshima J. Med. Sci., 22:83, 1973.
40. Tuli, S. M., Khanna, N. N., and Sinha, G. P.: Congenital macrodactyly. Br. J. Plast. Surg., 22:237, 1969.
41. Wood, V. E.: Macrodactyly. J. Iowa Med. Soc., 59:922, 1969.
42. Yaghmai, I., McKowne, F., and Alizadeh, A.: Macrodactylia fibrolipomatosis. South. Med. J., 69:1565, 1976.

CLEFT HAND

Cleft hand is characterized by congenital absence of the central ray and splitting of the hand into radial and ulnar segments (Fig. 2–72).[1-37] This anomaly is rare, constituting about 2 per cent of all hand malformations.[3, 12] It occurs predominantly in the male. Involvement is usually bilateral. Similar cleft malformation of the foot occurs in about 50 per cent of cases. Other associated anomalies are cleft lip and palate, cataract, deafness, absence of nails, congenital heart disease, and imperforate anus (Table 2–13).

The association of lobster claw deformities of the hands and feet with cleft lip and cleft palate is considered by Walker and Clodius to be a separate syndrome.[37]

The exact cause of cleft hand is not known. The teratogenic insult to the developing plate occurs around the seventh week of embryonic development. The centripetal suppressive theory as a progression of insult to the developing hand plate is proposed by Maisels to explain the various forms of lobster claw deformities: simple cleft of the hand with no absence of digit

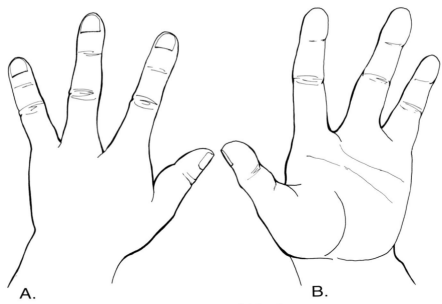

FIGURE 2–72. Cleft hand.

Note the V-shaped defect between the thumb-index finger and the ring-little fingers; the central ray is absent. **A.** Dorsal view. **B.** Palmar view.

Table 2–13. *Anomalies and Syndromes Associated with Split Hand, Lobster Claw Deformity or Monodactyly**

Anomalies
  Cleft lip and palate
  Ectodermal defects
    Anonychia
  Ear abnormality
    Deafness
  Eye abnormality
    Cataracts
    Cyclopia
    Nystagmus
  Limb abnormalities
    Cleft foot
    Clubfoot and other anomalies
    Bifid femur
    Tibial aplasia
    Radioulnar synostosis
  Gastrointestinal anomaly
    Imperforate anus
  Genitourinary anomalies
    Fusion
  Absence of pectoralis major muscle
  Pseudoarthrosis, clavicle
Syndromes
  Acral-renal association
  Aglossia-adactylia
  Ankyloglossia superior
  EEC
  Ives-Houston
  Mandibulofacial dysostosis
  Möbius
  Pseudothalidomide
  Unilateral ectromelia-ichthyosis

*From Poznanski, A. K.: The Hand in Radiologic Diagnosis. Philadelphia, W. B. Saunders Co., 1984, p. 255. Reprinted by permission.

is the mildest form; it is followed by absence of the long finger ray with progressive suppression of the radial rays and eventual involvement of the ulnar rays and total suppression of all digits (Fig. 2–73). Syndactyly of the marginal digits gives a typical lobster claw appearance.[25]

Cleft hand is a hereditary anomaly in which most pedigrees show a dominant transmission; incomplete penetrance and recessive inheritance can occur, and occasionally a generation may be skipped.[19, 35, 36]

Barsky has subdivided the split hand anomalies into two main groups—typical and atypical. The *typical* type presents with a deep V-shaped central defect and absence of the entire long finger ray. It is the typical form that is hereditary with bilateral involvement and frequent association with cleft foot anomalies. In the *atypical* type more than one central ray is absent, and there is a characteristic U-shaped defect between the remaining marginal fingers. In the atypical form involvement is unilateral, there are usually no associated foot anomalies, and it is nonhereditary, occurring sporadically and without involvement of other members of the family.[3] Flatt prefers to use the term *lobster claw hand* for the fully developed atypical type.[12]

Clinical Picture

The appearance of a cleft hand is obvious. Functionally, performance and dexterity of a

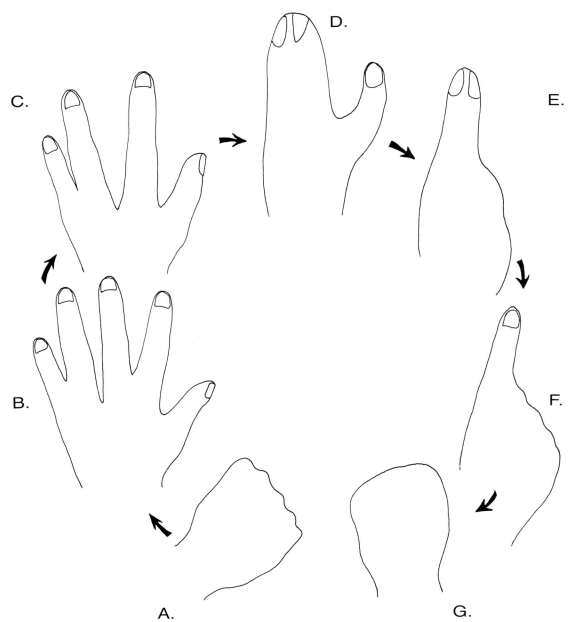

FIGURE 2–73. *Centripetal suppression theory as a progressive insult to the developing hand plate to explain the pathogenesis of lobster claw deformities.*

A. Insult to developing hand plate. **B.** Simple split of the hand with absence of tissue. **C.** Absence of long finger ray. **D.** Absence of long and index finger ray. **E.** Absence of long, index finger rays and thumb. The little and ring fingers are fused together. **F.** Absence of all rays except the little finger. **G.** Absence of all digits. (Redrawn after Maisels, D. O.: Theory of pathogenesis of lobster claw deformities. Hand, 2:79, 1970.)

cleft hand is amazingly good; these hands have excellent grasp and pinch. Syndactyly between the marginal digits and adduction contracture of the thumb, if present, may interfere with optimal function. Cosmetically, the appearance of a lobster claw hand is grotesque and objectionable. Often the affected teenager will hide his hand.

Treatment

The objective of treatment is to improve function. Attempts to improve appearance are unrewarding; substantial improvement in cosmesis cannot be achieved, and social acceptability of the deformity cannot be enhanced.

Treatment is carried out in stages. *First*, the syndactyly of border digits, if present, is separated; this is performed at one year of age. The technique is described in Plate 8. *Second*, the cleft in the hand is closed, usually six months later at about one and a half to two years of age. The goal of surgery is to prevent diasthesis of the repair later on. Osteotomy of adjacent metacarpals is ordinarily not required. On one finger, a diamond-shaped flap of skin with a broad base distally is fashioned and defatted. Later on it is sutured dorsolaterally to the adjacent finger to provide a transverse commissure. Any excessive tissue between the metacarpals is excised. The metacarpals are approximated and held together by soft-tissue and ligamentous repair or by tying with an unabsorbable suture such as Mersilene. The suture is inserted through fine drill holes in the metacarpal necks, avoiding injury to the physis, which is distal in the finger metacarpals. In severe cases if the metacarpals tend to spring apart, the capsule of the carpometacarpal joint is divided, and occasionally one may have to perform an incomplete osteotomy of one or both metacarpals. The chance of scar contracture is minimized by fashioning curvilinear and not straight-line skin flaps. The dorsal and palmar skin flaps are closed in a proximal-distal direction. Efforts should be made to provide a dorsopalmar slope and a normal commissure. An above-elbow cast is applied to protect the intermetacarpal repair for three to four weeks. The *third stage of treatment* of cleft hand is mobilization of the contracted thumb by rotating dorsal flaps into the thumb web to provide supple skin.

Occasionally the border fingers are unstable because of hypoplasia of the phalanges; usually the middle phalanges are affected. Arthrodesis of the distal or sometimes of the proximal interphalangeal joints will provide stability and improve function. If there is associated hypoplasia of the muscles controlling the border fingers, active motion and motor strength can be provided by tendon transfers. The extensors and flexors of the wrist are a good source of motors; adequate length of the tendons is provided by tendon grafts, a common source of supply being the plantaris tendon.

References

1. Ahstrom, J. P.: Surgical treatment of cleft hand. Orthop. Trans., *1*:92, 1977.
2. Ayer, A. A., and Rao, V. S.: Split hand and split foot. J. Indian Med. Assoc., *24*:108, 1954.
3. Barsky, A. J.: Cleft hand: Classification, incidence and treatment. J. Bone Joint Surg., *46-A*:1707, 1964.
4. Berndorfer, A.: Gesichtsspalten gemeinsam mit Hand- und Fussspalten. Z. Orthop., *107*:344, 1970.
5. Blankenburg, H.: Spalthand- und Spaltfussbildungen in typischen und atypischen. Beitr. Orthop. Traum., *14*:209, 1967.
6. Buck-Gramco, D.: Congenital malformations of the hand: Indications, operative treatment and results. Scand. J. Plast. Reconstr. Surg., 9:190, 1975.
7. Bujdoso, G., and Lenz, W.: Monodactylous split hand–split foot. A malformation occurring in three distinct genetic types. Eur. J. Pediatr., *133*:207, 1980.
8. Campbell-Reid, D. A.: Reconstruction of the thumb. J. Bone Joint Surg., *42-B*:444, 1960.
9. David, T. J.: The differential diagnosis of the cleft hand and cleft foot malformations. Hand, 6:58, 1974.
10. Der Koloustian, V. M., and Mnaymneh, W. A.: Bilateral tibial aplasia with lobster claw hands. A rare genetic entity. Acta Paediatr. Scand., *62*:77, 1973.
11. Dowd, C. N.: Cleft hand: A report of a case successfully treated by the use of periosteal flaps. Ann. Surg., *24*:211, 1896.
12. Flatt, A. E.: The Care of Congenital Hand Anomalies. (Cleft Hand and Central Defects). St. Louis, Mosby, 1977, pp. 265–285.
13. Flort, A. J. A.: Des difformités congénitales et acquises des doigts, et des moyens d'y remédier. Paris, Delahaye, 1869.
14. Godunova, G. S.: Operative treatment of congenital split hand. *In* Godunova, G. S. (ed.): Orthopaedics, Traumatology and the Application of Prostheses, No. 6, 1973. Summary in English I.C.I.B., *13*:14, 1974.
15. Gollop, T. R., Lucchesi, E., Martins, R. M. M., and Nione, A. S.: Brief clinical report: Familial occurrence of bifid femur and monodactylous ectrodactyly. Am. J. Med. Genet., 7:319, 1980.
16. Graham, J. B., and Badgley, C. E.: Split-hand with unusual complications. Am. J. Hum. Genet., 744, 1954.
17. Grebe, H.: Spalthande und Fusse. *In* Becker, P. E. (ed.): Humangenetik. Stuttgart, Thieme, 1964, pp. 304–316.
18. Holmes, L. B., and Remensnyder, J. P.: Hypoplasia of the second metacarpal in mother and daughter. J. Pediatr., *81*:1165, 1972.
19. Jaworska, M., and Popiolek, J.: Genetic counselling in lobster-claw anomaly: Discussion of variability of genetic influence in different families. Clin. Pediatr., 7:396, 1968.
20. Kelikian, H.: Congenital Deformities of the Hand and Forearm. Philadelphia, Saunders, 1974, pp. 467–489.
21. Kelikian, H., and Doumanian, A.: Congenital anomalies of the hand. Part I. J. Bone Joint Surg., *39-A*:1002, 1957.
22. Lees, D. H., Lawler, S. D., Renwick, J. H., and Thoday, J. M.: Anonychia with ectrodactyly: Clinical and linkage data. Ann. Hum. Genet., *22*:69, 1957.

23. Lewis, T., and Embleton, D.: Split-hand and split-foot deformities, their types, origins and transmission. Biometrika, 6:25, 1908.

24. Maisels, D. O.: Lobster claw deformities of the hands and feet. Br. J. Plast. Surg., 23:269, 1970.

25. Maisels, D. O.: Lobster claw deformities of the hand. Hand, 2:79, 1970.

26. Milford, L.: The hand. *In* Edmonson, A. S., and Crenshaw, A. H. (eds.): Campbell's Operative Orthopaedics. 6th Ed. St. Louis, Mosby, 1980, pp. 349–353.

27. Miura, T., and Komada, T.: Simple method for reconstruction of the cleft hand with an adducted thumb. Plast. Reconstr. Surg., 64:65, 1979.

28. Nutt, J. N., III, and Flatt, A. E.: Congenital central hand deficit. J. Hand Surg., 6:46, 1981.

29. Pearson, K.: On the existence of the digital deformity—so-called "lobster claw"—in the apes. Ann. Eugen., 4:339, 1931.

30. Poznanski, A. K.: The Hand in Radiologic Diagnosis. Philadelphia, Saunders, 1984, pp. 252–256.

31. Ribiero, A. L.: Lobster-claw hands. Br. Med. J., 1:1209, 1954.

32. Rudiger, R. A., Haasse, W., and Passarge, E.: Association of ectrodactyly, ectodermal dysplasia, and cleft lip-palate. Am. J. Dis. Child., 120:160, 1970.

33. Searle, A. G.: Hereditary "split-hand" in the domestic cat. Ann. Eugen., 17:279, 1953.

34. Snow, J. W., and Littler, J. W.: Surgical treatment of cleft hand. Transactions of the International Society of Plastic and Reconstructive Surgery, 4th Congress, Rome, 1967, Excerpta Medica Foundation, pp. 888–893.

35. Temtamy, S. A., and McKusick, V. A.: The genetics of hand malformations. Birth Defects, Original Article Series, 14:3, 1978.

36. Verma, I. C., Joseph, R., Bhargara, S., and Mehta, S.: Split hand and split foot deformity inherited as an autosomal recessive trait. Clin. Genet., 9:8, 1976.

37. Walker, J. C., and Clodius, L.: The syndromes of cleft lip, cleft palate and lobster claw deformities of hands and feet. Plast. Reconstr. Surg., 32:627, 1963.

HYPOPLASTIC HAND AND DIGITS

Hypoplasia of the distal phalanges is known as brachytelephalangy. Different digits are identified with different syndromes. For example, a short distal phalanx of the fifth finger is known as Senior syndrome.[18] Hypoplasia of the middle phalanges is known as brachymesophalangy, and that of the metacarpals as brachymetacarpalia. Poznanski has given an excellent description of various hypoplasias and aplasias of digits and metacarpals in the hand.[17]

Treatment

Short metacarpals can be lengthened.[9, 12, 13] The treatment of other hypoplasias should be individualized. It is crucial to have a realistic goal and not to subject the infant to multiple operations that fail to improve function and appearance. Toe-to-hand transfers by microsurgical technique are still in the developing stages.[3, 4, 7, 8, 11, 13, 14] The short digits in the hand may be elongated by insertion of the proximal

phalanx of a third or fourth toe into the hypoplastic digit.

References

1. Bass, H. N.: Familial absence of middle phalanges with nail dysplasia: A new syndrome. Pediatrics, 42:318, 1968.

2. Buckwalter, J. A., Flatt, A. E., Schurr, D. G., Dryer, R. F., and Blair, W. F.: The absent fifth metacarpal. J. Hand Surg., 6:364, 1981.

3. Buncke, H.: Toe digital transfer. Clin. Plast. Surg., 3:49, 1976.

4. Buncke, H. J., McLean, D. H., George, P. T., Breevator, J. C., Chater, N. L., and Commons, G. W.: Thumb replacement, great toe transplantation by microvascular anastomosis. Br. J. Plast. Surg., 26:194, 1973.

5. Carroll, R. E.: Insertion of toe phalangeal grafts in hypoplastic digits. *In* Flatt, A. E. (ed.): The Care of Congenital Hand Anomalies. St. Louis, Mosby, 1977, pp. 143–144.

6. Carroll, R. E., and Green, D. P.: Reconstruction of hypoplastic digits using two phalanges. J. Bone Joint Surg., 57-A:727, 1975.

7. Clarkson, P.: Reconstruction of hand digits by toe transfers. J. Bone Joint Surg., 37:270, 1955.

8. Cobbett, J. R.: Free digital transfer: Report of a case of transfer of a great toe to replace an amputated thumb. J. Bone Joint Surg., 51:677, 1955.

9. Cowen, N. J., and Loftus, J. M.: Distraction, augmentation, manoplasty: Technique for lengthening digits for the entire hand. Orthop. Rev., 7:45, 1978.

10. Crawford, H. H., Horton, C. E., and Adamson, J. E.: Congenital aplasia or hypoplasia of the thumb and finger extensor tendons. J. Bone Joint Surg., 48-A:82, 1966.

11. Goldberg, N. H., and Watson, H. K.: Composite toe (phalanx with epiphysis) transplants in the reconstruction of the aphalangic hand. Orthop. Trans., 5:98, 1981.

12. Kessler, I., Baruch, A., and Hecht, O.: Experience with distraction lengthening of distal rays in congenital anomalies. J. Hand Surg., 2:394, 1977.

13. Matev, I. B.: Thumb reconstruction in children through metacarpal lengthening. Plast. Reconstr. Surg., 64:665, 1979.

14. May, J. W., and Daniel, R. K.: Great toe–to–hand free tissue transfer. Clin. Orthop., 133:140, 1978.

15. Murray, J. F., and Shore, B.: The use and disuse of prostheses in children with unilateral congenital absence of the hand. J. Bone Joint Surg., 54-A:902, 1972.

16. O'Brien, B. McC., Black, M. J. M., Morrison, W., and MacLeod, A. M.: Microvascular great toe transfer for congenital absence of the thumb. Hand, 10:113, 1978.

17. Poznanski, A. K.: The Hand in Radiological Diagnosis. Philadelphia, Saunders, 1984, p. 209.

18. Senior, B.: Impaired growth and onychodysplasia. Short children with tiny toenails. Am. J. Dis. Child., 122:7, 1971.

19. Strauch, B.: Microsurgical approach to thumb reconstruction. Orthop. Clin. North Am., 8:319, 1977.

20. Tajima, T., Watanabe, Y., and Uchiyama, J.: Treatment and study of the hypoplastic thumb. Jpn. J. Plast. Reconstr. Surg., 10:227, 1967.

21. Tamai, S., Hori, Y., Tatsumi, Y., and Okuda, H.: Hallux-to-thumb transfer with microsurgical technique: A case report in a 45-year-old woman. J. Hand Surg., 2:152, 1977.

22. Tsuge, K.: Congenital aplasia or hypoplasia of the finger extensors. Hand, 7:15, 1975.

23. Van Beek, A. L., Wavak, P. W., and Zook, E. G.: Microvascular surgery in children. Plast. Reconstr. Surg., 63:457, 1979.

FINGER DEFORMITIES

Camptodactyly*

Camptodactyly ("bent finger" in Greek) is characterized by flexion deformity of a digit. It commonly occurs at the proximal interphalangeal joint of the little finger; next in frequency, in the ring finger. In the other digits from the ulnar to the radial side there is progressively marked decrease of its incidence and of the severity of the flexion contracture. Flexion deformity of the distal interphalangeal joint is rare. Compensatory hyperextension of the metacarpophalangeal joint may develop, especially when the flexion deformity of the proximal interphalangeal joint is very severe. The overall incidence of camptodactyly in the general population is less than 0.1 per cent.

The deformity usually increases with skeletal growth, especially during the adolescent growth spurt. Progression is insidious and often the date of its onset is unknown. It appears in two forms: the *infantile type*, which is noted in the first six months of life and occurs equally in males and females, and the *adolescent type*, developing between 12 and 14 years of age and being more common in the female.

ETIOLOGY

Although the exact cause is unknown, several pathogenic factors have been implicated in the production of the deformity: muscle imbalance between flexors and extensors of the finger, abnormal insertion of lumbricals, faulty development of the dorsal extensor aponeurosis, some anomaly of the flexor digitorum sublimis and profundus tendons, contracture of the collateral ligaments, and ischemic fibrosis of the intrinsic muscles. Camptodactyly may occur sporadically or be of autosomal dominant inheritance. It is frequently associated with congenital malformation syndromes and disorders (Table 2–14).

DIAGNOSIS

The deformity is not painful. There is no increased local temperature, erythema, or tenderness.

The affected joint, usually the proximal interphalangeal of the little finger, presents in varying degrees of flexion contracture (Fig. 2–74). From the fixed flexion posture the involved joint can be flexed almost fully. In the younger child, on hyperflexion of the wrist and metacar-

---

Table 2–14. *Disorders Associated with Camptodactyly†*

Chromosomal disorders
  Monosomy 21*
  Trisomy 8*
  Trisomy 13
  Other
Craniofacial syndromes
  Ankyloglossia superior
  Emery-Nelson*
  Gordon*
  Lenz microphthalmos
  Oculodentodigital*
  Orofaciodigital I*
  Trismus pseudocamptodactyly*
Other congenital malformation syndromes
  Aarskog*
  Arthrogryposis
  Camptobrachydactyly*
  Cerebrohepatorenal
  Congenital contractural arachnodactyly
  Distal arthrogryposis*
  Fetal alcohol
  Goltz focal dermal hypoplasia*
  Manzke
  Marfan
  Osteo-onychodysplasia
  Pena-Shokeir I*
  Pena-Shokeir II*
  Pectoral aplasia dysdactyly (Poland)
  Roberts*
  Spondylothoracic
  Weaver*
Acquired
  Burns
  Digital fibromas
  Trauma
  Tumors

*Frequent
†From Poznanski, A. K.: The Hand in Radiologic Diagnosis. Philadelphia, W. B. Saunders Co., 1984, p. 290. Reprinted by permission.

---

pophalangeal joints, range of extension of the affected interphalangeal joint is increased; in the older patient, however, flexion contracture becomes so fixed that hyperflexion of the wrist will not decrease the degree of flexion deformity. The skin on the ulnar surface of the interphalangeal joint will be shortened. Camptodactyly is not a local manifestation of a generalized disorder; by a detailed history and physical examination, one can rule out generalized affections such as arthrogryposis multiplex congenita, rheumatoid disease, or collagen diseases. The metacarpophalangeal joint, not the proximal interphalangeal joint, is affected in congenital absence of the extrinsic extensor mechanism. Stenosing tendovaginitis (trigger finger) primarily affects the thumb in infants and children.

Radiographic features are best depicted in the lateral projection. The flexed posture of the proximal interphalangeal joint is obvious. The

---

*See references 1–3, 8, 9, 11, 14–17, 19, 23, 24, 28, 29, 38, 41, 44, 46, 49, 51, 58, 59.

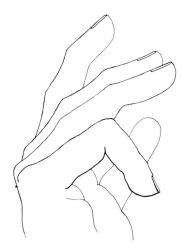

FIGURE 2–74. *Camptodactyly of the little finger.*

Note the flexion contracture of the proximal interphalangeal joint.

base of the middle phalanx is subluxated volar to the head of the proximal phalanx; the latter is flattened and narrowed. In long-standing cases a depression in the neck of the proximal phalanx may be produced by pressure of the base of the middle phalanx.

TREATMENT

Mild deformities do not require surgical treatment; there is no functional improvement, and the patients can learn to live with the problem. Because of the possibility of progression with growth, it is best to perform passive stretching exercises several times a day. If the deformity increases, splinting at night is indicated. For splinting to succeed, the splint should be manufactured, fitted, and applied correctly. First, the wrist should be included, i.e., a wrist-hand-finger orthosis is ordered for night use. There should be no extension force on the distal phalanx because it will simply push the distal interphalangeal joint into hyperextension. The three points of pressure are the *volar surface of the proximal and middle phalanges* and the *dorsum of the proximal interphalangeal joint*. A Velcro strap or in the older child a padded strap with a buckle is used to push the proximal interphalangeal joint into hyperextension. Parents should be carefully instructed in proper fitting of the splint. The period of splinting is long, possibly several years. It should be explained to the parents that even if the finger is operated on, postoperative splinting is recommended for one to two years to prevent recurrence of the deformity.

If the flexion deformity is marked and cannot be improved or controlled by these conservative

measures, surgical intervention is indicated. Severe flexed posture of the little or other fingers will cause functional impairment in activities such as playing musical instruments, typing, or sports. Surgery should be performed at a young age before structural changes develop in the joints.

Soft-tissue release is performed when there are no structural joint changes. The best procedure is release of the flexor digitorum sublimis tendon; it may be performed in the forearm or wrist by sliding or Z-lengthening or, usually in the more severe case, at its insertion. In the latter instance the flexor sublimis is transferred as an intrinsic transfer to provide extension of the proximal phalanx. The volar plate may be released and advanced distally. Surgical approach is palmar. A Z-plasty or full-thickness skin graft may be necessary to provide coverage of the extended joint. It is wise to use a smooth Kirschner wire to ensure that the proximal interphalangeal joint is kept in extension and to protect the finger in a below-elbow (or in the young child an above-elbow) cast.

Extension dorsal wedge osteotomy of the neck of the proximal phalanx is indicated when the flexion deformity of the proximal interphalangeal joint is severe and there are structural fixed joint changes (Fig. 2–75). The finger is made straighter, but range of motion of the proximal interphalangeal joint does not improve because it is in a different arc. Some degree of diminution of strength of the ulnar grasp is the price tag for a straighter-appearing little finger.

Clinodactyly

This simple deformity is characterized by varying degrees of inclination or curving of a digit in the radioulnar plane (Fig. 2–76 A). It is caused by shifting in the alignment of the articular surfaces of either the proximal or the distal interphalangeal joint away from its normal position perpendicular to the long axis of the digit. It is very common, occurring in 1.0 to 19.5 per cent of normal children; it appears this wide range of reported prevalence depends upon the thoroughness of the examiner. Clinodactyly is a hereditary condition with autosomal dominant transmission. There is a greater incidence in Down's syndrome (35 to 79 per cent). It may also occur in other syndromes and congenital malformations (Table 2–15).

The small finger is the most commonly affected, although any finger may curve. Often there is no functional impairment; it is the cosmetic appearance that is objectionable to the parents.[5, 7, 18, 27, 31–33, 45–47]

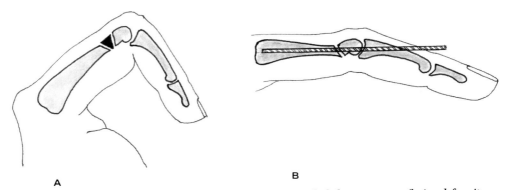

A   **B**

FIGURE 2–75. Extension osteotomy of the neck of the proximal phalanx to correct flexion deformity.

A. The wedge to be resected based dorsally. **B.** Internal fixation with threaded Steinmann pin.

TREATMENT

Surgery is not justified unless the affected finger overlaps its neighbor when the child makes a fist. Splinting is ineffective in correcting the deformity. In the rare case in which surgery is indicated, angular deformity is corrected by a closing wedge osteotomy taken from the convex (usually the ulnar) side of the phalanx immediately proximal to the affected joint. In the little finger the wedge is usually taken from the middle phalanx. The osteotomy is fixed with two crisscross threaded Kirschner wires,

inserted from the ulnar side in the horizontal plane, avoiding the dorsal extensor mechanism (Fig. 2–76 B and C). A below-elbow cast incorporating the little and ring fingers is applied for further immobilization. The osteotomy usually heals in four to six weeks, at which time the cast and wires are removed.[7]

Kirner Deformity

In this deformity, described by Kirner in 1927, the terminal phalanx of the little finger is

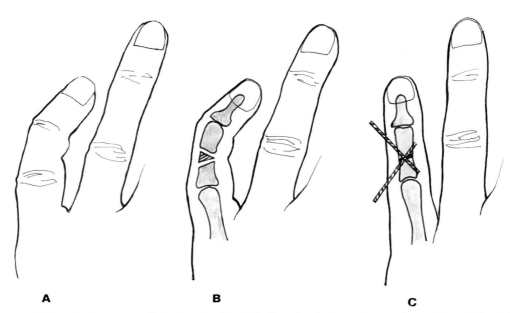

A   **B**   **C**

FIGURE 2–76. Surgical correction of clinodactyly of the little finger by closing wedge osteotomy of the middle phalanx.

A. The deformity. Note the radial inclination. The distal interphalangeal joint is shifted radially from its normal alignment of 90 degrees to the long line of the digit. **B.** Closing wedge osteotomy is taken from the convex ulnar side. **C.** Internal fixation with two threaded Kirschner wires. Note they are placed from the ulnar side in a horizontal plane. Avoid penetration of the dorsal extensor mechanism.

Table 2–15. *Disorders Associated with Clinodactyly of the Fifth Finger†*

Hand and foot syndromes	Cerebrohepatorenal
Brachydactyly A-1	De Lange*
Brachydactyly A-2	EEC*
Brachydactyly A-3*	Fetal alcohol*
Brachydactyly C	Fetal aminopterin*
Symphalangism	Fibrodysplasia ossificans progressiva
Chromosomal disorders	Goltz focal dermal hypoplasia
Triploidy	Hand-foot-genital*
Trisomy 8*	Hollister-Hollister*
Trisomy 9p*	LADD*
Trisomy 18	Marfan
Trisomy 21*	Noonan*
4p −	Osteo-onychodysplasia*
13q −	Pancytopenia-dysmelia
XXY	Pectoral aplasia dysdactyly (Poland)
XXXXY*	Popliteal pterygium
XXXX and XXXXX	Prader-Willi
Craniofacial syndromes	Pseudothalidomide*
Ankyloglossia superior	Reiger
Cohen*	Roberts*
Lenz microphthalmos	Robinow*
Mandibulofacial	Seckel
Oculodentodigital*	Shwachman*
Orofaciodigital, type I*	Silver
Otopalatodigital*	Spherophakia brachymorphia
Other congenital malformations	Taybi-Linder*
Aarskog*	Thrombocytopenia–absent radius*
Bloom*	Trichorhinophalangeal
Cardiomelic (Holt-Oram)*	Williams*

*Frequently
†From Poznanski, A. K.: The Hand in Radiologic Diagnosis. Philadelphia, W. B. Saunders Co., 1984, p. 288. Reprinted by permission.

deviated *palmoradially* (Fig. 2–77). It is also referred to in the literature as dystelephalangy. Involvement is almost always bilateral. It is a hereditary affliction transmitted as an autosomal dominant trait. The deformity is not present at birth. It presents as a painless tumefaction on the dorsoulnar aspect of the distal interphalangeal joint of the little finger; the distal phalanx progressively deviates palmarly and radially, and usually by ten years of age the deformity is evident. It is found in association with various syndromes such as Silver and Cornelia de Lange.

Radiograms show the typical palmoradial deviation of the distal phalanx of the little finger. In the differential diagnosis one should consider frostbite of the digits.* Extreme cold will injure the growth plates, which will become angular and close prematurely; the result is a characteristic deviation of the digits. In frostbitten fingers, other digits besides the little finger are usually involved, and the physes of the middle phalanges may also be affected.

Treatment is seldom indicated. The deformity is a cosmetic rather than a functional disability. Surgical correction consists of an osteotomy performed through a midlateral incision and internal fixation with two threaded Kirschner wires or one intramedullary threaded Steinmann pin.

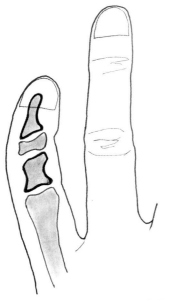

FIGURE 2–77. *Kirner deformity of the little finger.*

*See references 4, 6, 10, 12, 13, 26, 33–37, 46, 50, 54–55.

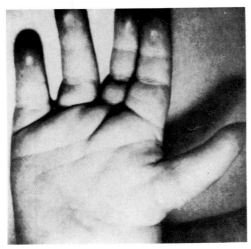

FIGURE 2–78. *Congenital absence of the flexor pollicis longwise and the intrinsic muscles innervated by the median nerve—flexor pollicis brevis, opponens, and abductor pollicis brevis—in an infant.*

Note the characteristic flattening of the thenar eminence and absence of the thumb's interphalangeal crease. (From Strauch, B., and Spinner, M.: Congenital anomaly of the thumb: absent intrinsics and flexor pollicis longus. J. Bone Joint Surg., 58-A:115, 1976. Reprinted by permission.)

Congenital Absence of Flexor Pollicis Longus and Median-Innervated Intrinsic Muscles (Abductor Pollicis Brevis, Opponens and Short Flexors)

This rare anomaly was first described by Fromont in 1895.[20] Su and associates reported a case in 1972.[53] Strauch and Spinner reported 11 hands in eight patients. In one family three members were involved; the inheritance in this family pedigree was probably by autosomal dominant transmission.[52] The condition is characterized by flattening of the thenar eminence, absence of interphalangeal creases of the thumb, and an adduction contracture of the first web space due to the unopposed action of the adductor pollicis (Fig. 2–78). There may be a dorsal dimple at the metacarpophalangeal joint. In the absence of the flexor pollicis longus the interphalangeal joint of the thumb may be stiff in extension. Flexion of the thumb of up to 20 to 25 degrees may be possible—in some patients by the action of the deep head of the flexor pollicis brevis and by means of the ad-

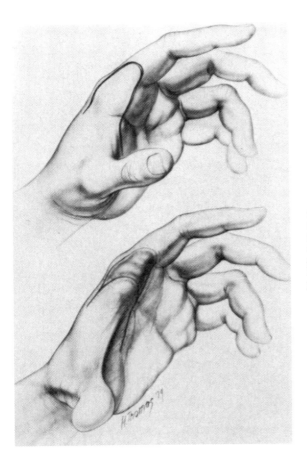

FIGURE 2–79. *Release of adduction contracture of the first web space by use of the sliding flap (Brand).*

Note the dorsal and volar incisions extend to the level of the junction of the thumb and index metacarpals so that subsequently the soft tissue can be released at the apex of the web space. The defect is covered with a full-thickness skin graft. (From Strauch, B., and Spinner, M.: Congenital anomaly of the thumb: absent intrinsics and flexor pollicis longus. J. Bone Joint Surg., 58-A:115, 1976. Reprinted by permission.)

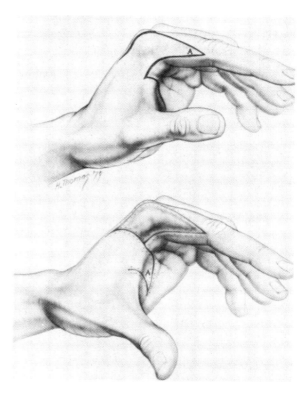

FIGURE 2–80. Transposition flap to release adduction contracture of the first web space.

The resultant defect on the index finger and metacarpal is covered with full-thickness skin graft. (From Stracuh, B., and Spinner, M.: Congenital anomaly of the thumb: absent intrinsics and flexor pollicis longus. J. Bone Joint Surg., 58-A:115, 1976. Reprinted by permission.)

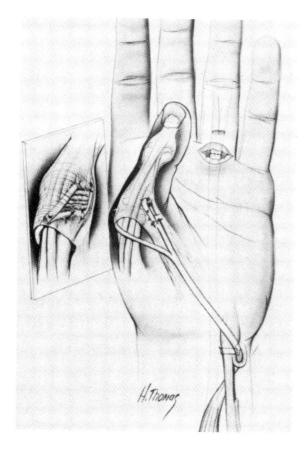

FIGURE 2–81. Transfer of flexor sublimus of ring finger of the thumb to provide opposition.

Note one slip is attached to the normal insertion of the abductor brevis and the other is used to reinforce and plicate the ulnar collateral ligament of the metacarpophalangeal joint of the thumb. (From Strauch, B., and Skinner, M.: Congenital anomaly of the thumb: absent intrinsics and flexor pollicis longus. J. Bone Joint Surg., 58-A:115, 1976. Reprinted by permission.)

ductor attachment of the extensor mechanism. Functionally there is marked impairment or lack of opposition, fine pinch, key pinch, and grasp.

Treatment consists of adduction contracture release by either a sliding flap, shown in Figure 2–79, or a transpositional flap, shown in Figure 2–80. The defect in the index finger and metacarpal is covered with full-thickness skin graft. The opposition is restored by transfer of the flexor sublimis tendon of the ring finger to the thumb with one slip attached to the normal insertion of the abductor brevis and the other used to plicate the ulnar collateral ligament of the thumb metacarpal joint (Fig. 2–81). The result of the surgery is significant improvement in pinch and grasp.

References

1. Baraitser, M.: A new camptodactyly syndrome. J. Med. Genet., *19*:40, 1982.
2. Barinka, L.: Kampylodaktylie (predbezne sdeleni). Acta Chir. Orthop. Traumatol. Cech., *28*:279, 1961.
3. Barletta, L. P. A.: Campilodactilia. Prensa Med., *46*:758, 1959.
4. Blank, E., and Girdany, B. R.: Symmetric bowing of the terminal phalanges of the fifth fingers in a family (Kirner's deformity). A. J. R., *93*:367, 1965.
5. Burke, F., and Flatt, A. E.: Clinodactyly. A review of a series of cases. Hand, *3*:269, 1979.
6. Carstam, N., and Eiken, O.: Kirner's deformity of the little finger. J. Bone Joint Surg., *52-A*:1663, 1970.
7. Carstam, N., and Theander, G.: Surgical treatment of clinodactyly caused by longitudinally bracketed diaphysis. Scand. J. Plast. Reconstr. Surg., *9*:199, 1975.
8. Courtemanche, A. D.: Camptodactyly: Etiology and management. Plast. Reconstr. Surg., *44*:451, 1969.
9. Currarino, G., and Waldman, I.: Camptodactyly. A. J. R., *92*:1312, 1964.
10. David, T. J., and Burwood, R. L.: The nature and inheritance of Kirner's deformity. J. Med. Genet., *9*:430, 1972.
11. DeHaas, W. H. D.: Camptodactylie. Ned. Tijdschr. Geneeskd., *101*:2121, 1957.
12. Dutta, P.: The inheritance of the radially curved little finger. Acta Genet., *15*:70, 1965.
13. Dykes, R. G.: Kirner's deformity of the little finger. J. Bone Joint Surg., *60-B*:58, 1978.
14. Edwards, J. A., and Gale, R. P.: Camptobrachydactyly: A new autosomal dominant trait with two probable homozygotes. Am. J. Hum. Genet., *24*:464, 1972.
15. Engber, W. M., and Flatt, A. E.: Camptodactyly: An analysis of sixty-six patients and twenty-four operations. J. Hand Surg., *2*:216, 1977.
16. Fevre, M.: Camptodactylie (lésions anatomiques d'un doigt surnuméraire atteint de camptodactylie). Ann. Anat. Pathol., *13*:1018, 1936.
17. Flatt, A. E.: The Care of Congenital Hand Anomalies. St. Louis, Mosby, 1977, p. 147.
18. Flatt, A. E.: The Care of Congenital Hand Anomalies. St. Louis, Mosby, 1977, p. 154.
19. Forral, G.: Gehauftes Verkommen von Kamptodaktylia und Leinersher Krankheit in derselben Familie. Wien. Klin. Wochenschr., *77*:259, 1965.
20. Fromont: Anomalies musculaires multiples de la main. Absence du fléchisseur propre du pouce; l'éminence thenar; lombricaux supplémentaires. Bull. Soc. Anat. Paris, *70*:395, 1895.
21. Gellis, S. S., and Feingold, M.: Male Turner's syndrome. Am. J. Dis. Child., *112*:63, 1966.
22. Gerald, B., and Umansky, R.: Cornelia de Lange syndrome: Radiographic findings. Radiology, *88*:96, 1967.
23. Goodman, R. M., Katznelson, M. B. M., and Manor, E.: Camptodactyly: Occurrence in two new genetic syndromes and its relationship to other syndromes. J. Med. Genet., *9*:203, 1972.
24. Gordon, H., Davies, D., and Berman, M.: Camptodactyly, cleft palate, and club foot: A syndrome showing the autosomal-dominant pattern of inheritance. J. Med. Genet., *6*:266, 1969.
25. Harle, T. S., and Stevenson, J. R.: Hereditary symphalangism associated with carpal and tarsal fusions. Radiology, *89*:91, 1967.
26. Hefner, R. A.: Inheritance of crooked little finger (streblomicrodactyly). J. Hered., *20*:395, 1929.
27. Hersh, A. H., Dearinis, F., and Stecher, R. M.: On the inheritance and development of clinodactyly. Am. J. Hum. Genet., *5*:257, 1953.
28. Hoefnagel, D., and Gerald, P. S.: Hereditary brachydactyly. Ann. Hum. Genet., *29*:377, 1966.
29. Iselin, F., Levame, J., and Afanassief, A.: Les camptodactylies congénitales (Soc. Med. Chir. des Hôpitaux Libres de Fourier, 1966). Arch. Hôp., *5*:1, 1966.
30. Jaeger, M., and Refior, H. J.: Congenital triangular deformity of tubular bones in hand and foot. Clin. Orthop., *81*:139, 1971.
31. Jurgens, H. W.: Zur Problematik der Klinodaktylie. Arztl. Jugenkd., *52*:341, 1960.
32. Katz, G.: A pedigree with anomalies of the little finger in five generations and seventeen individuals. J. Bone Joint Surg., *52-A*:717, 1970.
33. Kaufmann, H. J., and Taillard, W. F.: Bilateral incurving of the terminal phalanges of the fifth fingers. A. J. R., *86*:490, 1961.
34. Kelikian, H.: Congenital Deformities of the Hand and Forearm. Philadelphia, Saunders, 1974, pp. 220–221.
35. Kirner, J.: Doppelseitige Verkrümmungen des Kleinfingerendgliedes als selbständiges. Fortschr. Gen. Röntgen., *36*:804, 1927.
36. Kirner, J.: Doppelseitige verkrümmung der Endglieder bei der Kleinfinger. Fortschr. Gen. Röntgen., *78*:745, 1953.
37. Lee, F. A.: Generalized overconstriction of long bones and unilateral Kirner's deformity in a de Lange dwarf. Am. J. Dis. Child., *116*:599, 1968.
38. Littman, A., Yates, J. W., and Treger, A.: Camptodactyly. A kindred study. J.A.M.A., *206*:1565, 1968.
39. Lundblom, A.: On congenital ulnar deviation of the fingers of familial occurrence. Acta Orthop. Scand., *3*:393, 1932.
40. McArthur, R. G., and Edwards, J. H.: De Lange syndrome: Report of 20 cases. Can. Med. Assoc. J., *96*:1185, 1967.
41. Millesi, H.: The pathogenesis and operative correction of camptodactyly. Chir. Plast. Reconstr., *5*:55, 1968.
42. Millesi, H.: Camptodactyly. *In* Littler, J. W., Cramer, L. M., and Smith, J. W. (eds.): Symposium on Reconstructive Hand Surgery. St. Louis, Mosby, 1974, pp. 175–177.
43. Moseley, J. E., Moloshok, R. E., and Freiberger, R. H.: Silver syndrome: Congenital asymmetry, short stature and variations in sexual development: Roentgen features. A. J. R., *97*:74, 1966.
44. Oldfield, M. C.: Camptodactyly: Flexor contracture of the fingers in young girls. Br. J. Plast. Surg., *8*:312, 1956.
45. Pol, P.: Brachydaktylie-Klinodaktylie-Hyperphalangie und ihre Grundlagen. Arch. Pathol. Anat. Klin. Med., *229*:388, 1921.

46. Poznanski, A. K., Pratt, G. B., Manson, G., and Weiss, L.: Clinodactyly, camptodactyly, Kirner's deformity, and other crooked fingers. Radiology, 93:573, 1969.

47. Roche, A. F.: Clinodactyly and brachymesophalangia of the fifth finger. Acta Paediatr. Scand., 50:387, 1961.

48. Sengupta, A.: Multiple congenital contracture of fingers. J. Indiana State Med. Assoc., 43:285, 1964.

49. Smith, R. J., and Kaplan, E. B.: Camptodactyly and similar atraumatic flexion deformities of the proximal interphalangeal joints of the fingers. J. Bone Joint Surg., 50-A:1187, 1968.

50. Staheli, L. T., Clawson, D. K., and Capps, J. H.: Bilateral curving of the terminal phalanges of the little fingers, report of two cases. J. Bone Joint Surg., 48-A:1171, 1966.

51. Stoddard, E. E.: Nomenclature of hereditary crooked fingers: Streblomicrodactyly and camptodactyly—are they synonyms? J. Hered., 30:511, 1939.

52. Strauch, B., and Spinner, M.: Congenital anomaly of the thumb: Absent intrinsics and flexor pollicis longus. J. Bone Joint Surg., 58-A:115, 1976.

53. Su, C. T., Hoopes, J. E., and Daniel, R.: Congenital absence of the thenar muscles innervated by the median nerve. Report of a case. J. Bone Joint Surg., 54-A:1087, 1972.

54. Sugiura, Y., Ueda, T., Umezawa, K., Tajima, Y., and Sugiura, I.: Dystelephalangy of the fifth finger. Dystrophy of the fifth finger. J. Jpn. Orthop. Assoc., 34:1573, 1961.

55. Taybi, H.: Bilateral incurving of the terminal phalanges of the fifth fingers, (osteochondrosis). J. Pediatr., 62:431, 1963.

56. Todd, A. H.: Case of hereditary contracture of the little fingers. Lancet, 2:1088, 1929.

57. Urban, M. D., Rogers, J. G., and Meyer, W. J., III: Familial syndrome of mental retardation, short stature, contractures of the hands, and genital anomalies. J. Pediatr., 94:52, 1979.

58. Welch, J. P., and Temtamy, S. A.: Hereditary contractures of the fingers (camptodactyly). J. Med. Genet., 3:104, 1966.

59. Wilhelm, A., and Kleinschmidt, W.: New etiologic and therapeutic viewpoints on camptodactyly and tendovaginitis. Chir. Plast. Reconstr., 5:62, 1968.

CONSTRICTION RING SYNDROME

Constriction ring syndrome is a rare abnormality that manifests itself as ringlike constriction bands in the upper and lower limbs and occasionally in the trunk. In the literature it is also referred to as Streeter's dysplasia, annular defects of the limbs, and congenital constriction band.[42] The use of the term *syndrome* is preferable because of the common association of the constriction rings with either acrosyndactyly or transverse arrest of the digits, or both.[24]

Etiology

The exact cause is not known. Intrinsic and extrinsic factors have been incriminated. Patterson proposed that the development of constriction bands is similar to that of cleft lip, in that they both result from failure of development of the mesodermal masses under the skin.[36, 37] Selective lack of development in the mesodermal mass destined to produce the subcutaneous tissues results in the normal skin crease. Abnormal failure of this process will cause constriction ring; the more severe the mesodermal failure, the deeper the ring.

The proponents of the theory that extrinsic factors are responsible in the pathogenesis of constriction ring syndrome propose that the probable cause is premature rupture of the amniotic sac and sudden reduction of amniotic fluid volume, and that this precipitates abnormally strong uterine muscle contraction with resultant formation of amniotic bands. The distal portions of the limb may even penetrate the amnion. This is supported by the observation that constriction rings in the short marginal digits are the least common.[24]

The syndrome is nonhereditary. The cases occur sporadically. The incidence is reported by Patterson to be one in 15,000.[36]

Clinical Picture

The extent and depth of the ring constrictions vary; they may be shallow, including only the skin and subcutaneous tissue, as shown in Figure 2–82, or they may be deep, extending to the fasciae and as far as the bone (Fig. 2–83).

The circular grooves are at right angles to the long axis of the digit or limb. On the dorsum of the digit the grooves are usually deeper than the volar aspect. The deeper fibrous bands may

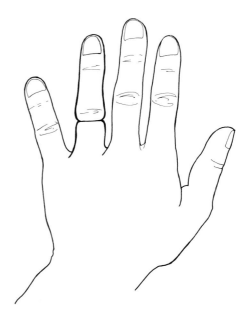

FIGURE 2–82. *Simple constriction ring on the ring finger.*

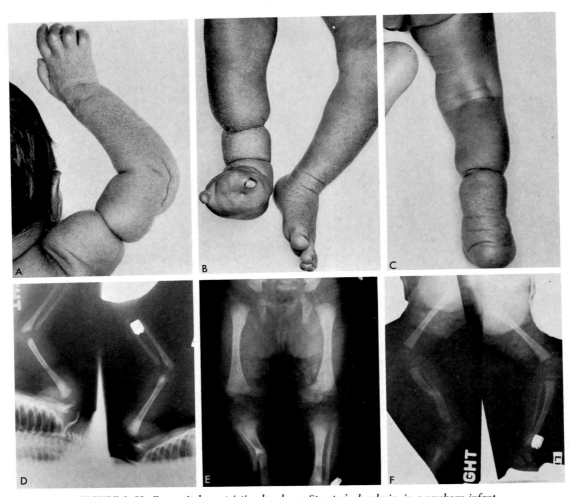

FIGURE 2–83. Congenital constriction bands, or Streeter's dysplasia, in a newborn infant.

A. Note the deep concentric fibrous band in the upper arm, which had caused ulnar and median nerve paralysis. **B** and **C.** Lower limbs of same patient. Note the concentric band on the right leg and associated syndactyly of the toes. Part of the limb distal to the concentric band is enlarged and edematous owing to interference with venous and lymphatic return. **D** to **F.** Radiograms of both the upper and lower limbs. Note the healing fracture in the middle third of the right tibia.

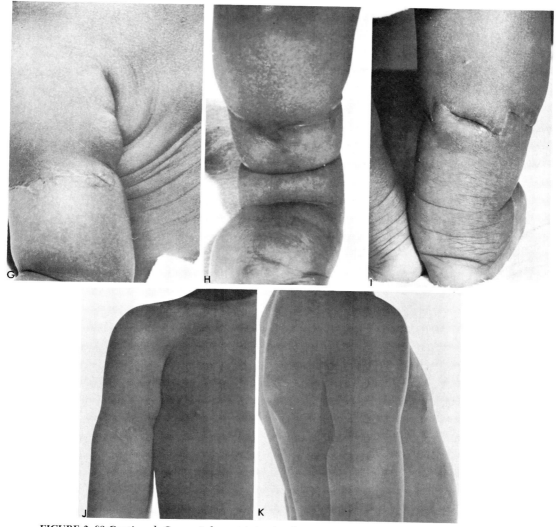

FIGURE 2–83 Continued. Congenital constriction bands, or Streeter's dysplasia, in a newborn infant.

G to I. Immediate postoperative photographs showing release of concentric constriction bands on the right arm and right leg. Deep fibrous bands were excised through a Z-plasty incision in two successive stages to minimize circulatory embarrassment. **J** and **K.** Healed scars on right upper arm four years postoperatively.

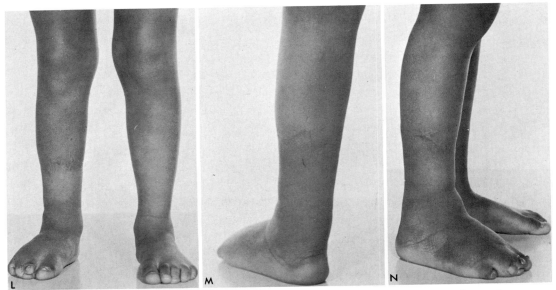

FIGURE 2–83 Continued. Congenital constriction bands, or Streeter's dysplasia, in a newborn infant.

L to N. Both legs showing healed scars four years postoperatively. A partial separation of syndactyly of the right foot was performed.

interfere with the lymphatic and venous return, causing edema, enlargement, cyanosis, and decreased capillary refill of the part distal to the ring. The part distal to the constriction ring may balloon (Fig. 2–84). Sensation, such as to pin prick and light touch, may be decreased distal to the constriction band. If local circulation is markedly disrupted, that part of the limb distal to the constriction band may undergo amputation in utero (Fig. 2–85). Single or multiple amputations of the digits can occur. The nails may be hypoplastic or absent.

Concomitant anomalies in the hand include syndactyly, acrosyndactyly, phalangeal hypopla-

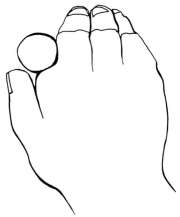

FIGURE 2–84. Constriction ring with a marked balloon swelling of the distal part.

sia, and brachydactyly; occasional anomalies of the digits are symphalangia, symbrachydactyly, and camptodactyly. Other associated anomalies are talipes equinovarus and cleft lip and palate. In the series of patients reported by Flatt, 80 per cent had concomitant hand anomalies, 40 per cent had a combination of hand and foot anomalies, and 11 per cent had oral cavity anomalies.[12]

Distal parts of the limbs, such as the fingers and toes and hands and feet, are affected more often than the forearms and legs and arms and thighs. The longer digits in the hand, i.e., the long, index, and ring fingers, are involved most commonly. There is no definite pattern of deformity; involvement is asymmetrical. Association with anomalies varies from the hand of one limb to the contralateral side. In severe cases the trunk may also be involved.[14]

In the newborn and rapidly growing infant the constriction rings have granulated tissue in their depths; progressive constriction and circulatory embarrassment may occur with healing of the granulated tissue. The dynamic nature of the constriction ring with growth and the importance of frequent observation cannot be overemphasized.

Treatment

Patterson gave the following classification of constriction ring syndrome: (1) simple constriction ring; (2) constriction ring with deformity of

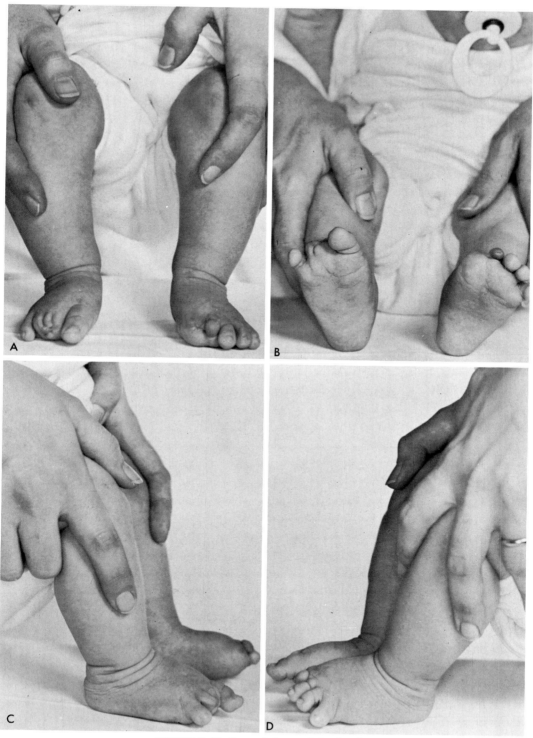

FIGURE 2–85. Congenital constriction bands.

A to **D.** Clinical appearance. Note the intrauterine autoamputation of the big toe on the left and amputation of distal phalanges and syndactyly of the proximal phalanges of the middle three toes on the right.

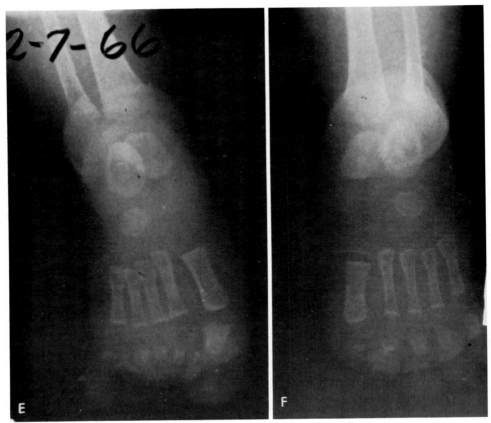

FIGURE 2–85 Continued. Congenital constriction bands.

E and F. Radiograms of both feet.

the distal part, such as swelling, lymphade-noma, or cyanosis; (3) constriction ring with fusion of the distal parts ranging from simple syndactyly to acrosyndactyly; and (4) intrauter-ine amputations. Treatment modalities and in-dications for surgery vary in different sub-groups.[36, 37]

Simple shallow grooves, especially the incom-plete rings and those that do not interfere with circulation or lymphatic drainage, do not re-quire treatment. With absorption of the infant's subcutaneous fat, the shallow grooves will be-come less conspicuous and cosmetically more acceptable. The deeper bands are surgically divided and excised down to normal structures through the use of Z-plasty transposition flaps.

The following technical points should be ob-served: Stage surgery in two or three successive steps performed several months apart in order to minimize circulatory involvement. Do no more than 50 per cent of the circumference of the digit at one operation. Z-plasty flaps should be large and at an angle of about 60 degrees. Do not simply excise the circumferential ring

and utilize everting interrupted sutures; this will result in a contracted scar that will constrict the digit. In the forearm or the finger of an older child use two or more pairs of transposable Z-flaps for each step. Excise the constricted band; do not simply incise it. Exercise great caution when excising the ring; do not injure digital vessels and nerves (they closely abut the undersurface of the band). Undermine the flaps, carefully transpose them, and close them by everting mattress sutures. When the constric-tion rings are associated with acrosyndactyly, separation of the digits takes priority; it is performed early in the first six months of life to permit parallel longitudinal growth. The fingers are drawn together; carefully identify the ap-propriate tip of each finger; use split-thickness skin grafts and Z-plasty flaps to close the skin.

References

1. Artz, T. D., and Posch, J. L.: Use of cross-finger flap for treatment of congenital broad constricting bands of the fingers. Plast. Reconstr. Surg., 52:645, 1973.

2. Bagg, H. J.: Hereditary abnormalities of the limbs, their origin and transmission. II. A morphological study with special reference to the etiology of club-feet, syndactylism, hypodactylism, and congenital amputation in the descendants of x-rayed mice. Am. J. Anat., 43:167, 1929.
3. Baker, C. J., and Rudolph, A. J.: Congenital ring constrictions and intra-uterine amputations. Am. J. Dis. Child., 121:393, 1971.
4. Barenberg, L. H., and Greenberg, B.: Intrauterine amputations and constriction. Am. J. Dis. Child., 64:87, 1942.
5. Blackfield, H. M., and Hause, D. E.: Congenital constricting bands of the extremities. Plast. Reconstr. Surg., 8:101, 1951.
6. Brindeau, A., Lantuejoul, P., and Chappaz, G.: Des malformations d'origine amniotique: (Arrets de développement ou maladies de la membrane amniotique). Sem. Hôp. Paris, 28:2769, 1952.
7. Browne, D.: The pathology of congenital ring constrictions. Arch. Dis. Child., 32:517, 1957.
8. Collins, R. J., and Nichols, D. H.: Congenital fetal anomalies: Intra-uterine amputation and annular constriction bands. N.Y. State J. Med., 50:1403, 1950.
9. Diamond, L. S.: Ring constrictions. *In* Bergsma, D. (ed.): Birth Defects Atlas and Compendium. Baltimore, Williams & Wilkins, 1973, p. 795.
10. Field, J. H., and Krag, D. O.: Congenital constricting bands and congenital amputation of the fingers: Placental studies. J. Bone Joint Surg., 55-A:1035, 1973.
11. Fischl, R. A.: Ring constriction syndrome. Transactions of the International Society of Plastic and Reconstructive Surgeons, 5th Congress. Australia, Butterworth, 1971, pp. 657–670.
12. Flatt, A. E.: The Care of Congenital Hand Anomalies. St. Louis, Mosby, 1977, pp. 213–227.
13. Gellis, S. S.: Constrictive bands in the human. Birth Defects, Original Article Series, 13:259, 1977.
14. Gupta, M. L.: Congenital annular defects of the extremities and the trunk. J. Bone Joint Surg., 45-A:571, 1963.
15. Higginbottom, M. C., Jones, K. L., Hall, B. D., and Smith, D. W.: The amniotic band disruption complex: Timing of amniotic rupture and variable spectra of consequent defects. J. Pediatr., 95:544, 1979.
16. Holtmann, B., Wray, R. C., Lowrey, R., et al.: Restoration of elbow flexion. Hand, 7:256, 1975.
17. Inoue, G.: An angiographic study of congenital hand anomalies. Nippon Seik. Gakkai Zasshi, 55:183, 1981.
18. Kato, T., and Yamane, H.: Experimental studies on the development of malformations of the extremities. J. Jpn. Orthop. Assoc., 42:379, 1968.
19. Kelikian, H.: Congenital Deformities of the Hand and Forearm. Philadelphia, Saunders, 1974, pp. 496–554.
20. Khudr, G., and Benirschke, K.: Discordant monozygous twins associated with amnion rupture. A case report. Obstet. Gynecol., 39:713, 1972.
21. Kino, Y.: Developmental disturbance in the rat fetus caused by amniocentesis. Kanken Nenpo (Japan), 21:225, 1969.
22. Kino, Y.: Morphogenesis of congenital limb defects. Clin. Orthop. Surg. (Japan), 6:664, 1971.
23. Kino, Y.: Reductive malformation of the limbs in the rat fetus following amniocentesis. Congen. Anom. (Japan), 12:35, 1972.
24. Kino, Y.: Clinical and experimental studies of the congenital constriction band syndrome, with an emphasis on its etiology. J. Bone Joint Surg., 57-A:636, 1975.
25. Kohler, H. G.: Congenital transverse defects of limbs and digits ("intra-uterine amputation"). Arch. Dis. Child., 37:263, 1962.
26. Kohler, H. G.: Die intra-uterine Amputation. Eine medizine-historische und biographische Betrachtung.
Part I, Med. Monatschr., 17:696, 1963. Part II, Med. Monatschr., 18:18, 1964.
27. Lenz, W., and Knapp, K.: Die Thalidomid-Embryopathie. Dtsch. Med. Wochenschr., 87:1232, 1962.
28. Losch, G. M., Schrader, M., and Eckert, P.: Malformation syndrome with constriction rings, pseudoligaments, acral defects and syndactylism: Diagnosis and treatment. Z. Kinderchir. Grenzgeb., 30:85, 1980.
29. Miura, T.: A clinical study of congenital anomalies of the hand. Hand, 13:59, 1981.
30. Mohan, V., Gupta, S. K., and Sharma, O. P.: Streeter's dysplasia. J. Postgrad. Med., 26:132, 1980.
31. Montgomery, W. F.: Observations on the spontaneous amputation of the limbs of the foetus in utero, with an attempt to explain the occasional cause of its production. Dublin J. Med. Chem. Sci., 1:140, 1832.
32. Moses, J. M., Flatt, A. E., and Cooper, R. R.: Annular constricting bands. J. Bone Joint Surg., 61-A:562, 1979.
33. Murakami, R.: Acrosyndactyly. Clin. Orthop. Surg. (Japan), 7:1047, 1972.
34. Opgrande, J. D.: Constriction ring syndrome—unusual case report. J. Hand Surg., 7:11, 1982.
35. Ossipoff, V., and Hall, B. O.: Etiologic factors in the amniotic band syndrome: A study of 24 patients. Birth Defects, Original Article Series, 13:117, 1977.
36. Patterson, T. J. S.: Congenital ring-constrictions. Br. J. Plast. Surg., 14:1, 1961.
37. Patterson, T. J. S.: Ring constrictions. Hand, 1:57, 1969.
38. Peet, E. W.: *In* Rob, C., and Smith, R. (eds.): Operative Surgery, Part X. London, Butterworth, 1959, p. 10.
39. Pillay, V. K., and Hesketh, K. T.: Intrauterine amputations and annular limb defects. J. Bone Joint Surg., 47-B:514, 1965.
40. Ramakrishnan, M. S., and Nayak, V. S.: Congenital constriction bands of lower extremities. Indian J. Pediatr., 30:191, 1963.
41. Street, D. M., and Cunningham, F.: Congenital anomalies caused by intra-uterine bands. Clin. Orthop., 37:82, 1964.
42. Streeter, G. L.: Focal deficiencies in fetal tissues and their relation to intra-uterine amputation. Contribution to Embryology., Vol. 22, No. 126. Publication No. 414. Carnegie Institution of Washington, 1930.
43. Temtamy, S. A., and McKusick, V. A.: Digital and other malformations associated with congenital ring constrictions. Birth Defects, 14:547, 1978.
44. Torpin, R.: Amniochorionic mesoblastic fibrous strings and amnionic bands. Am. J. Obstet. Gynecol., 91:65, 1965.
45. Torpin, R.: Fetal Malformations Caused by Amnion Rupture During Gestation. Springfield, Thomas, 1968, pp. 1–165.
46. Trasler, D. C., Walker, B. E., and Fraser, F.: Congenital malformations produced by amniotic puncture. Science, 124:439, 1956.
47. Turner, E. J.: Intra-uterine constriction band. J. Pediatr., 57:590, 1960.
48. Waterman, J. A.: Amputation of fingers in utero. Caribbean Med., 15:31, 1953.

CONGENITAL DYSPLASIA OF THE HIP

Embryology

In order to understand the etiology and pathology of congenital dysplasia of the hip, it is imperative to have a knowledge of the embryology of the hip joint.

At the age of four weeks (5 mm. embryo length, crown to rump), limb buds arise as folds of skin on the anterolateral aspect of the body at the proximal and distal limits of the peritoneal cavity. The development is craniocaudal, the upper limb making its appearance two to three days ahead of the lower limb bud. In the proximal and central portion of the distal limb buds, there is a condensation of highly cellular blastema composed of uniform, dense, packed cells. This is to form the cartilage model of the hip joint (Fig. 2–86 A).

At the age of eight weeks, the early cartilage model of the acetabulum and femoral head has commenced (Fig. 2–86 B).

The femur is formed by the differentiation of the primitive chondroblasts in the shape of a club. The anlagen of the ilium, ischium, and pubis develop as disc-shaped masses (Fig. 2–86 C).

At the age of 11 weeks (5 cm. fetal length), the femoral head is fully formed with a spherical configuration, a short femoral neck, and a primitive greater trochanter (Fig. 2–86 D and E). The musculoskeletal structures of the hip are completely formed. The femoral head is spherical, and the femoral anteversion is 5 to 10 degrees. The joint articular cartilage space is completely formed with good differentiation of the articular cartilage and acetabular anteversion of about 40 degrees. The hip joint capsule, ligamentum teres, glenoid labrum, and transverse acetabular ligament are well-defined structures. The fetal posture of the hip is one of flexion, adduction, and lateral rotation (left greater than right) (Fig. 2–86 F). This is the most stable position for the hip joint. Femoral antetorsion increases during the second half of fetal life, reaching 35 degrees at the time of birth. The acetabular inclination increases with the medial rotation attitude of the hips. With extension of the hips, the hip joints become unstable and susceptible to dislocation.

Definition

Congenital dysplasia of the hip comprises a wide spectrum of abnormalities ranging from simple hip instability with capsular laxity to complete displacement of the femoral head out of an anomalous acetabular socket. The term *dysplasia* connotes a developmental abnormality of the hip joint in which the capsule, the proximal femur, and the acetabulum are all defective. It emphasizes the dynamic nature of the alterations of the growing chondro-osseous components of the infant's hip and their re-

sponse to abnormal biomechanical forces. With restoration of normal articular relations between the femoral head and acetabulum, the anatomic changes are reversible in time with growth. Congenital dislocation of the hip should be regarded as a progressive deformation of a previously normally formed structure during the fetal period of development and not related to the embryonic period; it is not a malformation arising during the embryonic period of organogenesis.

Classification

It is essential to differentiate between two main groups of congenital dislocation of the hip: *teratologic* and *typical*. *Teratologic* dislocation of the hip is characterized by its association with other severe malformations (such as lumbosacral agenesis), chromosomal abnormalities, and neuromuscular disorders (such as arthrogryposis multiplex congenita and myelomeningocele). It develops early in utero with severe contracture of soft tissues and marked displacement of the femoral head. At birth the dislocation cannot be reduced by the Ortolani maneuver.

Typical congenital dislocation of the hip occurs in an otherwise normal infant; it may take place in utero (fetal, antenatal, or prenatal), occur at birth (perinatal), or develop after birth (postnatal). The time of onset of dislocation affects the severity of anatomic changes, the clinical and radiographic findings, and the type and course of treatment.

Typical dislocation of the hip can be subdivided into three types—the dislocated hip, the dislocatable hip, and the subluxatable hip. In the *dislocated* hip the femoral head is completely out of the acetabulum, riding superolaterally. In the newborn period the perinatal typical dislocated hip can be easily reduced by simple flexion-abduction of the hip, producing a clunk—the positive Ortolani test. In the *dislocatable* hip the femoral head is in the acetabulum but can be easily displaced out of it by Barlow's provocative test. The *subluxatable* hip is marked by ligamentous hyperlaxity, and the femoral head can be passively displaced partially out of the acetabulum but not completely dislocated by the Palmen subluxation provocation test. The examiner feels a "giving" sensation, but there is no clunk. The *unstable* hip may be dislocatable or subluxatable. The *subluxated* hip, by definition, has partially migrated laterally and upward in the joint but is not totally displaced out of the acetabu-

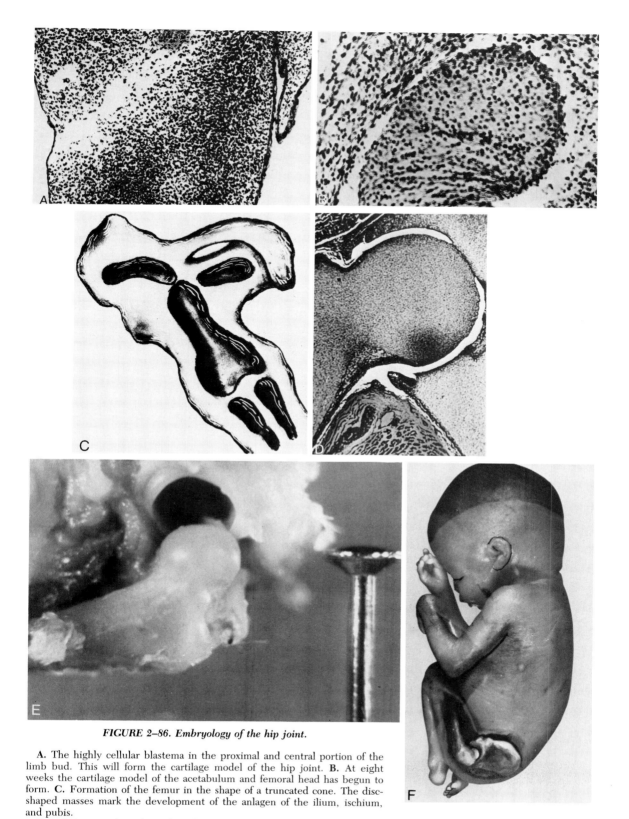

FIGURE 2–86. Embryology of the hip joint.

A. The highly cellular blastema in the proximal and central portion of the limb bud. This will form the cartilage model of the hip joint. **B.** At eight weeks the cartilage model of the acetabulum and femoral head has begun to form. **C.** Formation of the femur in the shape of a truncated cone. The disc-shaped masses mark the development of the anlagen of the ilium, ischium, and pubis.

D and **E.** Note the spherical configuration of the femoral head and acetabulum. The limbus and transverse acetabular ligament are well-formed structures. **F.** Note the posture of the lower limbs at 16 weeks of fetal life (100 mm.)—flexion, adduction, and lateral rotation.

Illustration continued on following page

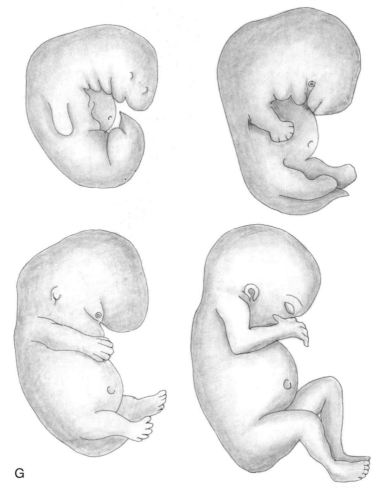

G

FIGURE 2–86 Continued. Embryology of the hip joint.

G. Development of the lower limb at different stages of the embryonic period. 1. Four weeks gestation. 2. End of fifth week of gestation. 3. Six weeks of gestation. 4. Eight weeks of gestation. (A to F from Watanabe, R. S.: Embryology of the human hip. Clin. Orthop., 98:8, 1974. Reprinted by permission.)

lum—there is still some contact between the two. The subluxated hip may be loose and reducible concentrically on flexion, abduction, and medial rotation of the hip, or it may be taut and irreducible.

Incidence

There is great geographic and racial variation in the incidence of congenital dislocation of the hip. Certain areas of the world have an endemically high incidence, whereas in other areas it is virtually nonexistent. Among 16,000 black African Bantu babies, Edelstein found not a single case of congenital dislocation of the hip, whereas in the Island Lake Region in Manitoba,

Canada, Walker reported an incidence of 188.5 per thousand.[248, 985] In New York, Artz and associates found the incidence of congenital dislocation of the hip to be 4.9 per thousand in Negroes as compared with 15.5 per thousand in Caucasians.[21]

The incidence of congenital dislocation of the hip is reported as 0.1 per thousand in Chinese children in Hong Kong (Hoaglund and associates, 1981); 1.5 per thousand in Salford, England, (Barlow, 1962); 1.7 per thousand in Sweden (von Rosen, 1962), and 75 per thousand in Belgrade, Yugoslavia (Klisic, 1975).[33, 416, 499, 788] Some other reports of the incidence of congenital dislocation of the hip are 1:50, by Coleman in 1956; 1:50, by Hiertonn and James in 1968;

1:60, by Dunn in 1971; 1:100, by Stanisavljevic in 1961; and 1:160, by Paterson in 1976 (Table 2–16).[152, 238, 408, 716, 890]

This difference in incidence of congenital dysplasia of the hip among disparate groups is explained by genetic and environmental factors. Another important consideration is the age of the infant at the time of examination. The congenitally dysplastic hip is observed more frequently in the newborn than in the four-week-old infant. Barlow found that about one infant in 60 was born with instability of one or both hips, and that of these 60 per cent recovered in the first week of life, and 88 per cent in the first two months. The remaining 12 per cent, an incidence of 1.55 per thousand, were typical congenital dislocations and persisted. These findings of Barlow indicate that unstable and dislocatable hips have a tendency to stabilize themselves spontaneously by tautening of the lax capsule. The age of the baby at the time of examination is, therefore, an important factor affecting the reported incidence of congenital dislocation of the hip.[33]

The experience and ability of the examiner and the clinical signs used for criteria in making the diagnosis are other factors that determine the reported incidence of congenital hip dislocation.

Etiology

Many factors are involved in causing congenital dislocation of the hip: ligamentous hyperlaxity, mechanical forces resulting from anatomic instability of the hip and intrauterine malposture, genetic influences, and postnatal environmental factors.

PERIODS AT WHICH THE HIP MAY BE DISLOCATED

In the *intrauterine life* of the fetus there are three periods during which the hip is at risk for dislocation: around (1) the twelfth week, (2) the eighteenth week, and (3) the final four weeks of gestation.[895]

The period *around the twelfth week* of in utero development is the *first period* of risk for hip dislocation because the first major positional change of the lower limb takes place—the limb rotates medially, using the hip joint as the pivot point. The joint capsule is weak, providing little resistance to lateral displacement of the femoral head, and the femoral neck is short and retroverted. Failure of synchronized development of neuromuscular units will result in abnormal muscle pull, and this coupled with an insufficiency of the acetabular labrum will result in an unstable hip that is unable to tolerate the torque of medial rotation of the lower limb. As a result the femoral head is displaced out of the acetabulum and remains dislocated until birth. In utero relocation of the femoral head into the acetabulum does not take place because the necessary anatomic and dynamic factors do not exist. With rapid growth all elements of the hip joint quickly become abnormal: the acetabulum becomes shallow, the capsule distends, the femoral head and greater trochanter remain small because compressional loading is lacking, and a false acetabulum develops. Pathologic changes observed at birth are the most severe.

During the *eighteenth week of gestation (the second period)*, the musculature around the hip joint is fully developed, and active motion of the hip begins. If there is anatomic instability of the hip joint—such as capsular weakness, insufficiency and shallowness of the acetabulum, or abnormal muscle pull due to nonsynchronous development of neuromuscular units—the femoral head will be drawn out of the acetabulum. During this period the pull of the iliopsoas muscle may displace the femoral head anteriorly.

The *third period* is the last four weeks of gestation, when the hip joint with all its muscles is fully developed. The factors producing hip

Table 2–16. Incidence of Congenital Dysplasia of the Hip

Authors	Year	Geographic Area	Incidence per Thousand
Walker	1973	Island Lake Region (Manitoba, Canada): Canadian Indians	188.5
Klisiç	1975	Belgrade, Yugoslavia	75.1
Coleman	1956	Utah	20.0
Hiertonn and James	1968	Akademiska Sjulchuset, Uppsala, Sweden	20.0
Stanisavljevic	1961	Detroit, Michigan	10.0
Paterson	1976	Adelaide, Australia	6.2
Barlow	1962	Salford, England	1.5
Von Rosen	1962	Malmö, Sweden	1.7
Hoaglund et al.	1981	Chinese Hong Kong	0.1
Edelstein	1966	Africa: Bantus	0.0

dislocation at this time are abnormal mechanical forces due to intrauterine malposture of the fetus such as breech position with extended knees or oligohydramnios (lack of the normal amount of amniotic fluid). This is the type of congenital hip dysplasia most commonly encountered at birth. The hip joint may also be dislocated at birth and postnatally.

LIGAMENTOUS LAXITY

Laxity and insufficiency of the capsule of the hip joint and its associated ligaments are the prime factors in the pathogenesis of typical congenital dislocation of the hip. This observation is based on experiments on animals, anatomic studies at operation and at autopsy, and clinical experience. The capsular and ligamentous laxity may be hereditary, hormonal, or mechanical.

Smith and associates, in an experimental study using young dogs, reported hip dislocation in a high percentage of the animals when both the capsule and ligamentum teres were removed during the growth period. Controlled mechanical stretching of the hip capsules of puppies caused dislocation or dysplasia or both. A shallow acetabular socket surgically produced in dogs soon after birth did not result in dislocation of the hip. Experimentally produced increased anteversion and retroversion in the postnatal phase in puppies had no significant effect on the acetabulum.[874]

Michelsson and Langenskiöld, in their experimental studies of causation of dislocation of the hip in the rabbit, supported the findings of Smith's group.[632]

On a clinical basis and from observations at open surgery, Howorth postulated a prime causal relation between capsular laxity and congenital dislocation of the hip.[431] Andrèn has demonstrated abnormal laxity of the pelvic ligaments in infants born with congenital dislocation of the hip, as shown by distraction of the symphysis pubis twice as great as in normal control cases.[10] The phenomenon is thought to result from the action of maternal sex hormones responsible for the physiologic prenatal relaxation of the maternal ligaments in preparation for labor. A change in the hormonal pattern of newborn infants with congenital dislocation of the hip has been demonstrated by Andrèn and Borglin, who found an increase in the urinary excretion of estrone and estradiol-17 during the first three days of life, as compared with that in normal newborns.[15] This has not, however, been supported by Aarskog and associates, who studied urinary estrogen excretion in newborn infants with congenital dislocation of the hip.[1]

Also, Thieme and associates found no significant difference in estrogen output in 24 urine samples collected from 16 patients with congenital dislocation of the hip and 19 matched controls during the first six days of life.[924] These results did not support the hypothesis that congenital dislocation of the hip is a result of an inborn error in estrogen metabolism in the newborn. The exact cause of excessive joint laxity and its predominance in the female has not yet been determined.

A decrease in the collagen content of connective tissue of children with dislocated hips was found by Fredensborg in studying the umbilical cords of babies born with congenital dislocation of the hip and comparing them with those of normal babies.[307] The maturation of newly synthesized tropocollagen into collagen is blocked by estrogens, which affect the cross linkage.[391]

THE CONCEPT OF PRIMARY ACETABULAR DYSPLASIA

In the past there has been much discussion and controversy regarding the etiologic importance of acetabular dysplasia. Does it represent a primary feature of congenital dislocation of the hip or is it a secondary adaptive defect? In recent years the support for primary acetabular dysplasia has waned, and it has become evident that the dysplasia of the acetabulum is the result and *not* the cause of congenital dislocation of the hip. Acetabular dysplasia is minimal in the newborn with perinatal congenital dislocation of the hip. This is shown by findings at autopsy of newborn babies with the defect, observations at surgery during open reduction, and radiographic and arthrographic studies.[431, 892]

Reversal of acetabular dysplasia following concentric reduction contradicts the hypothesis of a primary developmental defect in the acetabulum.[859] Experiments in animals have further supported the secondary nature of the acetabular changes.[632, 815]

MALPOSITION IN UTERO AND MECHANICAL FACTORS

Breech Presentation. The incidence of breech presentation in infants born with congenital dislocation of the hip is 15.7 per cent in the neonatal series and 8.3 per cent in the late diagnosis series of Bjerkreim and Van Der Hagen; 17.3 per cent in that of Carter and Wilkinson; and 30 per cent in that of Hass.[61, 107, 388] The incidence of breech presentation in the general population is about 3 per cent.

Ramsey and associates, in a study of 25,000 newborns, reported the incidence of true congenital dislocation of the hip to be one out of 35 births in females born by breech presentation. A fetus in breech position in utero is at high risk for hip dislocation (Fig. 2–87).[769]

Breech position in utero is the critical factor rather than the trip down the parturient canal in breech position; this is affirmed by the finding that breech-position infants delivered by Caesarean section have the same strong predisposition to hip dislocation.[61]

Birth Order. There is greater incidence of hip dislocation in firstborn children.[106, 107, 195, 1037, 1038] This appears to be related to intrauterine malposture caused by conditions unique in the primagravida, i.e., an unstretched uterus and taut abdominal muscles, oligohydramnios, and the increased likelihood of breech presentation.

Bjerkreim and Van Der Hagen observed that if the probands with breech presentation are excluded, the greater number of firstborn probands with congenital dislocation of the hip is eliminated. They proposed, therefore, that the higher frequency of firstborn status among patients with congenital hip dislocation is most probably due to the high degree of association between firstborns and breech presentations.[61]

Oligohydramnios. Amniotic fluid protects the fetus from pressure and permits it mobility and freedom of exercise. As the fetus gets longer and larger, the volume of amniotic fluid diminishes, and the fetus is subjected to mechanical pressure from the uterus and abdominal wall (Fig. 2–88).

There is an invariable association between facial and musculoskeletal postural deformities and congenital renal anomalies (Potter's syndrome). Most of the amniotic fluid in late pregnancy is derived from fetal urine. In congenital malformations of the kidney, oligohydramnios is usually found because of fetal oliguria and anuria. Dunn noted that oligohydramnios causes postural deformities of the fetus because of mechanical pressure. He observed 30 infants with Potter's syndrome—all of them were deformed at birth, and 19 (63 per cent) had congenital dislocation of the hip. Dissection of the hip joint showed a spectrum of pathologic changes ranging from unstable hip to the changes seen in late congenital dislocation of the hip that has remained untreated for two or more years.[238]

Congenital dislocation of the hip is extremely rare in fetuses aborted before 20 weeks' gestation.[236] Before 20 weeks, the fetus is very small and not subject to intrauterine pressure sufficient to produce a mechanical effect on the developing hip. Congenital dislocation of the hip is a late fetopathy.

Side Involved. The left hip is dislocated at birth three times as often as the right hip (approximately 60 per cent of congenital dislocations of the hip are on the left, 20 per cent are on the right, and in 20 per cent involvement is bilateral). The great frequency of left-side involvement is due to the fetus's tendency to lie with its back toward its mother's left side twice as often as it does toward her right side. The fetal lower limb lying posteriorly against the mother's back is much more likely to be dislocated than that lying anteriorly, whether the presentation is by vertex or by breech.

Wilkinson experimentally produced atrau-

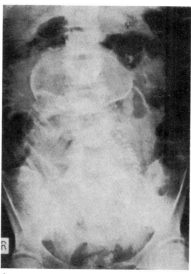 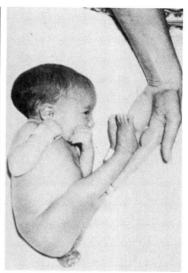

FIGURE 2–87. *The fetus presenting by the breech with extended knees is at high risk for hip dislocation.*

A. Radiogram showing the breech presentation. The baby's bottom is sunk into the mother's rigid bony pelvis. Note the knees are extended. The fetus is unable to move. **B.** The same infant six days after cesarean delivery at 35 weeks. Note the dolicocephalic shape of the molded head and the extended knees. Both hips are dislocated. (From Dunn, P. M.: Perinatal observations on the etiology of congenital dislocation of the hip. Clin. Orthop., *119*:17, 1976. Reprinted by permission.)

A   B

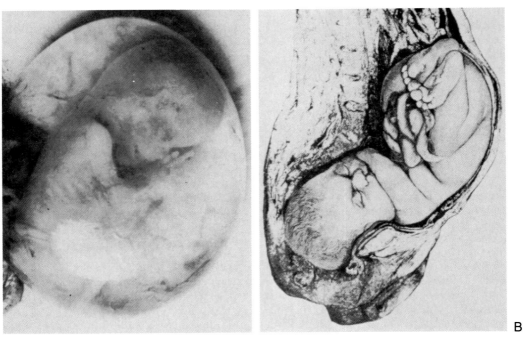

FIGURE 2–88. *The importance of amniotic fluid in protecting the fetus from pressure.*

A. A fetus of 13 weeks' gestation lying within amniotic sac removed at hysterectomy. Note the complete protection of the fragile fetus from mechanical pressure afforded by the abdominal musculature. **B.** Frozen sagittal section of abdomen of pregnant woman who expired during labor. The fetus is flexed laterally around the sacral promontory. (From Dunn, P. M. Perinatal observations on the etiology of congenital dislocation of the hip. Clin. Orthop., *119*:13, 1976. Reprinted by permission.)

matic dislocation of the hip in immature female rabbits by the combined effect of hormonal joint laxity and breech malposition. He induced joint laxity by injecting estrone and progesterone. Persistent breech malposition was obtained by splinting the hind limbs in the breech posture. When acting separately, neither factor dislocated the hip; i.e., dislocation did not occur in lateral rotation breech malposition in the absence of joint ligamentous laxity, nor did it occur as a result of hormonal joint laxity in the free hind limbs. Wilkinson also described the development of femoral retroversion and anteversion in the presence of joint laxity as well as other soft-tissue changes similar to those found in human congenital hip dislocation.[1022]

Salter, in an experimental study with newborn pigs, demonstrated the development of acetabular dysplasia and changes in the direction of the acetabulum as a result of maintaining the hips in extension for a period of six weeks. After the pigs were allowed to run free for ten weeks the condition corrected itself. Normal acetabuli developed when the hips were maintained in flexion and abduction.[808, 809, 815] In 85 growing rabbits, Michelsson and Langenskiöld immobilized one or both hind limbs with the knee in extension but the hip free and moveable. In almost all the younger rabbits, a subluxation, dislocation, or dysplasia of the hip joint developed. Dysplastic changes were typical of those seen in congenital dislocation of the hip in man. Development of the dislocation or dysplasia was due to immobilization of the knee in extension; if the hamstring muscles were sectioned either distally or proximally before the knee was immobilized in extension, neither dislocation nor obvious dysplasia of the hip developed (Fig. 2–89).[632]

The iliopsoas will become progressively short with flexed posture of the hip and rapid intrauterine growth of the fetus. Forcible extension of the unstable hip (due to excessive capsular laxity) may lever the femoral head out of the acetabulum.[207] Initially the femoral head will move anteriorly, and it will migrate upward and posteriorly as a result of capsular elongation.

GENETIC FACTORS

Familial Incidence. Wynne-Davies carried out a detailed survey of genetic and other etiologic factors in 589 index patients with congenital dislocation of the hip and their families. She especially investigated acetabular dysplasia

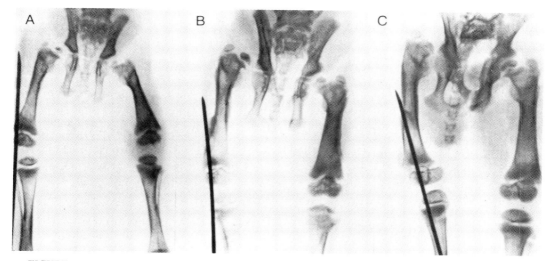

FIGURE 2–89. *Experimental production of dislocation of the hip by immobilization of the knee in extension in growing rabbits.*

A. Five days after immobilizing the knee in complete extension by inserting a metal pin in the soft tissues of the right hind limb. Note the hip is subluxated. **B.** Fifteen days postoperatively; the hip is completely dislocated. **C.** Twenty-one days postoperatively the rabbit was killed. The dislocation and dysplasia of the hip are visible in the roentgenogram of the specimen. (From Michelsson, J.-E., Langenskiöld, A.: Dislocation or subluxation of the hip. Regular sequels of immobilization of the knee in extension in young rabbits. J. Bone Joint Surg., *54-A*:1177, 1972. Reprinted by permission.)

and familial joint laxity and compared neonatal and late-diagnosed cases. According to her findings the risk to subsequent members of the family when dislocation is present is (1) normal parents with one affected child, risk to subsequent children 6 per cent, (2) one affected parent, risk 12 per cent, and (3) one affected parent with one affected child, risk 36 per cent. (These figures include both neonatal and late-diagnosed cases.) Wynne-Davies suggested that genetic predisposition operates through two separate heritable systems: the first is the development of *acetabular dysplasia*, which is inherited as a polygenic system and is responsible for a large proportion of the cases diagnosed late; the second system is generalized *joint laxity*, which is inherited as a dominant trait with incomplete penetrance and is responsible for a large proportion of neonatal cases.[1037] It is difficult to support the concept of acetabular dysplasia as a separate heritable system in view of the findings in numerous reports of series in which there were very few congenital hip dislocations diagnosed late and a large proportion of the unstable hips were diagnosed and treated neonatally.[34, 35, 769, 789, 790] The acetabular dysplasia in the parents of Wynne-Davies's second group can most probably be accounted for by the failure to detect and treat an unstable hip in the neonatal period.[1037]

Bjerkreim and Van Der Hagen studied the familial occurrence of congenital dislocation of the hip in 1147 probands in whom the condition was diagnosed neonatally and in 784 probands in whom the dislocation was diagnosed late. The proportions of affected siblings were 6 per cent in the former group and 8.5 per cent in the latter. The frequency in siblings of all probands was 7.1 per cent, which is 7.2 times the incidence of congenital dislocation of the hip reported in the general population. Congenital hip dysplasia occurred in 2.1 per cent of the parents of all probands, which is ten times the incidence in the general population. Heritability of congenital dislocation of the hip based on calculations on the Edward's model gave a phenotypic correlation of 37 per cent and a corresponding heritability of 74 per cent.[61, 251]

Idelberger investigated the incidence of congenital dislocation of the hip in 138 pairs of twins and found concordance (i.e., the likelihood that if one twin had congenital dislocation of the hip, the other twin did also) to be 42.7 per cent in monozygous pairs and 2.8 per cent in dizygous pairs. This greater incidence of congenital dislocation of the hip in twin pairs indicates that a genetic predisposition is an important etiologic factor.[443]

Sex Incidence. There is a definite preponderance of females affected by congenital dislocation of the hip, its incidence being four to six times as great in girls as in boys.

POSTNATAL ENVIRONMENTAL FACTORS

In the newborn and young infant the normal physiologic position of the hip is that of flexion and abduction (Fig. 2–90). In some areas of the world, such as Central Africa, China, and India, the hips of newborn infants are maintained in flexion and abduction, and the incidence of typical congenital dislocation of the hip is very low. In other areas, such as Northern Italy and Germany, where infants were customarily carried with the hips held in extension and adduction, the incidence was strikingly high. This variance in frequency seems to indicate that the infant is not developmentally prepared for a sudden transition from the intrauterine position of hip flexion to that of extension. With change of hip posture from extension-adduction to flexion-abduction the incidence of congenital dislocation of the hip has decreased remarkably.

SEASONAL INFLUENCE

More infants are born with congenital dislocation of the hip in the winter months—this is accounted for by the baby's heavy clothing holding the lower limbs in adduction and extension.[17, 61, 195, 1037]

Pathology

The spectrum of pathologic anatomy in congenital dislocation of the hip is dependent upon the type, grade, and age of dislocation. The longer the hip is dislocated the greater the degree of deformation of the acetabulum, proximal femur, capsule, and soft tissues.

In the unstable hip, which is subluxatable but not dislocatable, the joint capsule is loose and stretched out, and the ligamentum teres is elongated. The labrum is hyperelastic and everted. There are no inversion changes in the rim of the acetabulum, which is hypertrophied. The femoral head is normal in shape. There may be excessive antetorsion of the femur and acetabulum, making the hip joint anatomically unstable (Fig. 2–91). In the *dislocatable hip* the capsule is markedly stretched out and very loose. The ligamentum teres is elongated and may be attenuated. The labrum is definitely everted. In the older infant the posterosuperior portion of the acetabulum at its fibrocartilage-hyaline junction may show hypertrophic changes of inversion (Fig. 2–92). There may be chondro-osseous deficiency of the anterior part of the acetabulum due to abnormal pressure. The femoral head is spherical. Usually there is excessive antetorsion of both the proximal femur and the acetabulum.

In the *subluxated hip* the femoral head shows signs of loss of sphericity with varying degrees of posteromedial flattening. The femoral and acetabular antetorsion is excessive. The acetabulum has become shallower and begins to develop superoposterior marginal deformations. The fibrocartilaginous labrum is everted initially, but with time will show hypertrophic changes of gradual inversion at its fibrocartilaginous junction, especially in the superoposterior

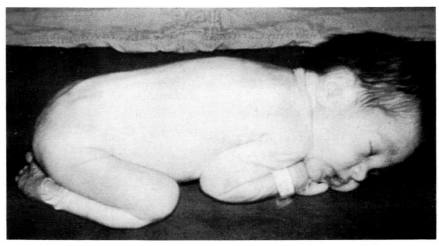

FIGURE 2–90. *Normal physiologic position of the hip in the newborn is flexion-abduction.*

Baby is prone, hips are flexed and abducted.

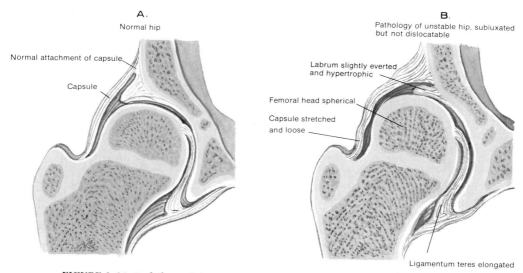

FIGURE 2–91. Pathology of the unstable hip that is subluxatable but not dislocatable.

A. Normal hip. **B.** The subluxatable hip. Note the loose hyperelastic capsule, the elongated ligamentum teres, and the slight eversion of the hypertrophied acetabular rim. The femoral head is normal in shape. Excessive femoral and acetabular antetorsion may be present, causing anatomic instability of the hip joint.

area of the acetabulum. In the early stages these inversional hypertrophic changes are reversible, but later on they become fixed. Inversion of the labrum is not a sudden event of "popping-in" but rather a gradual process of hypertrophy and ingrowth. Fibrofatty tissue may proliferate in the acetabulum. The subluxation may be irreducible because of intra-articular obstacles.

In the *dislocated hip* the femoral head is displaced upward and backward completely out of the acetabulum to lie on the lateral wall of the ilium (Fig. 2–93). The severity of the pathologic changes increases with age and progressive ascent of the femoral head.

Barriers to Reduction. The *capsule* of the hip joint and its associated ligaments are lax, as stated earlier—this is a major factor in the

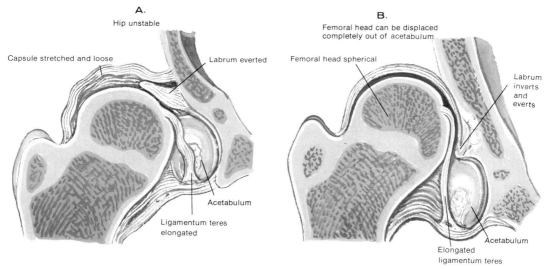

FIGURE 2–92. Pathology of the dislocatable hip.

The capsule is stretched out and very loose. The ligamentum teres is markedly elongated. The labrum is definitely everted. At the fibrocartilage-hyaline junction of the labrum with the acetabulum, there may be inversional hypertrophic changes. The femoral head is spherical. Femoral and acetabular antetorsion is usually excessive.

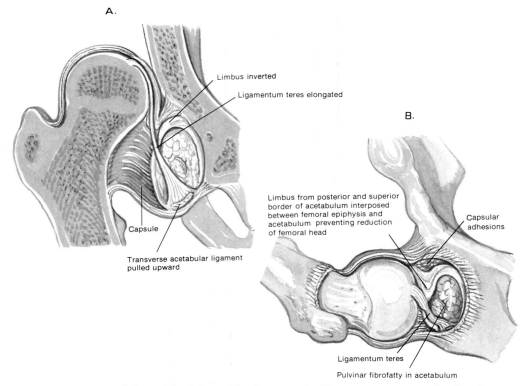

FIGURE 2–93. *Pathology of the dislocated hip that is irreducible owing to intra-articular obstacles.*

A. The hip is dislocated. **B.** It cannot be reduced on flexion, abduction, or lateral rotation. Obstacles to reduction are inverted limbus, ligamentum teres, and fibrofatty pulvinar in the acetabulum. The transverse acetabular ligament is pulled upward with the ligamentum teres.

pathogenesis of typical congenital dislocation of the hip. As the femoral head recedes out of the acetabulum the dilated capsule is elongated and drawn out into a tube. The lower half becomes tautly stretched upward across the acetabulum, closing its opening. Normally the transverse acetabular ligament is a heavy fibrous band that should be regarded as part of the fibrocartilaginous labrum that stretches across the acetabular notch in the lower part of the acetabulum. Attached only at its ends, the ligament completes the circle. Deep to it there is a foramen (between the ligament and bone) through which the acetabular branch of the obturator artery passes. With progressive upward displacement of the femoral head the transverse acetabular ligament is pulled upward with the capsule, becoming stretched and displaced into the acetabulum; in time the ligament hypertrophies and blocks the lower part of the acetabular cavity. The lesser trochanter moves upward with the lateral and upward displacement of the femoral head. Normally the iliopsoas tendon crosses the anterior aspect of the hip joint

capsule to reach to its insertion to the lesser trochanter. In the dislocated hip it compresses and indents and the attenuated, taut capsule across the mouth of the acetabular cavity is compressed and indented inferiorly and anteriorly by the tendon (Fig. 2–94). This hourglass constriction of the capsule and formation of the capsular isthmus markedly reduces the diameter of the acetabular mouth and acts as a definite obstacle to closed reduction. Adhesions may form between the capsule and the iliopsoas tendon and iliacus muscle.

The upper portion of the capsule, which closely covers the femoral head, is known as the capsular hood. With increasing femoral head displacement and under the stress of weight-bearing after walking age, the capsular hood becomes hypertrophic. The capsule may adhere to the lateral wall of the ilium or to the floor of the acetabulum, and may attach to the femoral head (pericephalic insertion of the capsule) (Fig. 2–95). These abnormal attachments and adhesions of the capsule will prevent complete repositioning of the femoral head in the

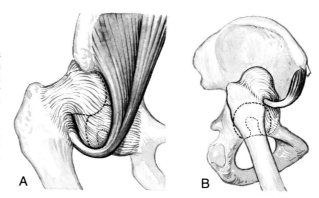

FIGURE 2–94. *The iliopsoas tendon as an obstacle to closed reduction.*

A. Anterior view. Note the iliopsoas tendon traverses the anteromedial aspect of the hip joint prior to its insertion to the lesser trochanter. With lateral and superior displacement of the femoral head and lesser trochanter, the iliopsoas tendon stretches tautly across the medial and anterior aspect of the hip capsule. **B.** Lateral view showing external pressure and indentation of the capsule by the iliopsoas tendon; this hourglass constriction of the capsule and formation of the capsular isthmus markedly reduces the diameter of the acetabular orifice and acts as a barrier to closed reduction.

acetabulum and concentric reduction of the dislocated hip. In the older child, soft-tissue planes are ill defined and poorly developed.

The ligamentum teres may be hypertrophic and abnormally long, and is usually flattened into a thick band, obstructing or even preventing reduction of the head in the acetabulum. At times, it may be attenuated, atrophic, or absent; most probably, however, it was present earlier but was torn or worn away during and after dislocation. In children up to seven years of age, circulation to the femoral head through the ligamentum teres is minimal if present at all. Histologic studies show that a few tiny blood vessels may be seen at its acetabular end, but that none are found at the femoral head.[963] Although blood enters the ligament, it does not traverse it to the femoral head. This is shown by dividing the ligamentum teres near its femoral end and demonstrating that blood flows from the distal, not from the proximal, part whereas when it is severed at its acetabular end, blood does flow from the ligament. *The*

pulvinar is a pad of fibrofatty tissue lining the base of the acetabular socket around the ligamentum teres, to which it is usually adherent. It hypertrophies with persistent dislocation and contributes to the flattening of the acetabular socket.

The limbus is a pathologic response to eccentric pressure. In the normal acetabulum the fibrocartilaginous labrum, triangular in cross section, is attached at its base to the edge of the acetabulum and, at its apex, is free. The free edge of the labrum forms the rim of the acetabular cavity and embraces the head of the femur closely. The concave deep surface of the labrum is in contact with the femoral head, and its convex external surface with that of the capsule and synovial membrane of the joint (Fig. 2–96). As the femoral head is dislocated superiorly, the fibrocartilaginous labrum everts and presses against the outer wall of the ilium, and the capsule and synovial tissue are interposed between it and the iliac bone. Mechanical stimulation from the dislocated femoral head

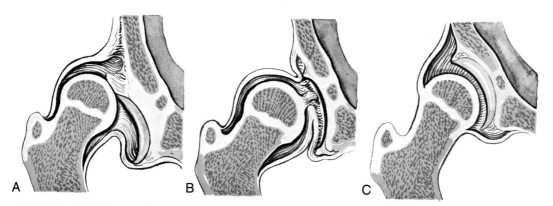

FIGURE 2–95. *Abnormal adhesions of capsule as barriers to closed reduction in congenital dislocation of the hip.*

A. Capsule adhering to lateral wall of ilium. **B.** Capsule adhering to floor of acetabulum. **C.** Pericephalic insertion of capsule. The capsular attachments on the femoral neck are displaced proximally and become attached to the femoral epiphysis, impeding complete placement of the femoral head in the acetabulum and concentric reduction.

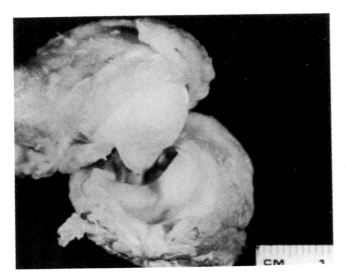

FIGURE 2–96. *Photograph of dissected dislocated right hip.*

Note the inverted limbus overlying the true acetabular fossa into which the elongated ligamentum teres passes. (From Milgram, J. W., and Tachdjian, M. O.: The pathologic anatomy of the limbus in untreated congenital dislocation of the hip. Clin. Orthop., *119*:107, 1976. Reprinted by permission.)

leads to formation of fibrous tissue, generated by the fibroblasts at the glenoid rim. The fibrocartilaginous acetabular rim is grossly and histologically distinct from the hyaline cartilage of the acetabulum. At their junction, these two distinct tissues merge imperceptibly without a tissue plane (Fig. 2–97).[637] The limbus forms as a result of gradual reactive ingrowth rather than abrupt mechanical inversion. Initially the limbus is biologically plastic and flattens out when the hip is reduced. In the older child, however, with up-and-down motion of the femoral head in walking, this fibrocartilaginous tissue hypertrophies and presents as a rigid semi-diaphragm interposed between the posterosuperior portion of the acetabulum and the femoral head. The cartilaginous rim of the acetabulum plays an important role in its growth and development; *it should not be excised.* The true limbus,

however, is hypertrophic fibrous tissue with overgrowth of cartilaginous elements from the labrum. Whenever the limbus prevents or hinders concentric reduction, it must be cautiously excised without disturbing growth zones of the acetabular rim.

Pelvifemoral Muscles. With progressive upward displacement of the femoral head, the fasciae and muscles about the hip joint become shortened and contracted, and their resistance makes it difficult to pull the head of the femur down to the level of the acetabulum. The contracted hip adductors also resist the abduction of the hip that is essential for reduction. With proximal displacement of the greater trochanter, the gluteus medius and minimus are shortened (Fig. 2–98). The piriformis muscle is contracted posteriorly. The iliopsoas muscle, prior to its insertion to the lesser trochanter, trav-

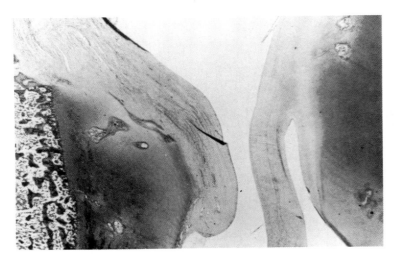

FIGURE 2–97. *Photomicrograph of a limbus.*

Note the fibrous structure covering the cartilaginous labrum and projecting toward the true joint cavity. Distinct tissue planes are lacking. Small blood vessels are present in the different layers of the limbus. (The femoral head and ligamentum teres are to the right of the illustration.) Hematoxylin and eosin, × 9. (Courtesy of the Armed Forces Institute of Pathology.)

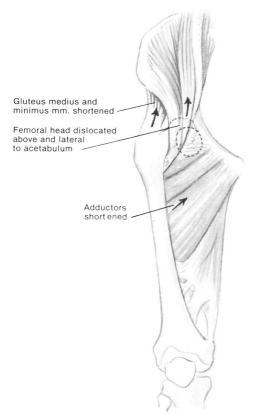

Gluteus medius and
minimus mm. shortened

Femoral head dislocated
above and lateral
to acetabulum

Adductors
shortened

*FIGURE 2–98. The pelvifemoral muscles become
shortened and contracted with progressive upward
displacement of the femoral head.*

erses the anteromedial surface of the hip joint, in close proximity to its capsule. As the femoral head is displaced laterally and superiorly from the acetabular socket, the lesser trochanter moves in the same direction and the contracted iliopsoas tendon is tightly stretched across the capsule, pressing it against the mouth of the acetabular cavity. With further superior migration of the femoral head, there is greater pressure and constriction of the capsule by the iliopsoas tendon. These barriers to reduction are extra-articular.

Vessels. The medial circumflex artery is displaced superiorly along with the iliopsoas tendon, passing in close proximity to the pubic ramus. The posteroinferior branch courses between the iliopsoas and the inferior aspect of the femoral neck, which makes it very susceptible to temporary occlusion.

Bony Changes

The Proximal Femur. Increased femoral anteversion is present to a varying degree in almost all cases of congenital dislocation of the hip and is a significant factor in instability of

reduction. It may increase up to 60 to 90 degrees. Often the contralateral normal hip will also have excessive femoral antetorsion. Excessive femoral antetorsion in itself does not prevent reduction, as all that is required is to rotate the hip medially sufficiently for the femoral head to be seated concentrically in the acetabulum. It causes instability, however, and leads to resubluxation or redislocation of the hip.

In an untreated dislocation the femoral head becomes flattened posteromedially and pear-shaped, making the hip joint incongruous. The incongruous joint is not adapted for perfect anatomic concentric reduction.

Acetabulum. Excessive acetabular antetorsion is common in congenital dislocation of the hip. In the last three months of gestation and at birth, the direction in which the entire acetabulum faces is more forward and more lateral than in adult life.[593, 766] With normal growth and development the position of the acetabulum changes as the hip changes from the intrauterine position of flexion and abduction to the erect position of extension and adduction. In congenital dislocation of the hip the corrective forces exerted by the proximal femur are not applied to the acetabulum; consequently, the acetabulum continues to face in a forward and lateral direction. This frontal inclination of the acetabulum was initially described by Langenskiöld and Laurent.[523]

When the entire acetabulum, instead of facing downward, is directed more anterolaterally than normal the femoral head is inadequately covered anteriorly when the hip is extended and laterally when the hip is adducted. This exaggerated acetabular antetorsion accounts for the stability of the reduced hip in flexion and abduction and explains why anterolateral resubluxation or redislocation occurs when the hip is adducted and extended in the position of weight-bearing.[805]

With the stimulation of growth lacking because of the absence of the concentric pressure of the femoral head, the acetabulum becomes progressively thick, shallow, and oblique. Its anterior wall and occasionally its posterior wall may become deficient. The appearance of antetorsion of the acetabulum may be exaggerated by the deficiency of its anterior wall and eversion and widening of its superolateral walls.

Dysplasia of the acetabulum results from hip dislocation with loss of the normal relationship between the head of the femur and the acetabulum. This has been experimentally shown by Smith, Ireton, and Coleman in dogs, and by Langenskiöld, Sarpio, and Michelsson in rabbits.[526, 872] Minimal in the newborn infant with typical dislocation of the hip, dysplasia of the acetabulum progressively increases with persistence of the luxation. Upon reduction and restoration of the femoral head's concentric pressure within the acetabulum, the acetabular roof ossifies and redevelops, especially within the first two years of life, when the dysplasia is reversible to a large extent.

Harris and associates studied 72 patients (85 hips) for development of the acetabulum in congenital dysplasia of the hip. The children were more than one year old on admission and over ten years of age at the time of assessment. These investigators found that if congruity is not obtained until after four years of age, the risk of producing a moderately or severely dysplastic acetabulum is more than doubled. If congruous reduction is obtained under four years of age, the acetabulum will grow and become normal in most patients by eight and in some by 11 years of age. If a patient is under four years of age, 95 per cent of the acetabuli will develop satisfactorily if three errors in management are avoided: namely, failure to obtain congruity, failure to maintain congruity, and ischemic necrosis secondary to manipulative reduction.[375, 377]

The chondro-osseous hip in the growing infant and child is a biologically dynamic structure and not a static unit. The time span of action of etiologic factors is the fourth dimension that should always be considered. Provision of a normal articular relationship between the femoral head and the acetabulum may reverse the deformations. The specific pathologic anatomy should be accurately defined prior to embarking on treatment.

TYPICAL PERINATAL CONGENITAL DISLOCATION OF THE HIP

Diagnosis

BIRTH TO TWO MONTHS OF AGE

Clinical Findings

In the *newborn* the diagnosis of congenital dislocation of the hip is made by clinical examination. Physical findings change with the age of the child. Dislocation of the hip in the newborn is determined by the Ortolani test, which was originally described by LeDamany in 1908.[540, 690, 691] It is a sign of *entry* of the femoral head from the dislocated position into the located position in the acetabulum, followed by exit of the femoral head out of the acetabulum into its dislocated position.

The infant is placed supine on a firm examination table or mattress. Examination of the child's hip on the mother's or nurse's lap is inadequate—avoid this pitfall! The Ortolani test must be performed with the baby relaxed; the muscles of a crying, struggling infant are taut. Resistance of the contracting muscles makes reduction difficult. Examine one hip at a time. With one hand stabilize the pelvis, and with the other hand bend the knee of the tested side acutely and flex the hip to 90 degrees (Fig. 2–99). The tips of the examiner's long and index fingers are placed over the greater trochanter on the lateral aspect of the upper thigh and the thumb across the knee. The thumb should *not* be placed over the lesser trochanter in the femoral triangle because pressure at this point is painful. There should be no digging in with fingertips. As the hip is *gently* abducted one can feel, and often hear, a *clunk* as the femoral head slides over the posterior rim of the acetabulum into the socket. The feeling is a more proprioceptive sensation. If a "clunk" is elicited it is recorded as a *"clunk of entry"*—it denotes a dislocated hip that can be reduced. Next, the hip is adducted and the femoral head displaced out of the acetabulum with a palpable "clunk"—this is recorded as a *"clunk of exit."*

Ortolani originally described a jerk or sudden movement when the femoral head snapped into the acetabulum when the flexed hip was abducted. He stated that the jerk of entry was not present in infants under three months of age. In the older infant in whom soft-tissue contracture provides resistance to reduction, the jerk of entry is a useful sign. In the newborn the posterolaterally displaced femoral head is easily located in the acetabulum, often without a jerk. To repeat, the feeling of reduction is a proprioceptive sensation felt by the examiner.

Another source of confusion about the Ortolani sign is the use of the term *click*; in the past it was often referred to as a hip "click." On examination of the infant's hips one may note a "click"—a short, dry, high-pitched sound or a dry crunching or crepitation. A *"click" is not a sign of congenital dislocation of the hip*; it is due to a vacuum phenomenon in the hip joint or ligamentous or myofascial "pops" and "snaps," e.g., the snapping of a taut iliotibial band or of the gluteal tendons over the greater trochanter. Sometimes a "click" comes from the knee because of a subluxating patella, ligamentous "popping," or a discoid lateral meniscus. The term *clunk* should be used (and not "click")

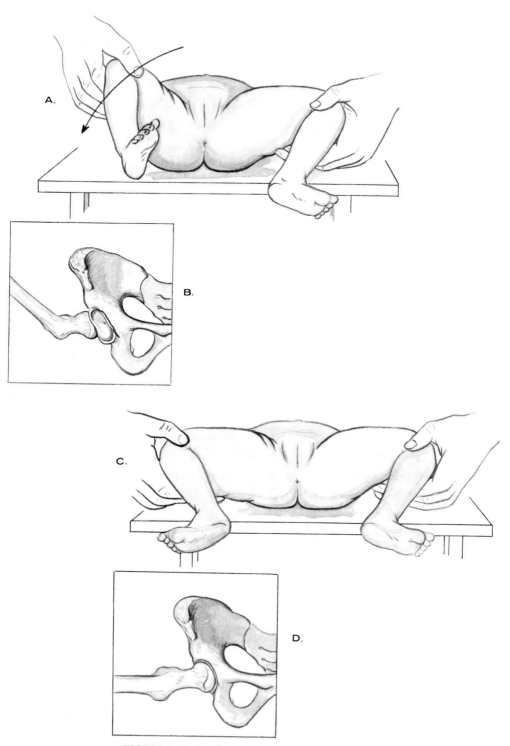

FIGURE 2–99. Ortolani test. See text for explanation.

to denote the deep feel and sound when the femoral head jumps into and out of the acetabulum.

The dislocated hip may be reduced on hyperflexion and redislocated on extension—a finding that emphasizes testing by Ortolani's and Barlow's methods in varying degrees of hip flexion. Extension posture increases instability of the hip, whereas hyperflexion enhances hip stability.[360]

Barlow's test is a maneuver to determine whether the hip is dislocatable—it is a *provocative test of dislocation* (Fig. 2–100).[33] Similar to Ortolani's test, the infant is placed supine on a firm mattress, and should be quiet and not crying. The examiner faces the infant. The examination is performed very gently. One hip is tested at a time. Both hips are flexed; the *untested hip* is in midabduction and 90 degrees of flexion, but the tested hip is in slight adduction and only 45 to 60 degrees of flexion because in less flexion and abduction the hip is in a more unstable position. This test is to demonstrate instability of the hip. With the tips of the long and index fingers over the greater trochanter on the lateral aspect of the upper thigh and the thumb over the medial aspect of the lower thigh (not in the lesser trochanter), the examiner attempts to displace the femoral head out of the acetabulum by gently pushing the upper femur posteriorly and laterally. In the dislocatable hip the femoral head can be felt to move completely out of the acetabulum with a clunk—the *"clunk of exit."* With release of thumb pressure and gentle abduction-flexion of the hip, the femoral head slips back into the acetabulum—the *"clunk of entry."*

In the *subluxatable hip* the femoral head is not completely displaced out of the acetabulum. In borderline cases it is best to position the tested hip in greater adduction and extension in a more unstable position and repeat Palmen's subluxation provocation test to ensure that the hip is not dislocatable.[705]

The *unstable hip* is characterized by a feeling of telescoping or sliding movement in the hip joint; the femoral head cannot, however, be pushed backward out of the acetabulum; there is no "clunk of exit." It is difficult to classify the anatomic state of the instability objectively. Experience is necessary. Overdiagnosis of hip instability may sometimes occur and is further complicated by the fact that in the newborn unstable hips become stabilized spontaneously (an observation made earlier by LeDamany in 1908 and later confirmed by Barlow in 1962).[33, 540] *Radiograms are normal in newborns with unstable hips.*

The future course of the unstable hip is dependent upon the degree of instability and upon environmental and genetic factors. An unstable hip may take one of the following courses if left untreated: it may become stable spontaneously by tautening of its capsule or ligaments and so become normal; it may proceed to subluxation; it may become dislocated; or it may persist into adolescence and adult life and manifest itself as hip dysplasia.

At birth it is impossible to predict which dislocations will resolve so that the hips become normal spontaneously, or to distinguish them from those that will not. It is best to regard all unstable hips as pathologic and treat them with the Pavlik harness. Failure to treat unstable hips with the Pavlik harness may lead to subluxation and luxation. Bjerkreim reports 2.1 per cent of unstable hips developed subluxation or dislocation due to failure of early treatment; other authors (von Klopfer, 1950; MacKenzie, 1972) have reported higher percentages.[57, 501, 578]

Normally a newborn baby has a 15- to 20-degree flexion contracture of the hips and knees; this neonatal flexion deformity gradually disappears by two to three months of age. In congenital dislocation of the hip, the Thomas test shows loss of the normal flexion contracture of the hip, while the knee extends fully or hyperextends (Fig. 2–101). This extension "looseness" of the hip and knee is easy to elicit (special experience is not necessary) and is a quite reliable suggestive sign for dislocation of the hip in the newborn. The diagnostic significance of full extension in the dislocated hip in the neonate cannot be overemphasized.

The classic signs of congenital dislocation of the hip seen in the older infant—asymmetrical thigh folds, limitation of hip abduction, and relative shortening of the femur (positive Galleazzi sign)—are not usually seen in the newborn unless the dislocation is antenatal, in which case the femoral head migrates out of the acetabulum in utero.

Pelvic obliquity and asymmetry of thigh folds can occur in the newborn; often, however, it is caused by abduction contracture of the contralateral hip and not by adduction contracture of the "dislocated" hip. Congenital pelvic obliquity due to abduction contracture of the hip may lead to overdiagnosis of congenital dislocation of the hip and overtreatment.

Green and Griffin studied 18 children with unilateral dysplasia of the hip and found them to have asymmetrical gluteal folds and an apparent lower limb length discrepancy secondary to pelvic obliquity caused by abduction contracture of the contralateral hip. The femoral head

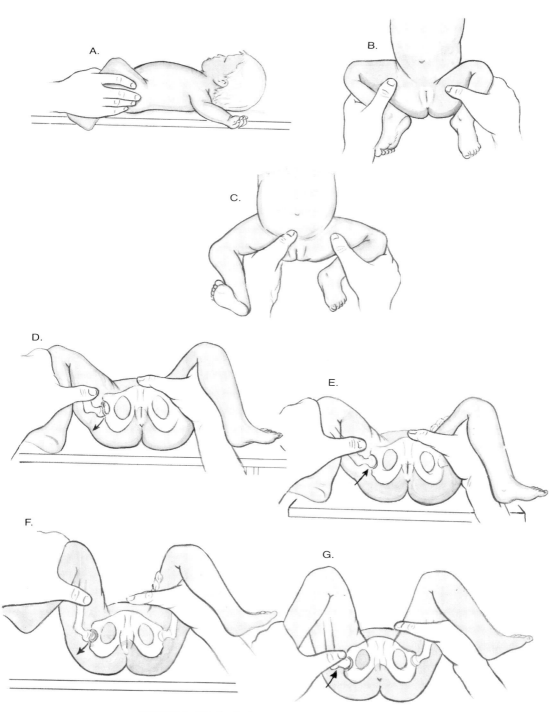

FIGURE 2–100. Barlow's test. See text for explanation.

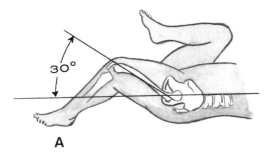

A

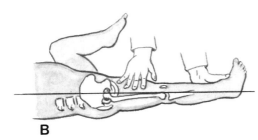

B

FIGURE 2–101. *Loss of normal knee flexion contracture in congenital dislocation of the hip.*

on the high side of the pelvis was directed superolaterally and not concentrically reduced. The acetabular dysplasia was on the left side in all but one patient. This can be explained by the position of the fetus in utero with its back toward the mother's left side. Such intrauterine posture places the fetus's left hip against the mother's rigid lumbosacral spine and the right hip against the more mobile anterior wall of the uterus; therefore, the right lower limb is more likely to be in abduction and the left lower limb in adduction.[357]

Associated Congenital Deformities

Bjerkreim and Van Der Hagen found concomitant anomalies in 9 per cent of patients with neonatal and 14 per cent of those with late-diagnosis congenital dislocation of the hip. Of the concomitant deformities, 7.7 per cent involved the musculoskeletal system in the neonatal group, as did 10.4 per cent in the late-diagnosis group.[61]

Intrauterine malposition will cause other deformities that are very easy to detect. Simple inspection should alert the examiner to the possible presence of congenital dislocation of the hip.

Torticollis. The possible relationship between congenital muscular torticollis and congenital hip dysplasia was first pointed out by Joachimsthal in 1908.[470] The incidence of congenital muscular torticollis in the newborn population is 4 per thousand and that of congenital

dislocation of the hip 1.5 per thousand; the probable incidence of coexistence of the two conditions is 0.06 per thousand. Iwahara and Ikeda, in 1962, reported that 14.8 per cent of their children with congenital muscular torticollis had dysplasia of the hip.[455] Hummer and MacEwen reported 20 per cent of children with torticollis had congenital hip dysplasia (5 per cent dislocation and 15 per cent subluxation).[441] This relationship between torticollis and congenital dislocation of the hip is significant; the presence of torticollis should serve as a warning to look for congenital dislocation of the hip. A careful clinical, ultrasonographic, and radiographic examination of both hip joints is in order.

Plagiocephaly. This condition was noted in 32 per cent of the patients with congenital dislocation of the hip by Wynne-Davies.[1037] The left and right sides were equally involved, and there was no correlation with the side of the dislocated hip.

Metatarsus Varus. Jacobs reported a much higher incidence of congenital hip dysplasia in infants with metatarsus varus than in the general population.[458]

Pes Calcaneovalgus. This deformity of the feet was found to be associated with congenital dislocation of the hip in 25 per cent of the cases by Paterson.[716, 717]

Generalized Laxity of Joints. Commonly found in patients with congenital dislocation of the hip, the lax ligaments as a rule tauten with skeletal growth; flexible pes planovalgus, however, is an almost universal problem in children with congenital dislocation of the hip.

Other Rare Musculoskeletal Deformities. Coexisting with congenital dislocation of the hip may be talipes equinovarus, congenital convex pes valgus (vertical talus), congenital defects (e.g., longitudinal deficiency) of upper and lower limbs, infantile scoliosis, congenital dislocation of the knee and shoulder, and radioulnar synostosis. *Some visceral anomalies* found concomitant with congenital dislocation of the hip include pyloric stenosis, patent ductus arteriosus, malformation of the urinary and gastrointestinal tracts, and undescended testicles.

It behooves the orthopedic surgeon and pediatrician to examine not just the hip but the entire infant. Conversely an infant that has a deformity or malformation of the musculoskeletal or visceral system should have a thorough examination of the hips to rule out congenital dislocation.

Newborn Infants at High Risk

A newborn infant subject to the following environmental factors, genetic composition, and clinical findings is more susceptible to congenital dislocation of the hip than the average infant: (1) positive family history; (2) female, firstborn, of breech presentation; (3) caesarean section because of breech presentation; (4) oligohydramnios—due often to renal malformations of the fetus or to premature rupture of the membranes; (5) intrauterine crowding due to twin or multiple pregnancy; (6) torticollis; (7) plagiocephaly; (8) infantile scoliosis; (9) absence of the normal flexion contracture with hyperextension of the hip and knee; (10) pelvic obliquity with abduction contracture of one hip and/or adduction contracture of the contralateral hip; (11) extension contracture of the knee; (12) metatarsus varus; or (13) calcaneovalgus deformity of the feet.

These infants should have very thorough sequential examinations of their hips at birth, at six weeks, at three months, and at six months. Routine radiograms are not recommended for all newborns at high risk because they give a false sense of security. The radiograms may be normal, but the hips dislocated. This author recommends ultrasonography of the hips after examination by a competent orthopedic surgeon.

Postnatal Dislocation of the Hip

Infants may have "normal" hips when examined at birth, but later present with dislocation. Seven such children were reported by Walker in 1971.[984] In 1984, Davies and Walker reported ten children who had clinically stable hips at birth; at one month of age their hips were radiographed because they had factors predisposing them to hip dislocation. In all ten of these cases one or both hips showed radiographic changes suggestive of hip dysplasia; four of these hips subsequently were dislocated.[203] Tredwell and Bell reported five hips that had been clinically normal at birth and presented later with acetabular dysplasia and adduction contracture; none of these five hips were dislocated, however.[95]

In neonatal screening programs late-diagnosed cases are referred to as "missed dislocations." These late-presented cases of congenital dislocation of the hip comprise a mixed group—true congenital dislocations of the hip associated with ligamentous laxity, and late dislocations secondary to hip dysplasia and marked instability of the hip due to excessive femoral and acetabular antetorsion. Hips that are stable at birth will *not* necessarily develop normally. Repeated examination of the hips is essential. Infants at high risk should routinely have ultrasonograms and radiograms of the hips at three months of age. The importance of sequential hip examinations at birth, at three weeks, at six weeks, at three months, and at six months cannot be overemphasized.

Radiographic Findings

Radiographic assessment of the newborn hip *if normal* may be misleading and deceptive (Fig. 2–102). A negative radiogram does not rule out the presence of dislocation. Much of the newborn pelvis is cartilaginous and therefore not visible on the routine radiogram; the

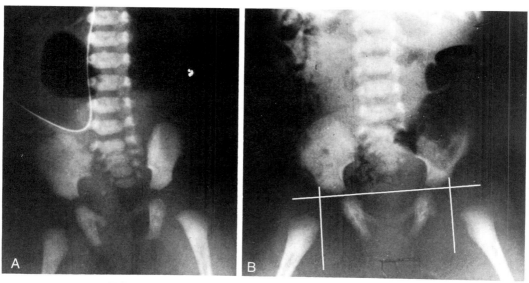

FIGURE 2–102. Congenital dysplasia of the left hip in a newborn.

A. An anteroposterior radiogram of both hips appears normal, giving a false sense of security. **B.** A radiogram of both hips made ten minutes later shows the left hip is dislocated. The medial metaphysis of the femoral neck is lateral to Perkins's line.

femoral head is not ossified at birth, and its exact relationship to the acetabulum is hard to determine. Because the usual bony landmarks are not seen distinctly, the acetabular index, Hilgenreiner's line, and Perkins's line are difficult to delineate accurately. Shenton's line may not be broken. Because dislocation of the hip is recent, the characteristic secondary radiographic changes have not had sufficient time to develop. There is no false acetabulum. Radiograms should not be relied upon to make the diagnosis of congenital dislocation of the hip.

In the newborn the femoral head will easily move into and out of the acetabulum. The dislocated hip may be reduced at the time the radiogram is made. Positioning for the Von Rosen view—which is made with the hips in abduction and medial rotation—may itself re-

duce the dislocation and make the radiographic study of no value. Another pitfall is to make radiograms in the frog-leg lateral position, a position of flexion-abduction that also reduces the dislocation. The radiograms show the hip reduced, but in neutral position it will be dislocated.

Improper positioning of the infant's hips may cause problems. A common mistake is to make the radiograms with the hips rotated laterally; this disrupts the radiographic landmarks.

Side-to-side tilting of the pelvis will give an abnormal acetabular index and cause the femoral head to appear uncovered. Posterior pelvic rotation decreases the acetabular index, whereas forward tilting of the pelvis may increase it. (The flexion contracture of the hips caused by pressing the thighs against the x-ray

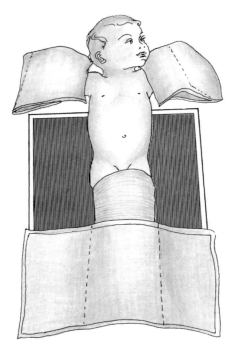

FIGURE 2–103. Coleman's technique for taking a true anteroposterior radiogram of the hips in the newborn.

A and **B.** The hips are stabilized in neutral rotation and abduction-adduction by holding or loosely binding the thighs together parallel with the hips in about 25 to 30 degrees of flexion. This flexion posture neutralizes the normal flexion contracture of the hips and prevents anterior tilting of the pelvis.

A.

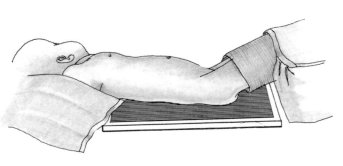

B.

plate causes the pelvis to tilt forward.) Contractures of the newborn hip must be taken into account when the infant is positioned for hip radiography. The hips are flexed 30 degrees so that the pelvis is positioned flat on the x-ray cassette (Fig. 2–103). A restrained, crying, feisty baby will automatically contract the hip abductor-flexor muscles and spontaneously reduce the dislocation.

In the newborn, radiograms of the hip are made if abnormal physical findings are present to suggest a pathologic condition of the hip. The technique of radiography is critical. A single true anteroposterior view of the pelvis made with the hips in 20 to 30 degrees of flexion will serve as a baseline examination and rule out other congenital deformities that may simulate congenital dislocation of the hip, such as developmental coxa vara, congenital short femur, or proximal femoral focal deficiency. A positive radiographic study is helpful, but a normal radiogram in the presence of a positive Ortolani or Barlow test is of no significance. Diagnosis of congenital dislocation of the hip in the newborn is made by clinical examination. Dynamic stress ultrasonography will confirm the diagnosis.

If the hip is dislocated at the time the radiogram is made in unilateral and even in bilateral cases, the radiographic signs will essentially be diagnostic; lateral and superior displacement of the upper femoral metaphysis can be visualized.

In the properly made anteroposterior radiogram of the hip one assesses the lateral and upward displacement of the head of the femur and the development of the acetabulum. Since ossification centers are not present, the following lines and determinations are made: *Hilgen-*

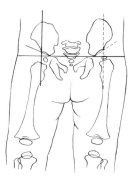

FIGURE 2–104. *Hilgenreiner's and Perkins's lines.*

Hilgenreiner's, or Y, line is a horizontal line drawn through the top of the triradiate cartilage. Perkins's, or Ombrédanne's, vertical line is drawn from the most lateral ossified margin of the roof of the acetabulum perpendicular and distal to the Y line to form quadrants. In the normal hip, the medial margin of the ossified proximal metaphysis of the femur is medial to Perkins's line.

reiner's line, or the Y line, is a horizontal line drawn through the top of the clear areas in the depth of the acetabula, which represents the triradiate or Y cartilage (Fig. 2–104).[409] *Ombrédanne's vertical line, or Perkins's line*, is drawn downward from the most lateral ossified margin of the roof of the acetabulum perpendicular to and through the Y line to form quadrants.[688, 724]

The medial margin of the ossified proximal metaphysis of the femur lies medial to Perkins's line; if it lies lateral to Perkins's line, the femoral head is laterally displaced and the hip is considered to be subluxated or dislocated (Fig. 2–105). In the newborn this is a very reliable diagnostic determinant in the radiographic assessment of the hip. According to Coleman, when this radiographic sign is present, a dislo-

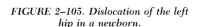

FIGURE 2–105. *Dislocation of the left hip in a newborn.*

Note the medial margin of the ossified metaphysis of the femoral neck lies lateral to Perkins's line.

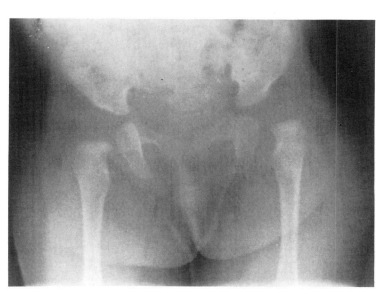

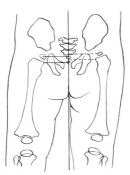

FIGURE 2–106. *Method of measuring lateral displacement of femoral head by the Y coordinate (Ponseti).*

The lateral displacement is the distance from the midsacrum to the ossified medial protruding tip of the metaphysis of the femoral neck, or the center of the ossific nucleus of the femoral head may be used as a lateral point of reference.

catable hip is found by careful physical examination in 50 per cent of the cases.[157]

Lateral displacement may be measured by the Y coordinate (Ponseti), which is the distance from the midsacrum to the center of the ossified nucleus of the femoral head; or the medial protruding tip of the ossified femoral neck may be used as a lateral point of reference (Fig. 2–106).[739] The inner border of the "teardrop" shadow (shown in Figure 2–107), the floor of the acetabular socket, or the lateral wall of the ischium may be used as the medial point of reference (Fig. 2–108). These reference points are altered by changes in position of the pelvis, and care should be taken to focus the x-ray tube directly over the middle of and a little above the symphysis pubis to ensure symmetry of both halves of the pelvis.

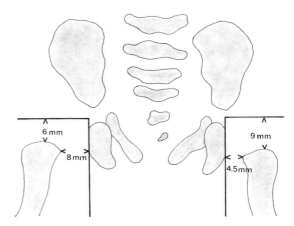

FIGURE 2–108. *Measurement of lateral displacement of the femoral head.*

A line drawn perpendicular to the lateral edge of the ischium is used as the medial point of reference.

Bertol and associates studied the radiographic features of 271 cases of clinically diagnosed congenital dislocation of the hip. They found the medial gap, a measure of the separation between the proximal femur and a line drawn perpendicular to the lateral margin of the ischium, to be significantly greater than normal in patients with unilateral or bilateral dislocations. A medial gap of over 5 mm. should be considered suspicious, and one of over 6 mm. is indicative of dislocation. A difference from the normal value of approximately 4 mm. was found to be highly significant when analyzed retrospectively.[51]

Superior displacement of the proximal femur is measured by *Shenton's* or *Menard's line*, which is drawn between the medial border of

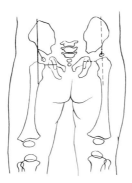

FIGURE 2–107. *Measurement of lateral displacement of the femoral head.*

The inner border of the tear-drop shadow is used as the middle point of reference. In this illustration the method of measuring the CE angle of Wiberg is shown.

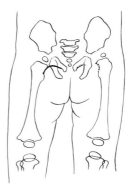

FIGURE 2–109. *Shenton's, or Menard's, line.*

A line is drawn between the medial border of the femoral neck and the superior border of the obturator foramen. In the normal hip this line is a continuous arc, whereas in the dislocated hip it is broken and interrupted.

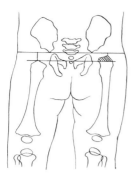

FIGURE 2–110. *Diagram illustrating a method of measuring superior displacement by the H distance.*

This is the distance between the proximal end of the ossified shaft and the Y line.

the neck of the femur and the superior border of the obturator foramen. In a normal hip, this line is an even arc of continuous contour; in the dislocated hip with proximal displacement of the femoral head, it is broken and interrupted (Fig. 2–109). Shenton's line may, however, be slightly interrupted if the x-ray films are taken with the hip in lateral rotation and adduction.

Superior displacement (H distance) may also be determined by measuring the distance between the proximal end of the ossified shaft (diaphyseal tip) of the femoral neck and the Y line of both hips (Fig. 2–110). This sign is helpful in unilateral dislocation; the H distance (the distance between the upper end of the femur and the Y line) is reduced in the dislocated hip as compared with the contralateral normal hip.

The position of the unossified femoral head

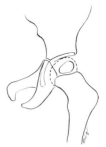

FIGURE 2–112. *Teardrop shadow of Koehler.*

is suggested by the location and direction of the proximal femur in relation to the acetabulum. Both hips are fully extended, abducted 45 to 50 degrees, and laterally rotated fully. The radiogram includes the femoral shafts. In the normal hip, a longitudinal line drawn through the center of the femoral shaft bisects the outer corner of the acetabulum, whereas in a dislocated hip, it points above the lateral edge of the acetabulum, bisecting the anterior superior iliac spine (Fig. 2–111).

In the Von Rosen view both hips are extended, abducted 45 to 50 degrees, and *medially rotated.*[787] As stated previously, medial rotation may reduce the dislocation; the Von Rosen view is therefore not recommended in the neonate or early infancy. Diagnostically it is much more helpful to rotate the hips laterally.[360]

The *U figure, or "teardrop" shadow of Koehler*, a normal radiographic appearance, becomes visible when the infant is a few months old (Fig. 2–112). It consists of three lines: an external semicircular line that corresponds to the wall of the acetabulum; a long, almost straight, medial line that corresponds to the wall of the lesser pelvis; and a short, connecting, curved line that corresponds to the semicylindrical cortex of the acetabular notch. It is interrupted in the middle by the Y line (acetabular synchondrosis). The teardrop shadow is an important landmark for measurements, provided the x-ray tube is focused exactly over the midline, the pelvis is not rotated, and the two halves of the pelvis are symmetrical. Delay in ossification of the teardrop will suggest lack of stimulus from a concentrically located femoral head in the acetabulum. In subluxation of one hip the width of the teardrop shadow is greater on that side than on the normal side. Upon concentric reduction and maintenance of reduction there will be progresive decrease in the width of the teardrop.

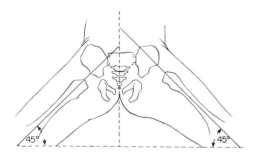

FIGURE 2–111. *Diagram of an anteroposterior radiogram showing both hips in extension, 45 degrees of abduction, and lateral rotation.*

A long line drawn through the center of the femoral shaft bisects the outer corner of the acetabulum in the normal hip, whereas in the dislocated left hip it points above the lateral edge of the acetabulum and bisects the anterior superior iliac spine.

Acetabular Index. The acetabular index is measured by the angle formed between the Y line and a line passing through the depth of the acetabular socket at the Y line to the most lateral ossified margin of the roof of the acetabulum (see Fig. 2–104). According to Kleinberg and Lieberman, the acetabular angle is a helpful index in measuring the development of the osseous roof of the acetabulum.[495] In normal newborns the acetabular index averages 27.5 degrees (30 degrees being the upper limit of normal) and decreases to 20 degrees by about two years of age. A dislocated hip will have an acetabular index of more than 30 degrees.

Caffey and colleagues, in a well-controlled radiographic study of 627 normal infants at birth, then at six months and at one year, found the mean acetabular index to vary between 25 and 29 degrees. The mean value for female infants was 30 degrees. They concluded that a diagnosis of hip dysplasia cannot be made solely by a high acetabular index.[98]

Coleman reported considerable variation in the range of acetabular indices. In a combined clinical and radiographic study of 150 newborn infants the mean acetabular index was found to be 30.86 degrees, with a range from 20 to 42 degrees. This was contradicted by the later report of Laurenson, in 1959, that the upper limit of normal is 30 degrees.[152, 530] Therefore, in 1968 Coleman reported a second study in 1155 Navajo neonates who were examined both clinically and radiographically: 77 of them had abnormal hips clinically and 1078 had clinically normal hips. During the first three months of life the acetabular index averaged 28.6 degrees in normal infants and 34.8 degrees in infants with abnormal physical findings. Coleman concluded that a single determination is of little value unless the acetabular index exceeds 40 degrees, and even then, in the absence of abnormal physical findings, the index, if solely abnormal, has little diagnostic value for hip dysplasia.[154]

The positioning of the patient significantly changes the acetabular index; rotation of a pelvis in both the axial and sagittal planes will convert a dysplastic appearance to a normal one, and rotation of a normal hip to the opposite direction may produce a dysplastic appearance.

Ultrasonographic Findings*

In infants and young children cartilaginous tissue cannot be visualized by plain radiogra-

phy. In the hip joint the cartilaginous parts of the acetabulum and femoral head-neck can be imaged indirectly by arthrography and poorly by computerized axial tomography (CT); these modalities of imaging will be discussed later. Magnetic resonance imaging (MRI) depicts the cartilaginous parts of the hip joint in great detail—but its routine clinical use is not practical and its cost is prohibitive. Ultrasound has recently become the primary imaging tool to assess the hip of the neonate and infant, gradually replacing plain radiography.

In 1981, Graf was first to report the use of ultrasound to study the hip in the neonate and infant.[354a] Since then numerous studies have been published on the utilization of ultrasound in the evaluation of the hip with congenital dysplasia. At present, two methods of assessing the dysplastic hip with ultrasound are available: (1) static nonstress technique (proposed by Graf), and (2) dynamic stress method (used by Novick, Keller, Harcke, Boal, and Clarke).[67a, 148a, 148b, 673a, 492, 492a–c]

The Static (Non-Stress) Technique of Graf.

The Graf evaluation of the hip is based on a direct single coronal image of each hip obtained with a linear array transducer. The infant is placed in lateral decubitus position with the hips flexed 30 to 45 degrees and medially rotated 10 to 15 degrees. The transducer is placed in the coronal plane (Fig. 2–113 A). It is vital to obtain reproducible images; pay careful attention to the following two anatomic landmarks: first, the configuration of the ossified ilium; it should be a straight linear white shadow extending superiorly from the hip joint. When the transducer is not in the proper plane the iliac line will flare laterally or medially. Second, the most distal point of the ilium is the roof of the acetabulum. In the image it appears very bright; interposition of fibrofatty tissue or ligamentum teres may obscure this point; one may have to slide the transducer anteriorly or posteriorly for proper identification of the center of the acetabulum. The following structures are identified (Fig. 2–113 B and C):

1. Iliac bone.
2. The most distal point of the ilium in the roof of the acetabulum.
3. Ossified medial wall of the acetabulum.
4. The inferior end of the iliac bone at the triradiate cartilage.
5. Triradiate cartilage.
6. Ossified ischium.
7. The cartilaginous femoral head.
8. Ossific nucleus of the femoral head.
9. Cartilaginous roof of the acetabulum.
10. Labrum.

---

*Written with Dr. James S. Donaldson, Assistant Professor of Radiology, Northwestern University Medical School and Attending Radiologist, Children's Memorial Hospital, Chicago, Illinois.

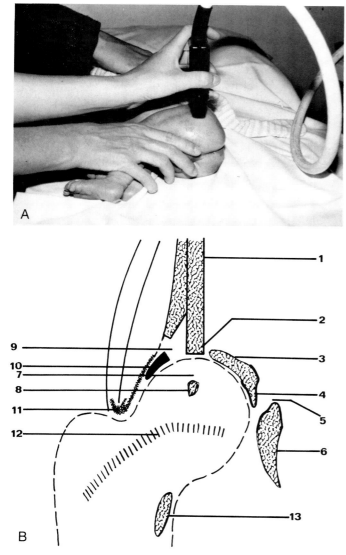

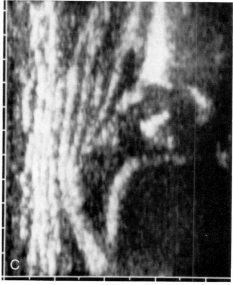

FIGURE 2–113. *Ultrasonography of the hip in congenital hip dislocation.*

A. Lateral decubitus position of the infant for ultrasonographic examination of the hip.

B. Diagram of structures identified during static non-stress ultrasonography of the hip: (1) Iliac bone. (2) The most distal point of the ilium in the roof of the acetabulum. (3) Ossified medial wall of the acetabulum. (4) The inferior end of the iliac bone at the triradiate cartilage. (5) Triradiate cartilage. (6) Ossified ischium. (7) The cartilaginous femoral head. (8) Ossific nucleus of the femoral head. (9) Cartilaginous roof of the acetabulum. (10) Labrum. (11) Intertrochanteric fossa. (12) Cartilaginous growth plate of the femoral head. (13) Ossified metaphysis of the femoral neck.

C. Ultrasonogram showing structures.

11. Intertrochanteric fossa.

12. Cartilaginous growth plate of the femoral head.

13. Ossified metaphysis of the femoral neck.

A visual impression is made of the position of the femoral head in the acetabulum. Three lines are drawn on the image (Fig. 2–114). First, a vertical line (base line) is drawn parallel to the ossified lateral wall of the ilium. Second, the cartilaginous roof line is drawn from the lateral bony edge of the acetabulum through the labrum, and third, a bony roof line from the inferior bony edge of the acetabulum at the roof of the triradiate cartilage to the most distal point of the ilium in the center of the hip joint. The *alpha angle* is the angle formed by lines one and three. According to Graf, 60 de-

grees is the upper limit of normal, but according to Exner, it should be 55 degrees.[267a, 354a] The smaller the angle, the greater the dysplasia of the hip. The *beta angle* is the angle formed by lines 1 and 2. An angle greater than 77 degrees indicates eversion of the labrum and subluxation of the hip.

Irreproducibility has been an objection to the Graf method. Whereas Graf claims reproducibility of one to two degrees when measuring the various angles, in our experience there is a variation of five degrees. When an inadequate image is obtained, the hip appears more dysplastic than it is in actuality. It is impossible to make a normal hip appear dysplastic. Therefore, the errors may occur as false positives but not false negatives. These authors do not adhere

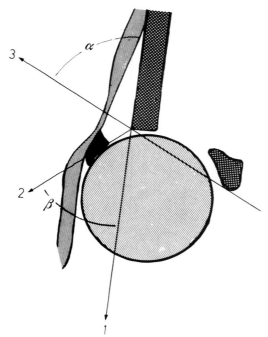

FIGURE 2–114. A diagram illustrating visual impression of the position of the femoral head in the acetabulum.

1. Base line parallel to the ilium. 2. Cartilage roof line from the bony edge of the acetabulum through the labrum. 3. Bony roof line from the bony edge of the acetabulum to the lowest point of the ilium in the center of the joint. α angle—between lines 1 and 3 (the smaller the angle, the more dysplasia present). β Angle—between 1 and 2 (eversion of the labrum and subluxation of the hip indicated by an angle > 77 degrees).

exclusively to the strict measurement criteria but also use a subjective visual impression.

The Graf method is rather easy to learn initially since the coronal anatomy is easy to recognize. Complicated cases, however, can cause trouble even for experienced examiners. The examination is a learned skill requiring practice and patience to master. Consistency is crucial.

The Dynamic Stress Method. The dynamic stress examination of the hip involves imaging in both axial and coronal planes and during part of the study, stressing the hip carefully. The femoral head is observed in real time for any abnormal motion within the acetabulum— whether it can be subluxated or dislocated.

The study is performed with the child supine instead of in a decubitus position. The first image obtained is a transverse view with the hip extended (Fig. 2–115). The position of the femoral head with respect to the ischium and pubic bones is determined. The hip is then flexed 90 degrees, maintaining the ultrasono-

graphic transducer in a transverse plane (with respect to the pelvis). The thigh is then gently "pistoned" by placing posterior stress on the knee. Any amount of motion is noted and can be measured. Keller noted that up to 6 mm. of motion on the left and 4 mm. of motion on the right is normal in the first few days of life, with no difference between males and females. This laxity is normal and diminishes after a few days.[492c] If a hip is subluxatable or dislocatable, it is noted and an attempt at reduction is made. A coronal image is then obtained and the position of the femoral head within the acetabulum is determined.

Anatomic landmarks in transverse neutral and transverse flexion views are at first confusing. The stress part of the examination requires care and expertise. With practice, however, the amount of gentle stress required to dislocate a dislocatable hip and the ability to reduce a dislocated hip can be readily learned.

Classification. Graf has classified the following hip types according to the ultrasonographic findings: Type I—normal hip (Fig. 2–116 A and B). The alpha angle is less than 60 degrees. The hip joint is stable when stressed by dynamic examination. Graf believes that such hips do not require follow-up. This author recommends sequential hip examination, particularly when the hips are at high risk. Type II—concentric

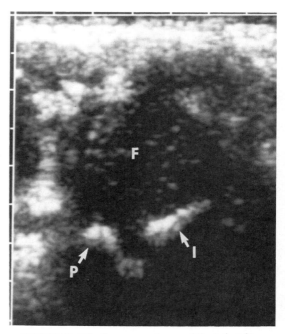

FIGURE 2–115. Transverse image of the infant hip.

The femoral head (F) is centered between the public bone and the ischium.

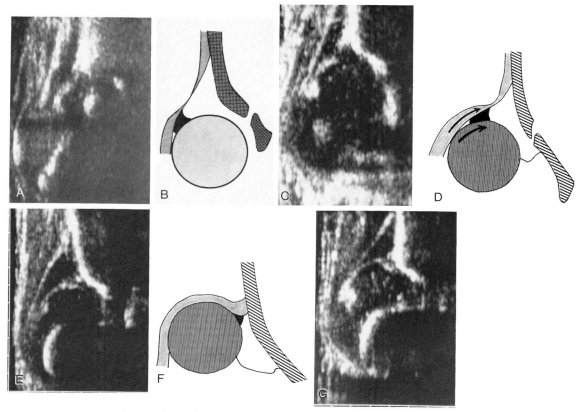

FIGURE 2–116. Four Graf hip types—diagram and corresponding images.

A. Type I—sharp angular acetabular rim and deep acetabular cup (see Fig. 2–113B for diagram). **B** and **C.** Type II, rounding of acetabular rim, thick cartilaginous roof, shallower acetabular cup. **D** and **E.** Type III—concentric position, labrum everted, shallow acetabulum. **F** and **G.** Type IV—high dislocation, labrum interposed between femoral head and acetabulum. Arrows mark position of labrum.

position. The beta angle is less than 77 degrees. Type IIa—skeletally immature with delayed ossification of the acetabulum (mild dysplasia). When the child is less than three months of age, the alpha angle is 50 to 60 degrees. Graf recommends that these hips be followed until they are Type I. Type IIb—have delayed ossification with an alpha angle greater than 50 to 60 degrees. These are encountered in children over three months of age. According to Graf, these hips required treatment by Pavlik harness (Fig. 2–116 B and C). Type IIc—the femoral head is contained concentrically in the acetabulum, which is very deficient with an alpha angle of 43 to 49 degrees. According to Graf, these hips require treatment by Pavlik harness. Type IId—these hips are subluxated with an alpha angle of 43 to 49 degrees and with the labrum everted and with a beta angle of greater than 77 degrees. According to Graf, these hips require definite treatment. Type III—low dislocation with a deficient acetabular bony roof with an alpha angle of greater than 43 degrees and an everted labrum (Fig. 2–116 D and E).

Type IV—high dislocation with an almost flat bony acetabulum and the alpha angle cannot be measured. The labrum is interposed between the head and the ilium. These hips often require open reduction (Fig. 2–116 F and G).

Screening. In some areas of Europe, ultrasound screening is performed on every newborn and some reported series suggest that this is valuable. Mass screening, however, has resulted in high false positive and high treatment rates.[915a, 1045] The amount of manpower, equipment, and monies required to screen all newborns is prohibitive.

Donaldson et al. screened 1772 consecutive newborns at high risk for congenital dislocation of the hip (family history, breech presentation, postural orthopedic abnormalities, and oligohydramnios) and identified 97 high-risk newborns. Ultrasonography was performed on 67 of these, and four girls with congenital dislocation of the hip were found. Three of these four girls had normal (two patients) or overlooked abnormal (one patient) physical examinations by their pediatricians at birth. This screening identified three clinically silent dysplasias that were originally missed.[990] Clarke also reported finding five clinically silent dysplasias out of eight total high-risk newborns with congenital dislocation of the hip.[148a] Although these series are small, they demonstrate the value of screening high-risk infants.

It is vital that the hips at risk be examined clinically by a competent orthopedic surgeon prior to ultrasonography being performed. The pediatrician should not be lulled into a false sense of security by a so-called normal ultrasound examination, particularly when the imaging is not properly performed and is inadequate.

Follow-up Examinations. By carefully obtaining a reproducible coronal image, dysplastic hips or physiologically immature hips can be followed for progressive development of the acetabulum. Graf angles can be measured, documenting improvement in the acetabulum while confirming concentric reduction of the hip. At our institution most children in a Pavlik harness remain so until the alpha angle meets Type I (normal) criteria.

Harness and Spica Cast Evaluation. When a child is initially placed in an abduction splint the reduced position of the hip should be verified. This can be done by examining transversely from a posterior approach.[360a] The position of the femoral head with respect to the position of the acetabulum is determined. A U

configuration is made up of the femoral metaphysis and the ischium when the femoral head is reduced. This view is simple to obtain and is very reliable in confirming satisfactory hip position.

Children immobilized in hip spica casts are evaluated by ultrasonography during cast changes. Verification of the position of the femoral head in the acetabulum is difficult when the child is in a hip spica cast.

An anterior approach can be used to obtain an axial image similar to a CT section. This requires a large perineal opening and may allow too much motion within the cast. Alternatively, a window can be cut in the side of the cast and replaced after scanning is complete. This risks allowing a reduced hip to dislocate, since the opening cut into the cast is exactly where the support is needed. Computed tomography with low mA is our preferred method of verifying the hip position in a spica cast. Sedation is not necessary, and CT is more reliable and much simpler than struggling with ultrasound through small openings in the cast.

BETWEEN THREE AND TWELVE MONTHS OF AGE

Clinical Findings

With lateral and upward displacement of the femoral head, suggestive physical findings develop: (1) The skin folds of the thigh and of the gluteal and popliteal creases will become asym-

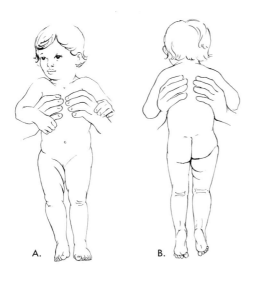
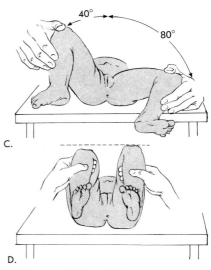

FIGURE 2–117. *Physical findings in congenital dislocation of the right hip.*

A and **B.** Asymmetry of the thigh folds and of the popliteal and gluteal creases with apparent shortening of the extremity on the right. **C.** Limited abduction of the right hip. **D.** Galeazzi's sign—apparent shortening of the femur as shown by the difference of the knee levels with the hips and knees flexed at right angles and the child lying on a firm table.

metrical, with apparent shortening of the dislocated lower limb, and a deep and more cephalad inguinal crease will appear on the affected side (Fig. 2–117 A and B). (2) Passive abduction of the affected hip will be limited in the 90-degree flexed position (Fig. 2–117 C). (3) There will be apparent shortening of the femur as shown by the difference in the knee levels with the knees flexed at right angles as the infant lies on a firm, flat examining table (Galleazzi sign) (Fig. 2–117 D). (4) The posture of the dislocated lower limb usually is 15 to 25 degrees of lateral rotation. The greater trochanter is prominent and the buttocks are flattened. (5) The abnormal laxity of the hip is manifested by excessive mobility of the femoral head during passive manipulation. There will be a piston mobility, or the telescoping sign, when the thigh is pushed in piston fashion with the adducted hip alternately in flexion and extension. To elicit this sign the examiner grasps the distal thigh and the knee with one hand, places the index finger of the other hand over the greater trochanter, and splays the thumb and other fingers over the ilium (Fig. 2–118). (6) The femoral head is absent from its normal site anteriorly in the groin beneath the femoral artery at about the middle of Poupart's ligament (Fig. 2–119). (7) When dislocation is complete, the tip of the greater trochanter lies proximal to Nélaton's line, which is a line drawn between the anterior superior iliac spine and the ischial tuberosity (Fig. 2–120).

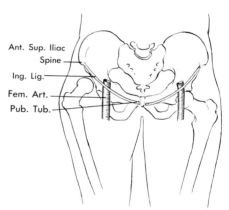

FIGURE 2–119. Absence of femoral head.

Absence of the femoral head from its normal site anteriorly in the groin beneath the femoral artery at about the middle of Poupart's ligament.

Radiographic Findings

In the growing child the degree of an abnormality of the hip as seen in the radiogram changes rapidly. Normally, the femoral head ossifies between four and six months of age. In the dislocated hip its ossification is delayed. It migrates upward and laterally, and it is usually easily detectable (Fig. 2–121). The acetabular index becomes progressively shallower, and the acetabular roof becomes bilabiated (furrowed). The structures producing the teardrop shadow are delayed in ossification, and often there is delay in maturation of the ischiopubic synchondrosis.

AFTER WALKING AGE

Clinical Findings

Despite the great emphasis that has been placed on the value of early diagnosis, the

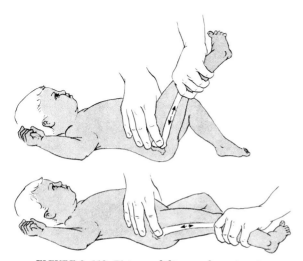

FIGURE 2–118. Piston mobility or telescoping sign.

There is abnormal mobility or a feeling of telescoping when the extremity is pushed in piston fashion with the adducted hip in alternate flexion and extension.

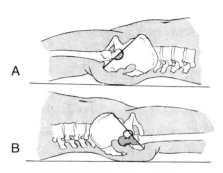

FIGURE 2–120. Nélaton's line.

In complete dislocation the tip of the greater trochanter lies proximal to Nélaton's line, which is a line drawn between the anterior superior iliac spine and the ischial tuberosity. **A.** Normal hip. **B.** Dislocated hip.

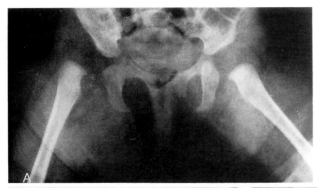

FIGURE 2–121. Radiograms of the pelvis and hips in dislocation of the left hip.

A. In a 2-month-old infant. **B.** In a 6-month-old girl. **C.** In a 12-month-old girl.

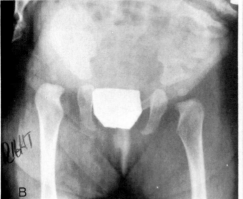

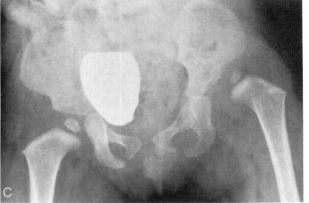

condition nevertheless may remain undetected until after the child has begun to walk. By this time there is a typical limp in her gait, characterized in the standing phase of each step on the dislocated hip by a contralateral tilt of the pelvis, lateral deviation of the spine toward the affected side, and a vertical telescoping movement of the affected lower limb. In bilateral

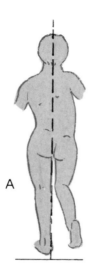

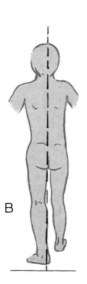

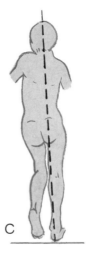

FIGURE 2–122. "Ducklike waddle" or "sailor's gait" in bilateral hip dislocation.

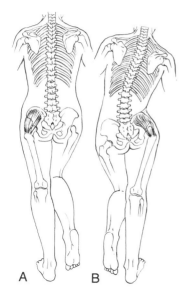

FIGURE 2–123. Trendelenburg lurch.

The Trendelenburg test is positive on the dislocated right side. **A.** As the child stands with his weight on the normal hip, the pelvis is maintained in the horizontal position by contraction and tension of the normal hip abductor muscles. **B.** As he stands with it on the dislocated hip, the pelvis on the opposite normal side drops owing to weakness of the hip abductor muscles.

dislocation the gait has been described as a "ducklike waddle" or a "sailor's gait" (Fig. 2–122).

The Trendelenburg test is positive; as the child stands on the dislocated hip, the pelvis drops on the opposite normal side because of the weakness of the hip abductors. In the normal hip, on standing, the pelvis is maintained in the horizontal position by contraction

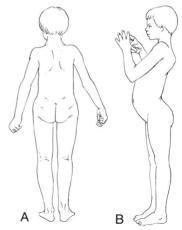

FIGURE 2–124. Bilateral hip dislocation.

A. The perineal space is widened, and the greater trochanters are prominent. **B.** Severe hyperlordosis.

and tension of the normal hip abductors (Fig. 2–123).

In bilateral hip dislocation the perineal space is widened and the greater trochanters are prominent, but the buttocks are broad and flat (Fig. 2–124 A). Hyperlordosis is present, caused by backward displacement of the femoral heads and increased forward inclination of the pelvis (Fig. 2–124 B).

Radiographic Findings

The radiographic findings become definite. With an ossified femoral head there is no problem in detecting dislocation (Figs. 2–125 and 2–126). The femoral head is displaced out of the acetabulum and migrates proximally and distally.

In the newborn with prenatal dislocation of

FIGURE 2–125. Radiogram of congenital dislocation of the hip in a two-year-old child.

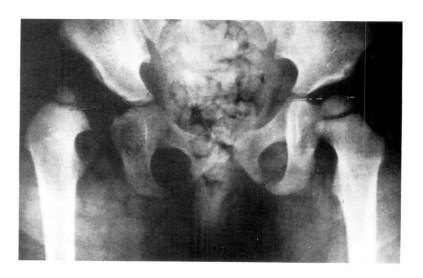

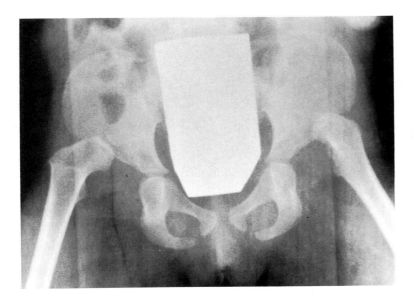

FIGURE 2–126. *Radiogram of a hip in a three-year-old child.*

the hip, the findings are different and distinctive; this is in contrast to the radiographic findings in the newborn. Marked upward and lateral displacement of the proximal femoral metaphysis is easily detectable, and there will be a false acetabulum (Fig. 2–127).

Treatment

Management of congenital dislocation of the hip depends on three factors: the *type* of dislocation—whether teratologic or typical; the duration of dislocation—whether antenatal, perinatal, or postnatal—and age of the patient; and the *degree* of displacement of the femoral head out of the acetabulum—whether the hip is

dislocated, dislocatable, or subluxatable. (The unstable hip may be dislocatable or subluxatable.) The following comments relate to typical, not to teratologic, dislocation; the latter is discussed separately. In this section treatment of *typical congenital dislocation of the hip* is discussed in relation to different age groups. It is important to commence treatment as soon as the condition is detected.

BIRTH TO TWO MONTHS OF AGE

The optimal solution to the problem of congenital dislocation of the hip is early diagnosis at birth or in the first few days of life and immediate correct treatment with meticulous

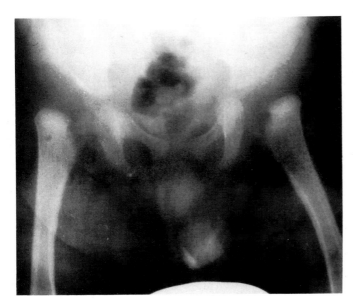

FIGURE 2–127. *Radiogram of the hips in a neonate with prenatal dislocation of both hips.*

Note the marked upward and lateral displacement of the upper femoral metaphysis and the false acetabula. These advanced radiographic changes are not seen in perinatal dislocation. This infant had arthrogryposis multiplex congenita.

attention to detail. It has been well documented that with such ideal management the results can be excellent and normal hips obtained in almost all cases. The problem is that not all dislocated hips in the newborn are perinatal; 1 to 2 per cent are antenatal. In *perinatal dislocation* in the newborn and young infant (up to two months of age), reduction can be easily accomplished by gently positioning the femoral head in the acetabulum by the Ortolani maneuver—the hip is flexed 90 degrees and abducted while traction is exerted in the longitudinal axis of the thigh, thereby lifting the femoral head gently over the posterior rim of the acetabulum into the hip socket. In antenatal dislocation closed reduction is difficult (requiring great force and extreme positions) if not impossible. The first step in treatment of congenital dislocation of the hip is to distinguish perinatal from antenatal dislocation. In antenatal dislocation, preliminary traction is applied prior to attempting closed reduction, often under general anesthesia, as described later, whereas in perinatal dislocation gentle reduction is achieved with the infant awake and without requiring prereduction traction. Occasionally as the infant gets older (reaching two to three months) and is getting heavy, a short period of traction to stretch contracted hip adductors may be advisable. The technique of closed reduction of the hip is described and illustrated in Plate 12. This is the first step in treatment of congenital dislocation of the hip.

Maintenance of Reduction of the Hip

The second step is to maintain the reduction dynamically in a physiologic position. In the literature a number of hip orthoses have been described to hold the hip in a position of flexion and abduction. If the device is properly applied in a physiologically safe human position, one can expect a satisfactory outcome. If it is improperly applied and the hip is forced into an unnatural nonphysiologic position of extreme abduction, avascular necrosis of the femoral head may ensue; or if it is loose and ineffective, the hip may become redislocated. A rigid position of the hip in a forced position is harmful. Some range of hip motion is desirable.

The Pavlik Harness. This device is simple in design, consisting of a shoulder harness with posteriorly crossed shoulder straps, lower limb stirrup straps, and booties with their heels cut out and straps and Velcro closures (Fig. 2–128 A and B). It is made of canvas, webbing, felt, Velcro closures, and metal buckles. The Pavlik harness is easy to apply, and it can be easily adjusted as the child grows. It can be used with the infant as an outpatient.

The harness was introduced by Pavlik in 1944, and in 1957 he reported the results of treatment in 1,912 hips, stating that successful reduction could be achieved with a very low

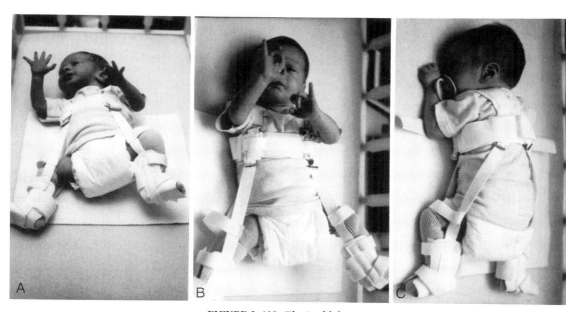

FIGURE 2–128. The Pavlik harness.

A and **B.** Anterior views. **C.** Posterior view.

Technique of Closed Reduction of Congenital Dislocation of the Hip

Manipulative reduction is best performed under general anesthesia (except in the newborn or young infant whose hips "clunk" in and out easily). It is crucial that the child be completely relaxed. At no time should excessive force be utilized. The principle is gentle repositioning of the femoral head in the acetabulum. Arrangements for radiographic confirmation of reduction are made ahead of time, and the child is not anesthetized until the x-ray technician is in the operating room. An image intensifier should be available for possible arthrography of the hip. Recently this author has employed ultrasonography to determine concentricity of reduction of the hip.

A. The anesthetized infant's position is supine. An assistant manually fixes the pelvis by exerting firm pressure upon it. The surgeon grasps the distal third of the involved thigh with one hand and places the fingers of the other hand posterolaterally over the greater trochanter.

B. The hip is then flexed to 90 to 110 degrees; this levers the femoral head from its superior position to the level of the acetabulum and immediately behind the posterior rim of the socket.

C. Next the flexed hip is abducted while moderate traction is exerted in the longitudinal axis of the thigh. In the older child one may have to hyperflex the hip and gently rotate it medially and laterally to free the femoral head and facilitate its entrance through the capsular isthmus.

D. Then pressure is applied over the posterior aspect of the greater trochanter, and the femoral head is gently lifted anteriorly over the posterior rim of the acetabulum into the socket. Upon reduction of the hip, a "clunk" will be felt and often heard—this is the most reliable sign of success of reduction. Disappearance of the hollow in the inguinal area, palpability of the femoral head in the middle of the groin beneath the femoral artery, longer appearance of the thigh, and development of tension in the hamstrings and flexion contracture of the knee are other physical signs of reduction. The success of the procedure is confirmed by anteroposterior and lateral radiograms of the hips and by ultrasonography, if available.

It is important to determine and record the stability of the reduction by reversing the preceding maneuver, testing the ease of dislocation, and checking the position of greatest stability. The degree of abduction and extension of the hip at which it will redislocate—the *zone of redislocation*—is recorded (Fig. 2–128). If the zone of stability of reduction (the safe zone of Ramsey[769]) is narrow or the reduction is nonconcentric, arthrography of the hip is performed. If hip adductor contracture is the cause of a narrow zone of reduction, myotomy of the hip adductors is performed to increase its stability.

Plate 12. Technique of Closed Reduction of Congenital Dislocation of the Hip

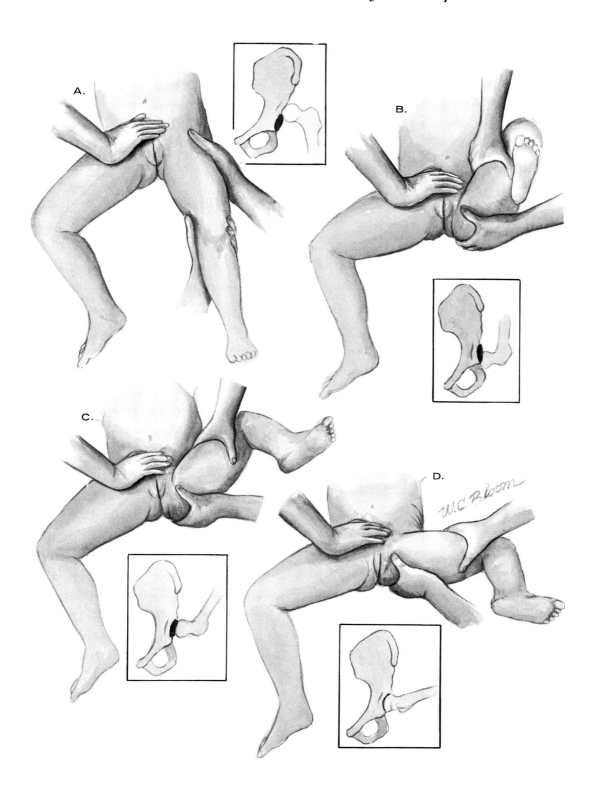

incidence of aseptic necrosis.[719] Soon afterward the device became very popular in Europe, Japan, and the United States. The harness is widely used because it is effective and relatively safe.

The Pavlik harness is a dynamic splint that allows active hip motion and avoids the rigid positions of immobilization in cast. It employs the principles of active hip flexion and free abduction to achieve and maintain reduction. The corrective and retentive forces are exerted gently. The original concept of Pavlik, *gewaltlose Selbsteinrenkung* (self reduction without force), has proved to be true. Normal development of the acetabulum and femoral head is stimulated when the hip moves in its reduced position.

Indications and Contraindications. The use of the Pavlik harness is *indicated* in an infant up to four to six months of age with typical perinatal dislocation of the hip that can be easily reduced by the Ortolani maneuver. It is also used to provide stability to the unstable hip that is dislocatable or subluxatable.

The Pavlik harness is *contraindicated* (1) when the infant is old enough to stand (usually nine months or older); (2) when the femoral head cannot be centered toward the triradiate cartilage with the hip in 90 to 110 degrees of flexion (when the hip must be forced into hyperflexion of 120 degrees for the upper femoral metaphysis to point toward the triradiate cartilage do not use the Pavlik harness—apply prereduction traction); (3) in fetal (antenatal) dislocation irreducible by the Ortolani maneuver (in these hips anatomic changes have occurred that obstruct concentric reduction by gentle repositioning of the femoral head in the acetabulum); (4) when the hip is stiff and muscle imbalance is present as in arthrogryposis and myelomeningocele; (5) in extension contracture of the knee as in congenital hyperextension or dislocation (provide mobility of the knee prior to reduction of the hip); (6) in connective tissue disorders with severe generalized ligamentous and capsular laxity such as Down's syndrome, osteogenesis imperfecta, or Marfan's syndrome (in which, because of the marked laxity of the capsule, the femoral head will move inferiorly [obturator dislocation] or anteriorly because of the lax capsule); or (7) for positioning of a septic hip after drainage—the femoral head will be dislocated anteriorly or inferiorly (Table 2–17).*

Mechanism of Reduction. As the hip flexes to

---

*See references 38, 225, 341, 342, 456, 483, 569, 662, 719, 769, 772, 777, 912–914, 962, 966.

Table 2–17. *Contraindications to Use of Pavlik Harness*

Inability to center the femoral head toward the acetabulum with the hip in hyperflexion

A child strong enough to attempt to stand—usually nine months and older

Fetal (antenatal) dislocation irreducible by Ortolani maneuver

Hip-knee joint stiffness and muscle imbalance such as in arthrogryposis and myelomeningocele (L-2, L-4 level)

Severe generalized capsular laxity—as seen in such connective tissue disorders as Down's syndrome, Marfan's syndrome, osteogenesis imperfecta (in these conditions the femoral head will become displaced inferiorly because of the lax capsule)

Positioning a septic hip after drainage (the femoral head will become displaced anteriorly or inferiorly)

---

90 to 100 degrees, the femoral head shifts from its superior position to the posterior aspect of the acetabulum; this is illustrated in the closed manipulative reduction of the hip joint in which the source of force is the power of the surgeon's hand, which lifts and levers the femoral head into the acetabulum. In the Pavlik harness the weight of the lower limbs is the source of the power. When the flexed hip falls into abduction the weight of the lower limb stretches the hip adductor muscles and permits the posteriorly displaced femoral head to slide anteriorly over the posterior acetabular margin into the acetabulum. The infant's supine posture during part of the day and at night will assist gravity to stretch the hip adductors. *Release of hip adduction contracture is indispensable for reduction.*

Method. Prior to application of the Pavlik harness the *zone of dislocation* is determined by the Ortolani and Barlow maneuvers. The harness should permit hip motion in the safe zone of reduction (the safe zone of Ramsey).[769] It should be noted, however, that in the zones of safety of Ramsey only abduction-adduction in 90 degrees of hip flexion is emphasized; it is crucial that the stability of reduction be determined in varying degrees of hip flexion-extension. How much can the hip can be extended with safety? When does dislocation occur (Fig. 2–129)?

The *anterior (flexor) strap* (or stirrup) prevents hip extension but allows hip flexion. Forced hyperflexion of the hip should be avoided. The infant should be able to kick the knees into semiextension. The anterior strap should be on the medial aspect of the child's knee and not on the middle or upper thigh. Upward migration on the thigh is prevented by a lateral strap at the knee. It is crucial that the anterior buckles for the anterior stirrup be at

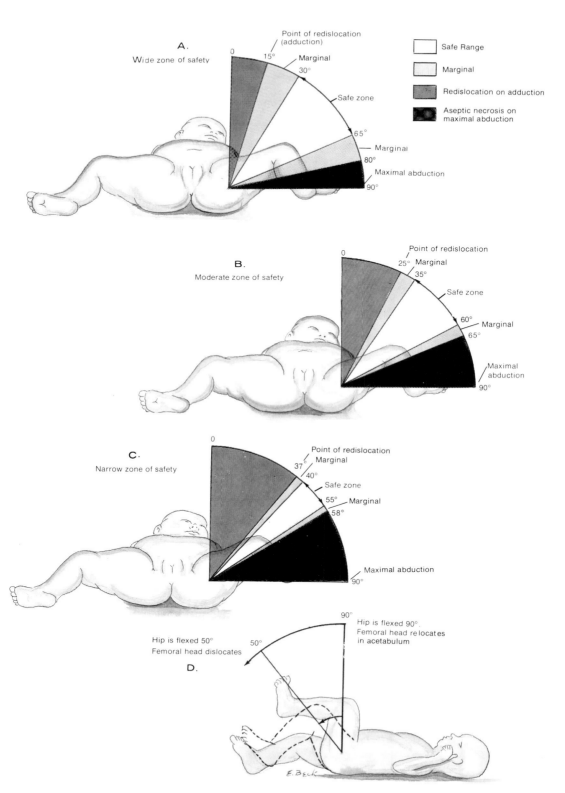

FIGURE 2–129. Zone of safety.

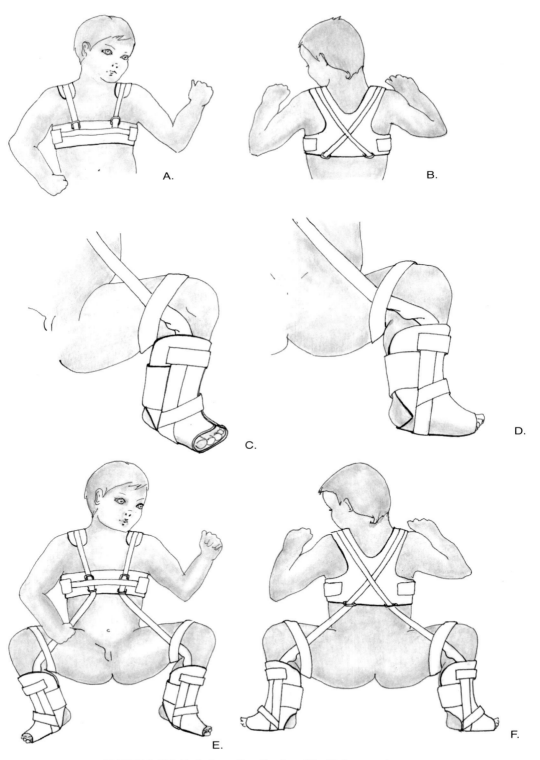

FIGURE 2–130. *Technique of application of Pavlik harness. (See text.)*

the anterior axillary line (Fig. 2–130). A common pitfall in the application of the Pavlik harness is placing the buckle of the anterior (flexor) stirrup strap too far medially; tautening the strap will then cause hip flexion and *adduction*. The result is failure to stretch the hip adductors. The proximal Velcro strap on the leg should be immediately distal to the popliteal fossa; positioning the strap at this level will ensure better control of hip flexion and abduction and will not cause excessive knee flexion.

The *posterior strap* (or stirrup) should be loose and not tight (Fig. 2–130 F); its purpose is *to control hip adduction* and prevent adduction to the point that will cause dislocation (out of the zone of safety). The hips are allowed to fall freely into comfortable abduction, pulled by the weight of the lower limbs. Pavlik's original recommendation was to tauten the posterior strap to force the hips into maximal abduction, but this forced "frog position" resulted in a high incidence of ischemic necrosis of the femoral head. The purpose of the anterior and posterior straps is to prevent the hip from entering the zone of redislocation and to permit its active motion in the zone of safety.

Anteroposterior radiograms of the hips are made with the Pavlik harness properly adjusted to ascertain the adequacy of reduction (Fig. 2–131). Inadequate hip flexion is the most common pitfall. The importance of routine radiography of the hips in the Pavlik harness to ensure proper hip flexion and concentricity of reduction cannot be overemphasized.

In the *intermediate hip*, i.e., the one that is in a transitional stage between the easily redu-cible and the definitely irreducible, one may attempt reduction with the Pavlik harness. In such an instance reduction in the harness is possible if the upper metaphysis of the femur is directed toward the triradiate cartilage. When 90 to 100 degrees of hip flexion will not redirect it toward the cartilage, the chances of reduction by the Pavlik harness are poor. The harness should *not* be used; apply prereduction traction.

During diaper change and perineal care the Pavlik harness can stay on the infant; this is a definite advantage. Parents accept the harness because of its simplicity; compliance usually is not a problem. Instructions to parents for proper application of the harness are crucial.

Technique of Application. First, place the chest halter on the infant, level with the nipple line, and close the Velcro straps; the chest halter is kept in secure position by the shoulder straps, which cross in the back to prevent them from sliding down the infant's shoulder (see Fig. 2–130 A and B).

Second, check the position of the buckles on the chest halter to which the lower limb straps (stirrups) are attached; the buckles for the posterior (abductor) straps should be located over the scapula, those for the anterior strap should be lateral, level with the child's anterior axillary line. Caution! If the anterior straps are placed too far medially, when tautened they will cause not only hip flexion but also hip adduction.

Third, the infant's legs and feet are placed in the stirrups; it is preferable that the stirrups have booties with their heels cut out, as they provide better control of the foot and ankle.

Fourth, fasten the two stirrup straps on the

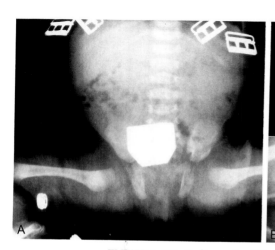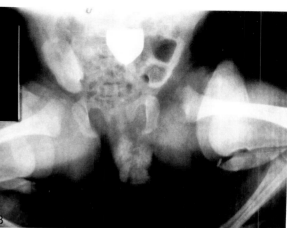

FIGURE 2–131. *Radiographs of the hips of a child wearing a Pavlik harness.*

An anteroposterior view is made to check adequacy of reduction. **A.** Hip is reduced. **B.** Inadequate hip flexion. The metaphyisis of the femoral head is not pointing to the triradiate cartilage. Avoid this pitfall!

leg. The site of the lower leg strap is one fingerbreadth above the ankle; the upper strap on the leg should be located immediately below the popliteal fossa. The upper strap prevents bowstringing of the anterior and posterior stirrup straps and controls and stabilizes the knee. If the stirrup straps form a bowstring when the posterior lower limb strap is tightened, the hip will rotate medially and adduct.

Fifth, the hip is flexed to 90 to 100 degrees and the anterior (flexor) stirrup strap is adjusted and attached to the anterior buckle on the chest halter. The anterior straps prevent hip extension and allow active hip flexion. The anterior strap should be on the medial aspect of the child's knee; it should not migrate upward on the thigh. Double-check the position of the buckle on the chest halter for the anterior strap—is it at the anterior axillary line?

Sixth, the posterior (or abductor) stirrups are attached to the chest halter—the buckle for the posterior strap should be over the scapula. The posterior harness strap should be loose; its purpose is to limit hip adduction, not to force the hip into abduction. Hip abduction is passively achieved by the weight of the child's lower limb, as shown in Figure 2–130.

After the harness is applied an anteroposterior radiogram of the hip is made with the child in the harness to confirm adequate hip flexion.

Treatment Regimen. This varies, depending on whether the hip is *dislocatable* with a good zone of safety of stability, whether it is *dislocated* but easily reducible, or whether it is an *intermediate hip*, not reducible but with potential to progress to a stable reduction in the Pavlik harness.

The *dislocatable hip with a good zone of safety*: Initially for the first three weeks of treatment, the infant is left in the harness 22 hours of the day. When the hip becomes stable, as shown by inability to dislocate it by the Barlow maneuver and confirmation of adequacy of reduction by anteroposterior radiograms made with the hips in neutral position, the infant is gradually weaned from the harness. Periods out of the harness are progressively increased at weekly or biweekly intervals to four, six, and eight hours per day. During the final two to four weeks, the infant sleeps in the harness at night only.

If *the hip is dislocated but easily reducible*, the infant wears the harness *full time* for the first three to four weeks. When the harness is initially applied an anteroposterior radiogram is made with the hips in the desired degree of flexion and abduction. The proximal femoral metaphysis should point toward the triradiate cartilage. Inadequate hip flexion will cause persistence or recurrence of the dislocation while the infant is in the harness. The hips are reexamined in two to three days, then in a week, and then two weeks later. It is not necessary to make radiograms of the hips at each visit. Usually within four to six weeks, the hip will be stable clinically and one cannot dislocate the femoral head out of the acetabulum by the Barlow provocation test. At this time anteroposterior radiograms of the hips are made to confirm the concentricity of reduction. The infant is then gradually weaned from the harness as described for the dislocatable hip. Radiograms of the hips are made at appropriate intervals. Crucial periods are during weaning and when the harness is discontinued. When the anteroposterior radiogram of the hips in neutral position shows lateral subluxation, it indicates premature weaning from the harness, and the full-time program of wearing the harness is resumed.

The use of the Pavlik harness in the *intermediate hip* requires considerable clinical judgment, and each case should be individualized. In the infant under three months of age a Pavlik harness may be applied with the hips in physiologic position of flexion and only mild abduction. Should one employ the harness if there is marked limitation of abduction due to severe hip adductor tautness? If, in 90 degrees of hip flexion and mild abduction, the proximal femoral metaphysis points toward the triradiate cartilage, the Pavlik harness may be tried. Some hips will become reduced spontaneously after the harness has been worn for one or possibly two weeks. If a hip cannot be reduced concentrically *within two weeks*, it should be placed in traction prior to attempted reduction. Some surgeons advocate four weeks of trial with the Pavlik harness before considering the harness program to be a failure.[394] This author does not concur with them. At no time should the hip be forced into abduction or forced hyperflexion. If in doubt, apply traction to stretch and elongate the contracted soft tissues.

Total duration of treatment in the Pavlik harness varies depending on whether the hip being treated is dislocated or dislocatable; if dislocated, whether it can be reduced easily; or if of the intermediate type, whether it cannot be easily reduced (because of associated hip adduction contracture) and requires too long a time to achieve reduction and clinical stability; and on the age of the infant when treatment is initiated.[483]

In perinatal typical dislocation when the hip is easily reducible, a safe estimate of length of treatment is twice the age (in weeks) of the infant when the Pavlik harness is first applied, with a minimum period of six weeks. The sooner the dislocation is detected and treated, the less severe are the adaptive anatomic changes to be corrected and the shorter is the duration of treatment required to achieve a stable and normal hip joint.

Problems of Treatment. Problems that may be encountered during the treatment regimen are listed in Table 2–18. *Hip adduction contracture* may persist and cause a narrow zone of safety of reduction. Often the adductor muscles will stretch out and the zone of safety of reduction will increase after two weeks of wearing the harness. If it does not, the infant is placed in traction, and if, after a two-week trial of traction, the hip adductor tautness persists and prevents reduction, adductor myotomy under general anesthesia will be required prior to reduction. In such an instance a hip spica cast is applied for four weeks, and then the infant wears the Pavlik harness to increase stability of the hip.

Failure to achieve concentric reduction after two to four weeks of wearing the harness requires that an arthrogram of the hip be performed to delineate the cause of the nonconcentricity. Intra-articular and extra-articular obstacles of reduction may require surgical intervention.

Failure of stabilization of the hip may be due to noncompliance by the parents, or the anatomic factors causing hip instability may be great. A period of immobilization in a hip spica cast is appropriate in such an instance. One may have to delineate the problem by arthrography and computed tomographic studies.

Complications of Treatment. These do occur, but they are very infrequent if the Pavlik harness is properly applied and appropriately adjusted for growth.

Table 2–18. *Problems and Complications of Pavlik Harness Treatment of Congenital Dislocation of the Hip*

Failure to achieve concentric reduction
Failure to stabilize hip
Failure to stretch taut hip adductors
Avascular necrosis
Femoral nerve palsy
Inferior dislocation of hip
Anterior dislocation of hip
Medial instability of knee joint
Failure of compliance by parents

Aseptic necrosis of the proximal femur following treatment with the Pavlik harness reportedly varies in incidence from 0 to 28 per cent. The higher incidence is usually associated with cases of dislocation. When the harness is used to treat the dislocatable or subluxatable unstable hip, aseptic necrosis is very rare. Originally Pavlik recommended that the hips be maintained in maximal abduction by tightening the posterior strap; the result was aseptic necrosis in a high percentage of cases. Later on the harmful effects of forced abduction were appreciated; the posterior strap was adjusted to be loose, serving to prevent the hip from adducting to the point of redislocation. In a multicenter study Tönnis reported 15 per cent incidence of avascular necrosis; Ueno and associates reported 9 per cent; Suzuki, 9 per cent; Pavlik, 5 per cent; and in the overall experience of Tsuyama and Sakaguchi the incidence of aseptic necrosis was approximately 0.9 per cent.[315a, 719, 913, 941, 961, 965] Kalamchi and MacFarlane treated 77 dislocated hips, 141 subluxated hips, and 105 hips with acetabular dysplasia with the Pavlik harness and reported the end results; there was not a single case of avascular necrosis.[483] In the personal experience of this author in the treatment of 140 *dislocated* hips with the Pavlik harness, the incidence of aseptic necrosis has been nil.

In order to minimize and probably eliminate the problem of avascular necrosis in treatment of congenital dislocation of the hip with the Pavlik harness, it is imperative to follow the indications and contraindications strictly and to be meticulous in the technique of application and adjustment of the harness. The hip should not be forced into abduction; the posterior strap should be loose. Prone sleeping posture may force the hips into extreme abduction. Alternate the sleeping position between supine and prone. A dislocated femoral head that cannot be lowered opposite the triradiate cartilage by flexion-abduction of the hip should not be treated by the Pavlik harness; it should be placed in traction prior to reduction.

Inferior or obturator subluxation or dislocation of the hip is caused by forced hyperflexion of a "loose" dislocation. Avoid extreme forced flexion of this hip.

Anterior dislocation is due to marked abduction and lateral rotation of the hip; a hip that becomes stiff and painful on passive motion should make the surgeon suspicious of this complication. On palpation of the groin, the femoral head is usually prominent. A true lateral radiogram of the hips and, if indicated, a computed tomographic scan will confirm the diagnosis of anterior displacement of the femoral head. Immediately the infant is taken out of the Pavlik harness and placed in traction with the hips in progressively increasing flexion and abduction. After reduction of the anterior dislocation it is best to immobilize the hip in a spica cast and not take the chance of recurrent anterior dislocation.

Femoral nerve palsy is caused by excessive hip flexion and entrapment of the nerve under the inguinal ligament; it is transient, with universal recovery as a rule. At each outpatient visit it should be routine to remove the booties and check quadriceps muscle function. Ask the parents if the baby can kick its legs straight. If femoral nerve paresis develops, it is treated by decreasing the amount of hip flexion. Obese babies are more prone to stretching of the femoral nerve.

Medial knee joint instability can occur if the harness is too small for the infant (Fig. 2–132). The taut posterior strap will exert valgus stress on the flexed knee as the infant kicks a medially rotated hip. Repeated, the stress will stretch the medial collateral ligament and result in gross medial knee joint instability. This complication can be avoided by the proper application of the harness and its periodic adjustment for amount of growth.

Other Retentive Hip Positioning Devices

The Von Rosen (or Malmö) Splint. This splint, shown in Figure 2–133, is the next most frequently used retentive device, particularly in Scandinavian countries and in Great Britain. Made of flexible metal and covered by soft padding, it extends over the shoulders and around the thighs and can be appropriately bent and molded to the child. In it the hips can be placed in the desired degree of flexion and abduction, and extreme abduction can be prevented. The shoulder extensions prevent the device from sliding down the infant's leg. Some degree of mobility of the hips is allowed by having the device fitted loosely. It allows diaper changes without removing the splint. Caution! Be sure that the metal extending over the shoulders is well padded. The newborn infant with poor head control will tilt the head to one side; pressure by the metal near the mastoid process will cause facial nerve paralysis. This author has seen two such cases.

The Craig, or Ilfeld, Splint. This device, shown in Figure 2–134, maintains the hips in flexion and abduction, but tends to slide distally (because it is not secured over the shoulders),

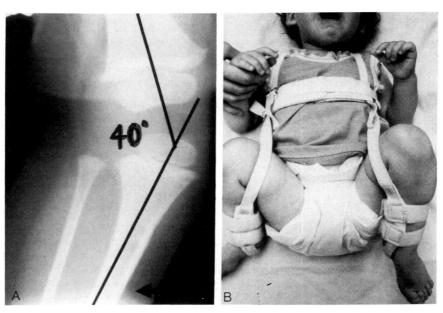

FIGURE 2–132. Knee joint instability.

A. Radiogram of right knee at age 14 months with valgus stress applied at the knee. Note the instability. **B.** Photograph of the patient in the Pavlik harness. The knee joint instability was discovered after eight months of treatment with the harness. The right hip is held in flexion, abduction, and medial rotation. Valgus stress to the knee was exerted as the child kicked her knee into extension. (From Schwentker, E. P., Zaleski, R. J., and Skinner, S. R.: Medial knee instability complicating the Pavlik harness treatment of congenital hip subluxation. J. Bone Joint Surg., 65-A:679, 1983. Reprinted by permission.)

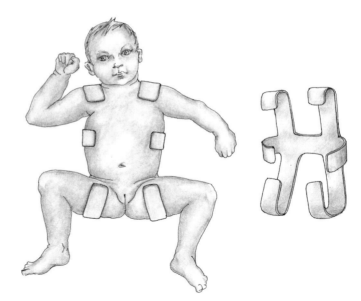

FIGURE 2–133. Von Rosen splint.

thereby forcing the hips into abduction and extension with the consequent risk of redislocation. It requires constant adjustment for growth. The perineal opening avoids the necessity of removing the splint frequently for diaper change.

The Denis Browne Hip Abduction Splint. This splint consists of a sacral piece with a posterior bar, thigh straps, and a shoulder harness with posteriorly crossed straps (Fig. 2–135). The degrees of hip flexion and abduction are controlled; a certain degree of hip mobility

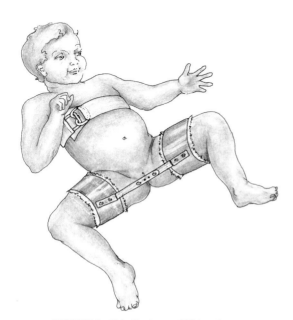

FIGURE 2–134. Craig, or Ilfeld, splint.

is permitted, and the problem of frequent reapplication is avoided, as diaper change and perineal care can be provided with the device in place. This author recommends its use in children after they have begun to sit or stand; at this age the Pavlik harness is no longer suitable.

The Frejka Pillow. Consisting of a bulky device covered with a nonabsorbent material, the Frejka pillow keeps the hips in abduction and flexion (Fig. 2–136). Its danger is that it forces the hips into marked abduction, and an additional drawback is that it has to be reapplied with each diaper change. It should not be used in the treatment of congenital dislocation of the hip. Because of the risk of excessive hip abduction and aseptic necrosis, this author also discourages its use in the management of the unstable (subluxatable or dislocatable) hip.

The application of *triple diapers*, illustrated in Figure 2–137, is a very unreliable and ineffective means of maintaining flexion and abduction of the hips. This author does not recommend its use in the treatment of congenital hip dysplasia. The use of triple diapers may be indicated on occasion when a hip is minimally unstable and the surgeon wishes to keep the parents under control and to provide continuous observation to recheck the hips.

THREE TO TWELVE MONTHS OF AGE

In this age group the femoral head becomes progressively displaced laterally and upward, and contractures of the iliopsoas, hip adductors, and other pelvifemoral muscles develop. The initial stage of treatment is to place the infant's

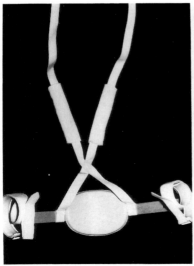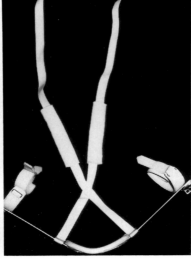

FIGURE 2–135. Denis Browne hip abduction splint.

This splint is utilized to maintain the hip in moderate flexion, abduction, and lateral rotation. It controls the degree of hip abduction and flexion, and provides freedom of mobility of the hip.

lower limbs in traction to pull the displaced femoral head down to a level opposite or below the center of the acetabulum.

Preliminary Traction

The importance of preliminary traction prior to closed or open reduction cannot be overemphasized. There is overwhelming evidence in the literature that such preliminary traction markedly reduces the incidence and the degree of avascular necrosis of the femoral head.[321, 433]

Percutaneous or open myotomy of the hip adductors prior to traction is not recommended by this author because the myostatic contracture of these shortened muscles prevents sudden stretching of the retinacular vessels.

The *type* of traction employed among surgeons varies: it may be in the form of overhead Bryant's traction, split Russell's traction with the hip in semiflexion, straight Buck's unilateral traction, or skeletal traction with a threaded pin through the distal femur. (Skeletal traction should never be applied with a pin through the proximal tibia.)

Split Russell's traction, with the hips flexed

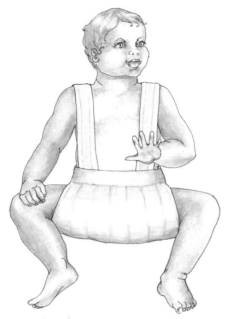

FIGURE 2–136. Frejka pillow.

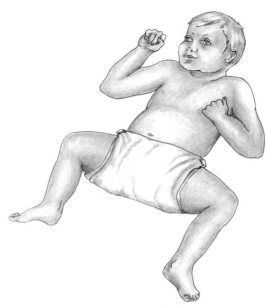

FIGURE 2–137. Triple diapers.

30 to 60 degrees and the knees flexed 20 to 30 degrees, is the type recommended by this author (Fig. 2–138). Traction with the hips in complete extension will cause compression of the hip capsule by the taut iliopsoas tendon and, therefore, may interfere with the blood supply to the femoral head. The purpose of traction is to elongate the shortened pelvifemoral muscles; traction applied with the hips in 90 degrees of flexion will not stretch the hip flexors (especially the iliopsoas) and the hip adductors. These are the reasons why the hips should be in semiflexed position of 45 degrees (with a range from 30 to 60 degrees). Initially in a greater degree of flexion, the hips are extended into less flexion as the femoral heads are pulled down. The hips should not be abducted until the femoral heads have come to the level of the acetabulum. Premature abduction of the hips may lock the upwardly displaced femoral head against the lateral wall of the ilium. Another potential problem of early hip abduction is infolding of the superior portion of the hip capsule into the acetabulum. Inversion of the limbus is a gradual phenomenon and not a sudden "popping in." When the femoral heads are lowered distally to the level of the acetabulum, the hip abduction should never exceed 45 degrees. A strap between the foot plates to control hip rotation is not required. Some surgeons employ an upper thigh strap to lift the

posteriorly dislocated femoral head anteriorly into the acetabulum. This author finds it cumbersome and unnecessary.

The 20 to 30 degrees of knee flexion will relax the hamstrings; there is experimental evidence that immobilization of the knees in extension will dislocate the hips.[632] Hyperextension of the knee may cause circulatory embarrassment. Both lower limbs are placed in traction in order to control the pelvis.

Some authors apply Bryant's overhead traction with the hips in 90 degrees of flexion and the knees in extension (Fig. 2–139). Flexing the hips 90 degrees will lower the superiorly displaced femoral head to the level of the acetabulum and in back of its posterior rim, while the vertical traction will elevate the posteriorly dislocated femoral head anteriorly into the acetabulum. The drawbacks of Bryant's traction are the possibility that the hyperextended posture of the knees will cause vascular compromise of the lower limbs while in traction and the fact that traction with the hips in 90-degree flexion does not elongate the iliopsoas and the hip adductors.

Skeletal traction through the distal femur will exert greater and direct traction forces on the femur (Fig. 2–140). It has its definite drawbacks, however. Pin tract infection, disuse atrophy, and possible damage to the distal femoral

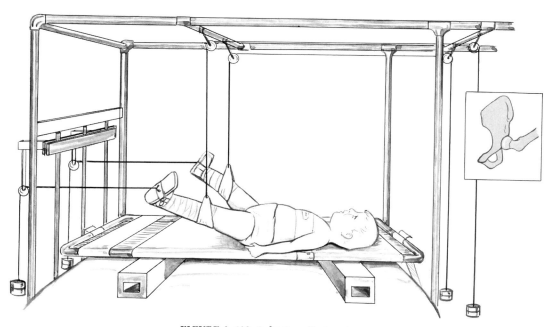

FIGURE 2–138. Split Russell's traction.

This is used to bring the femoral head to the level of the acetabulum. Note that the hips are in semiflexion. This method is preferred by the author. (From Tachdjian, M. O. (ed.) Congenital Dislocation of the Hip. New York, Churchill-Livingstone, 1982. Reprinted by permission.)

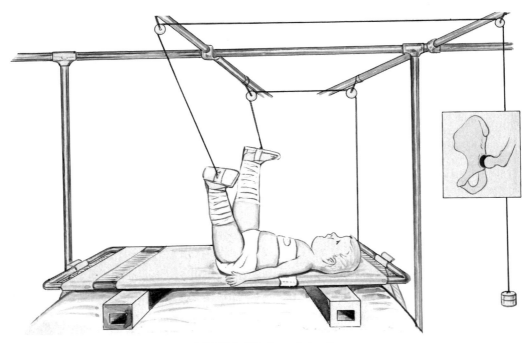

FIGURE 2–139. Bryant's traction.

The hips are in 90 degrees flexion and the knees are in extension. Flexing the hips 90 degrees will bring the femoral head down from its superior position to the level of the acetabulum and in back of the posterior rim of the acetabulum. The drawback is the completely extended posture of the knees. In the older child, vascular compromise is a definite hazard. (From Tachdjian, M. O. (ed.) Congenital Dislocation of the Hip. New York, Churchill-Livingstone, 1982. Reprinted by permission).

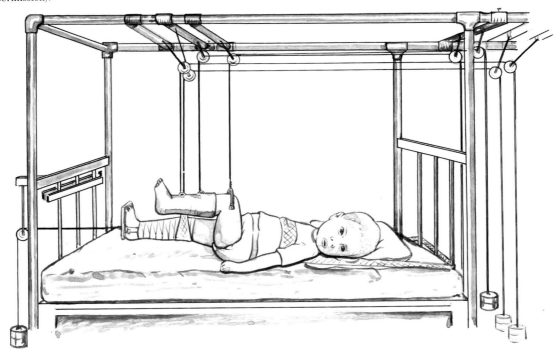

FIGURE 2–140. Skeletal traction pin through distal femur.

This permits greater distraction force by its direct pull on the femur; however, pin tract infection, disuse osteoporosis, and possible damage to the distal femoral physis are definite complications. In the modern era of femoral shortening, one should not employ skeletal traction to lower the femoral head in congenital dislocation of the hip. (From Tachdjian, M. O. (ed.) Congenital Dislocation of the Hip. New York, Churchill-Livingstone, 1982. Reprinted by permission.)

physis are complications of skeletal traction. If so much force is required to bring the femoral head down, subtrochanteric femoral shortening is indicated. In the modern era of treatment of congenital dislocation of the hip by femoral shortening, skeletal traction ordinarily is not indicated.

Usually the child must be hospitalized, and the parents must be informed that the period of traction may be two to three weeks. The duration of traction varies from one case to another; one should not employ a rigid approach to the duration of traction. As a rule of thumb, it should not exceed three weeks because of the risk of disuse atrophy and the possibility of fracture and problems with internal fixation when femoral shortening is performed. The objective of traction is to stretch and elongate the shortened pelvifemoral muscles and soft tissues, to bring the femoral head to the level of the acetabulum opposite the triradiate cartilage, and to facilitate gentle reduction of the hip without stretching retinacular vessels and compromising circulation to the femoral head. Periodic anteroposterior radiograms of the hip are made *while in traction* to document the level of the femoral head. The end point of traction is when the femoral head is opposite the triradiate cartilage. The length of time in traction is not a measure of the effectiveness of traction; the important determining factor in preventing avascular necrosis is how well the femoral head is pulled down distally to its normal position opposite the acetabulum.

Gage and Winter quantitated the effectiveness of traction by means of a series of *"traction stations,"* which relate the position of the femoral head to the acetabulum.[321] The medial ossified corner of the metaphysis of the femoral neck is used as a reference point; the ossific nucleus of the femoral head is unsatisfactory because the capital epiphysis may not be ossified (or ossification may be delayed), may be smaller, and can vary in size. The obturator foramen and Hilgenreiner's line are the reference points on the pelvis. In the normal hip Shenton's line is intact—i.e., a line drawn between the medial border of the neck of the femur and the superior border of the obturator foramen forms an even arc of continuous contour; this normal position is termed the *plus-one station* (Fig. 2–141 C). If the medial corner of the femoral neck is superior to Hilgenreiner's line, the hip is at *minus-one station* (Fig. 2–141 A). If it is between Hilgenreiner's line and the superior border of the obturator foramen, it is at the *zero station* (Fig. 2–141 B). If it is inferior to the upper border of the obturator foramen

(i.e., the normal position), it is at the *plus-two station* (Fig. 2–141 D).

Technique of Application of Skin Traction. It is best to utilize nonadhesive traction straps because adhesive straps may blister the skin and are painful to remove. The traction straps are secured on the medial and lateral aspects of both lower limbs with an elastic bandage. The skin pull should encompass the entire leg and thigh. A foot plate spreads the traction straps to keep them away from the malleoli of the ankles, preventing pressure sores. The elastic bandages and straps are removed and reapplied several times a day. Each time skin care is given. Wrapping of the elastic bandages must be meticulous; if they are too loose, traction will be ineffective and the bandages will gather about the ankle; if too tight, they may constrict vessels and nerves. The vascular and neuromuscular status of the foot and toes is assessed several times a day by a registered nurse and by the treating orthopedic surgeon. If there is any suggestion of neurovascular compromise the traction is removed immediately. This form of skin traction is not painful, and the infant should not be fussy or cry abnormally.

Another method of applying skin traction is to spray a nonallergenic adhesive such as Ace Adherent or tincture of benzoin on the skin of both lower limbs and then apply a snug stockinette smoothly on each lower limb. Medial and lateral adhesive straps are applied over the surface of the stockinette and secured in place by one or two layers of sheet wadding (to protect the bony prominences) and elastic bandages. Removal of the stockinette is painful and cumbersome; often the skin is not inspected frequently enough. This author has encountered skin problems more often with this technique.

Split Russell's traction with a vertical traction strap behind the upper third of the tibia ensures that the knees are in 20 to 30 degrees of flexion. The direction of longitudinal traction on the leg and thigh is such that the hips are in 30 to 60 degrees of flexion. The amount of weight varies with the weight and size of the child. Two pounds on the longitudinal traction straps and one to two pounds on the vertical traction straps is usually adequate and the maximum traction force that is safe for skin traction.

Downward pull of the traction should be counterbalanced by a pelvic restraint and by elevating the foot of the bed or the distal end of the Bradford frame; otherwise the infant will be pulled distally toward the foot of the bed. The pelvic restraint is well-padded and diaper-shaped to fit over the perineum; it is secured with cloth straps to the sides or the canvas of

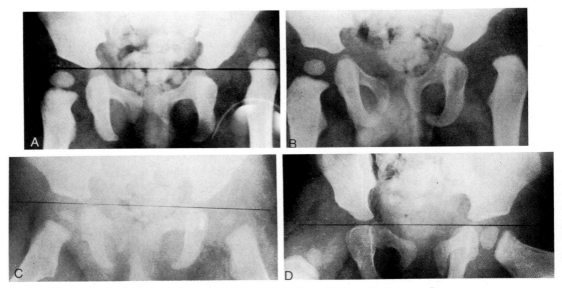

FIGURE 2–141. Gage and Winter's method of quantitating effectiveness of traction.

The position of the femoral head in relation to the acetabulum is determined by anteroposterior radiograms of the hip made with the infant in traction. The reference point on the upper femur is the ossifed medial corner of the femoral neck (the ossific nucleus of the femoral head is unsatisfactory becasue it may not be ossified or may vary in size because of delayed maturation). The reference points on the pelvis are the upper border of the obturator foramen and Hilgenreiner's line. **A.** A minus-one station of the dislocated left hip in a five-month-old girl. Note the ossified medial corner of the femoral neck is superior to Hilgenreiner's line. **B.** A zero station of the dislocated left hip in an 18-month-old boy. The medial corner of the femoral neck metaphysis is at the level of the triradiate cartilage between Hilgenreiner's line and the upper border of the obturator foramen. **C.** A plus-one station of the dislocated left hip in a five-month-old girl. Note the medial corner of the metaphysis of the femoral neck is level with the upper border of the obturator foramen. **D.** A plus-two station of the dislocated right hip, which is pulled down below the opposite normal left hip. The upper medial corner of the femoral neck is inferior to the upper border of the obturator foramen. (A to D from Gage, J. R., and Winter, R. B.: Avascular necrosis of the capital femoral epiphysis as a complication of closed reduction of congenital dislocation of the hi, J. Bone Joint Surg., 54-A:373, 1972. Reprinted by permission.)

the Bradford frame. It is vital that the width of the pelvic restraint at the perineum be correct; if too wide, it will force the hips into premature abduction and lock the femoral heads on the lateral wall of the ilium; it may also cause pressure irritation of the skin of the upper medial thighs. If the restraint is too narrow, the traction force will cause pressure on the perineum. A jacket-type restraint should not be used because of the potential for constricting the infant's neck if it is pulled into the restraint.

The infant is released from traction several times a day for brief periods for feeding, toilet, skin care, and affection and physical contact. Otherwise the infant should stay in traction continuously throughout the day and night.

Economic reasons may dictate the use of home traction. This may be tried with intelligent parents with medical background or with adequate home visiting nurse supervision. The potential for skin blistering and neurovascular problems is greater, however. For maximum effectiveness and the fewest problems, this author recommends traction in hospital.

Closed Reduction

In the child three months of age and older, closed reduction of the hips is best performed under anesthesia in the operating room. The technique is described and illustrated in Plate 12.

Arthrography. Plain radiograms demonstrate only osseous relationships. In the newborn and the infant up to six months of age, the femoral head is not ossified, and a large portion of the hip joint is cartilaginous. Therefore, arthrography of the hip should be performed. Arthrography will show and define the radiolucent portions of the hip and soft-tissue structures; it will depict the limits of the capsule, whether the capsule is stretched out, adherent to the lateral wall of the ilium or to the floor of the acetabulum, or indented externally by a taut iliopsas tendon with hourglass constriction. With image intensifier radiographic control, arthrography will dynamically determine the zone of safety of reduction, concentricity of reduction, and anatomic factors of instability of the hip. An arthrogram will provide information

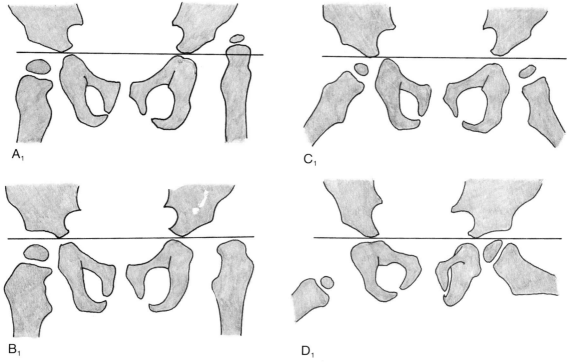

A₁

C₁

B₁

D₁

FIGURE 2–141 *Continued*

Diagram showing traction stations in congenital dislocation of the hip. A₁ = minus-one station. B₁ = zero station. C₁ = plus-one station. D₁ = plus-two station.

regarding the depth of the acetabular socket and the thickness of the cartilage of the femoral head and acetabulum. It will depict the intrinsic barriers to concentric reduction such as an inverted limbus or hypertrophied and redundant ligamentum teres and pulvinar.*

Technique. Arthrography is performed under general anesthesia. This author prefers to carry out the procedure in the operating room under strict aseptic conditions and image intensifier radiographic control. Before the child is anesthetized, it is wise to check whether the image intensifier is working and whether the x-ray technician is immediately available. In some centers arthrography is performed in the radiography department where aseptic conditions and anesthesia back-up support tend to be less satisfactory than in the operating room. Anaphylactic reaction to the radiopaque dye may very occasionally occur (about one in 100,000).

The patient is placed in supine position, and the perineum is shielded with Steri-Drapes. The skin is prepared with Betadine soap and paint, and the hip is draped carefully with sterile towels and sheets. The surgeon should wear a mask, hat, sterile gown, and gloves.

Lackadaisical performance of sterile technique should not be tolerated. Sepsis of the hip joint is a definite complication that could be disastrous.

A 20- or 18-gauge lumbar puncture needle with a stylet inside is used to puncture the hip joint. The radiopaque dye may be injected into the hip joint through different routes: superior, lateral, anterior, or inferior (adductor).

The adductor (inferior) route is preferred by this author (Fig. 2–142). With the patient in supine position both hips are flexed 90 degrees, maximally abducted, and laterally rotated. The needle is introduced in the *horizontal plane* immediately posterior to the tendon of the adductor longus. The needle is pointed upward medially toward the ipsilateral shoulder and directed toward the inferior capsule of the hip joint. (The tendency of the novice surgeon is to introduce the needle anteriorly and perform a psoasgram instead of an arthrogram [Fig. 2–143].) A sensation of resistance is felt upon touching the capsule. The needle is advanced under slight pressure, and the joint is entered. At this time the position of the point of the needle is confirmed by screening with an image intensifier. Then the hip is gently rotated medially and laterally, and the touch of the needle against the femoral head is felt by the surgeon

*See references 26, 102, 355, 356, 440, 553, 554, 640, 699.

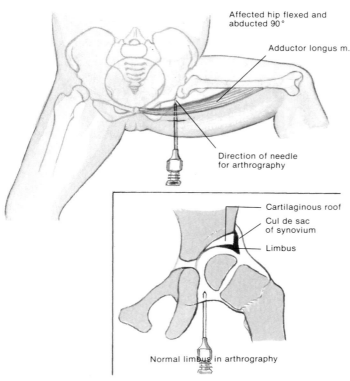

Affected hip flexed and
abducted 90°

Adductor longus m.

Direction of needle
for arthrography

Cartilaginous roof

Cul de sac
of synovium

Limbus

Normal limbus in arthrography

FIGURE 2–142. Adductor approach for insertion of the needle for arthrography of the hip.

and seen on the image intensifier screen. If the needle appears to be in the joint, 1 ml. of sterile normal saline solution is injected; free flow of the water indicates the needle is in the joint; upon release of pressure on the plunger of the syringe the fluid will readily flow back into the syringe. At this point some surgeons prefer to use a small amount of air to further confirm with the image intensifier whether the needle has entered the joint. This author recommends the use of air in doubtful cases but not routinely. A few drops of the contrast medium (25 per cent Hypaque diluted half and half with sterile water) is injected, and its presence (or absence) in the joint is confirmed by the image intensifier. When the needle point is definitely positioned intra-articularly, 1 to 3 ml. of the dye is slowly injected. Avoid injecting too much or too heavy a concentration of the dye, as it will obscure the anatomic features of the hip. Conversely, too little dye will not provide sufficient information. Extravasation of the dye should be avoided, as it will obscure the picture. Injection of the dye into the vascular system can be prevented by checking whether blood can be aspirated. Occasionally an overzealous surgeon may force the dye into the femoral head or neck.

The dye will first appear in the inferior part of the joint; the injection is continued under image intensifier control until the entire femoral head and the lower, medial, and upper parts of

the hip joint are clearly outlined. Rotation of the hip and intermittent traction on the lower limb will disperse the dye within the joint. The amount of dye injected should not exceed 3 ml. An excessive amount of dye will mask filling defects, obscure the free edge of the limbus, and cause painful distention and irritation of the hip joint. Withdrawal of the needle will cause extra-articular extravasation of the dye.

With the needle in situ, the following radiograms are made: anteroposterior projection with the hip in neutral weight-bearing position (Fig. 2–144); anteroposterior projection with the hips in abduction, extension, and medial rotation (shows relation of articular structures with antetorsion corrected); anteroposterior radiogram with the hips in 90 degrees of flexion, maximal abduction, and lateral rotation (demonstrates the joint in position of reduction); and true lateral projection (depicts posterior or anterior subluxation).

The degree of laxity of the capsule may be determined by applying traction on the lower limb, and stability of reduction assessed by performing Barlow's test and observing on the screen of the image intensifier. Video recording of the arthrogram is possible by connecting a video recorder to the image intensifier.

The dosage of radiation should be kept to a minimum; the child, surgeon, and anesthesiologist should be protected by appropriate lead attire. The surgeon should not forget to wear a

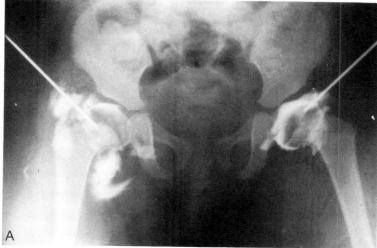

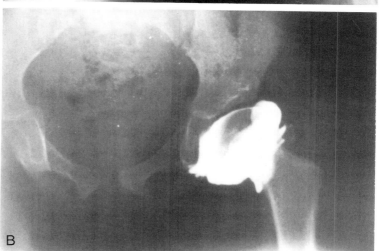

FIGURE 2–143. Pitfalls to avoid in arthrography of the hip.

A. Arthrogram of both hips. In the right hip the dye has escaped from the joint, obscuring detail. The satisfactory arthrogram of the left hip shows blunting of the rose thorn, pooling of the dye medially, and a suggestion of an inversion of the limbus. **B.** In this arthrogram, too much dye has been injected, obscuring detail.

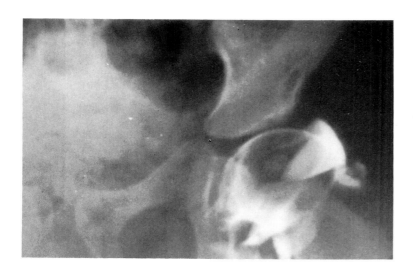

FIGURE 2–144. Anteroposterior arthrogram of a normal hip in neutral position.

thyroid shield. Routine arthrography of a normal contralateral hip should not be performed.

Mitchell prefers the superior approach, introducing the needle ½ inch posterior to the anterior superior iliac spine, then pointing it distally and medially toward the ilium.[640] The needle is slowly advanced until it makes contact with the roof of the acetabulum; then it is tilted laterally and, on slight pressure, enters the capsule of the joint.

Hughes utilizes the anterior approach. With the patient supine and the hip in neutral position, he marks the anterior iliac spine, the symphysis pubis, and the femoral artery with indelible ink. The fingers of one hand are placed over the greater trochanter and the thumb over the midinguinal region immediately lateral to the vessels (avoid puncturing the femoral artery and the femoral nerve, which courses immediately lateral to the artery). As an assistant rotates the limb, the surgeon can feel the femoral head rotating under his thumb. When the hip is in lateral rotation (when the femoral head is most superficial) a 2½-inch short lumbar puncture needle (with the stylet inside) is introduced perpendicularly into the hip joint. The surgeon can feel the needle touch the femoral head; then the hip is rotated medially and laterally, and the surgeon feels the femoral head rotating against the needle. The position of the needle is verified by the image intensifier prior to injection of the dye.[440]

The needle may also be introduced from the lateral aspect of the hip joint immediately anterior to the greater trochanter and directed along the anterior aspect of the femoral neck until the capsule is pierced. The surgeon should be familiar with all routes for introducing the needle into the hip joint.

In the normal infant hip joint the following anatomic features are studied: (1) the shape and size of the femoral head; (2) the cartilaginous rim of the acetabulum; (3) the orbicular zone (i.e., the area surrounding the hip joint capsule, which reinforces it and consists of thickened circular fibers), seen as a radiolucent zone that encompasses the femoral neck and divides the opaque medium in half; (4) the transverse ligament, manifest as a depression in the inferior and medial margins of the radiopaque medium; and (5) the ligamentum teres, not seen in the normal hip, but identified in its site of origin by two small prongs of contrast medium (see Fig. 2–144).

The various arthrographic changes in congenital dislocation of the hip are discussed next.

The Capsule. The arthrogram will depict the limits of the capsule, which in congenital dislocation of the hip is stretched, permitting the femoral head to migrate posterolaterally and upward. In the subluxated hip the arthrogram will show pooling of the dye medial to the femoral head (Fig. 2–145). When reduction of the femoral head is concentric there will be a thin meniscus of the dye superiorly, medially, and inferiorly outlining the femoral head and separating it from the floor, and concavity of the floor of the acetabulum without any pooling or filling defect in the dye shadow (see Fig. 2–144). When the hip is in neutral weight-bearing position the femoral head is laterally displaced, and upon flexion–abduction–medial rotation of the hip, concentric reduction is achieved (i.e., the subluxation is reducible by changes in position of the femur alone). This finding indicates femoral antetorsion and excessive acetabular antetorsion (maldirection) as the cause of subluxation. If subluxation cannot be reduced by

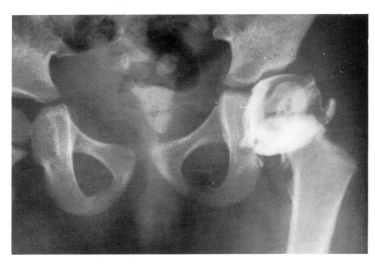

FIGURE 2–145. Pooling of the dye medially.

The rose thorn appears to be normal.

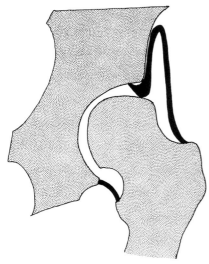

FIGURE 2–146. *Diagram of extension of injected dye into a superior recess (thin pouch) lateral to the labrum indicates adhesion of the capsule to the lateral wall of the ilium.*

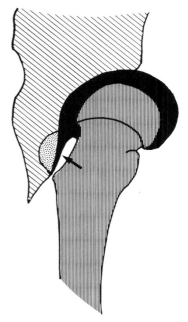

FIGURE 2–147. *Closure of the lower part of the acetabular cavity by the upwardly pulled and adherent capsule and transverse acetabular ligament.*

changes in position of the femur, an intrinsic obstacle to concentric reduction exists.

When the capsule is adherent to the lateral wall of the ilium the injected dye passes into a superior recess lateral to the labrum (Fig. 2–146).

The capsule with the transverse acetabular ligament may be pulled up and adherent to the inferior half of the acetabulum, closing the lower half of the introitus of the acetabular socket (Fig. 2–147).

Hourglass constriction of the capsule is clearly depicted on the arthrogram—the femoral head is in a separate pouch of the capsule in a false acetabulum and separated from the true acetabulum by a narrow isthmus through which passes the attenuated ligamentum teres (Fig. 2–148).

Labrum and Limbus. In the anteroposterior projection the normal fibrocartilaginous labrum is depicted as a triangular area surrounded by contrast material; its apex is lateral and inferior, and its base continuous with the roof of the acetabulum. A "rose thorn" appearance is given by the contrast material outlining the labrum (Fig. 2–149). The labrum constitutes not only

FIGURE 2–148. *Congenital dislocation of the hip in a four-year-old.*

A. Anteroposterior radiogram. **B.** Arthrogram showing the hourglass constriction of the capsule.

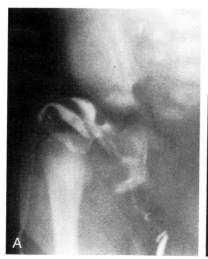

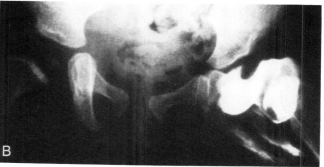

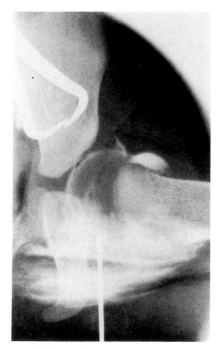

FIGURE 2–149. The "rose thorn" on the arthrogram marking the superolateral margin of a normal fibrocartilaginous labrum.

Note the dye in the inferior part of the acetabulum marking the inferior transverse ligament. The line between the two delineates the introitus to the acetabulum and clasps the greatest diameter of the femoral head.

the superior rim of the acetabulum but also the anterior and posterior rims; the latter are visualized in the lateral projection of the hip.

Normally the limbus thorn clasps the largest diameter of the femoral head; if it does not, either the acetabulum is dysplastic or the hip is subluxated—the reduction is nonconcentric and incongruous.

When an inverted limbus is present the normal "rose thorn" is not seen; instead there is a crescent-shaped filling defect in the superoposterior margin of the joint with the injected dye passing medial to and below its free border (Fig. 2–150).

The pulvinar will be depicted in the arthrogram as an irregular filling defect in the floor of the acetabulum (Fig. 2–151).

The ligamentum teres, if intact and closely investing the femoral head, cannot be seen in the arthrogram. If the hip is subluxated, the redundant and hypertrophied ligamentum teres can be visualized as a space-filling defect.

The femoral head, instead of being spherical, may be flattened posteromedially and become conical or egg-shaped. The arthrogram will show deformation of the femoral head. Thickening of the floor of the acetabulum and deficiency of its wall can also be visualized by arthrography.

Retention of Reduction in Hip Spica Cast. If reduction of the hip is concentric and stable with a wide zone of safety, the hips are immobilized in a bilateral hip spica cast.

Proper positioning of the hip is *crucial.* The reduced hip should be maintained in a physiologic position. Extreme positions of abduction and rotation should be avoided. The ideal position of hip flexion is 90 degrees. Occasionally the hips may require greater flexion to 100 to 110 degrees to provide greater stability of reduction. Such hyperflexed posture of the hip causes no harm; it simulates intrauterine fetal posture. Of course, extreme hyperflexion of the hip may force the femoral head below the socket, into the area of the obturator foramen. Severe hip hyperflexion is an extreme position—avoid it.

Forced extreme abduction of the hips should

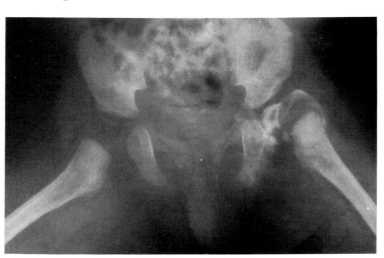

FIGURE 2–150. Inverted limbus.

Note the crescent-shaped defect in the superoposterior part of the joint; the injected dye has passed inferior and medial to the free margin.

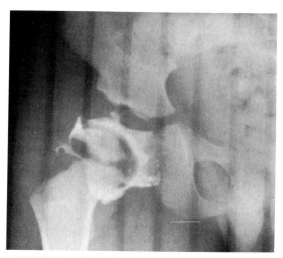

FIGURE 2–151. *Arthrogram of the right hip showing marked laxity of the capsule.*

There is an irregular defect in the floor of the acetabulum caused by the pulvinar.

not be employed, since it may be a factor in avascular necrosis of the femoral head. In regional stress angiography of the hip in autopsy material, Nicholson and associates have demonstrated that the frog-leg position interferes with arterial filling in the hip area. The arteries most affected by this position were the medial femoral circumflex, the lateral femoral circumflex, and the profunda femoris. The effect on the circulation of the hip area was aggravated by hip adductor contracture, while adductor tenotomy abolished it.[670] This work emphasized the advisability of avoiding forced abduction of the hip.

In an experimental study in newborn pigs, Salter produced adduction contracture by immobilizing the hips in adduction for a period of three weeks; then he immobilized the hips for another three weeks in a position of forced abduction. Injection studies disclosed compression of the vessels within the resilient preosseous cartilage of the femoral head and a varying degree of avascular necrosis in all animals. In another group of pigs, Salter prevented development of avascular necrosis by dividing hip adductor muscles prior to placing the hips in forced abduction.[815, 817] His results stress the wisdom of correcting tightness of the hip adductor muscles prior to reduction. A position of extreme flexion (much more than 90 degrees) and mild to moderate abduction was also emphasized by Salter as being much safer and

equally stable for maintenance of reduction in young children.

The Technique of Cast Application. First, the infant is positioned on the infant fracture table (Fig. 2–152 C). An assistant (or preferably the surgeon) holds the lower limbs, maintaining the hips in the predetermined position of flexion, abduction, and rotation. Another assistant applies counter pressure to the shoulders and pushes the baby against the well-padded perineal post. This serves to steady the infant and prevent cephalic migration and extension of the hips. It is vital to allow for abdominal distention following feeding; therefore, a 2-inch-wide stockinette or a towel is folded crisscross on the chest and abdomen (Fig. 2–152 D). The stockinette or towel is removed after the cast sets. The child is appropriately padded with sheetwadding and felt or commercially available self-adhering sponge (such as Reston) (Fig. 2–152 E and F). One or two layers of plaster of Paris are applied and carefully molded over the bony prominence, particularly the greater trochanters and sacral region, and then reinforced with synthetic tape. There should be a definite waistline above the iliac crests. The posterior part of the pelvic portion of the cast is lifted up and smoothly molded over the sacrum. When the infant is young and reduction is stable, the hip spica cast extends only to the knees; but in the older infant, especially if control of hip rotation is crucial to stability of reduction, the cast should extend below the knees with the knees in moderate flexion (Fig. 2–153). Whether the foot and ankle should be included in the cast varies with the preference of the surgeon. Some leave the feet out in order to allow for growth while the infant is in cast. This author includes the feet and ankles, placing them in neutral position because it is more comfortable for the infant to lie prone. The use of synthetic cast tape makes the cast much lighter and stronger.

Following cast application, anteroposterior and, if possible, true lateral radiograms of the hip are made to confirm maintenance of concentric reduction in the cast. Radiographic visualization can be improved by removal of the cast over the hip. If in doubt this author recommends a computed tomographic scan to ensure that the hip is concentrically reduced (Fig. 2–154). If computed tomography is not available, a single-cut laminagram (50 per cent penetration) will assist in visualization of the hip; it is made at the level of the urethra in the female and at the penoscrotal angle in the male. The

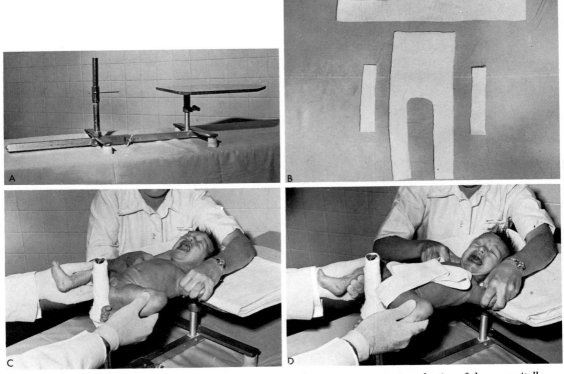

FIGURE 2–152. *Technique of applying bilateral above-knee hip spica cast to retain reduction of the congenitally dislocated left hip in an infant.*

A gentle closed reduction was performed and the success of reduction was confirmed by taking radiograms before the plaster of Paris cast was applied. **A.** Infant fracture table. **B.** Strips of white felt to be used for padding. **C.** Position of infant on the fracture table. Note the surgeon holds the hips in the desired position; the nurse steadies the infant by holding her shoulders and arms, and pushes her against the well-padded perineal post. **D.** Two-inch-wide stockinette is folded criss-cross on the chest and abdomen to allow space for abdominal distention following feeding. (The stockinette is removed after the cast sets.)

cast is trimmed. The perineal opening should be adequate to facilitate toilet, cleansing, and diapering. Soiling of the cast should be prevented. A soiled cast will be odoriferous, and it will soften and cause skin irritation and superficial infection. It is best for the first day or two following cast application for the infant to lie and sleep on a small Bradford frame that is fitted to the crib with the head end elevated. Because water runs downhill, the cast is kept dry. The cast is securely fixed to the Bradford frame and the crib with a restraint (see Fig. 2–152 H). The perineum should be kept dry and clean. The diapers should be changed frequently; urine- and feces-soiled and saturated diapers spell trouble. The parents should be educated to use smaller diapers that are plastic covered and to tuck them beneath the cast edges. Powder should never be placed beneath the cast. Food debris and other objects should not be allowed to fall beneath the cast. A hair

dryer is used to dry the cast if it is inadvertently wetted. Normal activity of the child in the cast should be encouraged. A cast that becomes softened or cracked should be repaired or changed. With adequate care, a hip spica cast should last for six to eight weeks. The importance of parent education in the care of the child and the cast prior to discharge from the hospital cannot be overemphasized.

The period of immobilization in the plaster cast depends on age at diagnosis. A simple rule of thumb is a minimum of six weeks with one month of immobilization added for each month of delay in diagnosis. The total period of immobilization in the cast should not exceed six months. Under this regimen, normal development of the femoral head and acetabulum can be expected.

The initial cast is changed at six to eight weeks postreduction; the change is performed as an outpatient procedure in the hospital and

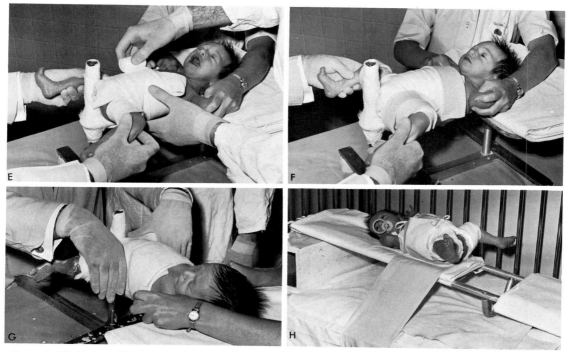

Figure 2–152 *Continued* **E.** System of application of sheath wadding. **F.** The strips of white felt are laid for padding. **G.** Method of molding the plaster of Paris cast above the iliac crests. **H.** Bradford frame fitted to the crib with the head end elevated. Water runs downhill; the cast is kept dry. Note how the infant is securely fixed on the frame with a hip spica cast restrainer.

under general anesthesia. The affected hip is *gently* examined for stability of reduction. Anteroposterior and lateral radiograms of the hips are made out of the cast to verify the maintenance of concentricity of complete reduction. The skin is cleaned thoroughly with soap and lukewarm water, and another hip spica cast is applied. If the stability of the hip is adequate with a wide zone of safety, the position of the hips can be changed to a lesser degree of flexion

and abduction; the cast may extend to only above the knee.

The second cast is changed in six to eight weeks, again under general anesthesia and as an outpatient procedure in the hospital. Depending on the age of the infant at diagnosis and treatment (usually three to four months of age), this may be the last cast. In an older child, a third cast may be required for an additional eight weeks to enhance stability of reduction.

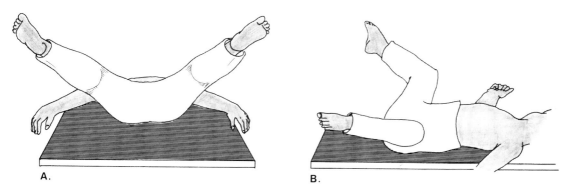

A.   **B.**

FIGURE 2–153. A bilateral below-knee hip spica cast.

Note the hips are in 90 degrees of flexion and only 50 degrees of abduction. The infant is in the human position, not the frog position.

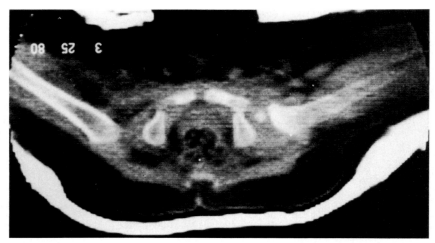

FIGURE 2–154. Computed tomographic scan showing hip dislocated posteriorly in cast.

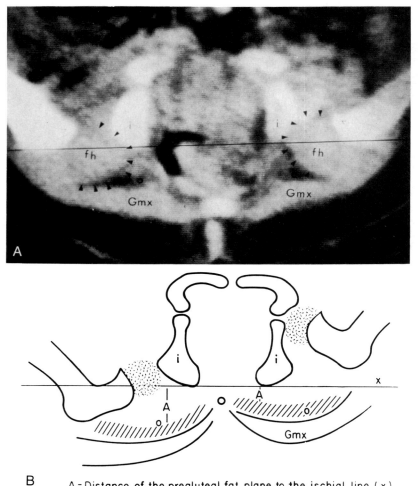

A = Distance of the pregluteal fat plane to the ischial line (x)

FIGURE 2–155. Computed tomography of both hips to determine concentricity of reduction.

A. CT scan of the pelvis through the cast. Note the left femoral head (fh) is dislocated posteriorly (the arrowheads outline the cartilaginous femoral head), projecting posterior to the ischial line; i, ischium. The backward displacement of the pregluteal fat plane (o) is evident. Gmx, gluteus maximus. **B.** Diagram of CT scan illustrating the posterior dislocation of the left hip.

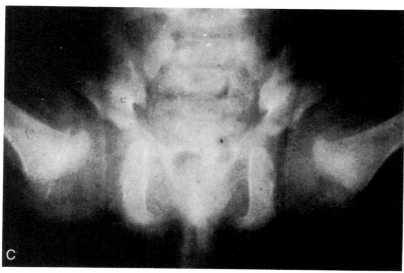

Figure 2–155 *Continued* **C.** Plain anteroposterior radiograms of the hips of the same patient made before the hip spica cast was applied. The left hip was thought to be reduced concentrically.

Following removal of the final cast, a removable containment device is utilized to maintain the hip in moderate flexion, abduction, and lateral rotation. The type of device varies according to the surgeon's choice. This author prefers a Denis Browne hip abduction splint because it controls the degree of hip abduction and flexion and provides a certain degree of controlled mobility (see Fig. 2–135). Motion is life. In the infant under sitting and crawling age, one may use a Pavlik harness. Other surgeons may prefer a rigid posterior hip-knee-ankle orthosis custom-made for the patient, the posterior half of a hip spica cast, a bivalved hip spica cast, or even a Scottish-Rite brace as used for Legg-Perthes disease. The child is gradually weaned from the removable orthosis. Initially the child is out of the brace for two hours twice a day; then after a few weeks, the periods out of the brace are increased to three to four hours twice a day. After that it is worn only at night. The transition to normal activity is gradual. Radiograms of the hips are made periodically to determine the maintenance of concentric reduction and the development of the femoral head and acetabulum.

If the hips are normal, the night splinting is discontinued. Most children require the splint (a removable device) for a period of three to nine months with an average of six months.

Computed Tomography

Because of the transverse orientation of the hip, computed tomography (CT) is of great help in the assessment of the pathologic anatomy of congenital dislocation of the hip and in the planning of its treatment.

Concentricity of Reduction. After closed or open reduction and cast application, the relationship of the femoral head to the acetabulum is determined by anteroposterior and true lateral radiograms of the hips (the latter is sometimes difficult to obtain). Even with good visibility through the cast, this is difficult and sometimes inaccurate (Fig. 2–155). Linear tomography may be misinterpreted because of pelvic obliquity; in bilateral involvement, asymmetry of appearance of the hips will be difficult to detect. A CT scan of the hips is indicated when asymmetry suggests nonconcentric reduction or when there is a question of the adequacy of the reduction because of instability of the hips.

In the CT scan the cartilaginous femoral head may be difficult to visualize because of problems in distinguishing between cartilage and soft tissue such as muscle. The new generation of scanners, however, is providing sufficient resolution to permit visualization of cartilage and the various contents of the acetabulum. The location of the unossified femoral head can be detected as follows: when a section of the femoral neck is made with the hip in flexion–abduction–lateral rotation it has the appearance of a foot in a clog (a "wooden shoe"). The upturn (the hook) of the femoral neck metaphysis indicates the position of the femoral head (Fig. 2–156). It looks like a ball being kicked by a foot with a clog. The anterior boundary of the

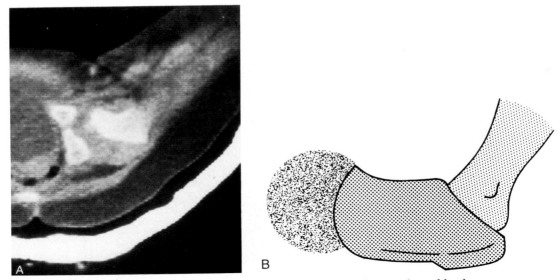

FIGURE 2–156. *Determination of the location of the cartilaginous femoral head.*

A. CT section through the proximal femoral metaphysis with the hip in flexion, abduction, and lateral rotation. Note the contrast material outlining the cartilaginous femoral head. The cartilaginous upper femoral epiphysis has the appearance of a ball being kicked by a foot in a wooden shoe. The tip of the ossified femoral neck metaphysis indicates the most anterior boundary of the femoral neck. **B.** Diagram illustrating the preceding CT section.

femoral head is level with the tip of the upturn of the femoral neck metaphysis. These findings also indicate that the section made is appropriate—through the level of the femoral neck metaphysis. The distance of the hook of the femoral neck from the floor of the acetabulum measures the degree of *lateral displacement* of the femoral head (Fig. 2–157).

Superior displacement is detected by the appearance of the femoral head of the dislocated hip before that of the opposite normal hip as the scan cuts move inferiorly from above. *Posterior displacement* of the femoral head is determined as follows: first draw the *ischial line*, which is a horizontal line tangent to the ischial spines (Fig. 2–158). In the normal hip the

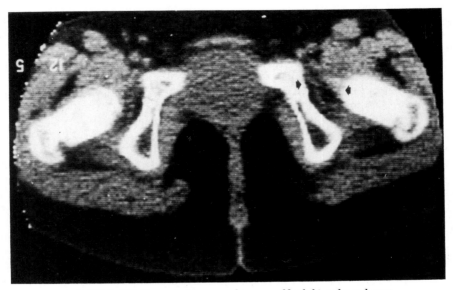

FIGURE 2–157. *Computed tomographic scan of both hips through cast.*

Note the lateral displacement of the hook of the right femoral neck metaphysis (*arrows*).

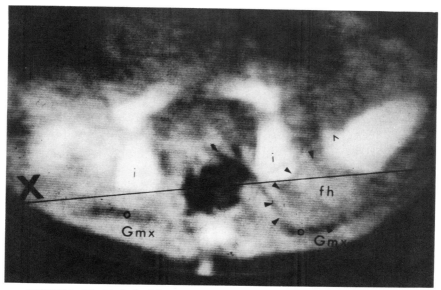

FIGURE 2–158. Method of determining posterior displacement of the femoral head.

The unossified femoral head (fh) outlined by arrowheads is posterior to the ischial line (X), which is a line tangent to the posterior margin of the ischium (i). The pregluteal fat plane (o) in front of the gluteus maximus (Gmx) is displaced and deformed by the unossified femoral head. The location of the femoral head is indicated by the upward hook of the femoral metaphysis (∧).

radiolucent pregluteal fat pad is located anterior to the soft-tissue shadow of the gluteus maximus and immediately posterior to the ischial line (Fig. 2–159). When the femoral head is dislocated posteriorly the pregluteal fat plane is displaced posteriorly and the distance between it and the ischial spine is increased. In unilateral dislocations the asymmetry is evident. The upturned hook of the metaphysis of the femoral neck is displaced posteriorly from its normal position in the acetabulum. This is difficult to detect in even clear plain anteroposterior radiograms.

In posterior dislocation, the femoral head is projected posterior to the ischial line, and the fat plane anterior to the gluteus maximus is displaced backward.

Constriction of the Capsule by the Taut Iliopsoas. The iliopsoas is the most medial of the muscles anterior to the hip joint, apposing closely to the capsule (Fig. 2–160). The CT scan will visualize the indentation and hourglass constriction of the capsule by the psoas tendon, caused by the lateral and upward displacement of the femoral head (Figs. 2–161 and 2–162).

Intra-articular Barriers to Concentric Reduc-

FIGURE 2–159. Diagram of computed tomographic findings in posterior dislocation of the hip.

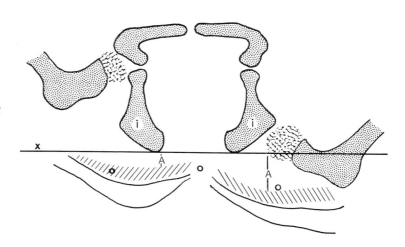

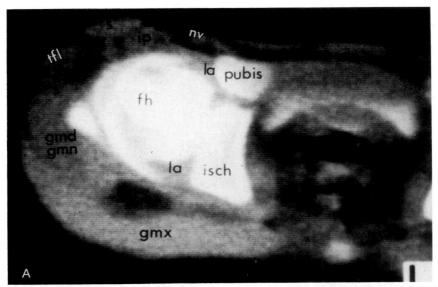

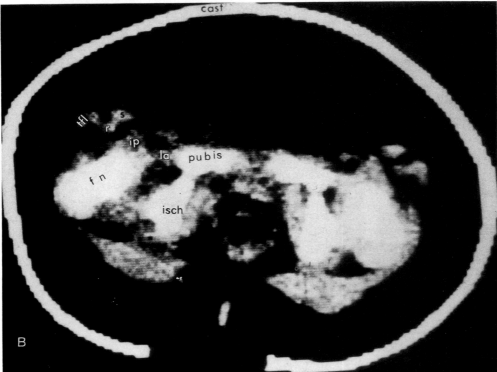

FIGURE 2–160. *Computed tomography of hip demonstrating constriction of the capsule by the contracted iliopsoas tendon.*

A. Normal hip after arthrogram. Note the iliopsoas *(ip)* is the most medial of the muscles anterior to the hip joint; *fh*, femoral head; *la*, labrum; *nv*, neurovascular bundle; *s*, sartorius; *tfl*, tensor fascia latae; *gmd*, gluteus medius; *gmn*, gluteus minimus; *gmx*, gluteus maximus. **B.** Indentation of the capsule by a taut iliopsoas tendon (ip). The acetabular and the capital parts of the capsule are connected by the isthmus *(arrowhead)*.

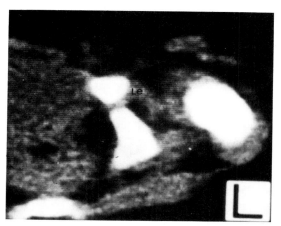

FIGURE 2–161. Computed tomography of hip showing marked constriction of the capsule by a taut iliopsoas tendon.

Note the inverted limbus (Le).

tion. The pulvinar is a fibrofatty tissue, and because of its adipose content, it can be clearly visualized on the CT scan (Fig. 2–163). The hypertrophic ligamentum teres and inverted limbus usually are not adequately depicted; their visualization can be improved by a combination of CT scan and arthrography.

Pin protrusion into the hip joint following Salter or other innominate osteotomy can be detected on the CT scan (Fig. 2–164).

Femoral Torsion. Determination of femoral torsion by CT scan is simple and accurate. It measures the angle directly and obviates the need for trigonometric calculation. The radiation dose with computed tomography is comparable to that with the radiographic method and is probably less than with fluoroscopy. This author recommends the method of Hernandez because it makes use of an immobilization board, which increases its accuracy.[395] There should be no motion between the scans of the upper and lower segments of the femur. The child is immobilized in a specially designed footboard (Fig. 2–165). The board is fitted to the table curvature by shelf brackets attached to one side of the board. Its other side is covered with Velcro. Several sizes of shoes (front ends cut open) are used to fit different foot sizes, and the bottoms of the shoes are also covered with Velcro. The thighs and legs are wrapped to check hip rotation or flexion between scans of femoral necks and condyles. The CT technologist watches carefully that the child does not move. The uncooperative feisty child may have to be sedated. The board is stabilized by placing a heavy object such as a folded lead apron or a sandbag on it.

The *proximal section* is made to visualize the femoral neck. It is usually level with the symphysis pubis. For an ideal section of the femoral neck to determine femoral torsion, the tip of the greater trochanter should be seen in the CT scan. The *distal section* is made to visualize the femoral condyles; it is level with and immediately inferior to the upper pole of the patella. Additional sections are made at increments of 5 to 10 mm. if indicated. CT scans of both sides can be obtained in one section except in lower limb length disparity or pelvic obliquity, in which case separate CT sections of each femur must be obtained.

Next, the sections are depicted on a wide window. The soft tissues are eliminated by making sections at the appropriate levels to provide only bony outline. The image is reversed so that the bone appears black; the

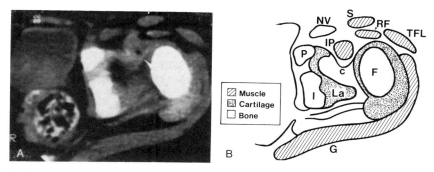

FIGURE 2–162. Computed tomography of hip showing indentation and infolding of capsule by taut iliopsoas tendon.

A. CT scan: the arrowhead points at site of indentation of capsule. **B.** Diagram illustrating the scan. IP, iliopsoas tendon; C, capsule; NV, neurovascular bundle; S, sartorius; RF, rectus femoris; TFL, tensor fasciae latae; La, fibrocartilaginous labrum; F, femoral head; P, pulvinar; I, ischium. (From Hernandez, R., and Poznanski, A.: CT Evaluation of pediatric hip disorders. Orthop. Clin. North Am., *16*:521, 1985. Reprinted by permission.)

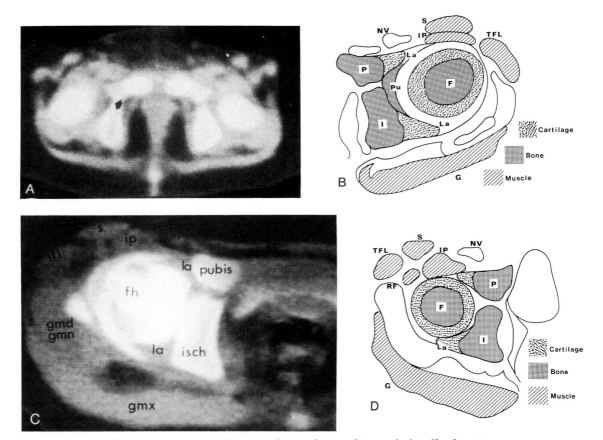

FIGURE 2–163. *Computed tomography visualizing pulvinar, which is fibrofatty tissue.*

A and **B.** CT scan and corresponding diagram of the left hip, showing the pulvinar *(arrow)* in the acetabular cavity; low-attenuation material is the pulvinar. Pu, pulvinar; F, femoral neck; P, pubis; I, ischium; La, labrum; NV, neurovascular bundle; S, sartorius; Tfl, tensor fasciae latae; IP, iliopsoas tendon; G, gluteus maximus; RF, rectus femoris. **C** and **D.** CT scan and the corresponding diagram of the opposite *normal* hip. Pu, pulvinar; F, femoral neck; fh, femoral head; P, pubis; I, ischium; La (la), labrum; NV, neurovascular bundle; S, sartorius; TFL (tfl), tensor fasciae latae; IP (ip), iliopsoas tendon; G (gmx), gluteus maximus; gmd, gluteus medius; gmn, gluteus minimus.

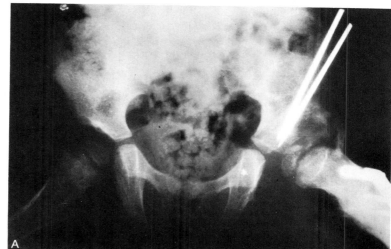

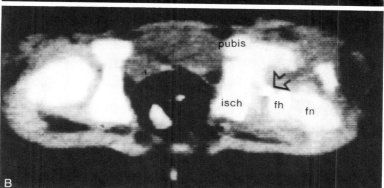

FIGURE 2–164. *Intra-articular protrusion of pins in a child with Salter's innominate osteotomy.*

A. Plain radiogram of the hips. Note the lateral displacement of the left femoral head. **B.** CT scan of the hips. Note the pin *(arrow)* in the joint, keeping the femoral head (fh) displaced posterolaterally.

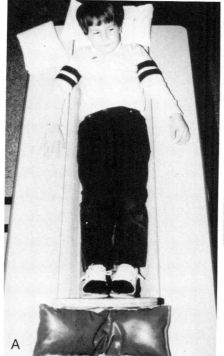

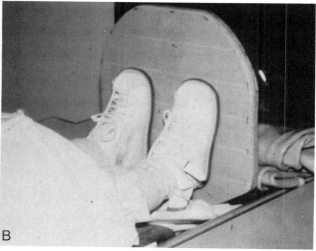

FIGURE 2–165. *Footboard used to immobilize child for computed tomographic determination of femoral torsion.*

There should be no motion between the scans of the upper and lower segments of the femur. The patient is fitted with shoes with velcro-covered soles that are attached to the velcro-covered board. Note the wrapping around the thighs and legs to prevent hip rotation and flexion.

visibility of the bony outline is thereby increased. Expose the section of the femoral neck and condyles on the same film, with the neck section above and the condylar section below (Fig. 2–166). The axis of the femoral neck is drawn (line *D* in Fig. 2–166). In the neonate with a short ossified portion of the femoral neck, it may be less clearly defined. Vertical correction of the femoral neck because of lateral rotation of the hips or severe coxa valga may cause inaccuracies in determination of the femoral neck axis and femoral torsion.

The *transcondylar axis* is determined as follows: first draw tangents to the anterior (line *a*) and posterior (line *b*) borders of the femoral condyles. Then the *transcondylar line* (line *C*) is drawn by drawing a line bisecting the angle between lines *a* and *b*. The degree of torsion of the femur is the angle between the axis of the femoral neck (line *D*) and the transcondylar axis (line *C*). If the lines *C* and *D* meet lateral to the hip, the femur is anteverted (femoral antetorsion); if they meet medially toward the symphysis pubis, there is retrotorsion. A true lateral radiogram of the hip will show femoral retrotorsion (Fig. 2–167).

Configuration of the Acetabulum. The CT scan will determine the depth of the acetabulum, the thickness of its floor, and the size of its anterior and posterior walls (Fig. 2–168). In congenital dislocation of the hip, blunting and failure of development of the acetabulum decrease the capacity of the socket. The scan will also determine the degree of *acetabular torsion*, which is the angle of inclination of the acetabulum in reference to the sagittal plane. Acetabular torsion is determined as follows: first, draw a line tangent to the anterior and posterior lips of the acetabulum; second, draw a vertical line perpendicular to a horizontal line drawn through the center of the triradiate cartilage. The angle formed between the vertical and the tangent lines is the degree of acetabular torsion; if it falls forward of the vertical line the acetabulum is anteverted (Fig. 2–169).

Open Reduction

If a concentric and stable reduction cannot be achieved by the closed method, an open reduction should be carried out. *In the child under walking age*, if the obstacles to concentric reduction are medial and inferior, such as an iliopsoas tendon contricting the capsule and a transverse acetabular ligament, then open reduction by the medial approach may be indicated.

Open Reduction Via the Medial Approach

This was originally described by Ludloff in 1908, and was popularized in the 1970's by Mau and associates and by Ferguson.[285, 572, 625]

The advantages of the medial approach are that it is simple, requiring minimal dissection; blood loss is minimal; and it provides the most direct approach to the obstacles that prevent concentric reduction of the hip, i.e., the iliopsoas tendon, transverse acetabular ligament, and contracted inferoanterior capsule of the hip joint. It does not, however, allow thorough exploration and visualization of the hip, and one cannot adequately expose the redundant capsule. Therefore, plication of the lax capsule to

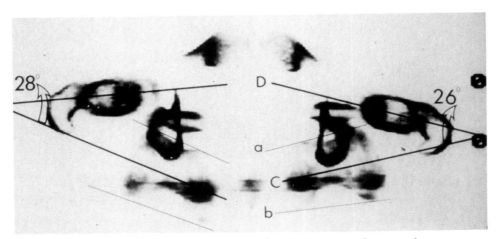

FIGURE 2–166. Determination of femoral torsion by computed tomography.

Reversal of the polarity (so that the bones appear black) and elimination of soft tissues improve the visibility of the bony outline. Line D represents the axis of the femoral neck. Line C is the transcondylar axis—it is drawn by bisecting the angle between the anterior tangent (line a) and the posterior tangent (line b) of the margins of the femoral condyles. Femoral torsion is the angle between line D (femoral neck axis) and line C (transcondylar axis). In this case they meet lateral to the hip. The femur is anteverted—the antetorsion measures 28 degrees on the right and 26 degrees on the left.

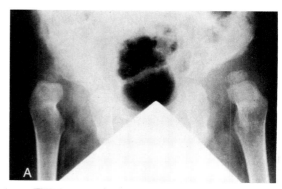

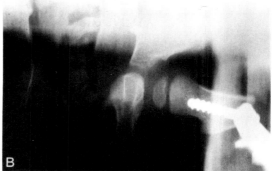

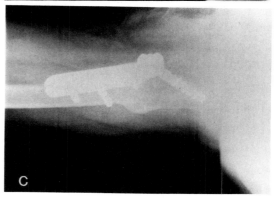

FIGURE 2–167. Femoral retrotorsion following derotation osteotomy.

A. Preoperative anteroposterior radiogram of both hips. Note the dislocated hips. **B.** Lateral radiogram of left hip showing the antetorsion. **C.** Lateral radiogram of right hip showing the retrotorsion.

In the CT scan the transcondylar axis and femoral neck axis will meet medial to the hip joint toward the symphysis pubis, indicating retrotorsion.

prevent redislocation is not feasible. Consequently the capsular hyperlaxity persists, resulting in residual subluxation and failure of development of the acetabulum. A high percentage of the cases (about 40 per cent) require secondary operative procedures such as innominate or femoral osteotomy.[888]

The incidence of avascular necrosis following open reduction by the medial approach is about 10 per cent.[1005] If preliminary traction is not applied, that incidence may be much higher.

In the early 1970's the medial approach for open reduction of congenital dislocation of the hip did achieve great popularity, but recently the enthusiasm has waned, and in some insti-

tutions the procedure has been totally abandoned.[484]

Contraindications. In general the author does not recommend the medial approach for open reduction after walking age; in these hips the capsule will be markedly distended, and capsulorraphy is a very important part of the operation. This approach is also contraindicated in the prenatal dislocation—in these hips the femoral head is riding high and cannot be pulled down easily, there are capsular adhesions between the lateral wall of the ilium and the femoral head, and thorough exposure of the pathologic changes in the capsule and its meticulous repair and plication with femoral short-

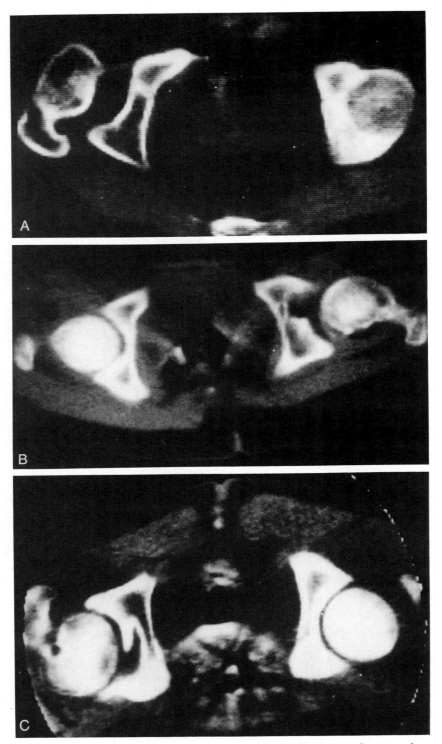

FIGURE 2-168. Configuration of the acetabulum as depicted by computed tomography.

A. The anterior lip of the acetabulum is markedly deficient. **B.** The acetabular capacity is decreased by hypertrophy of the posterior wall of the acetabulum. **C.** Note the bony projection from the posterior lip of the acetabulum, giving the appearance of a double-floor acetabulum.

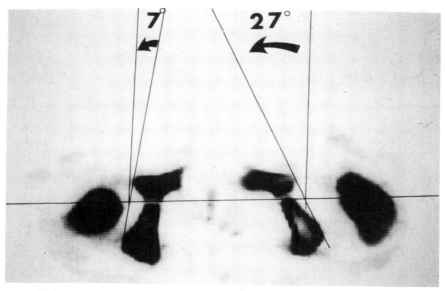

FIGURE 2–169. *Determination of acetabular torsion by computed tomography.*

First draw lines tangent to the anterior and posterior lips of the acetabula. Then draw a horizontal line through the center of the triradiate cartilage and a vertical line perpendicular to it. The angle formed between the vertical and the tangent lines shows the degree of acetabular torsion. If the angle faces forward the acetabulum is anteverted. In this case antetorsion in the left hip is excessive (27 degrees), and in the right normal hip is 7 degrees.

ening are necessary. Teratologic dislocations (such as in arthrogryposis or myelomeningocele) and redislocations of hips that were previously operated on are other contraindications.

Indications. Open reduction via the medial approach is appropriate in typical perinatal dislocation of the hip in a child under 12 months of age (preferably 9 months old, before standing and weight-bearing) when preliminary traction has brought the femoral head down to the level of the acetabulum and when, after a closed reduction performed under general anesthesia, it is discovered that reduction is unstable and nonconcentric, and when arthrography shows that the obstacle to reduction is the iliopsoas tendon constricting the capsule anteroinferiorly or a taut transverse acetabular ligament. It should be explained to the parents that preliminary traction should precede all open reductions via the medial approach and that the excessive femoral and acetabular antetorsion may require subsequent derotation osteotomy of the femur or Salter's innominate osteotomy. It is difficult to perform an adequate capsulorraphy via the medial approach.

The operative technique of open reduction via the medial approach is described and illustrated in Plate 13.

This author prefers to detach the origin of the adductors longus and brevis. This facilitates surgical exposure, and chances of inadvertent division of the medial circumflex artery are minimized. The adductor longus is reattached later to provide better cosmesis, especially in the female.

Ludloff, who described a single case in 1908, three more patients in 1913, and 15 patients in 1914, reported good results in all.[572–574] Chiari, in 1957, reported the results of the medial approach in 43 hips; Salzer and Zuckriegl, in 1967, in 250 hips; and Dorr, in 1968, in 24 hips.[127, 227, 819] In general these authors were favorably impressed by the results of the medial approach. Mau and associates, in 1971, reported 36 good results in a series of 46 hips. Severe avascular necrosis developed in two cases, and there were "transient roentgenographic changes in the femoral head"—which indicates avascular necrosis—in 16 hips. One hip was redislocated. Subsequently 10 hips required innominate osteotomy and 15 required derotation varus osteotomy.[625]

Ferguson, in 1973, reported the results in 32 hips—there were no cases of avascular necrosis, no subsequent operations, and two redislocations. He modified the Ludloff exposure by going posterior to the adductor longus. He also stressed the importance of postoperative im-

Text continued on page 378

Medial (Adductor) Approach for Open Reduction of the Congenitally Dislocated Hip

The patient is placed in supine position, and the ipsilateral hip, hemipelvis, and entire lower limb are prepared and draped in the usual fashion, allowing free mobility of the limb during surgery.

There are two alternative skin incisions, longitudinal and transverse. This author prefers the transverse incision because of its better cosmesis. The iliopsoas tendon and hip joint capsule may be reached by an approach posterior to the adductor brevis, anterior to the adductor brevis and posterior to the pectineus, or anterior to the pectineus.

LONGITUDINAL SKIN INCISION WITH SURGICAL APPROACH POSTERIOR TO ADDUCTOR BREVIS

A. With the hip flexed 70 to 80 degrees, abducted, and laterally rotated, the adductor longus muscle tendon is palpated, and a straight longitudinal incision is made immediately behind the adductor longus muscle for a distance of 6 to 8 cm. It begins at the adductor tubercle and extends distally along the course of the muscle.

B and **C.** The subcutaneous tissue is divided in line with the incision. The deep fascia is divided. The anterior and posterior margins of the adductor longus muscle are delineated, and the muscle is sectioned over a blunt elevator at its origin and retracted distally. The adductor brevis muscle is retracted anteriorly, and the anterior branches of the obturator nerve and vessels are visualized but not disturbed. By blunt digital dissection the interval posterior to the adductor brevis is developed; the lesser trochanter is easily palpated in the intermuscular interval. The iliopsoas tendon is exposed, and the fatty tissue and the bursa over the tendon are elevated. A curved hemostat is inserted beneath the iliopsoas tendon; the tendon is divided by a transverse incision and allowed to retract proximally.

D. Dissection is carried proximally until the femoral head is palpated. Two curved retractors are placed around the femoral neck and capsule, one superolaterally and the other inferomedially to expose the capsule of the hip joint. Next the capsule is divided by a T incision with the longitudinal limb along the long axis of the femoral neck and the transverse limb along the margin of the acetabulum.

Plate 13. Medial (Adductor) Approach for Open Reduction of the Congenitally Dislocated Hip

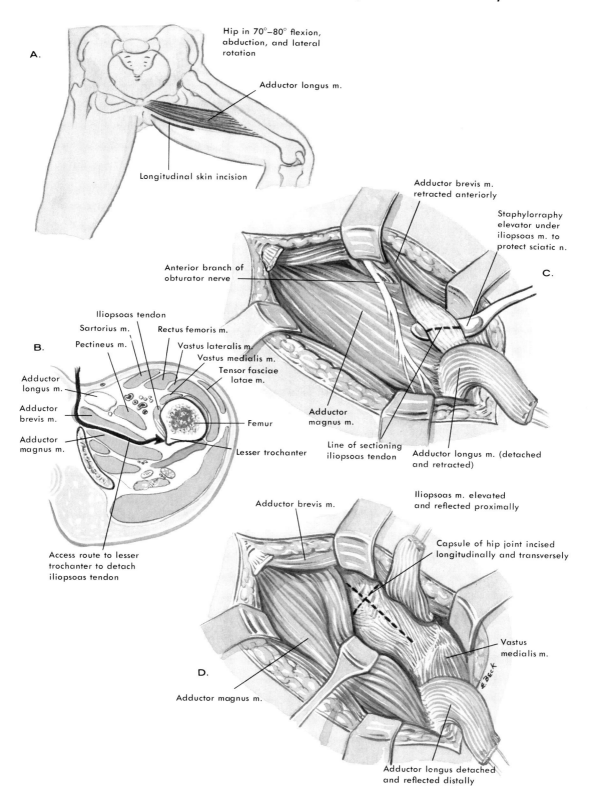

A.

Hip in 70°–80° flexion, abduction, and lateral rotation

Adductor longus m.

Longitudinal skin incision

B.

Iliopsoas tendon

Sartorius m.

Pectineus m.

Rectus femoris m.

Vastus lateralis m.

Vastus medialis m.

Tensor fasciae latae m.

Adductor longus m.

Adductor brevis m.

Adductor magnus m.

Femur

Lesser trochanter

Access route to lesser trochanter to detach iliopsoas tendon

Anterior branch of obturator nerve

Adductor brevis m. retracted anteriorly

Staphylorraphy elevator under iliopsoas m. to protect sciatic n.

C.

Adductor magnus m.

Line of sectioning iliopsoas tendon

Adductor longus m. (detached and retracted)

Iliopsoas m. elevated and reflected proximally

Adductor brevis m.

Capsule of hip joint incised longitudinally and transversely

Vastus medialis m.

D.

Adductor magnus m.

Adductor longus detached and reflected distally

Medial (Adductor) Approach for Open Reduction of the Congenitally Dislocated Hip (Continued)

TRANSVERSE SKIN INCISION WITH SURGICAL APPROACH ANTERIOR TO ADDUCTOR BREVIS AND MEDIAL TO PECTINEUS

E. An alternative surgical approach is through a transverse oblique skin incision about 5 to 7 cm. long centered over the anterior margin of the adductor longus about 1 cm. distal and parallel to the inguinal crease.

F. The deep fascia is divided. One should take care not to injure the saphenous vein, but if necessary it may be ligated and sectioned.

G. The adductor longus muscle is sectioned at its origin and reflected distally. At the anterior margin of the adductor longus the fibers of the pectineus muscle are identified.

Plate 13. Medial (Adductor) Approach for Open Reduction of the Congenitally Dislocated Hip

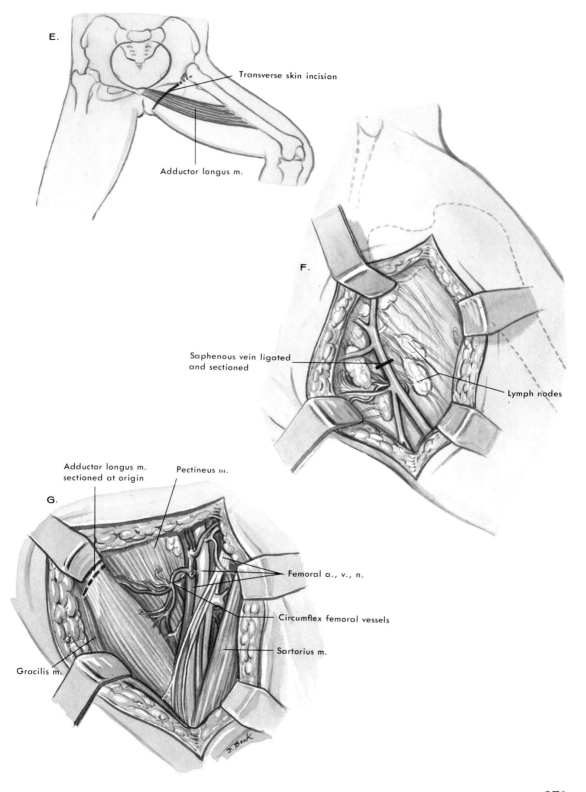

E.

Transverse skin incision

Adductor longus m.

F.

Saphenous vein ligated and sectioned

Lymph nodes

G.

Adductor longus m. sectioned at origin

Pectineus m.

Femoral a., v., n.

Circumflex femoral vessels

Sartorius m.

Gracilis m.

E. Beck

Medial (Adductor) Approach for Open Reduction of the Congenitally Dislocated Hip (Continued)

H and **I.** One can approach the lesser trochanter by a route medial to the pectineus muscle to release the iliopsoas tendon. The pectineus muscle is retracted laterally, protecting the femoral vessels and nerve, and the adductor brevis muscle is retracted medially, bringing the iliopsoas tendon into view at its insertion to the lesser trochanter. A Kelly clamp is passed under the iliopsoas tendon and opened slightly, and the tendon is sectioned.

TRANSVERSE SKIN INCISION WITH SURGICAL APPROACH LATERAL TO THE PECTINEUS

J and **K.** Another route to the lesser trochanter to release the iliopsoas tendon is lateral to the pectineus muscle. In this approach, the pectineus muscle is retracted medially and inferiorly, and the femoral vessels and nerve are retracted laterally, exposing the iliopsoas tendon at its insertion to the lesser trochanter.

Plate 13. Medial (Adductor) Approach for Open Reduction of the Congenitally Dislocated Hip

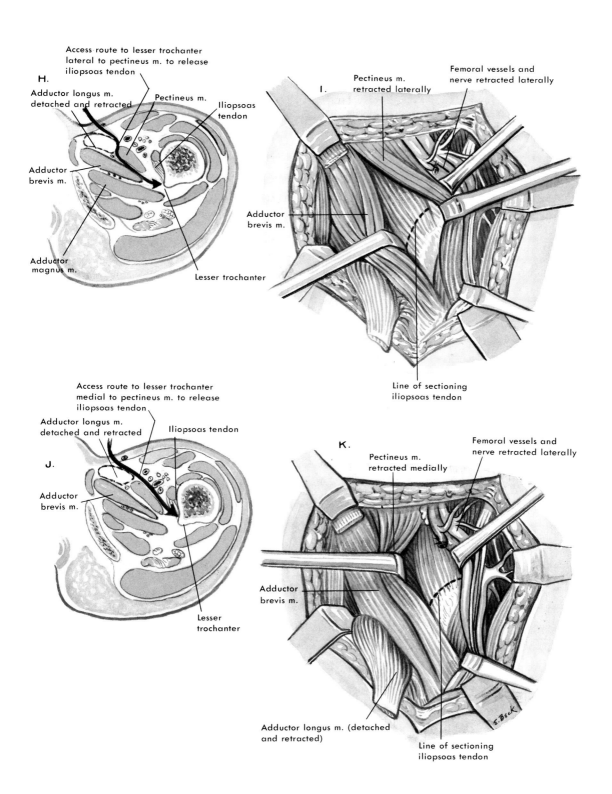

H.

Access route to lesser trochanter lateral to pectineus m. to release iliopsoas tendon

Adductor longus m. detached and retracted

Pectineus m.

Iliopsoas tendon

Adductor brevis m.

Adductor magnus m.

Lesser trochanter

I.

Pectineus m. retracted laterally

Femoral vessels and nerve retracted laterally

Adductor brevis m.

Line of sectioning iliopsoas tendon

J.

Access route to lesser trochanter medial to pectineus m. to release iliopsoas tendon

Adductor longus m. detached and retracted

Iliopsoas tendon

Adductor brevis m.

Lesser trochanter

K.

Pectineus m. retracted medially

Femoral vessels and nerve retracted laterally

Adductor brevis m.

Adductor longus m. (detached and retracted)

Line of sectioning iliopsoas tendon

Medial (Adductor) Approach for Open Reduction of the Congenitally Dislocated Hip (Continued)

L. In all these surgical approaches the psoas tendon is sectioned and allowed to retract proximally, and the iliacus muscle fibers are gently elevated from the anterior aspect of the hip joint capsule.

M and N. The inferior part of the capsule and the transverse ligament are pulled upward with the femoral head. The capsule may adhere to the floor of the acetabulum, and the ligamentum teres may be hypertrophic.

O. The capsule is opened with a longitudinal incision along the long axis of the femoral neck and a transverse cut near the acetabular margin. Incisions in the capsule should be thorough, obtaining joint fluid and visualizing the femoral head. In the drawing a cruciate cut is shown; this author, however, recommends a T-shaped cut as illustrated in Plate 14.

Plate 13. Medial (Adductor) Approach for Open Reduction of the Congenitally Dislocated Hip

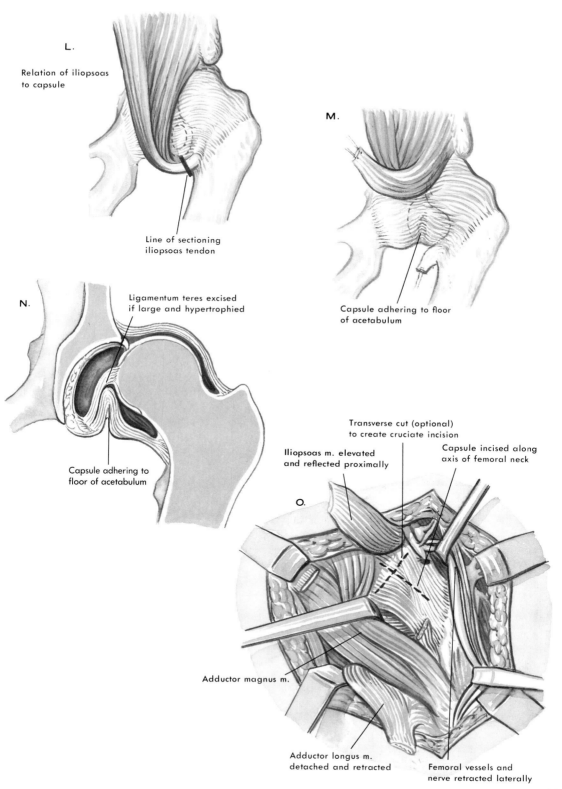

L.

Relation of iliopsoas
to capsule

Line of sectioning
iliopsoas tendon

M.

Capsule adhering to floor
of acetabulum

Ligamentum teres excised
if large and hypertrophied

N.

Capsule adhering to
floor of acetabulum

Transverse cut (optional)
to create cruciate incision

Iliopsoas m. elevated
and reflected proximally

Capsule incised along
axis of femoral neck

O.

Adductor magnus m.

Adductor longus m.
detached and retracted

Femoral vessels and
nerve retracted laterally

375

Medial (Adductor) Approach for Open Reduction of the Congenitally Dislocated Hip (Continued)

P. The transverse acetabular ligament is sectioned, and the ligamentum teres is excised if large and obstructive. The hypertrophied pulvinar is also removed.

Q. Following this, the femoral head can be easily reduced underneath the limbus, and reduction can be maintained by holding the hip in 30 degrees of abduction, 15 degrees of flexion, and 20 degrees of medial rotation. According to Ferguson, it is not necessary to repair the capsule. This author strongly recommends its repair by plication as illustrated in Steps L and M of Plate 14. This author also recommends reattaching the adductor longus tendon to its origin because it is esthetically more pleasing, preventing an ugly depression on the upper medial aspect of the thigh. Tubes are inserted for closed Hemovac suction, and the wound is closed in the usual fashion.

R. A one–and–one half hip spica cast is applied with the hip in 30 degrees of flexion, 30 degrees of abduction, and 10 to 25 degrees of medial rotation. During application and setting of the cast, medially directed pressure is applied over the greater trochanter with the palm.

POSTOPERATIVE CARE

Ferguson recommends that the cast be changed at six-week to two-month intervals with total duration of cast immobilization of about four months. This author believes, however, that with repair of the capsule such prolonged immobilization in cast is unnecessary, and in about six to eight weeks the cast is removed. After removal of the cast, the patient is gradually mobilized. Initially a Denis-Browne hip abduction splint is utilized to maintain the hip abduction and flexion.

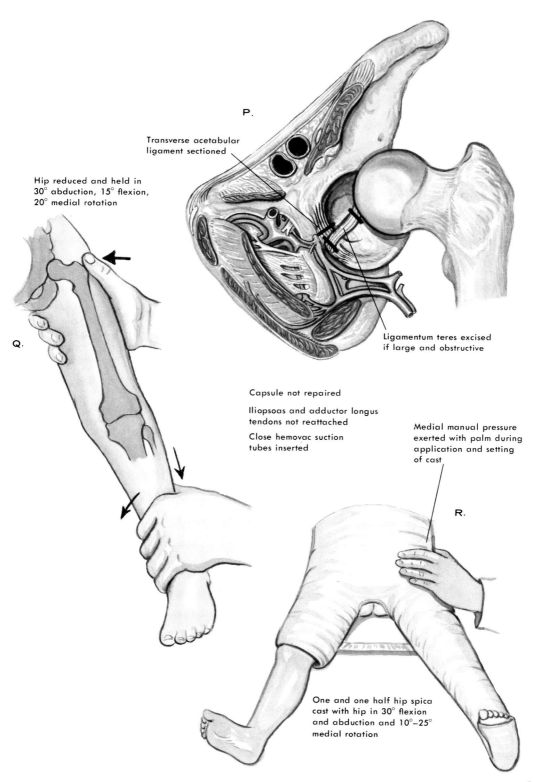

P.

Transverse acetabular ligament sectioned

Hip reduced and held in 30° abduction, 15° flexion, 20° medial rotation

Q.

Ligamentum teres excised if large and obstructive

Capsule not repaired

Iliopsoas and adductor longus tendons not reattached

Close hemovac suction tubes inserted

Medial manual pressure exerted with palm during application and setting of cast

R.

One and one half hip spica cast with hip in 30° flexion and abduction and 10°–25° medial rotation

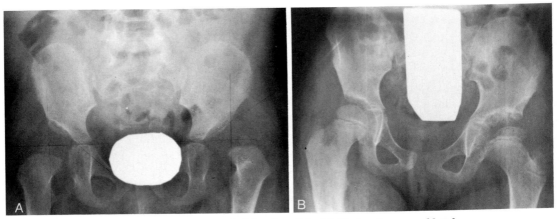

FIGURE 2–170. *Congenital dislocation of the left hip in a two-year-old girl.*

A. Preoperative radiograms. **B.** Postoperative radiograms following open reduction.

mobilization in "functional position" for four months.[285] Weinstein and Ponseti, in 1979, reported the results in 22 hips—two subluxations and 10 per cent avascular necrosis.[1005]

Staheli, in 1982, reported the results in 40 hips. There was avascular necrosis in 8 hips (in 2 clearly due to previous treatment), and residual subluxation and failure of development of the acetabulum in 16 hips (13 of which had iliac or femoral osteotomy).[888]

Open Reduction Via Anterolateral Approach

After walking age, with weight-bearing and progressive upward displacement of the femoral head, sequential pathologic changes take place that act as obstacles to concentric reduction. These barriers to reduction were described in the pathology section. Pelvifemoral muscles

(the iliopsoas, hip adductors, the gluteals, and the rectus femoris) will become shortened and prevent lowering of the femoral head to the level of the acetabulum. These muscles should be elongated to allow reduction without increased tension. The older the child and the higher the dislocation, the greater is the severity of myostatic contractures and the more resistance to pulling down of the femoral head. In addition, the capsule may be adherent to the lateral wall of the ilium. Therefore, it is imperative to apply preoperative traction prior to closed or open reduction.

In high dislocations, one may combine open reduction with femoral shortening. There is controversy whether prereduction traction should be applied if femoral shortening is per-

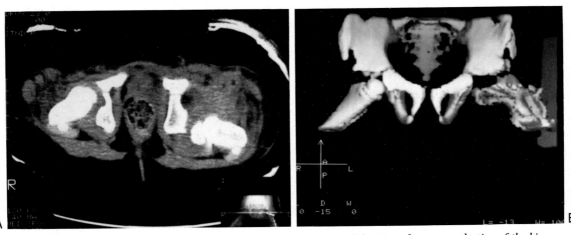

FIGURE 2–171. *Retrotorsion of the left proximal femur and posterior dislocation after open reduction of the hip.*

The retrotorsion is due to excessive derotation osteotomy. Determine the exact degree of antetorsion before derotating the femur. **A.** CT scan through the cast showing posterior dislocation of the left hip. **B.** Three-dimensional reconstruction of CT scan.

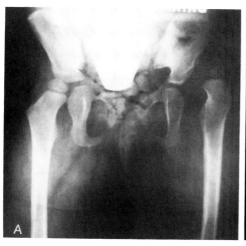 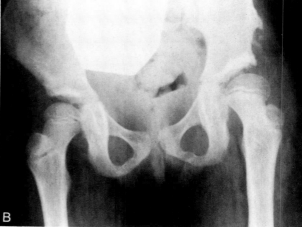

FIGURE 2–172. Congenital dislocation of the hip in a three-year-old child.

A. Preoperative anteroposterior radiogram. **B.** Postoperative radiogram following open reduction with femoral shortening.

formed with an open reduction. This author recommends that all patients be placed in skin *(not skeletal)* traction prior to surgery. It will minimize, if not obviate, the risk of vascular complications.

Indications. The indications for open reduction are a hip dislocation that cannot be reduced, a hip that requires extreme positions to maintain reduction, an unstable reduction, or a nonconcentric reduction. Any of these circumstances demand that an open reduction of the hip be performed. After walking age, the open reduction should be performed by the anterolateral approach. The operative technique is described in Plate 14. An illustrative case is shown in Figure 2–170.

A high dislocation and a dislocation that cannot be reduced after preliminary traction will require femoral shortening combined with open reduction of the hip. It is crucial that prior to surgery a CT scan be performed to determine the exact degrees of femoral antetorsion and acetabular antetorsion.

Routine derotation of the femur with femoral shortening may cause retrotorsion and posterior displacement of the femoral head (Fig. 2–171). The technique of femoral shortening with derotation osteotomy combined with open reduction of the hip is illustrated in Plate 15. An illustrative case is shown in Figure 2–172.

Antenatal Dislocation of the Hip

Hip dislocation in utero may occur at varying periods of gestation: in the twelfth or the eighteenth week, or during the final four weeks. The severity of pathologic findings varies according to the fetal age at dislocation. The longer the duration of dislocation, the more severe the pathologic changes.

Ordinarily, in prenatal dislocation, the acetabulum is small, very shallow and flat in its upper half, filled with fibrofatty tissue, and often not large enough to contain the femoral head (Fig. 2–173 C). The ligamentum teres is hypertrophic; the capsule is markedly thickened, dilated, and adherent to the femoral head. Soft-tissue planes are ill-defined, and the muscle contractures are so taut that they preclude any manipulative reduction. The femoral head is displaced high, articulating in a secondary acetabulum in the lateral wall of the ilium. The femoral head is distorted in shape, flattened medially, and hypoplastic (Fig. 2–173 F). The degree of antetorsion may be normal or increased, or there may be no antetorsion at all or retrotorsion. The femoral neck is often short (Fig. 2–173 I). Femoral antetorsion may be lacking with early dislocation at the twelfth week of gestation.

Treatment of prenatal dislocation is operative, often reduction with femoral shortening. Reconstruction of the acetabulum may be required (Fig. 2–174). This author prefers that acetabular reconstruction be staged as a subsequent procedure and not be performed concurrently with open reduction.

Problems and Complications

Resubluxation or Redislocation. Anatomic factors that cause instability of reduction are excessive laxity of the capsule, increased femoral antetorsion, excessive acetabular antetorsion, and insufficiency of the acetabulum.

In the pathogenesis of typical congenital dis-

Text continued on page 391

Open Reduction of Congenital Hip Dislocation Through Anterolateral Approach

OPERATIVE TECHNIQUE

A. The patient is placed in lateral position, and the entire lower limb, affected half of the pelvis, and lower part of the chest are prepared and draped to allow free motion of the hip. Then the patient is turned to lie in completely supine position. Image intensifier radiographic control should be available.

The skin incision extends from the junction of the posterior and middle thirds of the iliac crest to the anterior superior iliac spine and then distally into the thigh for about 7 to 10 cm. in the groove between the tensor fasciae latae and the sartorius muscles.

B. The deep fascia is incised over the iliac crest, and the fascia lata is opened in line with the skin incision.

The lateral femoral cutaneous nerve is identified; it crosses the sartorius muscle 2.5 cm. distal to the anterior superior iliac spine and lies close to the muscle's lateral border. A longitudinal incision is made over the medial part of the fascia covering the tensor fasciae latae; this 1 cm.-wide strip of fascia is mobilized by sharp dissection and used to protect the lateral femoral cutaneous nerve while the nerve is retracted medially with Silastic tubing or a hernia tape.

C. Blunt dissection is used to open the groove between the tensor fasciae latae muscle laterally and the sartorius and rectus femoris muscles medially, and the fatty layer of tissue that covers the front of the capsule of the hip joint is exposed. The ascending branches of the lateral femoral circumflex vessels cross the midportion of the wound. If they are in the way, they must be isolated, clamped, cut, and ligated.

D. With a scalpel, the cartilaginous iliac apophysis is split through the middle down to bone from the junction of its posterior and middle thirds to the anterior superior iliac spine. With a broad periosteal elevator, the lateral part of the apophysis and the tensor fasciae latae and the gluteus medius and minimus muscles are subperiosteally stripped and reflected as a continuous sheet to the superior rim of the acetabulum anteriorly and the greater sciatic notch posteriorly.

Plate 14. Open Reduction of Congenital Hip Dislocation Through Anterolateral Approach

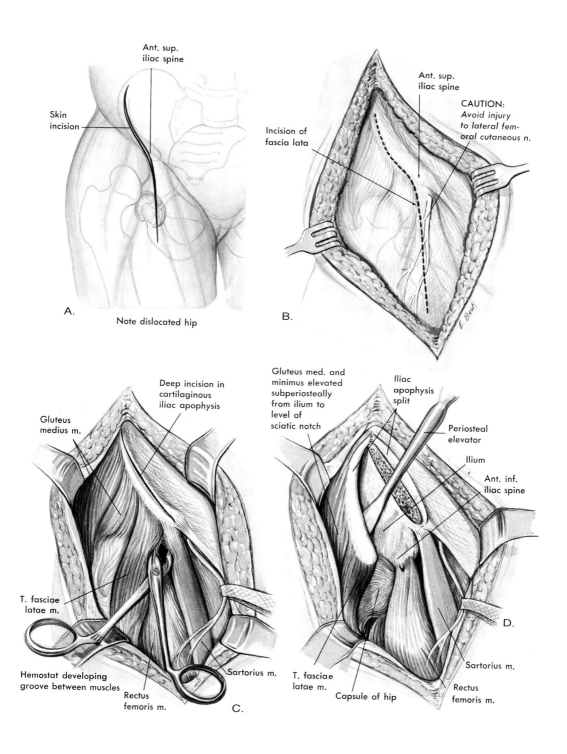

A.

Ant. sup.
iliac spine

Skin
incision

Note dislocated hip

B.

Ant. sup.
iliac spine

Incision of
fascia lata

CAUTION:
*Avoid injury
to lateral fem-
oral cutaneous n.*

E. Beck

C.

Deep incision in
cartilaginous
iliac apophysis

Gluteus
medius m.

T. fasciae
latae m.

Hemostat developing
groove between muscles

Rectus
femoris m.

Sartorius m.

D.

Gluteus med. and
minimus elevated
subperiosteally
from ilium to
level of
sciatic notch

Iliac
apophysis
split

Periosteal
elevator

Ilium

Ant. inf.
iliac spine

T. fasciae
latae m.

Capsule of hip

Sartorius m.

Rectus
femoris m.

381

Open Reduction of Congenital Hip Dislocation Through Anterolateral Approach (Continued)

E. Next, the origin of the sartorius muscle is detached from the anterior superior iliac spine, and its free end is marked with 2-0 Mersilene whip sutures for later reattachment. The sartorius muscle is reflected distally and medially. The two heads of the rectus femoris—the direct one from the anterior inferior iliac spine and the reflected one from the superior margin of the acetabulum—are divided at their origin, marked with 2-0 Mersilene whip sutures, and reflected distally.

F. The hip is then flexed, abducted, and laterally rotated, exposing the iliacus muscle fibers, iliopsoas tendon, and lesser trochanter. A moist hernia tape is passed around the femoral nerve and gently retracted medially with the femoral vessels. With a moist sponge and a periosteal elevator, the iliacus muscle fibers are elevated and dissected free of the capsule, which is thus exposed superiorly, anteriorly, and inferiorly.

The iliopsoas muscle is usually short; it is lengthened by two transverse incisions of its tendinous fibers only. Care should be taken not to injure the medial circumflex artery. When the hip is hyperextended, the tendinous fibers will slide and separate on the muscle, lengthening the iliopsoas.

G. At this point an attempt is made to reduce the dislocated hip in order to determine the factors obstructing closed reduction. Manipulation should not be forcible. If reduction is not possible, either there are intracapsular factors in the obstruction or all obstructing extracapsular factors have not been relieved, or both.

H. Next, the capsule and synovium are incised parallel to the superior and anterior margins of the acetabulum. Enough of a brim (usually ¼ to ⅜ inch) of the capsule should be left medially with the acetabulum and marked with 2-0 Mersilene sutures for capsuloplasty later. Superiorly, a longitudinal incision is made parallel with the neck of the femur, converting the capsular incision into a T. The free edges of the capsule are marked with 2-0 Mersilene sutures for traction and later plication.

Plate 14. Open Reduction of Congenital Hip Dislocation Through Anterolateral Approach

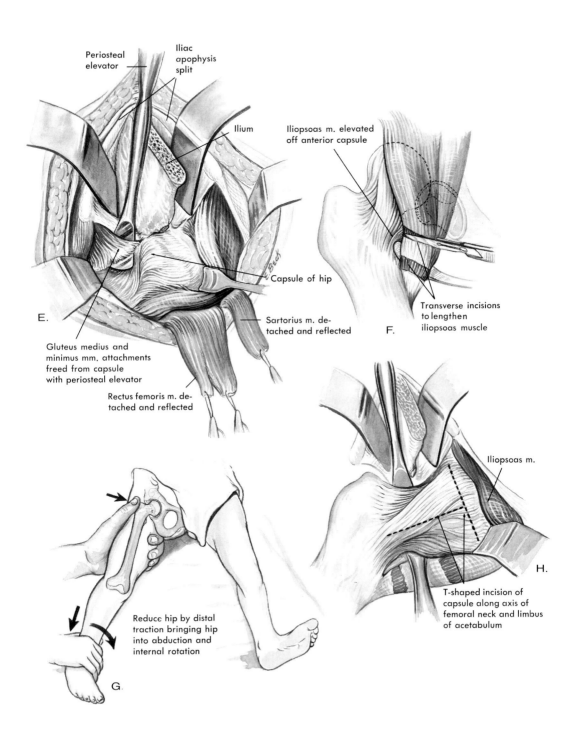

E.

Periosteal elevator

Iliac apophysis split

Ilium

Capsule of hip

Sartorius m. detached and reflected

Gluteus medius and minimus mm. attachments freed from capsule with periosteal elevator

Rectus femoris m. detached and reflected

F.

Iliopsoas m. elevated off anterior capsule

Transverse incisions to lengthen iliopsoas muscle

G.

Reduce hip by distal traction bringing hip into abduction and internal rotation

H.

Iliopsoas m.

T-shaped incision of capsule along axis of femoral neck and limbus of acetabulum

Open Reduction of Congenital Hip Dislocation Through Anterolateral Approach *(Continued)*

I. The hip joint is inspected for intra-articular factors obstructing reduction. The ligamentum teres is usually elongated and enlarged and may prevent anatomic reduction; if so, it should be excised. First, the femoral head end of the ligamentum teres is divided, and the opposite end is traced to the acetabular notch at the lower part of the true acetabulum, where it is divided by two cuts—one anterior and the other posterior. In this way injury to the acetabular branch of the obturator vessels is avoided, and one can easily release the transverse acetabular ligament, which is displaced superiorly with the inferior part of the capsule.

J. Next, the acetabulum is inspected. It may be filled with fibrofatty tissue, which may interfere with optimal seating of the femoral head within the socket; if so, it is excised with a sharp scalpel and curet. One should be cautious, however, not to remove articular cartilage with it.

K. The limbus may be inverted into the acetabulum, in which case its free edge is everted with a blunt hook and grasped with a hemostat. Its base is freed with either the tip of the hook or scalpel, and it is excised with strong curved scissors. It is important not to injure growth zones of the rim of the acetabulum.

Next, one inspects and determines (1) the depth of the acetabulum and the inclination of its roof, (2) the shape of the femoral head and the smoothness and condition of the articular hyaline cartilage covering it, (3) the degree of antetorsion of the femoral neck, and (4) the stability of the hip after reduction. The femoral head is placed in the acetabulum under direct vision by flexing, abducting, and medially rotating the hip while applying traction and gentle pressure against the greater trochanter. This maneuver is reversed to redislocate the hip. The position of the hip when the femoral head comes out of the acetabulum is determined and noted in the operative record. If necessary, sterile fine-mesh tantalum gauze is wrapped around the cartilaginous femoral head to delineate it, the hip is reduced, and radiographs are made. The tantalum gauze is then removed. If the hip joint is unstable or if, upon reduction under direct vision, the femoral head is insufficiently covered superiorly and anteriorly, one should decide whether to perform Salter's innominate osteotomy or a derotation osteotomy of the proximal femur at this time.

Plate 14. Open Reduction of Congenital Hip Dislocation Through Anterolateral Approach

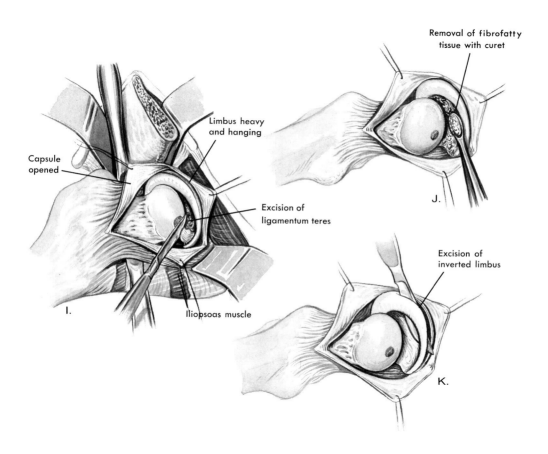

Capsule opened

Limbus heavy and hanging

Excision of ligamentum teres

Iliopsoas muscle

I.

Removal of fibrofatty tissue with curet

J.

Excision of inverted limbus

K.

Open Reduction of Congenital Hip Dislocation Through Anterolateral Approach (Continued)

L and **M.** A careful capsuloplasty is performed next and it is very important to keep the femoral head in its anatomic position in the acetabulum. With the femoral head reduced, the hip joint is held by a second assistant in 30 degrees of abduction, 30 to 45 degrees of flexion, and 20 to 30 degrees of medial rotation throughout the remainder of the operation. The degree of medial rotation depends on the severity of antetorsion.

The large, redundant superior pocket of capsule should be obliterated by plication and overlapping of its free edges. The capsule should also be tightened medially and anteriorly by a vest-over-pants closure. If it is too lax and redundant, a portion may be excised. First, the medial part of the capsule that was left attached to the margin of the acetabulum is everted by pulling the previously placed Mersilene sutures anteriorly and superiorly. Next, the superolateral segment of the T is brought inferomedially and sutured with interrupted sutures to the inner surface of the capsule there. Then the inferolateral segment is brought up and over the superolateral segment and sutured with interrupted sutures to the inner superoposterior surface of the medial part of the capsule. Next, the capsule is tautened anteriorly and medially, bringing the medial segment over the lateral segments and suturing it to them by interrupted Mersilene sutures. Skeletal fixation (e.g., a Steinmann pin to fix the proximal femur to the innominate bone) is unnecessary because the hip joint will be very stable following capsuloplasty as just described. The two halves of the iliac apophysis are sutured together over the iliac crest. The rectus femoris and sartorius muscles are resutured to their origins. The wound is closed in the routine manner. An anteroposterior radiograph of the hips is taken to double check the concentricity of reduction before a one–and–one half spica cast is applied with the hip in about 45 degrees of abduction, 60 to 70 degrees of flexion, and 20 to 30 degrees of medial rotation. The knee is always flexed at 45 to 60 degrees to relax the hamstrings and to control rotation in the cast.

POSTOPERATIVE CARE

Immobilization in a hip spica cast following open reduction and capsuloplasty is for four to six weeks. When a simultaneous derotation femoral osteotomy or Salter's innominate osteotomy is also performed, the cast is kept on for six weeks. Following these periods, the cast is bivalved, and radiographs of the hips are taken with the cast off. The child is allowed to move his lower limbs actively. Passive exercises should be avoided, as they stretch the shortened retinacular vessels. A bivalved hip spica cast, such as a hip abduction splint, is used at night. As soon as functional range of motion of the hips is obtained, partial weight-bearing with a three-point crutch gait is begun. It may be difficult to teach this to the young child. Full weight-bearing is started in four to six weeks, following removal of the solid cast. The bivalved hip spica cast or a hip abduction splint is used at night for 6 to 12 months, depending on the age of the patient, the degree of femoral antetorsion, and the adequacy of the acetabular roof.

Plate 14. Open Reduction of Congenital Hip Dislocation Through Anterolateral Approach

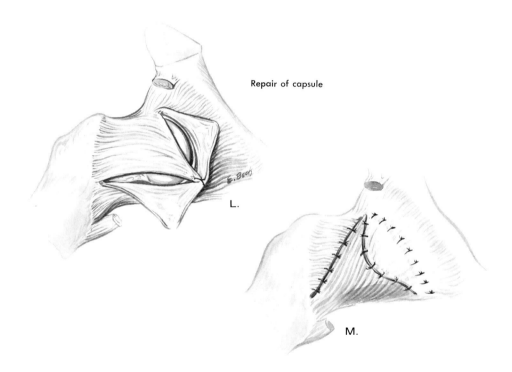

Repair of capsule

L.

M.

Femoral Shortening and Derotation Osteotomy Combined With Open Reduction of the Hip

This author performs femoral shortening and derotation osteotomy through a separate lateral longitudinal incision (See Plate 16, Steps **A** and **B**). (Coleman employs the iliofemoral approach and a large skin incision that begins at the midpart of the iliac crest, extends forward to the anterior superior iliac spine, then distally for 5 to 7 cm. over the upper thigh, paralleling the interval between the tensor fasciae latae and the sartorius muscles, and then curves posteriorly over the lateral aspect of the upper thigh, ending at the midlateral part of the upper femur. It is deepened, the tensor fasciae latae muscle is cut transversely, and the underlying vastus lateralis muscle is exposed by reflecting the divided tensor fasciae latae laterally. The tendinous insertion of the gluteus maximus, identified posteriorly, is left intact. The vastus lateralis muscle is detached at its origin, elevated, and reflected distally to expose the anterior and lateral surfaces of the intertrochanteric region and upper femoral shaft.)

Exposure of the upper femoral shaft through a separate longitudinal incision of the upper thigh is technically simpler, bleeding is less, and the scars esthetically more attractive. It is vital to expose a sufficient length of the upper femoral shaft subperiosteally.

In irreducible dislocation, femoral shortening facilitates reduction and, when reduction is difficult because of increasing pressure on the femoral head, decompresses the hip.

OPERATIVE TECHNIQUE

A. The amount of shortening is determined preoperatively by measuring the distance between the inferior margin of the femoral head and the floor of the acetabulum. The roof of the true acetabulum may be oblique and deficient, and measuring from it to the top of the femoral head may pose problems. Insufficient femoral shortening should be avoided. If inadequate, it will not permit positioning of the femoral head in the true acetabulum, and postoperatively, pressure on the femoral head leads to cartilage necrosis and a stiff hip joint.

Another method of determining the amount of femoral shortening desired is to reduce the femoral head in the acetabulum and measure the overlap of the osteotomized segments.

Next, a "score" of adequate length is made on the anterior aspect of the femur parallel to its longitudinal axis to serve as an orientation mark to determine the degree of rotation after osteotomy and resection. As an added safety measure this author recommends insertion of threaded Steinmann pins of appropriate diameter, one in the upper femoral segment and another in the distal segment.

B. Next, the femur is shortened by two parallel transverse osteotomies; the first immediately distal to the inferior pole of the lesser trochanter and the second distal to it. The osteotomies are performed with an oscillating power saw. This author prefers to make a four-fifths osteotomy first at each of the two levels. Then the four-hole plate of appropriate size is applied on the lateral aspect of the upper femoral shaft and firmly fixed with two screws to the upper segment. The osteotomies are completed, the segment of femur is resected, the distal segment is rotated laterally, and the bone surfaces are apposed.

C. Then the lower two screws are inserted, fixing the plate to the distal segment.

After the femoral osteotomy is firmly fixed, the femoral head is repositioned in the acetabulum. The stability of reduction is determined, and the adequacy of "decompression" of the hip is double checked. As a rule the degree of hip decompression is adequate if one can distract the reduced femoral head from the socket for about 3 to 4 mm. without much tension.

The lateral thigh wound is closed in the usual manner. Repair of the hip joint capsule and other steps are illustrated and described in Plate 14.

POSTOPERATIVE CARE

Care is like that for open reduction of the hip. The plate is removed three to six months postoperatively when the osteotomy is solidly healed.

Plate 15. Femoral Shortening and Derotation Osteotomy Combined With Open Reduction of the Hip

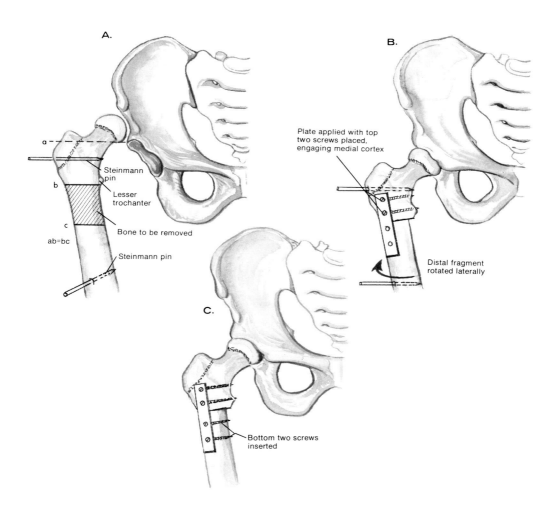

A.

a

Steinmann pin

b

Lesser trochanter

c

Bone to be removed

ab=bc

Steinmann pin

B.

Plate applied with top two screws placed, engaging medial cortex

Distal fragment rotated laterally

C.

Bottom two screws inserted

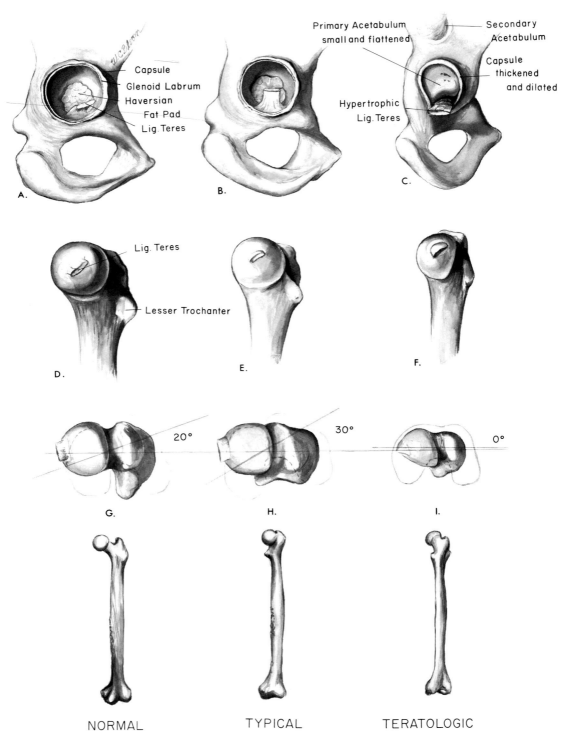

NORMAL   TYPICAL   TERATOLOGIC

FIGURE 2–173. Pathologic findings in typical and teratologic dislocation of the hip in the newborn.

A, D, and **G.** The normal for comparison. **B.** In typical dislocation the acetabulum may be smaller in circumference, but is normal in shape and depth. Significant pathologic findings include abnormal laxity of the capsule and elongation of the ligamentum teres. **C.** The acetabulum in teratologic dislocation of the hip is considerably smaller than normal, shallow and flat in its upper half, and filled with fibrofatty tissue. The capsule is markedly dilated and thickened. Note also the thickened ligamentum teres. **E.** In typical dislocation the femoral head may be smaller than normal, but it is of normal configuration. **F.** In teratologic or antenatal dislocation it is flattened medially, distorted in shape, and considerably smaller than normal. **H.** In typical dislocation of the hip the angle of anteversion is usually greater than normal, about 30 degrees. **I.** In teratologic dislocation the femoral neck is shortened and shows almost no antetorsion. (Redrawn from Hass, J.: Congenital Dislocation of the Hip. Springfield, Ill., Charles C Thomas, 1951.)

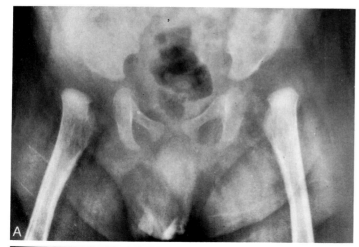

FIGURE 2–174. *Prenatal dislocation of the hip in a three-month old child treated with open reduction and femoral shortening.*

A. Preoperative radiograms. **B.** Postoperative radiograms. **C.** After removal of the plates four years later.

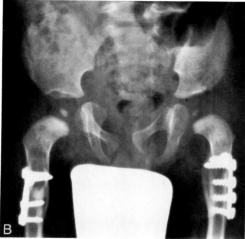

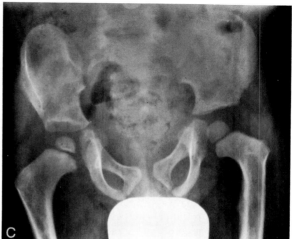

location of the hip, excessive laxity of the hip capsule and its associated ligaments is a major factor. After closed treatment, if the capsule does not tauten or, in cases treated with open reduction, if repair of the capsule is inadequate or if, after adequate repair, the capsule restretches, subluxation and dislocation of the hip will recur, especially if this situation is coupled with excessive femoral antetorsion and acetabular insufficiency.

The second anatomic factor in resubluxation of the hip is excessive femoral antetorsion. In almost all cases of typical congenital dislocation of the hip, there is increased femoral anteversion. After closed reduction of the hip the forces exerted by the acetabulum and the muscles on the proximal femur tend to correct the excessive antetorsion, especially in the infant and young child. In some children, femoral antetorsion persists and will cause resubluxation of the hip joint. The third anatomic factor in hip instability

is persisting antetorsion and insufficiency of the acetabulum. Subluxation of the hip may be reducible or irreducible.

When a hip joint resubluxates, it is crucial that arthrography and CT studies be performed to determine whether concentric and complete reduction can be accomplished and which factors are causing the subluxation. Is it excessive capsular laxity, excessive femoral antetorsion, excessive acetabular antetorsion, or deficiency and inadequacy of the acetabulum? All four factors may be operative singly or, often, in combination in the production of hip subluxation.

Treatment depends on whether the subluxation is reducible or irreducible. An irreducible subluxation requires open reduction.

Concentric reduction is the primary step in treating congenital dislocation of the hip. Femoral or innominate osteotomy should never be performed unless concentric reduction has been obtained. The second step is to maintain the reduction and enhance stability of the hip. An important factor in treatment is the age of the patient. Treatment of reducible subluxation will depend on the patient's age. In the infant and the young child up to two or three years of age, splinting the hip in abduction, flexion, and lateral rotation will tauten the capsule and will also decrease femoral antetorsion and acetabular antetorsion. This author therefore recommends full- or part-time dynamic splinting of the hip in infancy and early childhood. Initially, a solid hip spica cast may be required for three months. Once the patient reaches three years or more of age, femoral osteotomy or innominate osteotomy may be required to increase stability of the hip joint.

Femoral Osteotomy to Correct Excessive Antetorsion and Valgus Deviation of the Proximal Femur

Indications. The principal indications for proximal femoral osteotomy in congenital dislocation of the hip are instability of the hip joint and retardation of normal development of the acetabulum caused by femoral antetorsion, valgus deviation of the proximal femur, or both. Correction of these abnormalities will increase stability of the hip, and concentric reduction will stimulate normal growth and development of the acetabulum. The purpose of femoral osteotomy is to correct an axial deformation of the proximal femur and not to create one—i.e., if the upper femur is of normal configuration, a proximal femoral osteotomy in an effort to provide hip joint stability is contraindicated because, in such an instance, the dysplastic acetabulum and the laxity of the capsule are the most probable causes of the hip joint instability.

Prerequisites. *First*, there must be concentric and stable reduction of the femoral head in the acetabulum when the hip is medially rotated (to neutralize antetorsion) and abducted (to compensate for coxa valga). If the femoral head cannot be placed concentrically in the acetabulum and stabilized by abducting and medially rotating the lower limb, the stability of the hip joint will not be increased by femoral osteotomy and the hip will be subluxated after osteotomy. *Second*, there should be functional or adequate range of hip motion (preferably an arc of 50 to 60 degrees' abduction-adduction and 50 to 60 degrees' rotation). Femoral osteotomy in the presence of restricted range of motion will cause a deformity in attitude. When medial rotation of the hip is limited, lateral rotational osteotomy will result in a laterally rotated hip, whereas when abduction of the hip is restricted, varus

osteotomy will cause an adducted attitude of the hip. The *third* prerequisite is the presence of deformation of the proximal femur. In the absence of femoral antetorsion there is no sense in performing derotation osteotomy and causing femoral retrotorsion and possibly posterior subluxation of the hip. In the absence of coxa valga, varus osteotomy should not be performed. The author disagrees with Chuinard and Logan, who recommend varus osteotomy routinely in the treatment of congenital dislocation of the hip in children 18 months of age or older. Chuinard claims the varus angle is corrected gradually with skeletal growth; this is unpredictable, however, especially in children over five or six years of age.[138, 139, 142, 143] An important factor in spontaneous correction is the health of the capital physis. Varization osteotomy is contraindicated in the presence of total necrosis of the femoral head. Another consideration is limb length. Varization osteotomy will shorten the limb, and the shortening may be temporary or permanent.

Preoperative Assessment. Often apparent valgus deformity of the femoral neck is due to excessive antetorsion. Anteroposterior radiographs of the upper femur with the hip in varying degrees of medial rotation will demonstrate that the "coxa valga" is only apparent— the femoral neck-shaft angle will decrease with increasing medial rotation of the hip. It is important to distinguish true from apparent valgus deformity.

Prior to surgery, thorough radiographic studies should be carried out to determine the degree of deformation of the proximal femur and acetabulum and to demonstrate articular relations between the femoral head and acetabulum that can be anticipated after femoral osteotomy. The following radiographic studies are recommended.

First, an anteroposterior projection of both hips with the hips in neutral position (as to abduction-adduction, medial-lateral rotation, and flexion-extension); this will provide information about the position of the femoral head in the acetabulum in the normal weight-bearing posture of the lower limbs (Fig. 2–175 A).

Next, anteroposterior radiographs are made with the hips in carefully measured degrees of medial rotation and abduction to position the femoral head concentrically in the acetabulum. The amount of medial rotation determines the degree of derotation angle required, and the amount of abduction determines the degree of varus angle necessary for concentricity of the hip in weight-bearing position (Fig. 2–175 B).

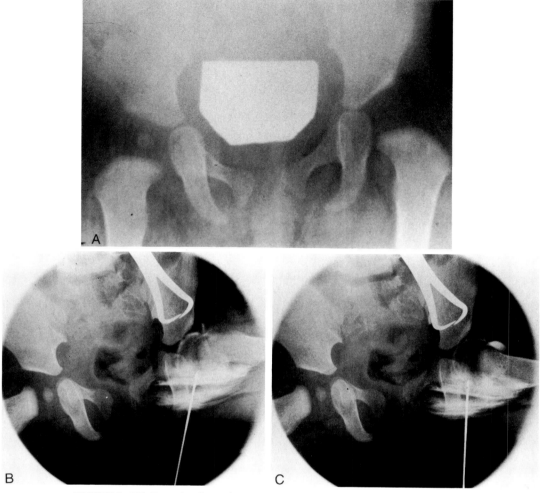

FIGURE 2–175. *Excessive femoral antetorsion as a cause of resubluxation of the hip.*

A. Anteroposterior radiogram of both hips in neutral weight-bearing position. Note the left hip is subluxated. **B.** Abduction and medial rotation of the hip. The subluxation can be reduced. **C.** CT scan showing excessive femoral antetorsion and concentricity of reduction. This child was treated by splinting the hips in flexion, abduction, and lateral rotation.

Often arthrography is performed in the young immature skeleton to determine the degree of concentricity of reduction (Fig. 2–175 C).

Finally, the degree of femoral antetorsion is determined accurately by computed tomography.

Level of Osteotomy. The choice of the correct *level of osteotomy* is important. In the literature, the osteotomy has been reported as performed at the intertrochanteric, subtrochanteric, and supracondylar levels.[121, 143, 581, 827–829] The author strongly recommends the intertrochanteric level, i.e., above the level of the lesser trochanter and the insertion of the iliopsoas and gluteus maximus muscles, for the following reasons. First, the objective of derotation osteotomy is to correct excessive femoral antetorsion, which means that when the femoral head is concentrically seated in the acetabulum the lesser trochanter is located posteriorly in relation to the center of rotation of the femoral head. Therefore, the hip has a strong tendency to rotate laterally owing to the pull of the iliopsoas muscle. If the level of derotation osteotomy is subtrochanteric (i.e., below the lesser trochanter) and the distal fragment is rotated laterally, the iliopsoas muscle will rotate the thigh further laterally. In other words, subtrochanteric osteotomy creates a pathologic retrotorsion of the lesser trochanter. If the

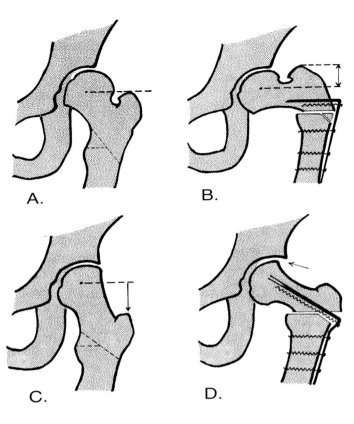

A.   **B.**

C.   **D.**

FIGURE 2–176. Effects of intertrochanteric osteotomy on the biomechanics of the hips.

A and **B.** Varus osteotomy will elevate the greater trochanter. **C** and **D.** Congruity of the hip will alter with changes in the femoral neck axis. (From Tachdjian, M.O. (ed.): Congenital Dislocation of the Hip. New York, Churchill-Livingstone, 1982. Reprinted by permission.)

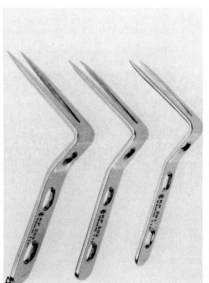

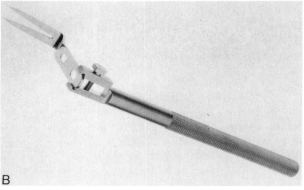

FIGURE 2–177. Wagner bifurcated blade-plate with special holding instrument.

A. Oblique views of the three different sizes of the plate. **B.** Blade-plate holding instrument.

derotation osteotomy is performed at the inter-trochanteric level, it will displace the lesser trochanter anteriorly, decrease the lateral rotatory force of the iliopsoas and gluteus maximus muscles, and preserve the medial rotatory power of the hip adductors and other pelvi-femoral muscles. Second, intertrochanteric osteotomy permits simultaneous effective correction of valgus deformity of the proximal femur (if indicated) without changing the axis of the femoral shaft. Third, at the intertrochanteric level, opposing surfaces of the osteotomized segments are broader, and the greater area of bony contact expedites rapid healing.

Biomechanical Considerations. Intertrochanteric femoral osteotomy has definite effects on the *biomechanics* of the hip.[978] First, the lever arm of the hip abductor muscles is changed by altering the direction and length of the femoral neck axis. Second, varization will elevate the greater trochanter and adversely influence the tension of hip abductor muscles (Fig. 2–176 A and B). Third, changes in the femoral neck axis will alter congruity of the femoral head in relation to the acetabulum (Fig. 2–176 C and D). Finally, lines of stress will change with alterations in the femoral neck axis with ensuing remodeling of bone structure.

Methods of Controlling the Fragments. This may be a matter of preference of the surgeon. A number of methods of osteosynthesis of the upper femoral osteotomy are described in the literature, such as simple encircling wires, crossed Kirschner wires or Steinmann pins, bent plate with screws, angled blade-plates, and nail plates. Regardless of which technique is utilized, it is vital to avoid the physis of the greater trochanter and femoral head. The screw blades in the femoral neck should not protrude from the cortex, and pins or screws should *not* cross the hip joint.

The Wagner technique of intertrochanteric osteotomy employs a bifurcated blade-plate for fixation (Fig. 2–177). The operation is illustrated and described in Plate 16.

The Lloyd Roberts technique of intertrochanteric oblique osteotomy and internal fixation with Coventry lag screw and plate is sometimes used by this author and frequently preferred by other surgeons. The operative technique is illustrated and described in Plate 17.

The Coventry apparatus was developed as a new device for internal fixation for varus-valgus osteotomies of the proximal femur in children by Raymond J. Brigden. It was made for Mr. J. H. Penrose at Warwickshire Hospital in

Coventry, England, and was manufactured by the Howse Company. It provides an acceptable level of secure internal fixation when combined with a hip spica cast, and it is easy to apply. The Coventry lag screw, however, has the following deficiencies: it is a small-diameter screw with less than adequate depth of the threads for secure purchase in the femoral neck canal, attachment of the screw to the side plate with a self-locking nut is bulky, the side plate lacks adequate strength, and the system cannot be used as a compression device.

The new pediatric lag screw (Howmedica) and the Campbell pediatric lag screw (Zimmer) diminish the problem of lateral prominence and provide better fixation. Currently in progress is development of other devices for internal fixation of proximal femoral osteotomies in children.

Canale and Holand reviewed the results of proximal femoral osteotomies fixed with the Coventry lag screw in 38 hips in 29 patients. The ages of the children ranged from 2 to 15 years with an average of 7.3 years. All the osteotomies united, averaging 10.5 weeks to union. The results were satisfactory in 31 of the 38 hips (81.6 per cent). The complications included two malunions, one fracture distal to the plate, one nonunion that required grafting before the osteotomy healed, and three cases of subcutaneous prominence of the screw.[101]

Correction of Acetabular Antetorsion

If the problem is excessive femoral antetorsion, then Salter's innominate osteotomy is indicated to derotate the maldirected acetabulum.

Salter, in 1961, described his procedure of innominate osteotomy based on observations that in congenital hip dislocation the major deformation of the acetabulum is a maldirection or excessive antetorsion. The acetabulum, instead of facing downward, is twisted and faces more anteriorly and laterally than normal. This acetabular maldirection or excessive torsion accounts for the stability of the reduced hip in the position of abduction and flexion and for its instability (i.e., lateral and anterior subluxation of the femoral head) when the lower limb is adducted and extended to the functional position of weight-bearing and walking.[804]

The objective of Salter's innominate osteotomy is to derotate the maldirected acetabulum and correct excessive acetabular antetorsion and thereby to improve stability of reduction by providing anatomic coverage of the femoral head by the anterior and superolateral portions of the acetabulum in the weight-bearing posi-

Text continued on page 404

Wagner Technique of Intertrochanteric Oblique Osteotomy and Internal Fixation With Bifurcated Blade-Plate

OPERATIVE TECHNIQUE

A. The operation is performed with the patient in the supine position on a radiolucent operating table. It is imperative to have image intensifier radiographic control. Some surgeons prefer to operate on an older child on a fracture table because it is technically easier to make a lateral roentgenogram of the hip. A straight midlateral longitudinal incision is made, beginning at the tip of the greater trochanter and extending distally parallel with the femur for a distance of 10 to 12 cm. The subcutaneous tissue is divided in line with the skin incision.

B. The fascia lata is exposed by deepening the dissection and is first divided with a scalpel and then split longitudinally with scissors in the direction of its fibers. Division of the fascia lata should be posterior to the tensor fasciae latae in order to avoid splitting its muscle.

C. By retraction, the vastus lateralis muscle is visualized. Next, the anterolateral region of the proximal femur and the trochanteric area are exposed. It is vital not to injure the greater trochanteric growth plate. The origin of the vastus lateralis muscle is divided transversely from the inferior border of the greater trochanter down to the posterolateral surface of the femur. The vastus lateralis muscle fibers are elevated from the lateral intramuscular septum and the tendinous insertion of the gluteus maximus.

Plate 16. Wagner Technique of Intertrochanteric Oblique Osteotomy and Internal Fixation With Bifurcated Blade-Plate

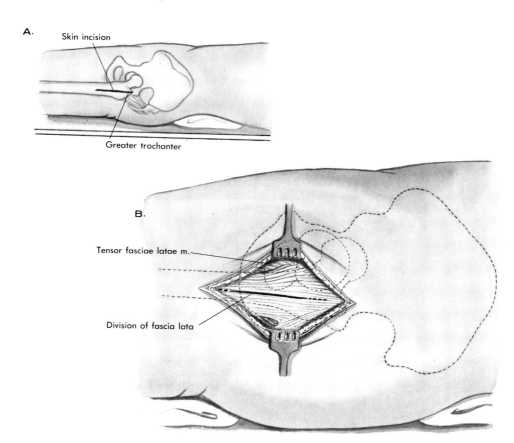

A.

Skin incision

Greater trochanter

B.

Tensor fasciae latae m.

Division of fascia lata

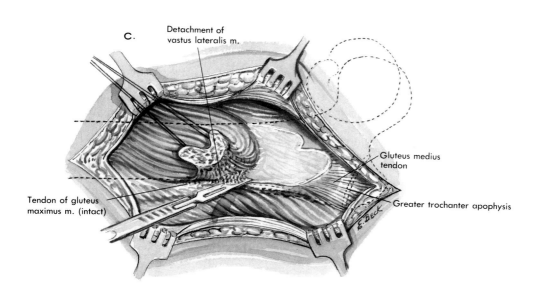

C.

Detachment of vastus lateralis m.

Tendon of gluteus maximus m. (intact)

Gluteus medius tendon

Greater trochanter apophysis

E. BECK

Wagner Technique of Intertrochanteric Oblique Osteotomy and Internal Fixation With Bifurcated Blade-Plate
(Continued)

D. To expose the posterior surface of the femur, a curved wide osteotome is used to cut a thin cortical shell from the linea aspera. This technique avoids bleeding from the perforating vessels. The anterior, lateral, and posterior surfaces of the femur are exposed by insertion of Chandler or Cobra retractors anteromedially and posterolaterally.

E and F. The femoral head is centered concentrically in the acetabulum by abduction and medial rotation of the hip; its position is checked by image intensifier. Immediately distal to the apophyseal growth plate of the greater trochanter, a 3-mm. Steinmann pin is inserted through the lateral cortex of the femoral shaft parallel to the floor of the operating room and at right angles to the median plane of the patient. The pin is drilled medially along the longitudinal axis of the femoral neck, stopping short of the capital femoral physis. This position of the proximal femur can be reproduced at any time during the operation by placing the Steinmann pin horizontally parallel to the floor and at 90 degrees to the longitudinal axis of the patient—a very dependable, simple method for proper orientation of the proximal femur.

G. With a slow oscillating saw, the intertrochanteric osteotomy is made parallel to the Steinmann pin and level with a point just below the inferomedial corner of the femoral neck. It is important to avoid and not enter the medial cortex of the femoral neck. The cut surfaces should be smooth to permit their accurate apposition and stable contact. It is best to be gentle and refrain from manipulating the proximal fragment by levering the Steinmann pin because the bone may be atrophic and easily cut through; instead the distal segment is manipulated. A wide flat osteotome is inserted into the osteotomy site, and the osteotomy cleft is opened by adducting and laterally rotating the lower limb into neutral position (with respect to adduction-abduction and medial-lateral rotation). Next, with an oscillating saw, a small wedge is removed from the medial peak of the distal segment. Removal of a full wedge will sacrifice too much bone.

H. With the proximal fragment in the corrected position (i.e., the Steinmann pin parallel to the floor and at right angles to the median plane of the patient), the distal fragment is displaced medially about half the diameter of the shaft. The site of insertion of the bifurcated blade of the Altdorf hip clamp will determine the degree of medial displacement. More medial insertion of the blade will increase the amount of medial displacement of the distal fragment, which has a definite advantage. Varization osteotomy without medial displacement moves the greater trochanter and femoral shaft laterally away from the median line. This varus position of the limb axis subjects the proximal end of the femur to bending force, which interferes with bone healing. By displacing the distal fragment medially and bringing it closer to the center of hip rotation, the weight-bearing lever arm is shortened, bending force is decreased, and compression force is increased. Biomechanically, the medial displacement of the distal fragment stimulates bone healing and provides better bony support.

Next, the appropriate size blade-plate is chosen. The proximal end of the blade is bifurcated, and the blade itself is bent to make an angle of 130 degrees with the plate (see Fig. 2–177). The metal of the plate is flexible enough to allow bending with instruments to change the blade-plate angle if necessary. Immediately below the angulation of the blade and plate there is a round hole through which a screw is inserted into the proximal fragment. The plate has two oval screw holes, which provide leeway for compression. The blade should be placed in the center of the femoral neck and not protrude from its cortices, nor should the points of its bifurcated end penetrate and injure the capital femoral physis. The blade-plate is held securely in a special holding instrument, and by careful hammer blows, the bifurcated end is inserted into the osteotomy surface of the proximal fragment parallel to the longitudinal axis of the femoral neck. The position of the blade is checked by image intensifier radiography.

Plate 16. Wagner Technique of Intertrochanteric Oblique Osteotomy and Internal Fixation With Bifurcated Blade-Plate

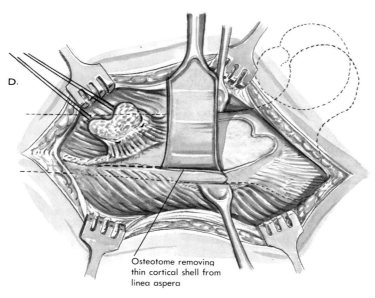

D.

Osteotome removing thin cortical shell from linea aspera

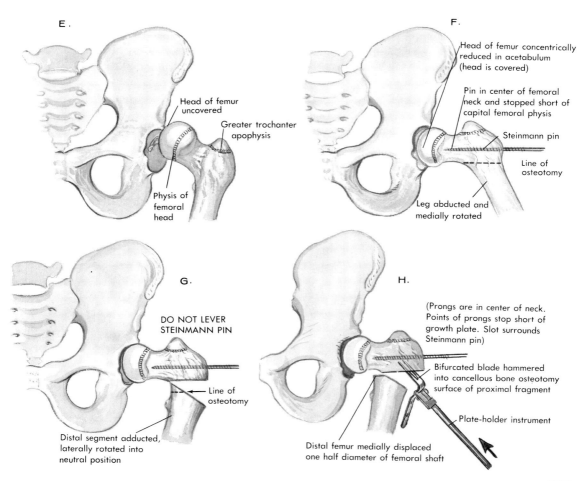

E.

Head of femur uncovered

Greater trochanter apophysis

Physis of femoral head

F.

Head of femur concentrically reduced in acetabulum (head is covered)

Pin in center of femoral neck and stopped short of capital femoral physis

Steinmann pin

Line of osteotomy

Leg abducted and medially rotated

G.

DO NOT LEVER STEINMANN PIN

Line of osteotomy

Distal segment adducted, laterally rotated into neutral position

H.

(Prongs are in center of neck. Points of prongs stop short of growth plate. Slot surrounds Steinmann pin)

Bifurcated blade hammered into cancellous bone osteotomy surface of proximal fragment

Plate-holder instrument

Distal femur medially displaced one half diameter of femoral shaft

Wagner Technique of Intertrochanteric Oblique Osteotomy and Internal Fixation With Bifurcated Blade-Plate
(Continued)

I and **J.** The blade is driven proximally into the osteotomy surface and buried almost to the angle with the plate. The holding instrument is removed, and the blade is impacted further with a punch. Next, a drill hole is made for the compression screw in the proximal fragment (small-fragment screws are used for the small and medium-sized blade plates and standard AO cortical screws are used for the large size). The screw is inserted into the proximal fragment, securely anchoring the bifurcated blade to the femoral neck. This type of fixation provides tremendous stability, which is essential in atrophic bone. (If the bone is not atrophic, some surgeons prefer to put the screw in the neck of the femur later.)

K and **L.** Next, interfragmentary compression is achieved. First, the osteotomy surfaces are fitted together in the desired position, paying meticulous attention to keeping the Steinmann pin parallel to the floor and at right angles to the longitudinal axis of the patient and the distal fragment in neutral position as to abduction-adduction and medial-lateral rotation. Second, the osteotomized fragments are deliberately placed in slightly overcorrected position, the distal fragment brought into further medial displacement and the proximal fragment into further valgus displacement, so that only the distal tip of the plate touches the femoral shaft. This maneuver keeps a cleft 4 to 6 mm. wide at the osteotomy site, allowing impaction as the plate is anchored to bone. A screw of appropriate size is inserted through the most distal hole of the plate first, and then another screw through the next proximal hole. By tightening the second screw, the distal fragment is pulled laterally against the plate, which in turn lowers the proximal fragment into varus position. By this technique the buttress point of the two fragments is compressed. If further compression is desired, the blade is impacted further into the proximal fragment and the screws are tightened. The bone wedge removed earlier is placed between the two femoral fragments and the previously inserted lag screw in the femoral neck is tightened, further compressing the fragments.

M. The vastus lateralis muscle is reattached to the tendinous insertion of the gluteus medius and minimus. Continuity of muscle structure of the gluteus medius and vastus lateralis takes much of the force on the lateral aspect of the upper femur and transforms bending force to compression force. One cannot overemphasize the importance of careful reattachment of the vastus lateralis to the gluteus medius insertion. A suction drainage tube is inserted underneath the free posterior margin of the vastus lateralis muscle. The fascia lata is sutured, and the subcutaneous tissues and skin are closed in the usual fashion. Skin closure should always be by a running subcuticular suture.

POSTOPERATIVE CARE

This type of osteosynthesis is so stable that it is safe not to apply a hip spica cast. Partial weight-bearing with crutches (three-point) is permitted on the fourth or fifth postoperative day when the child is comfortable. The osteotomy usually heals in about eight weeks, at which time crutch protection is discontinued. A hip spica cast is applied only when the femoral osteotomy is combined with open reduction of hip dislocation in which the cast is needed to maintain the stability of concentric reduction until the capsule and soft tissue heal.

Plate 16. Wagner Technique of Intertrochanteric Oblique Osteotomy and Internal Fixation With Bifurcated Blade-Plate

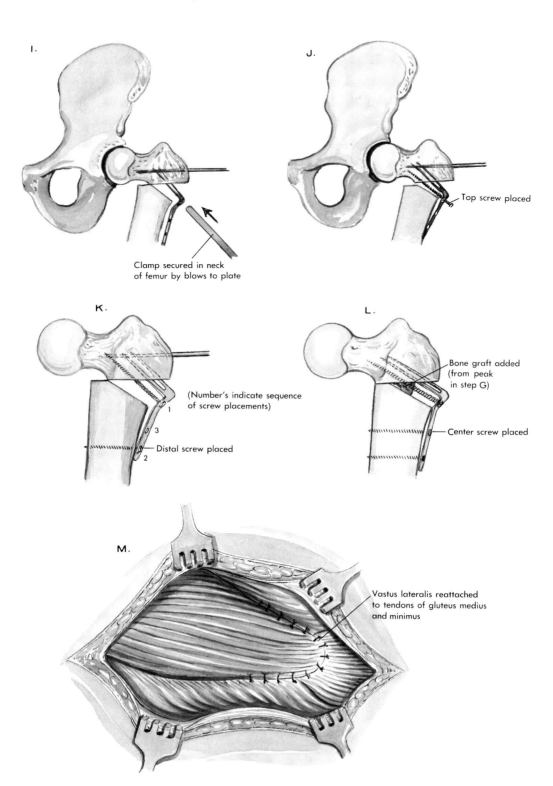

I.

Clamp secured in neck
of femur by blows to plate

J.

Top screw placed

K.

(Number's indicate sequence
of screw placements)

Distal screw placed

L.

Bone graft added
(from peak
in step G)

Center screw placed

M.

Vastus lateralis reattached
to tendons of gluteus medius
and minimus

Lloyd Roberts Technique of Intertrochanteric Oblique Osteotomy of Proximal Femur And Internal Fixation With Coventry Apparatus (Lag Screw and Plate)

The patient is placed supine on a radiolucent operating table. The operation is performed under image intensifier radiographic control. The iliac region, hip, and entire lower limb are prepared sterile and draped so that the limb can be manipulated freely.

OPERATIVE TECHNIQUE

A. The incision begins 1 cm. posterior and inferior to the anterior superior iliac spine, curves across to the top of the greater trochanter, and continues distally along the femoral shaft for a distance of 6 to 8 cm. The subcutaneous tissue is divided in line with the skin incision. The deep fascia is incised and the interval between the tensor fasciae latae anteriorly and the gluteus medius posteriorly is developed by blunt dissection. The vastus lateralis is divided longitudinally by an L-shaped or U-shaped incision, and the part of it that originates from the anterior aspect of the intertrochanteric area is detached. With a periosteal elevator, the intertrochanteric region and the upper femoral shaft are exposed. At this time the calcare femorale is visualized, and the femoral head can be palpated within the capsule. A sturdy stainless steel pin of appropriate diameter, usually 0.062 inches, is chosen; be sure its diameter fits the hole in the lag screw. With the hip in full medial rotation, a 3-mm. hole is drilled through the center of the lateral cortex of the upper femoral shaft, 0.75 to 1.0 cm. below the growth plate of the greater trochanter. Avoid injury to the growth plate of the apophysis; verify its site with an image intensifier radiogram. Next, insert the guide pin into the femoral neck parallel to the floor in a proximally inclined oblique plane parallel to the long axis of the femoral neck. The tip of the pin should stop immediately distal to the capital femoral physis. The proper placement of the guide pin is crucial; it is confirmed by anteroposterior and lateral image intensifier radiography.

B. A cannulated reamer (with a "stop" to prevent more than ½ inch penetration) is fitted over the guide pin; the lateral cortex of the upper femoral shaft is reamed to permit firm fixation of the lag screw in the cancellous bone.

C. Next, with the special lag screw inserter, a lag screw of appropriate length is inserted into the femoral neck. It should stop short of the capital physis. Avoid growth injury. Confirm the position of the screw by anteroposterior and lateral radiograms.

D. With an oscillating saw the femoral osteotomy is performed at the intertrochanteric level parallel to the calcare; use the guide pin, which protrudes from the lag screw, to guide the direction of osteotomy and verify it by image intensifier radiography. (Drill holes may be used to mark the line of osteotomy.) Once the osteotomy is completed, gently strip the adjacent periosteum to mobilize the bone fragments and permit free rotation of the femoral shaft.

E. The side plate is bent to the appropriate angle. The guide pin is removed and the top hole of the side plate is engaged to the protruding end of the lag screw. A cannulated lever with a handle is attached to the lag screw for firm control of the upper fragment. The distal fragment is adducted and rotated laterally to the desired degree. The oblique line of the osteotomy will often make a triangle of bone at the upper end of the femoral shaft that will protrude anteriorly; this is excised and used as a local bone graft. The osteotomized fragments are apposed and secured by attaching the side plate to the femoral shaft with screws and a nut at the top of the lag screw and the proximal fragment. Final radiograms are made to double check security of the fixation device. A one–and–one half hip spica plaster of Paris cast is applied.

POSTOPERATIVE CARE

The child is usually sent home three to four days postoperatively and readmitted to hospital six weeks later. The plaster cast is removed, and the hip and knee are mobilized. When able to ambulate with crutches (three-point partial weight-bearing on the affected limb), the patient is discharged, usually within two to four days.

The plate and screws are removed six months postoperatively.

Plate 17. Lloyd Roberts Technique of Intertrochanteric Oblique Osteotomy of Proximal Femur and Internal Fixation With Coventry Apparatus (Lag Screw and Plate)

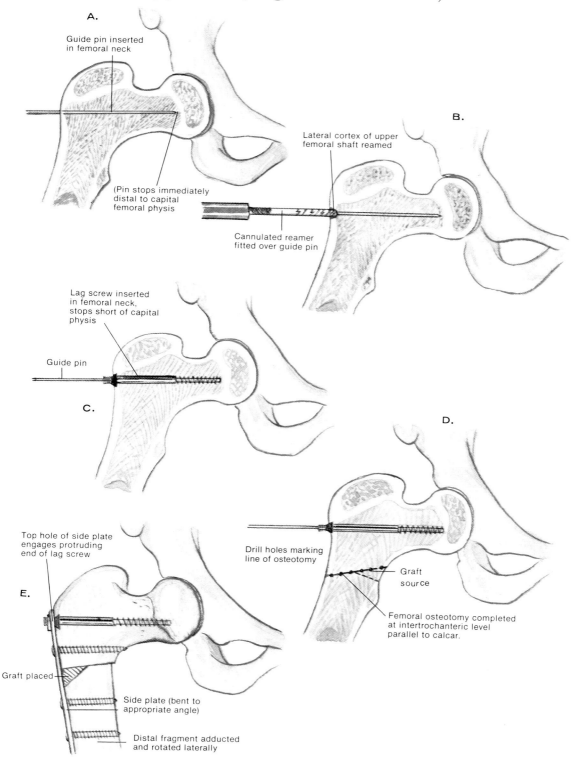

A.

Guide pin inserted in femoral neck

(Pin stops immediately distal to capital femoral physis

B.

Lateral cortex of upper femoral shaft reamed

Cannulated reamer fitted over guide pin

Lag screw inserted in femoral neck, stops short of capital physis

Guide pin

C.

D.

Drill holes marking line of osteotomy

Graft source

Femoral osteotomy completed at intertrochanteric level parallel to calcar.

Top hole of side plate engages protruding end of lag screw

E.

Graft placed

Side plate (bent to appropriate angle)

Distal fragment adducted and rotated laterally

403

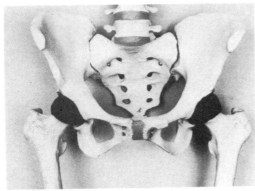

A

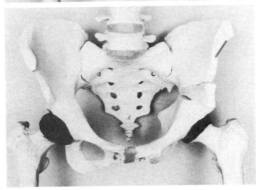

B

*FIGURE 2–178. Model of a pelvis, illustrating the design
of Salter's innominate osteotomy.*

A. Both femoral heads are inadequately covered by the
normal acetabula with the hips in the functional position of
weight-bearing. **B.** The left innominate bone has been
completely divided from the sciatic notch to the anterior
inferior iliac spine, and the distal fragment is rotated
downward, forward, and laterally through the flexible symphysis pubis. Note that the acetabulum is redirected,
covering the femoral head adequately in the functional
position of weight-bearing. (From Salter, R. B., and Dubos,
J. P.: The first fifteen years' personal experience with
innominate osteotomy in the treatment of congenital dislocation of the hip. Clin. Orthop., 98:73, 1974. Reprinted
by permission.)

tion (Fig. 2–178). The osteotomy is performed
via a transverse linear cut above the acetabulum
at the level of the greater sciatic notch and the
anterior inferior iliac spine. The whole acetabulum (with the distal fragment of the innominate bone) is tilted inferiorly and laterally by
rotating it around a pivot through the flexible
symphysis pubis and the greater sciatic notch.
The new position of the distal fragment is
maintained by inserting a triangular bone graft
taken from the proximal portion of the ilium
into the open wedge osteotomy site. Internal
fixation is secured by two threaded Kirschner
wires that traverse the proximal fragment, the
graft, and the distal fragment. Through this
rotation and redirection of the acetabulum, the
femoral head is covered adequately with the
hip in normal weight-bearing position, i.e., the
reduced dislocation or subluxation, which was

previously stable in the position of flexion and
abduction, is now stable in the extended-neutral
position of weight-bearing. Stability of the hip
allows early weight-bearing, which stimulates
further growth and ossification of the hip.[806–814]
The operative technique of Salter's innominate
osteotomy is described and illustrated in Plate
18.

Advantages. First, the procedure provides
coverage of the femoral head with an acetabular
roof consisting of hyaline cartilage, which is
biologically physiologic and has optimal load-
bearing capacity.

Second, it does not disturb the growth of the
acetabulum; i.e., it does not damage the triradiate cartilage and the acetabular lip—especially the superior rim where perichondral and
periosteal ossification abut—the site where
modeling and growth of the acetabular roof
takes place. Injury to the acetabular lip will
result in cessation of growth of the acetabular
rim.[741, 742]

Indications. According to *this author*, the
indication for Salter's procedure is instability of
the reduced hip in weight-bearing position due
to excessive acetabular antetorsion; on flexion,
abduction, and medial rotation, the hip is stabilized. The femoral antetorsion should not
exceed 35 degrees as determined accurately by
CT scan.

The indications according to *Salter* for his
procedure are: (1) congenital dislocation—previously untreated (primary), ages 18 months to
six years; (2) congenital subluxation—no previous treatment (primary), ages 18 months to
adult life; (3) residual or recurrent dislocation—
due to failure of previous treatment, ages 18
months to six years; and (4) residual or recurrent
subluxation—due to failure of previous treatment, ages 18 months to adult life.[812–814]

There are certain gray areas in these criteria,
and controversial issues that require further
elaboration.

Age Limits. In the infant under 18 months of
age, when the acetabulum is very shallow,
Albee's shelf acetabuloplasty is performed. The
youngest age for Salter's innominate osteotomy
should be one and a half years, since in children
below this age the innominate bone and graft
are too thin, and because of problems of internal
fixation, loss of correction is likely to occur.[812]
Others advocate a minimum age of three years
for Salter's innominate osteotomy because in
younger children a high percentage of patients
will develop an adequate acetabulum by concentric reduction and containment by splints or
by femoral osteotomy.[715]

There is definite controversy about the *upper
age limit.* Salter proposes six years as the upper

age for correcting a complete dislocation, since in children over six years the degree of secondary acetabular dysplasia, the incongruity of the hip, and the contractural shortening of the pelvifemoral muscles are so severe that it is difficult to obtain a stable concentric reduction. In recent years, however, the combination of femoral shortening and innominate osteotomy with open reduction has allowed raising the upper age limit to 8 to 12 years (especially in cases of unilateral involvement).[498, 500] For correcting subluxation, according to Salter, there is no upper age limit provided that there is reasonable congruity of the joint and that concentric reduction is obtained by simple abduction, medial rotation, and flexion of the hip. There may be some controversy among surgeons as to the exact delineation of absence of significant incongruity.[814] In the experience of this author, in children over ten years of skeletal age, inflexibility of the symphysis pubis hinders rotation of the distal segment, and adequate coverage of the femoral head is anatomically difficult. In the adolescent and the young adult the indications for Salter's innominate osteotomy should be individualized and the operation performed only by the experienced hip surgeon.

Combination of Open Reduction and Innominate Osteotomy. Salter performs open reduction and innominate osteotomy simultaneously following two weeks of preliminary traction if the child is over 18 months and under six years of age. This combination is fraught with problems and complications. Paterson reports a high risk of avascular necrosis.[716] It is inevitable that there will be some pressure on the articular cartilage when the femoral head is pulled down and located in the acetabulum, and if the innominate bone is rotated down over the femoral head, the intra-articular pressure will further increase. Consequently cartilage necrosis, bone necrosis, permanent joint stiffness, and growth disturbance are likely to follow. This author has taken the posture that open reduction of the hip in the older child should be combined with femoral shortening to unload the hip joint and facilitate removal of all intra-articular and extra-articular obstacles to concentric reduction. During femoral shortening, excessive femoral antetorsion is corrected to normal, thereby increasing the stability of reduction. Growth and development of the acetabulum are followed, and innominate osteotomy, if indicated, is undertaken six months to two years later.

Limitations and Drawbacks. There are certain drawbacks to Salter's innominate osteotomy. Studies by Salter have demonstrated that,

following his innominate osteotomy, there are no changes in the capacity or the contour of the acetabulum, provided that redirection of the distal part of the innominate bone containing the entire acetabulum is performed by rotation through the symphysis pubis, and that there is no medial or posterior displacement.[805] There is some controversy about this. Thomas states that Salter's innominate osteotomy produces a flattening of the posterior rim of the acetabulum. As the superior acetabular rim is displaced anteriorly and downward, the posterior rim is displaced upward. The anteroposterior radiograph shows the lowering of the superior rim but does not demonstrate the elevation of the posterior rim.[927] Coleman feels that Salter's innominate osteotomy uncovers the posterior portion of the acetabulum, which may cause difficulties in total joint arthroplasty later on if osteoarthritis develops in adult life.[159] This author's preliminary studies by computed tomography have shown that the posterior rim of the acetabulum is not uncovered, provided, first, that bony contact is maintained at the posterior osteotomy site and, second, that the femoral head is not enlarged relative to the acetabulum.

Anterior displacement of the distal segment will elevate the posterior rim of the acetabulum and uncover the femoral head posteriorly. When an enlarged femoral head is being covered anterolaterally by rotation of an insufficient acetabulum, the femoral head may be uncovered posteriorly. A curvilinear osteotomy parallel to the dome of the acetabulum and extending inferiorly into the body of the ischium will minimize the posterior uncovering of the femoral head.

Limitation on the Degree of Correction. The inferior displacement of the acetabulum is checked by the counterpressure exerted by the femoral head and the tension in the pelvifemoral muscles—iliopsoas, hip adductors, and glutei. Also, in the older child, inflexibility of the symphysis pubis restricts the degree of rotation and tilting at the symphysis. Rab, in a mathematical model of the Salter innominate osteotomy in an adult male pelvis, showed that the procedure extends and adducts the acetabulum by rotation and translation in space; the center of the hip joint moves distally, posteriorly, and medially. The practical maximum limit that can be obtained is probably 25 degrees of extension and 10 degrees of adduction of the acetabulum. The acetabulum extends by an angle roughly equivalent to the angle of the osteotomy opening. Diastasis at the posterior osteotomy site should be avoided. According to Rab, if a subluxated hip is unstable in 25

Text continued on page 412

Salter's Innominate Osteotomy

OPERATIVE TECHNIQUE

A to **D.** The Salter innominate osteotomy is based on redirection of the acetabulum as a unit by hinging and rotation through the symphysis pubis, which is mobile in children. It is performed by a transverse linear cut above the acetabulum at the level of the greater sciatic notch and the anterior inferior iliac spine. The whole acetabulum with the distal fragment of the innominate bone is tilted downward and laterally by rotating it. The new position of the distal fragment is maintained by a triangular bone graft taken from the proximal portion of the ilium and inserted in the open-wedge osteotomy site. Internal fixation is provided by two threaded Kirschner wires. Through the rotation and redirection of the acetabulum, the femoral head is covered adequately with the hip in normal weight-bearing position, i.e., the reduced dislocation or subluxation that was previously stable in the position of flexion and abduction is now stable in the extended and neutral position of weight-bearing.

E. The skin is prepared with the patient in the side-lying position so that the abdomen, lower part of the chest, and affected half of the pelvis can be draped to the midline anteriorly and posteriorly; the entire lower limb is also prepared and draped to allow free motion of the hip during the operation. Then the patient is turned on his back to lie completely supine. The range of abduction of the hip is tested. Maximum normal abduction must be present; if it is limited by contracted hip adductors, an adductor myotomy is performed first.

The skin incision is oblique, extending from the junction of the posterior and middle thirds of the iliac crest to a point 1 cm. below the anterior superior iliac spine, and then is extended medially to just below the midpoint of the inguinal ligament. The subcutaneous tissue is divided in line with the skin incision. The deep fascia is incised over the iliac crest. The wound edges are undermined, and pressure is applied with large sponges to minimize bleeding. Next the fascia lata is opened over the medial border of the tensor fasciae latae and lateral to the groove between it and the sartorius muscles—this 1-cm. strip of fascia protects the lateral femoral cutaneous nerve from inadvertent injury.

F. With a scalpel, the cartilaginous iliac apophysis is split in the middle down to bone from the junction of its posterior and middle thirds to the anterior superior iliac spine. By blunt dissection the groove between the tensor fasciae latae and the sartorius and rectus femoris muscles is opened and developed. With a broad, long-handled periosteal elevator, the lateral part of the iliac apophysis and the tensor fasciae latae and gluteus medius and minimus muscles are subperiosteally stripped and reflected as a continuous sheet to the superior rim of the acetabulum anterolaterally and the greater sciatic notch posteromedially.

Plate 18. Salter's Innominate Osteotomy

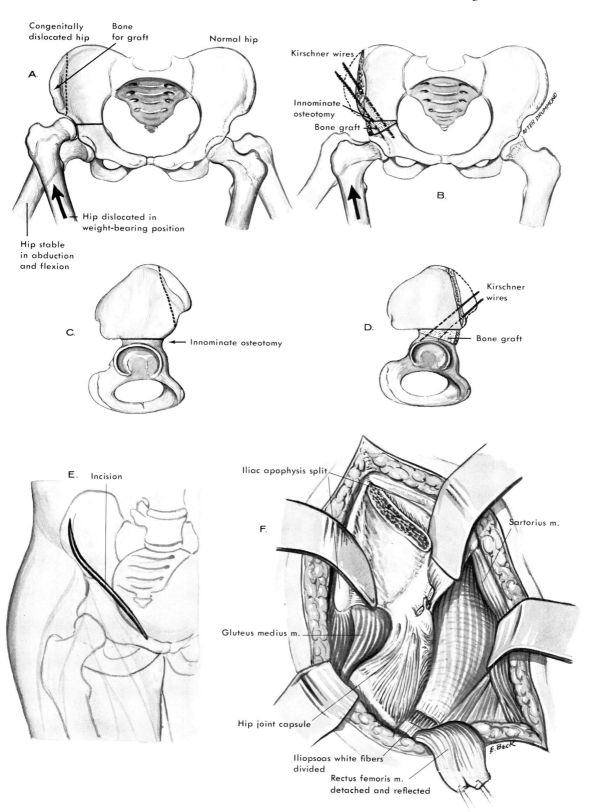

A. Congenitally dislocated hip. Bone for graft. Normal hip. Hip dislocated in weight-bearing position. Hip stable in abduction and flexion.

B. Kirschner wires. Innominate osteotomy. Bone graft. AFTER DRUMMOND

C. Innominate osteotomy

D. Kirschner wires. Bone graft

E. Incision

F. Iliac apophysis split. Sartorius m. Gluteus medius m. Hip joint capsule. Iliopsoas white fibers divided. Rectus femoris m. detached and reflected. E. BECK

Salter's Innominate Osteotomy *(Continued)*

G. Next, the periosteum is elevated from the medial and lateral walls of the ilium all the way posteriorly to the sciatic notch. It is vital to stay within the periosteum in order to prevent injury to the superior gluteal vessels and the sciatic nerve. A common pitfall is inadequate surgical exposure of the sciatic notch, making it difficult to pass the Gigli saw behind the notch. The space on the lateral wall of the ilium is packed with sponge to dilate the interval and to control oozing of blood. Next, the periosteum is elevated from the inner wall of the ilium in a continuous sheet, exposing the sciatic notch medially. Again, it is important to stay in the subperiosteal plane in order to avoid injury to vessels and nerves. The medial space is packed with sponge. The sartorius muscle usually can be reflected medially with the medial half of the cartilaginous iliac apophysis. If it is difficult to do so or if more distal exposure is desired, the origin of the sartorius muscle is detached from the anterior superior iliac spine, its free end is marked with whip sutures for later reattachment, and the muscle is reflected distally and medially. The two heads of origin of the rectus femoris, the direct one from the anterior inferior iliac spine and the reflected one from the superior margin of the acetabulum, are divided at their origin, marked with whip sutures, and reflected distally.

Next, on the deep surface of the iliopsoas muscle, the psoas tendon is exposed at the level of the pelvic rim. The iliopsoas muscle is rolled over so that its tendinous portion can be separated from the muscular portion. If identification is in doubt, a nerve stimulator is used to distinguish the psoas tendon from the femoral nerve. A Freer elevator is passed between the tendinous and muscular portions of the iliopsoas muscle, and the psoas tendon is sectioned at one or two levels. The divided edges of the tendinous portion retract and the muscle fibers separate; releasing contractures of the iliopsoas without disturbing the continuity of the muscle.

Two medium-sized Chandler elevator retractors, one introduced from the lateral and the other from the medial side of the ilium, are placed subperiosteally in the sciatic notch. This step is crucial; besides keeping neurovascular structures out of harm's way, the Chandler retractors maintain continuity of the proximal and distal innominate segments at the sciatic notch.

A right-angled forceps (Mixter or Negus) is passed subperiosteally from the medial side of the ilium and guided through the sciatic notch to the outer side with the index finger of the opposite hand. The Gigli saw is introduced from the lateral side, the loop of one end is grasped by the blades of the right-angled forceps, and the saw is passed through the sciatic notch from the lateral to the medial side.

H. The line of osteotomy extends from the sciatic notch to the anterior inferior iliac spine, perpendicular to the sides of the ilium. It is vital to begin the osteotomy well inferiorly in the sciatic notch; the tendency is to start too high. The handles of the Gigli saw are kept widely separated and at a continuous tension in order to keep the saw from binding in the soft cancellous bone. The osteotomy, which emerges anteriorly immediately above the anterior inferior iliac spine, is completed with the Gigli saw. Use of an osteotome may subject the superior gluteal artery and sciatic nerve to iatrogenic damage. A Midas power saw may be used instead of a Gigli saw, particularly if a curvilinear cut is planned.

I. The two Chandler retractors are kept constantly at the sciatic notch by an assistant to prevent posterior or medial displacement of the distal segment and loss of bony continuity posteriorly. A triangular full-thickness bone graft is removed from the anterior part of the iliac crest with a large, straight, double-action bone cutter. The length of the base of the triangular wedge represents the distance between the anterior superior and the anterior inferior iliac spines. The portion of bone to be removed as bone graft is held firmly with a Kocher forceps; be sure that it does not fall on the floor or get contaminated.

The proximal fragment of the innominate bone is held steady with a large towel clip forceps, and the distal fragment is grasped with a second stout towel forceps. The affected hip is placed in 90 degrees of flexion, maximal abduction, and 90 degrees of lateral rotation; a second assistant applies distal and lateral traction on the thigh. With the second towel clip placed well posteriorly on the distal fragment, the surgeon rotates the distal fragment downward, outward, and forward, thus opening the osteotomy site anteriorly. The site must be kept closed posteriorly. Leaving it open posteriorly displaces the hip joint distally without adequate rotation and redirection of the acetabulum at the symphysis pubis; furthermore, it will lengthen the lower limb unnecessarily. Another technical error to avoid is opening the osteotomy site with a mechanical spreader (such as a laminectomy spreader or a self-retaining retractor) because that will do nothing but move the proximal fragment upward and the distal fragment downward without rotating the distal fragment through the symphysis pubis. The acetabular maldirection will not be corrected unless such rotation of the distal fragment takes place. Posterior and medial displacement of the distal fragment should be avoided.

Plate 18. Salter's Innominate Osteotomy

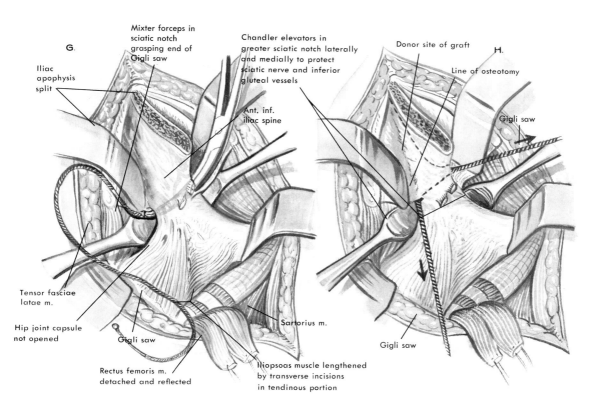

G.

Iliac apophysis split

Mixter forceps in sciatic notch grasping end of Gigli saw

Chandler elevators in greater sciatic notch laterally and medially to protect sciatic nerve and inferior gluteal vessels

Ant. inf. iliac spine

Tensor fasciae latae m.

Hip joint capsule not opened

Gigli saw

Rectus femoris m. detached and reflected

Iliopsoas muscle lengthened by transverse incisions in tendinous portion

Sartorius m.

H.

Donor site of graft

Line of osteotomy

Gigli saw

Gigli saw

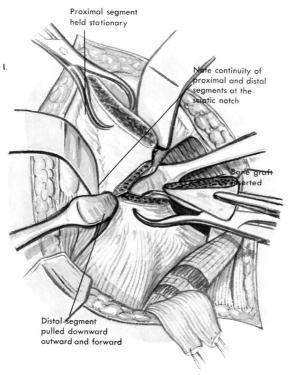

I.

Proximal segment held stationary

Note continuity of proximal and distal segments at the sciatic notch

Bone graft inserted

Distal segment pulled downward outward and forward

Salter's Innominate Osteotomy (Continued)

When the periosteum on the median wall of the ilium is taut, the cartilaginous apophysis of the ilium is divided as two or three levels; this will help to rotate the acetabulum.

J. Next, the bone graft is shaped with bone cutters to the appropriate size to fit the open osteotomy site. Ordinarily the graft is about the correct size for the size of the patient because the base of the triangular graft represents the distance between the anterior superior and anterior inferior iliac spines. Avoid using a large graft and hammering it in to fit snugly into the osteotomy site; this will open the site posteriorly. With the osteotomy site open anteriorly and the distal segment rotated, the bone graft is inserted into the opened-up osteotomy. The distal fragment of the innominate bone should be kept slightly anterior to the proximal fragment. When traction is released, the graft is firmly locked by the two segments of the bone.

A stout, threaded Kirschner wire is drilled from the proximal segment across the osteotomy site, through the graft, and into the distal segment posterior to the acetabulum, preventing any future displacement of the graft or the distal segment. The wire should never point in the direction of the hip joint. Radiographs are made to check the adequacy of correction of the acetabular maldirection and the position of the Kirschner wire. Then a second Kirschner wire is drilled parallel to the first to further stabilize internal fixation of the osteotomy. In the older patient this author uses a third threaded Kirschner wire or two cancellous positional screws to ensure security of internal fixation. Inadequate penetration of the wires into the distal fragment will result in loss of alignment of the osteotomy. They may bend or break, or if excessively heavy, they may fracture the graft or the innominate bone; the importance of choosing the correct diameter of wire or cancellous screw cannot be overemphasized. Penetration of the wires into the hip joint may cause chondrolysis of the hip or cause the wire to break at the joint level. They should not be inserted upward from below, since they may pass medial to the proximal segment and injure retroperitoneal or intraperitoneal structures. An anteroposterior radiograph of the hips is taken to check the depth of the Kirschner wires and the degree of correction obtained.

The two halves of the cartilaginous iliac apophysis are sutured together over the iliac crest. The rectus femoris and sartorius muscles are reattached to their origins. The wound is closed in the routine manner. Skin closure should be by continuous subcuticular 00 nylon. The Kirschner wires are cut so that their ends are in the subcutaneous fat and are easily palpable.

A one–and–one half spica cast is applied with the hip in stable weight-bearing position. Immobilization in forced or extreme position should be avoided because it will cause excessive and continuous compression of articular cartilage, osteonecrosis, permanent joint stiffness, and eventual degenerative arthritis. In the cast, the knee is bent to control the position of hip rotation. When there is excessive femoral antetorsion the hip is immobilized in slight medial rotation. A common pitfall is immobilization in marked medial rotation; this mistake will result in posterior subluxation or dislocation of the femoral head. In femoral retrotorsion the hip should be immobilized in slight lateral rotation. It is obvious that prior to Salter's innominate osteotomy it is vital to determine the degree of femoral torsion accurately.

A radiograph of the hips through the cast is made before the child is discharged from the hospital. Another set of radiographs is made two to three weeks postoperatively to ensure that the graft has not collapsed, that the pins have not migrated, and that there is no medial displacement of the distal segments. In the older cooperative patient, when cancellous screws are used for internal fixation, a hip spica cast is not necessary.

POSTOPERATIVE CARE

The hips remain immobilized in the spica cast for a total of six weeks, following which the cast is bivalved and radiographs of the hip are made with the cast off. It is best to readmit the child to the hospital, where bilateral split Russell's traction is applied, and gradual active exercises are performed to mobilize the lower limbs and develop muscle strength. An accidental fall during the first few weeks might result in collapse of the graft or stress fracture of the femur. When functional range of motion of the hips and knees is obtained, partial weight-bearing with a three-point crutch gait is begun. This may be difficult to teach to the two- or three-year-old child. Full weight-bearing is allowed 4 to 6 weeks following removal of the solid cast, or 10 to 12 weeks postoperatively. This author recommends removal of the Kirschner wires when there is complete consolidation and revascularization of the graft (usually three to six months postoperatively). Ordinarily this is performed under general anesthesia in the operating room as an outpatient procedure.

Plate 18. Salter's Innominate Osteotomy

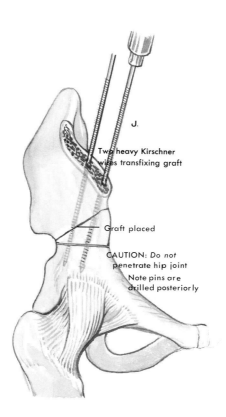

J.

Two heavy Kirschner wires transfixing graft

Graft placed

CAUTION: *Do not penetrate hip joint*
Note pins are drilled posteriorly

degrees of flexion and 10 degrees of abduction, the Salter innominate osteotomy will not provide the desired articular bony stability.[759] This does not take into account the joint capsule, which may be tautened by plication to provide additional stability of the hip. Also, these figures can be decreased by flexibility of the sacroiliac joint and the inevitable slight lowering at the posterior osteotomy site. Rab also showed in muscle studies that pelvifemoral muscles, especially the iliopsoas and hip adductors, tautened; thus they have to be released if they are contracted.[759, 760]

The following radiographic studies are recommended by Rab to determine the potential effectiveness of Salter's innominate osteotomy: The patient is placed in supine position and the affected hip is flexed 25 degrees and abducted 10 degrees while the femur is maintained in neutral position with the patella facing straight up. First a radiogram is made with the beam directed posteriorly and caudally, at an angle of 25 degrees to the coronal plane (Fig. 2–179). This projection will show the approximate relationship of the femoral head to the acetabulum on the anteroposterior radiograph after innom-

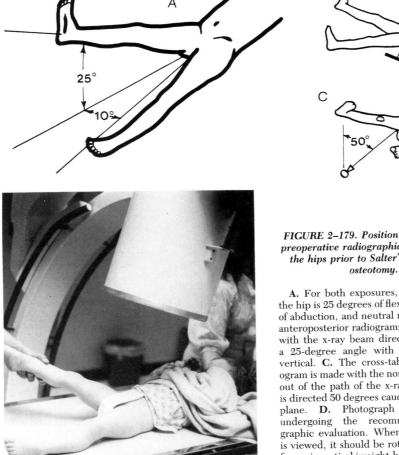

FIGURE 2–179. Position of patient for preoperative radiographic assessment of the hips prior to Salter's innominate osteotomy.

A. For both exposures, the position of the hip is 25 degrees of flexion, 10 degrees of abduction, and neutral rotation. B. The anteroposterior radiograms must be made with the x-ray beam directed caudally at a 25-degree angle with respect to the vertical. C. The cross-table lateral radiogram is made with the normal limb flexed out of the path of the x-ray beam, which is directed 50 degrees caudal to the frontal plane. D. Photograph of a patient undergoing the recommended radiographic evaluation. When the radiogram is viewed, it should be rotated so that the femur is vertical (weight-bearing position). (From Rab, G. T.: Preoperative roentgenographic evaluation for osteotomies about the hip in children. J. Bone Joint Surg., 63-A:306, 1981. Reprinted by permission.)

FIGURE 2–180. *Radiograms of the normal hip of an eight-year-old girl, made at autopsy.*

A. Standard radiograms with the femur in weight-bearing position. **B.** With the hip in 15 degrees of abduction and 15 degrees of internal rotation, the radiograms simulate a varus derotation osteotomy. **C.** Recommended roentgenograms of the hip, simulating innominate osteotomy. **D.** Appearance after an innominate osteotomy. Note the similar appearance of the hip in **C** and **D.** (From Rab, G. T.: Preoperative roentgenographic evaluation for osteotomies about the hip in children. J. Bone Joint Surg., 63-A:306, 1981. Reprinted by permission.)

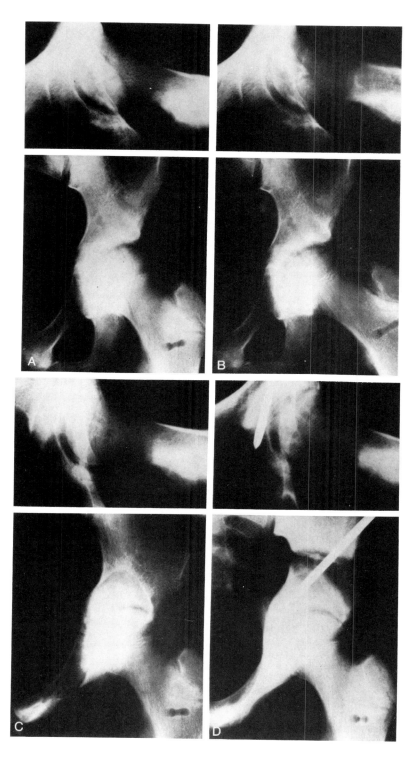

inate osteotomy. Then a true cross-table lateral radiogram is made with the hip in similar position and the roentgenographic beam directed at an angle of 50 degrees to the coronal plane; the opposite limb is flexed out of the way. Salter's innominate osteotomy is indicated if these special preoperative radiographs show reduction of subluxation and an acceptable center-edge angle; if not, a varus derotation–extension osteotomy of the proximal femur should be employed first (Figs. 2–180 and 2–181).[761]

The average improvement of acetabular index following Salter's innominate osteotomy is reported by Utterback and MacEwen to be 10 degrees, and by Morscher to be 6 to 12 degrees.[661, 967] Chapchal will perform the procedure with a maximum acetabular index of 30 degrees.[120] Morscher believes that, because of further improvement with the process of growth, the procedure is justified up to a maximum acetabular angle of 40 degrees between two and four or at most six years of age. If the

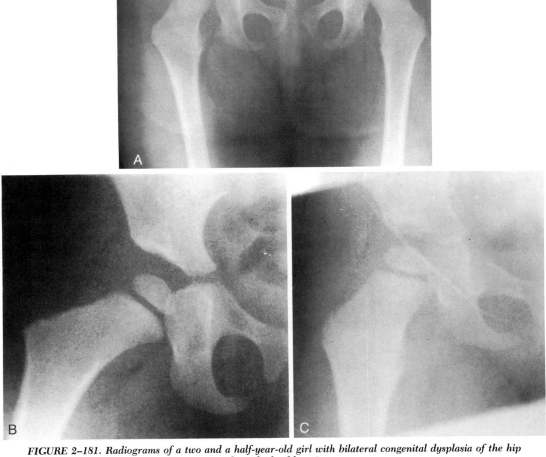

FIGURE 2–181. Radiograms of a two and a half-year-old girl with bilateral congenital dysplasia of the hip and residual subluxation.

A. Standard radiogram. B. Abduction—internal rotation radiogram to simulate varus derotational osteotomy. C. Radiogram to simulate innominate osteotomy. In this patient either procedure would resolve the subluxation, and the surgeon's technical preference would dictate the decision. Note that the radiogram is rotated so that the femur can be viewed in its weight-bearing position. (From Rab, G. T.: Preoperative roentgenographic evaluation for osteotomies about the hips in children. J. Bone Joint Surg., 63-A:306, 1981. Reprinted by permission.)

acetabulum is very shallow (i.e., the index is greater than 40 degrees), the recommendation is to perform an acetabuloplasty such as the Pemberton procedure.[661]

Metaizeau and Prevot studied dissected pelvises by axial radiography before and after Salter's innominate osteotomy. They found the osteotomy decreased excessive antetorsion of the acetabulum by rotating the distal fragment outward, but this movement seemed to increase the antetorsion of the opposite acetabulum. Anterior wall deficiency was not corrected. They recommended that when there was a greater anterior wall defect of the acetabulum or bilateral hip dysplasia, a triple pelvic osteotomy should be performed instead of Salter's osteotomy.[630]

This author recommends that an arthrogram of the hip be performed to depict the cartilaginous components of the acetabulum and its true adequacy. By combining arthrography of the hip with simultaneous computed tomography, one can determine the *chondro-osseous deficiency* of the acetabulum, whether it is posterior, anterior, superior, or all three. In addition, concentricity of reduction and the exact degrees of femoral antetorsion and acetabular antetorsion can be determined accurately by the same study.

Simple measurements of acetabular indices on the routine anteroposterior radiograph of the hips are not adequate to assess the true pathologic changes in hip dysplasia.

Salter's innominate osteotomy is designed to correct antetorsion of the acetabulum (Figs. 2–182 and 2–183). The procedure does not centralize the laterally placed femoral head, as shown in Figure 2–184, it does not medially displace the acetabulum, and it does not enlarge the acetabular cavity.

There is controversy about the degree of femoral antetorsion that can be accepted, i.e., that will correct itself spontaneously with growth. Should derotation osteotomy be performed prior to innominate osteotomy, or combined with it? Should one perform innominate

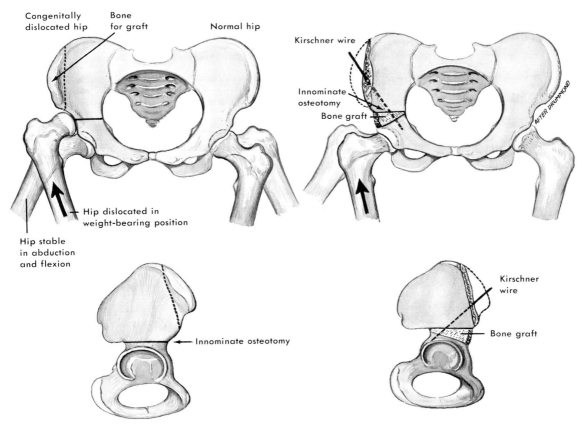

FIGURE 2–182. *Principle of innominate osteotomy.*

(Redrawn from Salter, R. B.: Innominate osteotomy in the treatment of congenital dislocation and subluxation of the hip. J. Bone Joint Surg., *43-B*:518, 1961.)

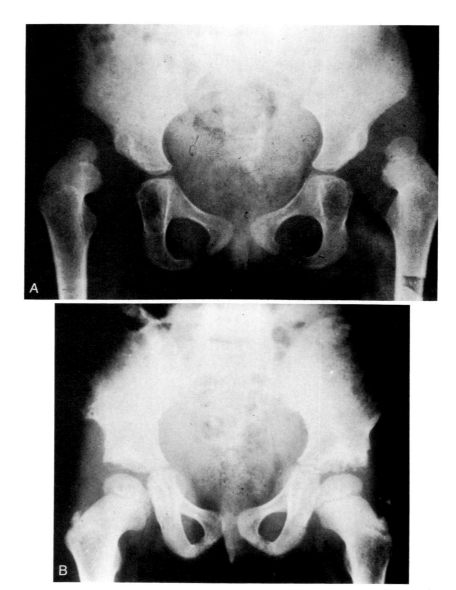

FIGURE 2–183. *Salter's innominate osteotomy in bilateral congenital dislocation of the hip.*

A. Preoperative anteroposterior view of both hips. **B.** Postoperative view after open reduction and Salter's innominate osteotomy. Note the change in the shape of obturator foramina, indicating derotation of the acetabulum. (From Tachdjian M. O. (ed.): Congenital Dislocation of the Hip. New York, Churchill-Livingstone, 1982. Reprinted by permission.)

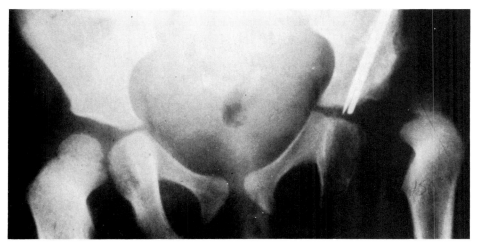

FIGURE 2–184. *Salter's innominate osteotomy is designed to redirect the acetabulum, not to reduce the dislocation of the hip.*

Anteroposterior radiogram of both hips. Note that left hip is still dislocated following the operation.
(From Tachdjian, M. O. (ed.): Congenital Dislocation of the Hip. New York, Churchill-Livingstone, 1982. Reprinted by permission.)

osteotomy first and then femoral osteotomy? These decisions have to be made following thorough study of the pathologic anatomy. Factors in decision-making are the age of the child, the degree of femoral antetorsion, the extent and site of deficiency of the acetabulum, the degree of acetabular torsion, and the severity of capsular ligamentous laxity.

Increased Intra-articular Pressure. The inferiorly and anteriorly tilted superior part of the acetabulum exerts increased pressure against the femoral head by the wedge-shaped bone graft. Therefore the procedure may cause restriction of hip motion. It is important to have good mobility of the hip prior to surgery.

Increased Tension of the Pelvifemoral Muscles. The caudal displacement of the lower segment of the innominate bone is opposed by the hip adductor, iliopsoas, and gluteal muscles. Following innominate osteotomy these muscles become shortened and taut. Therefore Salter recommends that routine tenotomy of the iliopsoas and myotomy of the hip adductors be performed at the same time as innominate osteotomy. Often in the child over three years of age, femoral shortening is carried out at the time of open reduction; this will relatively lengthen the tautened muscles and unload the hip.

Elongation of the Ipsilateral Limb. This is caused by caudal displacement of the acetabulum; this produces a functional pelvic obliquity in stance if the leg lengths were initially equal.

*Prerequisites.** *Complete and Concentric Reduction of the Hip.* The objective of the procedure is to stabilize a completely and concentrically reduced hip joint, not to achieve reduction. This same principle holds true for all the other types of innominate osteotomy discussed later. Failure to recognize this basic prerequisite is the most common pitfall. It is strongly recommended that arthrography of the hip be performed to confirm concentricity of reduction. In hip dislocation, when open reduction and innominate osteotomy are combined there should be a preliminary two-week period of traction, and the femoral head should be brought opposite the triradiate cartilage of the acetabulum. Failure to apply traction initially will cause tautness of muscles that cross the hip joint when the dislocation is reduced. The result will be excessive pressure between the femoral head and the acetabulum, and cartilage necrosis. A meticulous open reduction must precede innominate osteotomy.

Normal or Near-Normal Range of Motion. The reduced hip joint must have approximately normal range of motion, especially abduction, flexion, and medial rotation. Restriction of range of motion may be due to contracture of the soft tissues, intra-articular adhesions, or joint incongruity. If the hip is stiff, reduction of the acetabulum will change the position of the lower limb without providing better coverage

*See references 804–817.

of the femoral head. Reduction of the distal segment of the innominate bone will change only the arc of hip motion without increasing the range of motion. It is imperative that the stiff hip be mobilized by an initial period of traction (bilateral split Russell) and, if necessary, soft-tissue release.

Release of Myostatic Contracture of Iliopsoas and Hip Adductors. Such contractures must be released prior to innominate osteotomy, since they cause instability of the hip in weight-bearing position. This prerequisite must be met for both subluxation and dislocation. One cannot overemphasize the importance of releasing the deforming bowstring force of the iliopsoas by tenotomy.

A Congruous Hip Joint. Incongruity between the reduced femoral head and acetabulum will cause joint stiffness and an uneven gliding motion, and will lead to degenerative arthritis.

Correct Age of Patient. This has been discussed earlier.

Experienced Hip Surgeon. A good technique is essential for a satisfactory anatomic result.

Complications. Complications do occur. The best way to avoid them is to follow to the most minute detail the indications, prerequisites, technique, and postoperative care as described by Salter; departure from the original guidelines and technique is fraught with problems. Salter's innominate osteotomy is a specialized operation; it should not be performed by the inexperienced surgeon who is not trained in pediatric hip surgery.

Immediate Postoperative Problems. These are superficial or deep wound infection, wound dehiscence, and retroperitoneal hematoma. Curtail these problems by paying attention to sterility of technique, gentle handling of tissues, thorough hemostasis at the time of surgery, and closed suction drainage.

Sciatic Nerve Palsy. Nerve palsy can be caused by stretching or by inadvertent division of the nerve during surgery. It is vital to stay within the periosteum, to expose the sciatic notch adequately, and to use a Gigli saw for the osteotomy. Splintering of the thick cortex at the sciatic notch will injure the sciatic nerve.

Femoral Nerve Injury. Damage may be caused by stretching or by inadvertent division of the femoral nerve instead of the psoas tendon during surgery. The use of a nerve stimulator will assist in distinguishing the nerve from the tendon.

Wire Problems. Migration of the Kirschner wire or *Steinmann pin* can be prevented by using threaded instead of smooth wire. *Pin penetration of the hip joint* is avoided by never drilling the pin pointing toward the hip joint; it should be directed posteriorly and medially. The use of intraoperative radiography will prevent problems of overlong pins penetrating the hip joint or rectal mucosa. *Pin breakage* can be prevented by using stout pins.

Loss of Correction from Crushing of the Bone Graft. This is usually due to osteoporosis of disuse, to operating on children under 18 months of age, or to premature removal of the Kirschner wires. Prolonged immobilization beyond six weeks should be avoided. Unsupervised and unprotected ambulation during the first few weeks after removal of the solid cast may result in a fall and cause stress fracture of the graft or of the osteoporotic femoral shaft.

Medial Displacement of the Distal Segment. The cause may be faulty technique at the time of surgery or inadequate internal fixation at the osteotomy site. *Posterior slipping* of the distal segment should be avoided at the time of surgery.

Postoperative Stiffness of the Hip. Increased intra-articular pressure caused by failure to release the already contracted hip adductors and iliopsoas, or chondrolysis caused by penetration of the pins into the joint may result in stiffness of the hip. Full range of motion is essential prior to innominate osteotomy.

Avascular Necrosis. Usually avascular necrosis is the result of open or closed reduction. In the series of Roth and colleagues the three patients with avascular necrosis (out of 97 patients, 123 hips) had each undergone open reduction as well as innominate osteotomy; in cases in which only innominate osteotomy was performed avascular necrosis did not occur.[792] In the series of Paterson, 16 of the 143 hips developed avascular necrosis; in 5 of the hips reduction had been open, and in 11 hips the avascular necrosis was related to previous closed reduction.[715]

Progressive Lateral and Upward Resubluxation and Redislocation. A poorly executed Salter innominate osteotomy, excessive femoral antetorsion, or laxity of the capsule can lead to redislocation. It can be prevented by ensuring that reduction is complete and adequate prior to performing the innominate osteotomy, by performing a taut capsulorrhaphy at the time of open reduction, and by providing adequate protection during healing of the capsular repair. Femoral antetorsion, if in excess of 50 degrees, is best corrected prior to performing innominate osteotomy. This author strongly recommends the use of computed tomography to delineate the deficiency of the acetabulum. On several occasions the acetabular deficiency was posterior, and performance of Salter's innominate osteotomy would have caused the femoral head to be displaced posteriorly. In the young child CT scanning may be combined with simultaneous arthrography to delineate the chondroosseous deficiency of the acetabulum. A CT scan will also determine the degree of femoral antetorsion accurately.

Modifications of the Salter Innominate Osteotomy

Westin's Pember-Sal Osteotomy. Westin has described an acetabuloplasty combining some features of both the Pemberton and Salter procedures. The technique and results were published with Marafioti in 1980 and later with Perlik and Marafioti in 1985.[601, 725] The operation is performed through an anterior iliofemoral approach; the iliac apophysis is split, and the ilium is exposed subperiosteally. The tendinous portion of the iliopsoas is sectioned at the level of the triradiate cartilage. The anterior, superior, and posterior aspects of the hip joint capsule are exposed. The osteotomy begins in a manner similar to the Pemberton operation. A curvilinear cut of the ilium is made parallel to the dome of the acetabulum; it begins 10 to 15 mm. above the anterior inferior iliac spine, but instead of being directed toward the posterior limb of the triradiate cartilage (as in the Pemberton operation), it continues through the ischial limb of the cartilage across the inner brim of the true pelvis (as in the Salter procedure). Then, rather than completely sectioning the innominate bone at the greater sciatic notch, the osteotomy curves posteriorly into the body of the ischium, where it terminates (Fig. 2–185). Opening the osteotomy produces a greenstick fracture in the remaining portion of the body of the ischium. The hip is acutely flexed, abducted, and laterally rotated, and distal traction is applied on the thigh, thereby rotating the acetabulum forward, downward, and laterally about an axis that passes through the ischial fracture and the symphysis pubis. Some degree of inferolateral rotation of the acetabulum takes place through the hinge of the triradiate cartilage (Fig. 2–186). The advantage of the combination pelvic osteotomy (Westin's Pember-Sal) is that it reorients the acetabulum as in the Salter operation and deepens it as in the Pemberton procedure (Fig. 2–187). A triangular wedge of bone is used to maintain the new position of the acetabulum. Internal fixation by pins is not necessary.

A one and one half hip spica cast is applied for immobilization for six weeks, after which only partial weight-bearing is permitted for an additional six weeks. In the combined pelvic osteotomy inadvertent damage to the sciatic nerve or superior gluteal vessels is less likely to occur because the osteotomy line does not enter the sciatic notch, and—the aforementioned major advantage—the acetabulum is redirected by hinging at the symphysis pubis (as in the Salter procedure) and also can be cupped more deeply at the triradiate cartilage (as in the Pemberton operation). The author recommends Westin's combination pelvic osteotomy when both reorientation and deepening of the acetabulum are indicated in children over four years of age.

Kalamchi's Modification of the Salter Innominate Osteotomy. Salter's innominate osteotomy elongates the ipsilateral limb, the amount of added length depending on the size of the triangular graft inserted into the opened-up osteotomy site. When the lower limb lengths are equal preoperatively or if the ipsilateral limb is the longer one, the Salter innominate osteotomy can result in a noticeable lower limb

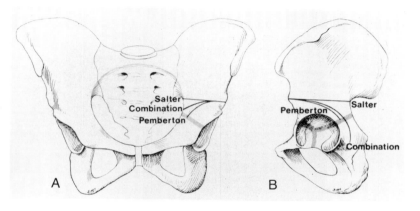

FIGURE 2–185. *Diagram of the lines of iliac cuts in the Westin combination pelvic osteotomy as compared with the Salter and Pemberton iliac osteotomies.*

A. Anteroposterior view. **B.** Lateral view. (From Perlik, P. C., Westin, G. W., and Marafioti, R. L.: Combination pelvic osteotomy for acetabular dysplasia in children. J. Bone Joint Surg., 67-A:842, 1985. Reprinted by permission.)

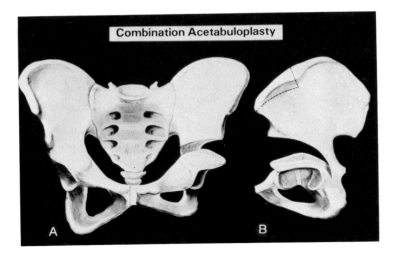

FIGURE 2–186. Westin's combination pelvic osteotomy.

Opening the osteotomy produces a greenstick fracture in the ischium. The rotation and displacement of the acetabulum takes place on the hinge of the fractured ischium and on the symphysis pubis. **A.** Anteroposterior view. **B.** Lateral view. The site of the graft from the ilium is shown by the broken line. (From Perlik, P. C., Westin, G. W., and Marafioti, R. L.: Combination pelvic osteotomy for acetabular dysplasia in children. J. Bone Joint Surg., 67-A:842, 1985. Reprinted by permission.)

length disparity and pelvic obliquity with a trunk list. Another problem of the Salter procedure is medial and posterior displacement of the osteotomized distal segment due to poor technical performance of the operation. This results in unsatisfactory rotation of the acetabulum and inadequate femoral head coverage. Kalamchi described a modification of Salter's innominate osteotomy in which a triangular piece of iliac bone is removed from the upper side of the osteotomy site. The distal segment is rotated and locked into the proximal segment, the triangular piece of bone is inserted anteriorly, and the osteotomized segments are fixed internally with two threaded pins (Figs. 2–188 and 2–189).[480] This provides greater stability, prevents medial and posterior displacement of the distal segment, and avoids the problem of limb elongation. The indications for surgery are

unilateral hip dysplasia and lower limb length discrepancy in which the affected limb is the longer. Details of the operative procedure are as follows:

Lateral and medial walls of the ilium are exposed subperiosteally according to Salter's technique. In order to allow free displacement of the distal segment, further subperiosteal exposure should be obtained distally. The iliac osteotomy is performed with a Gigli saw. A drill is used to mark the triangular wedge of bone to be removed from the upper segment of the ilium with the base of the wedge along the osteotomy line. The wedge is located posteriorly, immediately in front of the posterior cortex of the ilium. The posterior cortex should be left intact, and the triangular areas from the medial and lateral walls of the ilium should be of equal size. Uneven fit of the osteotomy

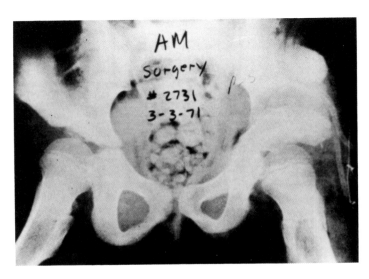

FIGURE 2–187. Radiogram after completion of combined pelvic osteotomy.

The asymmetry of the obturator foramen shows derotation of the acetabulum. Note the lateral coverage of the femoral head resulting from the deepening of the acetabulum. The gap in the pelvic rim is obvious. (From Perlik, B. C., Westin, G. W., and Marafioti, R. L.: Combination pelvic osteotomy for acetabular dysplasia in children. J. Bone Joint Surg., 67-A:842, 1985. Reprinted by permission.)

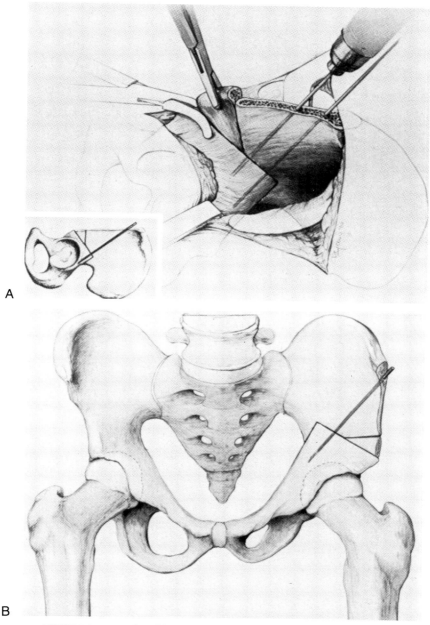

A

B

FIGURE 2–188. Kalamchi's modification of the Salter innominate osteotomy.

A and **B.** The completed osteotomy shown in lateral and anteroposterior views. A triangular wedge of bone is removed from the posterior part of the upper segment of the ilium, with its base along the osteotomy line. The posterior cortex is left intact. The distal segment is rotated and locked into the proximal segment. Internal fixation is with two threaded Steinmann pins. A triangular piece of bone graft is inserted anteriorly to fill the gap. (From Kalamchi, A.: Modified Salter osteotomy. J. Bone Joint Surg., *64-A*:183, 1982. Reprinted by permission.)

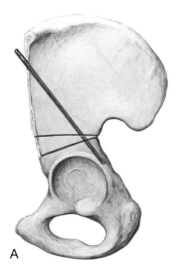 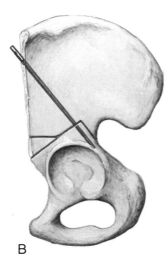

FIGURE 2–189. *Diagrams illustrating the difference between Salter's innominate osteotomy and Kalamchi's modification.*

A. Salter's innominate osteotomy. **B.** Kalamchi's modification.

A

B

should be avoided. Each side of the triangular wedge usually measures about 1 cm. in a five-year-old child; this varies with the degree of postoperative lower limb length disparity and the age of the child. The drill holes are connected with thin small osteotomes, the osteotomy is completed, and the triangular wedge is removed in one piece. In the older child the medial and lateral cortices may have to be removed separately; with a small rongeur or curet the intervening cancellous bone is excised. The angle of inclination of the osteotomy is about 30 degrees; if more rotation is desired, additional bone is removed with a rongeur. It is best to remove a small wedge initially. Next engage the posterior corner of the distal segment in the triangular slot of the proximal segment of the ilium, pulling the distal segment anterolaterally and rotating distally. Rotation takes place through the symphysis pubis. Upon engagement of the iliac segments, the osteotomy is very stable. An iliac bone graft is inserted into the triangular gap anteriorly, and the osteotomy is fixed internally with two threaded Steinmann pins as described by Salter. A one and one half hip spica cast is applied with the hip that was operated on in 30 degrees of flexion, 30 degrees of abduction, and neutral rotation. It is worn for six weeks. Then the cast and pins are removed, and active and passive range-of-motion exercises are performed to restore normal hip motion and muscle strength. An illustrative case is shown in Figure 2–190.

Correction of Deficient and Shallow Acetabulum in Children Under Six Years of Age

This can be carried out by two methods: The first, acetabuloplasty, and the second, Pember-

ton's pericapsular innominate osteotomy of the ilium.

Acetabuloplasty

In this procedure the acetabular roof is mobilized by a pericapsular curved dome osteotomy of the acetabulum. The procedure is extra-articular—the osteotomy does not violate the joint. The line of osteotomy is parallel to the acetabular roof—it begins 1 cm. superior to the margin of the acetabulum and extends from the iliopectineal prominence anteriorly to the posterior limb of the triradiate cartilage. It stops short of the growth plate of the Y-cartilage; physeal damage and growth arrest are thereby prevented. The osteotomy extends from the lateral wall of the ilium to its medial cortex. Acetabuloplasty differs from Pemberton's pericapsular innominate osteotomy in two ways: (1) Growth of the triradiate cartilage is not disturbed, and (2) the cortex of the medial wall of the ilium is left intact. The line of the osteotomy is curved in three planes: anteroposteriorly, laterally to medially, and superoinferiorly. The acetabulum is mobilized through cancellous bone of its roof. The cartilaginous and bony roof of the acetabulum is turned inferiorly and laterally, covering the concentrically reduced femoral head anteriorly, superiorly, and posteriorly. It is secured in place by wedges of cortical and cancellous bone taken from the crest of the ilium. Internal fixation with pins and screws is not required. In the literature, various forms of acetabuloplasty have been described, such as the Albee shelf, the Gill plastic reconstruction of the acetabulum and the Hughes acetabuloplasty.[2, 332, 438, 440]

Indications for acetabuloplasty are a deficient

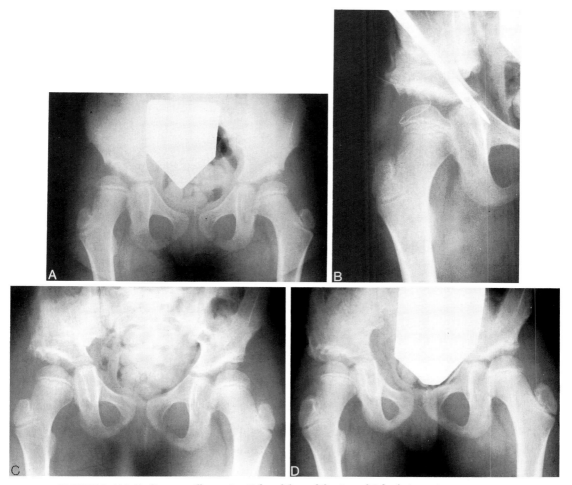

FIGURE 2–190. Radiograms illustrating Kalamchi's modification of Salter's innominate osteotomy.

A. Preoperative radiogram of a seven-year-old girl with bilateral congenital dislocation of the hip. Treated initially by closed reduction, she presented with pain and limp on the right. The right lower limb was 1 cm. longer than the left. **B.** Immediate postoperative radiogram of right hip. **C.** Five months postoperatively. Note the excellent coverage provided to the femoral head. **D.** One year postoperatively.

and shallow acetabulum in a child who is under three to four years of age. Requisites are a concentrically reduced hip that has functional range of motion. The procedure can be simultaneously performed during open reduction or staged six to ten weeks later depending upon the individual case. In the experience of this author, acetabuloplasty has been a very satisfactory method to correct a deficient acetabulum and fully cover a concentrically reduced femoral head in children under four years of age. Lately this author prefers acetabuloplasty over Pemberton's pericapsular innominate osteotomy.

Pemberton's Pericapsular Innominate Osteotomy of the Ilium

Pemberton, in 1958, described an iliac osteotomy in which the cut in the ilium begins between the anterosuperior and anteroinferior iliac spines and extends posteriorly around the acetabulum to the posterior limb of the triradiate cartilage, where it terminates.[721] In the Pemberton osteotomy the fulcrum of rotation and angulation takes place at the triradiate cartilage in contrast to the Salter osteotomy in which the rotation of the acetabulum occurs at the symphysis pubis. The Pemberton osteotomy requires an open triradiate cartilage, whereas the Salter osteotomy requires a flexible symphysis pubis.

The advantages of the Pemberton osteotomy are: First, the fulcrum of rotation is close to the hip joint; therefore it permits a greater degree of correction of the deficient acetabulum and better coverage of the femoral head than does the Salter innominate osteotomy. Second, the iliac osteotomy is incomplete, leaving the posterior and inferior segments of the acetabulum intact. The osteotomy is, therefore, relatively stable, and internal fixation is not required unless so desired by the surgeon. In the Salter innominate osteotomy the innominate fragments are unstable, and internal fixation is mandatory. Third, in the Pemberton procedure, the saw or osteotomes do not extend into the sciatic notch; therefore, the likelihood of damage to neurovascular structures is minimal. In the Salter osteotomy the Gigli saw is inserted through the greater sciatic notch, with potential for injury to the sciatic nerve and gluteal vessels.

The Pemberton osteotomy has, however, distinct *disadvantages* that should be seriously considered prior to performing the operation. First, the incomplete osteotomy distorts the configuration of the acetabulum, and the deformation of the acetabulum and the joint incongruity will cause stiffness of the hip; therefore, the procedure should be performed only in the young child (six years of age or under) who has considerable potential for biologic remodeling with skeletal growth. In contrast, the Salter innominate osteotomy does not change the configuration or the capacity of the acetabulum; it redirects and derotates it to correct excessive acetabular torsion. The second disadvantage of the Pemberton osteotomy is the possibility of growth disturbance because the cut may extend too far posteriorly as it hinges at the triradiate cartilage; this complication may be ominous. In contrast, the Salter innominate osteotomy does not disturb growth.

Age restrictions are more rigid with the Pemberton osteotomy than with the Salter innominate osteotomy. In Pemberton's operation the triradiate cartilage should be wide open—limiting the age span to between one and a half and six years. The procedure is contraindicated when the triradiate cartilage is thin or closing.

In contrast, the upper age limit for the Salter innominate osteotomy can be extended up to adolescence, especially in unilateral hip dysplasia. The Pemberton osteotomy is technically difficult, especially the visualization of the posterior limb of the triradiate cartilage. Image intensifier radiographic control is mandatory to determine the level, direction, and extent of the iliac cuts. It is easy to enter the hip joint and cause hyaline cartilage damage with consequent chondrolysis of the hip. Excess pressure by the bone graft on the rotated acetabular fragment may cause subchondral sclerosis of the roof of the acetabulum and possible avascular necrosis.

Indications. The primary indication for Pemberton's pericapsular iliac osteotomy is marked deficiency of the anterior and superolateral walls of the acetabulum in a child between two and six years of age with marked laxity of the capsule and hypermobility of the hip joint. It is vital to delineate the true deficiency of the cartilaginous walls and roof of the acetabulum by contrast arthrography. Computed tomography (combined with arthrography in the young child) will provide three-dimensional visualization of the cartilaginous acetabulum.

Prerequisites. The primary requirement is an open triradiate cartilage. Full range of hip motion is also important. Other prerequisites are similar to those for Salter's innominate osteotomy, i.e., concentric reduction of the femoral head in the acetabulum, a congruous hip joint with normal articular cartilage space, release of myostatic contracture of hip adductors and iliopsoas, and an experienced pediatric hip surgeon.

The operative technique of Pemberton's pericapsular iliac osteotomy is described and illustrated in Plate 19. An illustrative case is shown in Figure 2–191.

Complications

Ischemic Necrosis of Proximal Femur. A serious complication of treatment of congenital dislocation of the hip is ischemic necrosis of the femoral head and damage to growth of its physis. In the literature the terms *avascular necrosis* and *ischemic necrosis* are used interchangeably. From the semantic viewpoint, *ischemic necrosis* is more appropriate because the vascular compromise in congenital dislocation of the hip is partial, involving selected vessels, and is generally transient, whereas *avascular necrosis* denotes total absence of blood supply.[926] The ischemic necrosis in congenital hip dislocation is aseptic; it should be distinguished from the septic ischemic necrosis following pyogenic arthritis of the hip.

The incidence of avascular necrosis varies according to the method of treatment. In the past two decades, early diagnosis, the use of prereduction traction, gentle manipulation while reducing the dislocation under general anesthesia, immobilization of the hips in physiologic "human" position and not in extreme positions such as "frog" or marked medial rotation, as shown in Figure 2–192, and femoral shortening while open reduction is being performed have dramatically decreased its incidence—reportedly from 73 per cent to zero.[184, 555, 610, 817, 1046]

Ischemic necrosis of the hip follows treatment of congenital dislocation of the hip; it is iatro-

Text continued on page 433

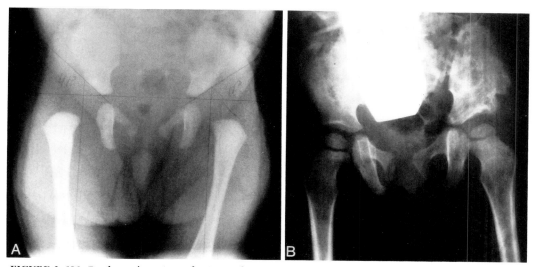

FIGURE 2–191. Pemberton's pericapsular incomplete osteotomy to correct a deficient and shallow acetabulum.

A. Preoperative anteroposterior radiograph of a three-year-old child. **B.** Postoperative radiograph showing excellent correction.

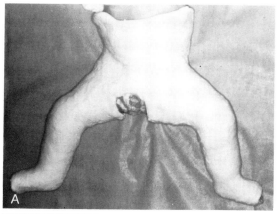

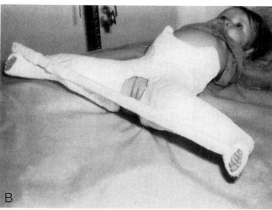

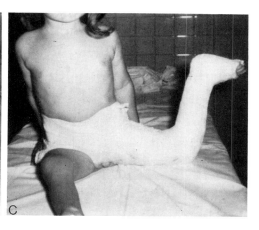

FIGURE 2–192. Immobilization of the hips in extreme positions in the hip spica cast.

These positions will compromise blood supply to the proximal femur. **A.** Frog-leg position. **B** and **C.** Extreme medial rotation.

Pemberton's Osteotomy

The skin of the affected side of the abdomen and pelvis and the entire lower limb is prepared with the patient lying on his side, and is draped to allow free hip motion during surgery. Then the patient is placed completely supine. The operation is performed on a radiolucent operating table. It is imperative to have image intensifier fluoroscopy and radiographic control.

OPERATIVE TECHNIQUE

A. The medial and lateral walls of the ilium and the hip joint are exposed through an anterolateral iliofemoral approach. The cartilaginous apophysis of the ilium is split according to Salter's technique. The sartorius muscle is sectioned at its origin from the anterior superior iliac spine, tagged with 2-0 Mersilene suture, and reflected distally. Both heads of the rectus femoris are divided at their origin and reflected. The iliopsoas tendon is lengthened by transverse incisions. Pemberton's iliac osteotomy lengthens the pelvis. Division of the psoas tendon (not the iliacus muscle) decreases the pressure over the femoral head.

B. The ilium is exposed subperiosteally all the way posteriorly. The interval between the greater sciatic notch and the hip joint capsule posteriorly is developed gently and cautiously. The periosteal elevator meets resistance at the posterior limb of the triradiate cartilage. Chandler elevator retractors are placed in the greater sciatic notch medially and laterally to protect the sciatic nerve and the gluteal vessels and nerves. On the inner wall of the pelvis the periosteum and the cartilaginous apophysis may be divided anteriorly to posteriorly at the level of the anteroinferior iliac spine as far as the sciatic notch; this will facilitate opening up of the osteotomy.

Plate 19. Pemberton's Osteotomy

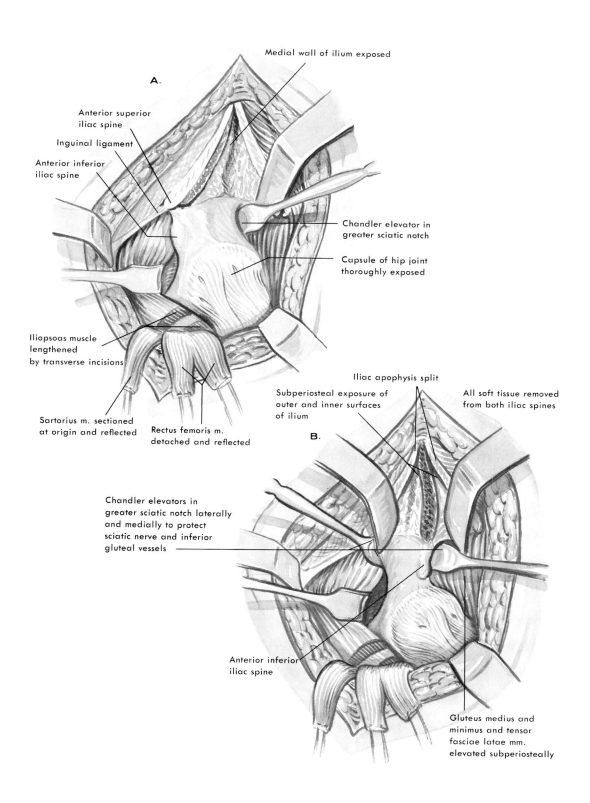

A.

Medial wall of ilium exposed

Anterior superior iliac spine

Inguinal ligament

Anterior inferior iliac spine

Chandler elevator in greater sciatic notch

Capsule of hip joint thoroughly exposed

Iliopsoas muscle lengthened by transverse incisions

Sartorius m. sectioned at origin and reflected

Rectus femoris m. detached and reflected

B.

Iliac apophysis split

Subperiosteal exposure of outer and inner surfaces of ilium

All soft tissue removed from both iliac spines

Chandler elevators in greater sciatic notch laterally and medially to protect sciatic nerve and inferior gluteal vessels

Anterior inferior iliac spine

Gluteus medius and minimus and tensor fasciae latae mm. elevated subperiosteally

427

Pemberton's Osteotomy (Continued)

C to E. The osteotomy is first performed on the outer table of the ilium. The cut is curvilinear, describing a semicircle around the hip joint on the lateral side at a level 1 cm. above the joint, between the anterosuperior and anteroinferior iliac spines. It is best to mark the line of osteotomy with indelible ink. The sharp edge of a thin osteotome is used to make the cut. The osteotomy ends at the posterior arm of the triradiate cartilage. This is most difficult to visualize if the exposure is inadequate. Image intensifier fluoroscopy with television control will help to determine the terminal point of the cut at the triradiate cartilage, which is anterior to the greater sciatic notch and posterior to the hip joint margin. The next cut is made on the inner wall of the ilium and should be inferior to the level of the outer cut. The more distal the level of the inferior cut, the greater the extent of lateral coverage. If more anterior than superior coverage is required, the medial and lateral cuts in the ilium are parallel. The importance of sectioning the ilium as far posterior and inferior to the triradiate cartilage as possible cannot be overemphasized. It is vital not to violate the articular cartilage of the acetabulum and enter the hip joint.

Plate 19. Pemberton's Osteotomy

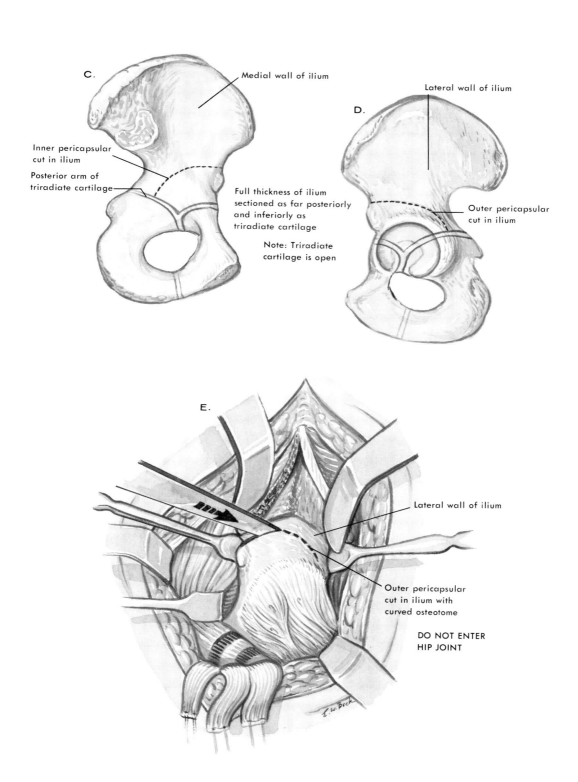

C.

Medial wall of ilium

Inner pericapsular cut in ilium

Posterior arm of triradiate cartilage

Full thickness of ilium sectioned as far posteriorly and inferiorly as triradiate cartilage

Note: Triradiate cartilage is open

D.

Lateral wall of ilium

Outer pericapsular cut in ilium

E.

Lateral wall of ilium

Outer pericapsular cut in ilium with curved osteotome

DO NOT ENTER HIP JOINT

E. W. Beck

Pemberton's Osteotomy (Continued)

F. With sharp curved osteotomes, the cuts of the inner and outer table of the ilium are joined. Periosteal elevators are used to mobilize the osteotomized fragments, and the inferior segment of the ilium is leveled laterally, anteriorly, and distally.

G. If necessary, a laminar spreader may be utilized to separate the iliac fragments. One should, however, be very gentle, and steady the upper segment of the ilium and push it distally. Care should be taken not to fracture the acetabular segment by forceful manipulation or crushing with the laminar spreader.

H and I. Next, a triangular wedge of bone is resected from the anterior part of the iliac wing. In the young child this author removes the wedge of bone more posteriorly and avoids the anterosuperior iliac spine. This gives greater stability to the iliac fragments. The wedge of bone graft may be shaped into a curve to fit the graft site. Pemberton and Coleman recommend that grooves be made on the opposing cancellous surfaces of the osteotomy. The graft is impacted into the grooves, and the osteotomized fragment is sufficiently stable to obviate the need for internal fixation. This author does not recommend cutting grooves because of problems with splintering and weakening of the acetabulum. The fragments are fixed internally with two threaded Kirschner pins or cancellous screws. The internal fixation allows one to remove the cast sooner, mobilize the hip, and prevent joint stiffness. The sartorius muscle is reattached to its origin, the split iliac apophysis is sutured, and the wound closed in the usual fashion. A one–and–one half hip spica cast is applied.

POSTOPERATIVE CARE

The cast is removed in four to six weeks, and the healing of the osteotomy is assessed by anteroposterior and oblique-lateral roentgenograms. The child is placed in bilateral split Russell's traction to mobilize the hip gradually. When joint motion and motor strength of the hip extensors, quadriceps, and triceps surae muscles are good, the child is allowed to ambulate. In the older patient, three-point crutch gait with toe touch on the limb that was operated on is used to protect the hip until the Trendelenburg test is negative.

Plate 19. Pemberton's Osteotomy

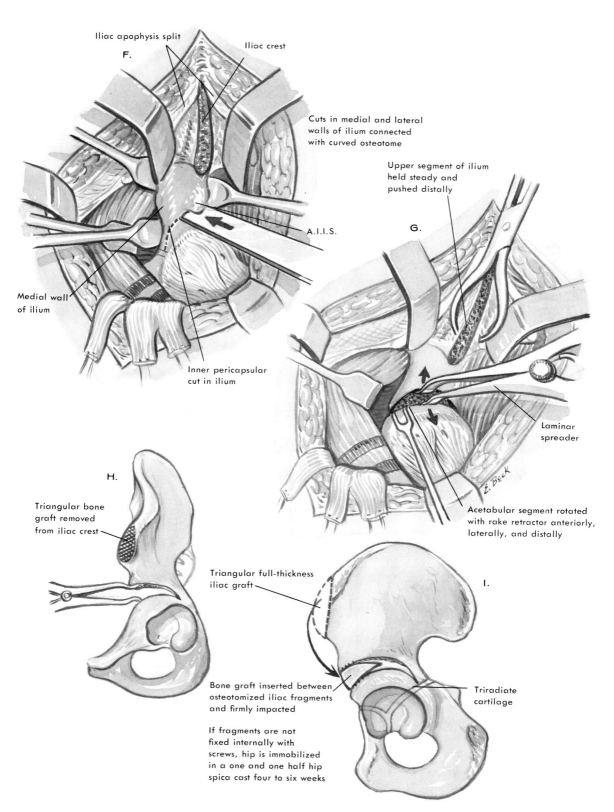

F.

Iliac apophysis split

Iliac crest

Cuts in medial and lateral walls of ilium connected with curved osteotome

A.I.I.S.

Medial wall of ilium

Inner pericapsular cut in ilium

G.

Upper segment of ilium held steady and pushed distally

Laminar spreader

Acetabular segment rotated with rake retractor anteriorly, laterally, and distally

E. Beck

H.

Triangular bone graft removed from iliac crest

Triangular full-thickness iliac graft

I.

Triradiate cartilage

Bone graft inserted between osteotomized iliac fragments and firmly impacted

If fragments are not fixed internally with screws, hip is immobilized in a one and one half hip spica cast four to six weeks

431

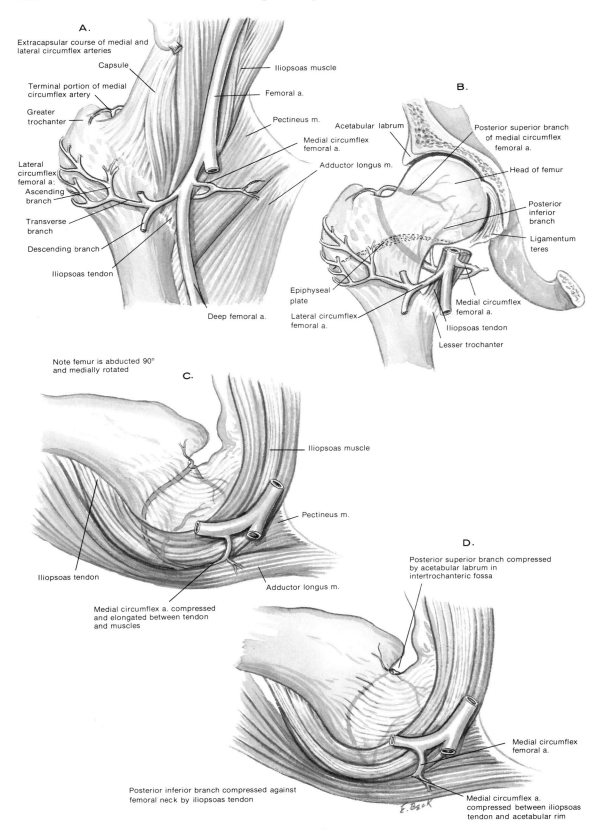

A.

Extracapsular course of medial and lateral circumflex arteries

Capsule

Terminal portion of medial circumflex artery

Greater trochanter

Lateral circumflex femoral a:
Ascending branch
Transverse branch
Descending branch

Iliopsoas tendon

Iliopsoas muscle

Femoral a.

Pectineus m.

Medial circumflex femoral a.

Adductor longus m.

Deep femoral a.

B.

Acetabular labrum

Posterior superior branch of medial circumflex femoral a.

Head of femur

Posterior inferior branch

Ligamentum teres

Medial circumflex femoral a.

Iliopsoas tendon

Lesser trochanter

Epiphyseal plate

Lateral circumflex femoral a.

Note femur is abducted 90° and medially rotated

C.

Iliopsoas muscle

Pectineus m.

Iliopsoas tendon

Adductor longus m.

Medial circumflex a. compressed and elongated between tendon and muscles

D.

Posterior superior branch compressed by acetabular labrum in intertrochanteric fossa

Medial circumflex femoral a.

Posterior inferior branch compressed against femoral neck by iliopsoas tendon

Medial circumflex a. compressed between iliopsoas tendon and acetabular rim

E. Beck

FIGURE 2–193 See legend on opposite page

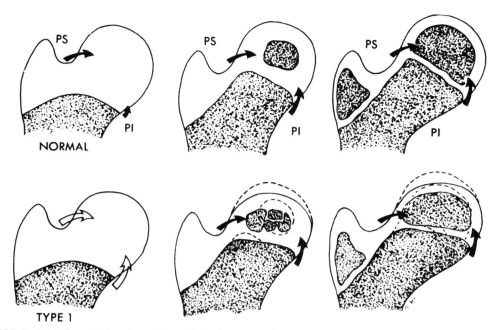

FIGURE 2–194. *Schematic drawings of normal development and Type I pattern of ischemic necrosis of the proximal femur following treatment of congenital dislocation of the hip.*

The normally developing hip *(above)* is compared with a hip with Type I pattern of ischemic necrosis *(below)* at two months, one year, and nine years of age. (From Bucholz, R. W., and Ogden, J. A.: Patterns of ischemic necrosis of the proximal femur in nonoperatively treated congenital hip diseases. *In* The Hip: Proceedings of the Sixth Open Scientific Meeting of the Hip Society. St. Louis, C.V. Mosby, 1978. Reprinted by permission.)

genic. The sequelae of ischemic necrosis of the proximal femur are serious; they include deformation of the femoral head, lateral subluxation, acetabular dysplasia, hip joint incongruity, relative overgrowth of the greater trochanter, lower limb length inequality, and later on in life, osteoarthritis of the hip. The prognosis and severity of residual structural deformities depend on the site of ischemic involvement, whether it be the femoral head or the capital physis or both, and also upon the extent and severity of ischemia. Various segments of the physis may be involved, producing different changes.

Vascular occlusion external to the capital chondroepiphysis may occur when, as the hip is abducted, the medial circumflex artery is compressed between the iliopsoas tendon and the adductor-pectineus group of muscles, especially if the latter are contracted, or when

the hip is maximally abducted, between the iliopsoas tendon and the pubic ramus. The course of the medial circumflex artery along the intertrochanteric notch is very hazardous; as the hip is maximally abducted the ring of the acetabulum impinges on the greater trochanteric fossa and occludes the posterosuperior vessels of the artery. Conversely, the artery is stretched when the hip is maximally abducted in flexion, and the medial rotation aggravates the undue stretching. Ogden has demonstrated that stretching of the medial circumflex vessels may take place in minimal abduction of the hip if the hip is in maximum medial rotation.[678] The posteroinferior vessels course beneath the iliopsoas tendon as they pass toward the lesser trochanter; these vessels may be compressed by the translocation of the iliopsoas tendon as the hip is flexed and abducted (Fig. 2–193).

It should be noted that the lateral circumflex

FIGURE 2–193. *Diagrammatic illustration of the various anatomic sites where compression of blood vessels to the proximal femur can occur.*

A and **B.** Normal blood supply of the upper end of the femur in an infant. **A.** Anterior view. **B.** Posterior view. **C.** The medial circumflex artery may be compressed between the iliopsoas tendon and the adductor and pectineus muscles, between the iliopsoas tendon and the pelvis. **D.** The posterior superior and medial circumflex vessels may be compressed by the acetabular rim, and the posteroinferior vessels may be compressed as they course behind the iliopsoas tendon and along the upper femoral metaphysis.

artery is minimally affected by the foregoing position of immobilization; therefore, the growth of the greater trochanter is unaffected, explaining the phenomenon of relative overgrowth of the greater trochanter.

Classification. Ogden and Bucholz and Ogden identified four radiographic patterns of ischemic necrosis in the proximal part of the femur caused by morphologic changes in the capital femoral epiphysis, the physis, and the proximal femoral metaphysis. Specific vascular occlusions result in characteristic morphologic patterns.[88, 674-678]

Type I is characterized by either temporary

fragmentation of the capital femoral ossific nucleus or delay in appearance of the ossific nucleus and mottling of the cartilage model (Fig. 2–194). It is caused by extracapsular occlusion of the main circumflex artery. Following ischemic necrosis, reossification is rapid and complete. The prognosis for Type I ischemic necrosis is good; loss of epiphyseal height is slight, and coxa magna is minimal, if any. At skeletal maturity the stigmata of the previous vascular compromise are radiographic findings of minor variations from the normal (Figs. 2–195 and 2–196). Hip function is excellent.

In *Type II* avascular necrosis, vascular occlu-

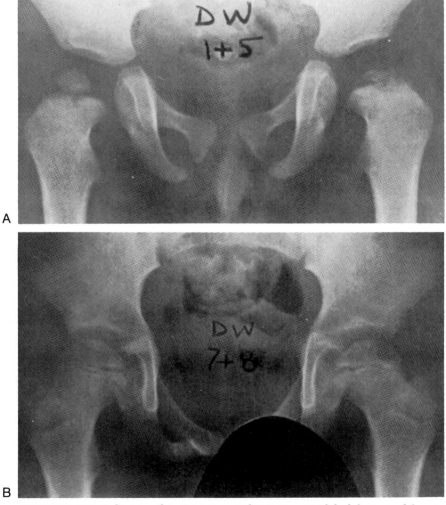

FIGURE 2–195. Radiogram of Type I pattern ischemic necrosis of the left proximal femur.

A. At 17 months of age. Note the smaller and irregular ossific nucleus of the femoral head on the left as compared with the right. **B.** At seven years and eight months of age. Note the epiphysis and physis of the left proximal femoral head are normal. (From Thomas C. L., Gage, J. R., and Ogden, J. A.: Treatment concepts for proximal femoral ischemic necrosis. J. Bone Joint Surg., 64-A:817, 1982. Reprinted by permission.)

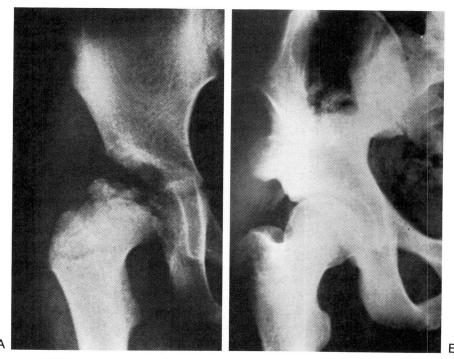

FIGURE 2–196. Group I (or Type I) Pattern of ischemic necrosis of right hip.

A. After closed reduction. Note the fragmentation and flattening of the femoral head. **B.** At 19 years of age the hip is normal. No residual deformity. (From Kalamchi, A., and MacEwen, G. D.: Avascular necrosis following treatment of congenital dislocation of the hip. J. Bone Joint Surg., 62-A:876, 1980. Reprinted by permission.)

sion of the posterosuperior branches of the medial circumflex artery results in localized radiographic changes in the lateral portions of the physis, epiphysis, and metaphysis (Fig. 2–197). Damage to the lateral part of the capital physis causes premature fusion of the superolateral part of the physis, whereas the medial parts of the femoral head and neck continue to grow normally. The roentgenographic signs that indicate damage to the lateral part of the capital femoral physis are lateral ossification, lateral physeal irregularity and bridging, lateral notching of the epiphysis, and a lateral metaphyseal defect (Fig. 2–198). The tethering effect of the lateral epiphyseodesis leads to growth retardation of the lateral segment of the femoral neck

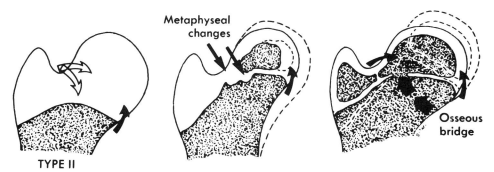

FIGURE 2–197. Type II pattern of ischemic necrosis of femoral head at two months, one year, and nine years old.

The open arrows represent the probable primary sites of vascular occlusion. Note the localized irregularity in the lateral portions of the metaphysis and physis and the subsequent premature epiphyseodesis in the same region. Both occur at the site of presumptive vascular ischemia to the epiphyseal vessels supplying this region of the physis. (From Bucholz, R. W., and Ogden, G. A.: Patterns of ischemic necrosis of the proximal femur in non-operatively treated congenital hip disease. *In* The Hip: Proceedings of the Sixth Open Meeting of the Hip Society. St. Louis, 1978. Reprinted by permission.)

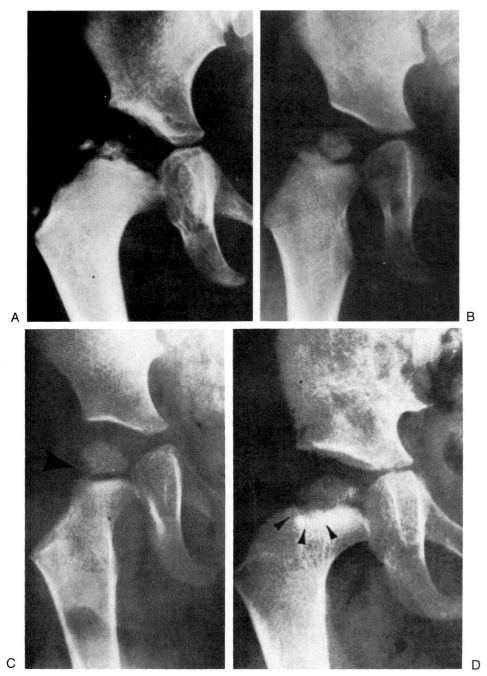

FIGURE 2–198. *Early radiographic signs of vascular damage, the lateral part of the capital femoral epiphysis.*

A. Lateral ossification. Note there is a radio-opaque fragment of the epiphysis beyond the normal femoral neck margin. **B.** Bridging and distortion of the lateral part of the capital physis. **C.** Notching of the lateral part of the epiphysis. **D.** Lateral metaphyseal cystic changes. (From Kalamchi, A., and MacEwen, G. D.: Avascular necrosis following treatment of congenital dislocation of the hip. J. Bone Joint Surg., 62-A:876, 1980. Reprinted by permission.)

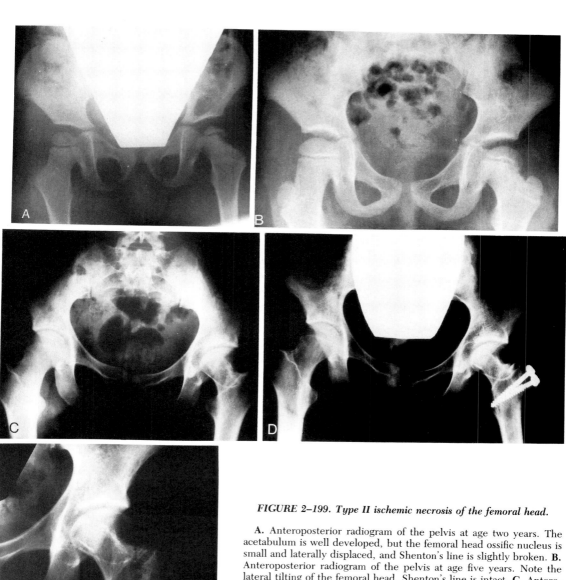

FIGURE 2–199. Type II ischemic necrosis of the femoral head.

A. Anteroposterior radiogram of the pelvis at age two years. The acetabulum is well developed, but the femoral head ossific nucleus is small and laterally displaced, and Shenton's line is slightly broken. **B.** Anteroposterior radiogram of the pelvis at age five years. Note the lateral tilting of the femoral head. Shenton's line is intact. **C.** Anteroposterior view of the pelvis at age 16 years. The femoral neck is short, and there is relative overgrowth of the greater trochanter. **D.** Immediate postoperative radiogram following distal and lateral transfer of the greater trochanter. **E.** One year postoperatively, showing an excellent result of the distal-lateral transfer of the greater trochanter.

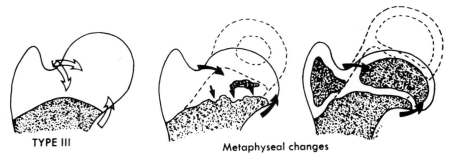

TYPE III   **Metaphyseal changes**

FIGURE 2–200. Type III pattern of ischemic necrosis.

Schematic diagram showing findings at two months, one year, and nine years of age. The open arrows represent the sites of temporary vascular occlusion, causing impaired longitudinal growth through the capital femoral physis as well as the intraepiphyseal physis. The trochanteric region continues relatively normal longitudinal growth. (From Bucholz, R. W., and Ogden, J. A.: Patterns of ischemic necrosis of the proximal femur in nonoperatively treated congenital hip disease. In the Hip: Proceedings of the Sixth Open Scientific Meeting of the Hip Society. St. Louis, C. V. Mosby, 1978. Reprinted by permission.)

and tilting of the head into a valgus posture. Eventually the central and medial parts of the physis will close prematurely. The outcome is a short femoral neck in valgus angulation with marked uncovering of the femoral head by the acetabulum (Fig. 2–199).

Thomas, Gage, and Ogden subclassified the Type II pattern of ischemic necrosis into two groups. The growth of the lateral portion of the physis is involved in both subgroups, but in Type II B there is central involvement of the ossific nucleus of the femoral head.[926]

Type III ischemic necrosis is the most severe vascular insult. The entire proximal part of the femur is involved, including the metaphysis, physis, and epiphyseal ossific nucleus (Fig. 2–200). The capital physis closes prematurely, which results in marked shortening of the femoral neck and severe relative overgrowth of the greater trochanter. The femoral head is flattened and deformed, and the hip joint is incongruous (Fig. 2–201).

Type IV ischemic necrosis is caused by the occlusion of the posteroinferior medial circumflex vessels (Fig. 2–202). The medial part of the capital femoral epiphysis and the subjacent medial metaphysis are involved. The resultant deformity is coxa breva and magna (Fig. 2–203).

Kalamchi and MacEwen reviewed 119 patients with congenital dislocation of the hip complicated by avascular necrosis, of whom 51 patients were skeletally mature. They classified the vascular disturbances into four groups depending on the damage involving the ossific nucleus and the physis.[481]

In *Group I* the vascular changes affected only the ossific nucleus of the femoral head. This is very similar to the Type I pattern of Bucholz and Ogden.

In *Group II* there was vascular damage to the lateral segment of the growth plate of the femoral head, and this group is quite similar to the Type II pattern of Bucholz and Ogden.

In *Group III* there was central closure of the physis of the femoral head. It caused symmetrical retardation and cessation of growth of the femoral head. A large central metaphyseal defect on the anteroposterior radiogram is the early sign of physeal damage (Fig. 2–204). The result is a short femoral neck; the head–neck shaft angle is not changed, and the femoral head is usually spherical and contained in the acetabulum. There will be relative overgrowth of the greater trochanter with functional coxa vara and a gluteus medius lurch. Lower limb length inequality will be moderate. Later on in life the

FIGURE 2–201. Type III ischemic necrosis of the right hip.

A. At two years and five months of age there is diffuse irregularity of the capital femoral epiphysis, physis, and metaphysis. **B.** At four years and two months of age, irregularity of the capital femoral epiphysis is marked. Note the epiphyseal deformity and the persistent metaphyseal irregularity. The femoral neck is short, and there is a varus tilt. **C.** At skeletal maturity height of the femoral head is decreased, it is severely deformed, and is not covered by the acetabulum. The hip joint is incongruous. The femoral neck is short with relatively severe overgrowth of the greater trochanter. (From Thomas, C. L., Gage, J. R., and Ogden, J. A.: Treatment concepts for proximal femoral ischemic necrosis. J. Bone Joint Surg., *64-*A:817, 1982. Reprinted by permission.)

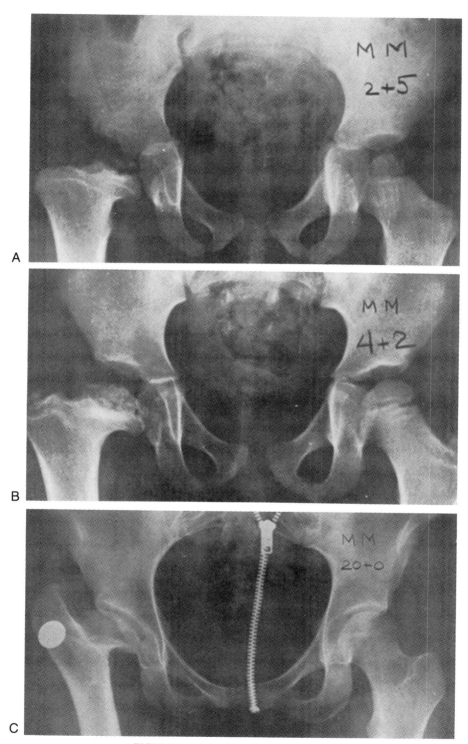

FIGURE 2-201 See legend on opposite page

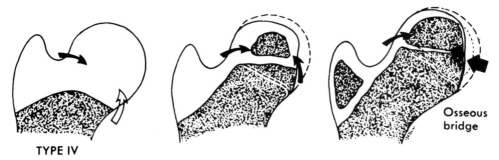

FIGURE 2–202. Type IV pattern of ischemic necrosis of proximal femur.

Schematic drawing showing findings at two months, one year, and nine years of age. The open arrow represents the site of temporary vascular occlusion, which corresponds to the region of impaired longitudinal and latitudinal growth and premature epiphyseodesis. (From Bucholz, R. W., and Ogden, J. A.: Patterns of ischemic necrosis of the proximal femur in nonoperatively treated congenital hip disease. *In* The Hip: Proceedings of the Sixth Open Scientific Meeting of the Hip Society. St. Louis, C. V. Mosby, 1978. Reprinted by permission.)

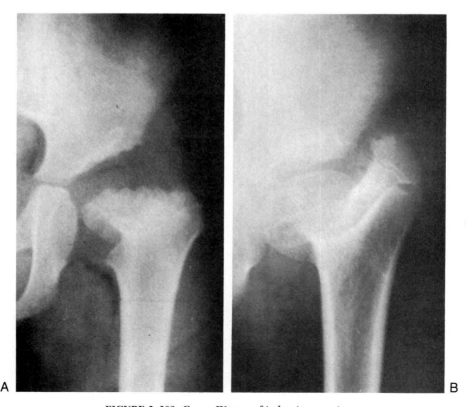

FIGURE 2–203. Group IV type of ischemic necrosis.

A. The entire femoral head is involved with gross metaphyseal irregularity and medial beaking. **B.** Same hip six years later showing closure of the growth plate, a deformed head, varus angulation of the femoral neck, relative overgrowth of the greater trochanter, and distortion of the acetabulum. (From Kalamchi, A., and MacEwen, G. D.: Avascular necrosis following treatment of congenital dislocation of the hip. J. Bone Joint Surg., 62-A:876, 1980. Reprinted by permission.)

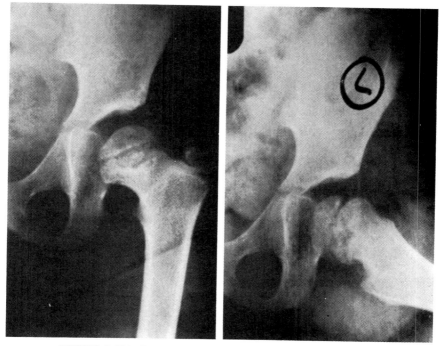

FIGURE 2–204. Group III avascular necrosis of the proximal femur.

Anteroposterior and lateral radiograms of the hip. There is central metaphyseal rarefaction and irregularity in the central part of the physis. (From Kalamchi, A., and MacEwen, G. D.: Avascular necrosis following treatment of congenital dislocation of the hip. J. Bone Joint Surg., 62-A:876, 1980. Reprinted by permission.)

Group III ischemic necrotic hip will develop dysplasia and early osteoarthritis.

In *Group IV* ischemic necrosis there is vascular insult involving the entire femoral head and the growth plates. Ossification of the femoral head is markedly delayed, with early joint incongruity, femoral head flattening, and coxa magna. The femoral neck will be short, widened, medially beaked, and tilted into true varus angulation. Development of the acetabulum is delayed with persistent hip dysplasia. Later on in life there will be progressive degeneration, increasing subluxation, and stiffness of the hip.

Distribution of the various groups in relation to the patient's age at initial treatment showed that Group IV, the severe type of avascular necrosis, was more common in the infants from birth to six months. Group I, the mild form, was much more common in the older children.[481]

Management varies according to type and pattern of avascular necrosis. In Type I of Bucholz and Ogden, or Group I of Kalamchi and MacEwen, no treatment is indicated. The hip is followed periodically with radiograms; the prognosis is excellent.

In Type II of Bucholz and Ogden, or Group II of Kalamchi and MacEwen, the prognosis is poor because of progressive uncovering of the femoral head, shortness of the femoral neck in valgus angulation, relative overgrowth of the greater trochanter, and lower limb length inequality. The deformity is progressive with growth. Treatment of each hip should be individualized. The goals of treatment are, first, to cover the femoral head by innominate osteotomy; second, to transfer the greater trochanter distally and laterally to restore functional physiologic length of hip abductors and normal biomechanics of the hip; and third, if the severity of the lower limb length inequality demands, to equalize limb lengths by an epiphyseodesis of the contralateral distal femur.

In Group III of Kalamchi and MacEwen, in which there is central closure of the physis of the femoral head, objectives of treatment should be directed to obtaining hip abductor motor strength. Initially this is achieved by side-lying hip abduction exercises, and later on, once it is unequivocally certain that there is no growth from the capital femoral physis, an apophyseodesis of the greater trochanter is performed following the Langenskiöld technique

(Plate 20). Greater trochanteric apophyseal arrest is ineffective in the child of six years or older because about 50 per cent of the growth of the greater trochanter occurs by appositional bone growth at its cephalic cartilaginous portion, where the hip abductors insert. The tip of the greater trochanter is not fused by greater trochanteric apophyseal arrest. In animal experiments Laurent and Salenius and Videman have demonstrated that only about half of the growth of the greater trochanter can be stopped by fusion of the greater trochanteric apophysis.[534, 802] Further growth and remodeling cannot restore the normal trochanter-head relationship. The results of greater trochanteric apophyseodesis in the older child in this author's series, as well as in those of Gage and Cary and of Langenskiöld and Salenius, are not satisfactory and confirm the foregoing postulate.[320, 525]

In addition, greater trochanteric growth arrest will not lateralize the greater trochanter or functionally lengthen the femoral neck.

Greater trochanteric apophyseodesis does not restore the neck-shaft angle if true coxa vara is present.[320] Severe or moderate coxa vara requires correction by valgus osteotomy of the proximal femur.

Should one perform stapling of the greater trochanteric growth plate when uncertain of the potential of growth from the capital physis? In the experience of this author, when unsure, it is best to wait until the child is older (age 10 or 12 years) and perform a distal and lateral transfer of the greater trochanter (Plate 21).

Lateral transfer of the greater trochanter is performed when the femoral neck is short and the tip of the greater trochanter is level with the center of the femoral head, i.e., there is no relative overgrowth of the greater trochanter (Plate 22).

Lower limb length inequality is corrected by epiphyseodesis of the contralateral distal femur.

In Group IV of Kalamchi and MacEwen, or Type III of Bucholz and Ogden, the prognosis is very poor. Femoral head coverage is provided by innominate osteotomy. If the femoral head is very deformed and irregular and the hip joint is incongruous, Chiari's pelvic osteotomy is indicated. The short femoral neck may be lengthened and its varus angulation corrected by the double intertrochanteric osteotomy of Wagner (Plate 23).[979] This is technically very difficult to perform. The varus angulation of the femoral neck may be corrected by the modified Pauwel's osteotomy of the proximal femur with simultaneous distal and lateral transfer of the greater trochanter (Plate 24).

Lower limb length inequality is corrected by epiphyseodesis of the contralateral lower limb.

Type IV ischemic necrosis of Bucholz and Ogden in general carries a good prognosis with minimal resultant deformity. Persistent subluxation and hip dysplasia may require innominate osteotomy, and residual limb length inequality may require equalization.

Lateral and Distal Advancement of the Greater Trochanter

The anatomic relationship between the greater trochanter and the femoral head is determined by the relative growth between the femoral capital physis and the greater trochanter, the femoral neck-shaft angle, and the length of the femoral neck. The center of the femoral head marks the center of its rotation.

In the normal hip the tip of the greater trochanter with the insertion of the hip abductor muscles is slightly distal to or level with the center of the femoral head, and the distance between them is two to two and one half times the radius of the femoral head (Fig. 2–205).[979] In the radiograph the articulotrochanteric distance (ATD) is used to assess the position of the tip of the greater trochanter in relation to the

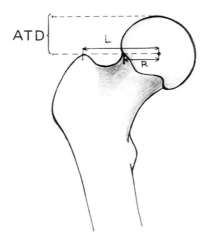

FIGURE 2–205. *Diagram showing the upper end of a normal femur.*

In the normal hip, the distance from the greater trochanter to the center of the femoral head is two to two and one half times the radius of the head (L = 2½ × R). The tip of the greater trochanter is at or slightly below the center of the femoral head. The articulotrochanteric distance (ATD) normally measures 10 to 25 mm. (From Kelikian, A. S., and Tachdjian, M. O.: Greater trochanteric advancement. *In* The Hip Society Award Papers. St. Louis, C. V. Mosby, 1983. Reprinted by permission.)

femoral head. It is measured in millimeters from the articular surface of the femoral head to the tip of the greater trochanter; the value is positive if the tip of the greater trochanter is distal to the center of the femoral head and neutral if the two are level. The trochanter-head relationship becomes negative if the tip of the greater trochanter is higher than the center of the femoral head.[249]

The height of the greater trochanter determines the tension of the gluteus medius and minimus muscles. According to Blix, muscle fiber tension is proportional to muscle fiber length at the moment of excitation.[63] The maximal tension is achieved at the normal resting length of the muscle fiber. As the muscle fiber shortens, the tension that the muscle fiber can produce decreases until it becomes zero when the fiber is approximately 60 per cent of its resting length.[253] The lever arm of the pelvifemoral musculature is determined by the relative height and lateralization of the greater trochanter. With relative overgrowth of the greater trochanter, the muscle fiber lengths of the gluteus medius and minimus shorten. Muscle tension of the hip abductors is important to balance body weight and provide pelvifemoral stability. With increasing elevation of the tip of the greater trochanter, Trendelenburg's sign becomes positive, and the patient walks with a gluteus medius lurch.[525]

With a short femoral neck the direction of pull of the hip abductor muscles is steeper and decreases the length of its lever arm.[718]

Avascular necrosis complicating congenital dislocation of the hip will damage the capital femoral physis and retard or completely arrest its growth. The results are a short femoral neck (coxa brevis) and relative overgrowth of the greater trochanter in relation to the center of motion of the femoral head. If the growth plate damage is central or complete, the growth arrest of the femoral neck will be symmetrical, whereas asymmetrical premature closure of the capital physis will lead to the deformity of coxa vara or coxa valga. Growth arrest of the medial part of the capital physis will tilt the femoral head to produce coxa vara; premature lateral arrest will result in lateral tilt of the head to produce coxa valga.[88, 481, 926]

Biomechanics of the hip joint and muscle physiology of the hip abductors are disturbed by the relative overgrowth of the greater trochanter, the shortening of the femoral neck, and the decreased or increased femoral neck-shaft angle.

Lateral and distal transfer of the greater trochanter has been described by Jani (in 1969, 44 cases) and Cohen (in 1971, a single case).[149, 463] In 1978 Wagner described the detailed techniques of the various types of trochanteric osteotomies, delineated their biomechanical advantages and indications, and presented the results.[979] Tauber and colleagues, in 1980, reported the results of distal transfer of the greater trochanter in nine hips (seven patients). Trendelenburg's sign diminished markedly or became negative; thus the gait improved. In three patients (four hips) operated on between the ages of 9 and 12 years the femoral neck-shaft angle increased 10 to 15 degrees, correcting the initial coxa vara to an almost normal valgus neck. In one patient early mobilization resulted in screw breakage and nonunion.[923]

Tachdjian and Kelikian and their associates reported excellent results in 39 of 40 hips and delineated the indications and prerequisites for the procedure.[491, 921] Lloyd Roberts and associates reported results in 17 hips (nine cases of Perthes disease and eight of congenital dislocation of the hip). The results in the Perthes patients were satisfactory in all, but less favorable results were obtained in congenital dislocation of the hip.[561]

The technique for distal and lateral transfer of the greater trochanter as described by Wagner is illustrated in Plate 21.[979] A typical case is shown in Figure 2–206.

Indications are: relative overgrowth of the greater trochanter with its tip at the joint line, a short femoral neck, a positive Trendelenburg's sign (immediate or delayed), and a lower age limit of eight years. There is no upper age limit.

Prerequisites are: congruous and concentric reduction of the hip joint, a femoral neck-shaft angle of at least 110 degrees (if it was less than this, a lateral closing wedge osteotomy of the proximal femur was combined with the greater trochanteric advancement), functional range of hip motion with a total arc of hip abduction-adduction in extension of at least 45 degrees, preoperative hip abductor muscle strength of at least fair minus, femoral antetorsion of less than 40 degrees, and a lower age limit of eight years.

Lateral Transfer of the Greater Trochanter

Lateral transfer of the greater trochanter, also described by Wagner, is indicated when the femoral neck is short and the tip of the greater trochanter is level with the center of the femoral head (i.e., there is no relative overgrowth of the greater trochanter).[979] The prerequisites are similar to those for lateral-distal transfer of the

Text continued on page 466

Greater Trochanteric Apophyseodesis (Langenskiöld)

OPERATIVE TECHNIQUE

A. The patient is placed supine with a sandbag under the ipsilateral hip. The entire lower limb, hip, and pelvis are prepared and draped to permit free passive motion of the hip. A 5- to 7-cm. long transverse incision is centered over the apophysis of the greater trochanter. If so desired, a longitudinal incision may be made, especially if distal transfer of the greater trochanter is anticipated in the future.

B. The site of origin of the vastus lateralis from the upper part of the intertrochanteric line, the anteroinferior border of the greater trochanter, the lateral tip of the gluteal tuberosity, and the upper part of the lateral tip of the linea aspera is shown.

C. Subcutaneous tissue is divided in line with the skin incision. The wound edges are retracted. A longitudinal incision is made in the fascia of the tensor fasciae latae muscle.

D. The tensor fasciae latae muscle is retracted anteriorly, and the origin of the vastus lateralis is detached and elevated extraperiosteally.

E. A Keith needle is inserted into the soft growth plate of the greater trochanteric apophysis. Anteroposterior radiograms are made to verify the position of the Keith needle and the growth plate.

Plate 20. Greater Trochanteric Apophyseodesis
(Langenskiöld)

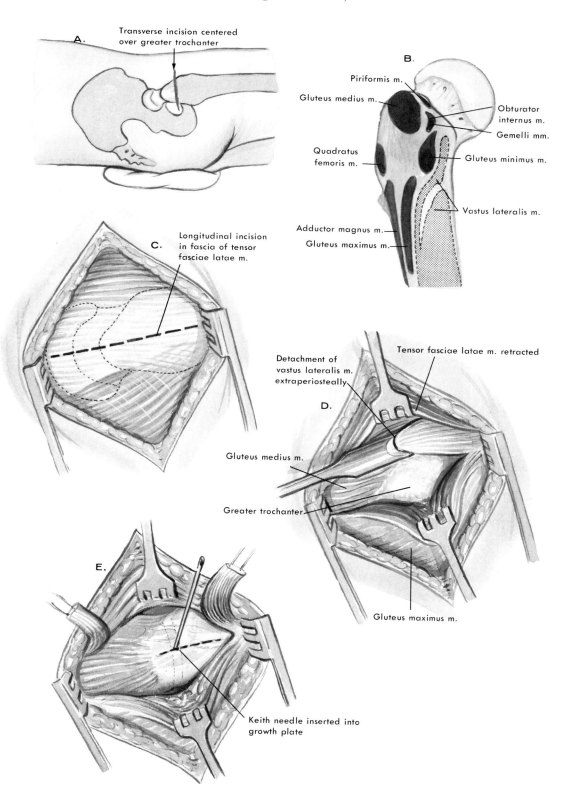

A. Transverse incision centered over greater trochanter

B.
Piriformis m.
Gluteus medius m.
Obturator internus m.
Gemelli mm.
Quadratus femoris m.
Gluteus minimus m.
Vastus lateralis m.
Adductor magnus m.
Gluteus maximus m.

C. Longitudinal incision in fascia of tensor fasciae latae m.

D.
Detachment of vastus lateralis m. extraperiosteally
Tensor fasciae latae m. retracted
Gluteus medius m.
Greater trochanter
Gluteus maximus m.

E. Keith needle inserted into growth plate

445

Greater Trochanteric Apophyseodesis (Langenskiöld)
(Continued)

F. The periosteum is divided by one longitudinal and two horizontal incisions. The dotted rectangle marks the bone plug to be removed and turned around. Note: it is 2 cm. long and 1.25 cm. wide. In the smaller child the rectangle is 3/8 inch (1 cm.) long and 1/4 inch (0.6 cm.) wide.

G and **H.** With straight osteotomes, the bone plug is removed. Note the growth plate is in the proximal third of the rectangle.

I. A diamond-shaped drill and curets are used to destroy the growth plate. One should be careful not to enter the trochanteric fossa and injure circulation to the femoral head.

Plate 20. Greater Trochanteric Apophyseodesis
(Langenskiöld)

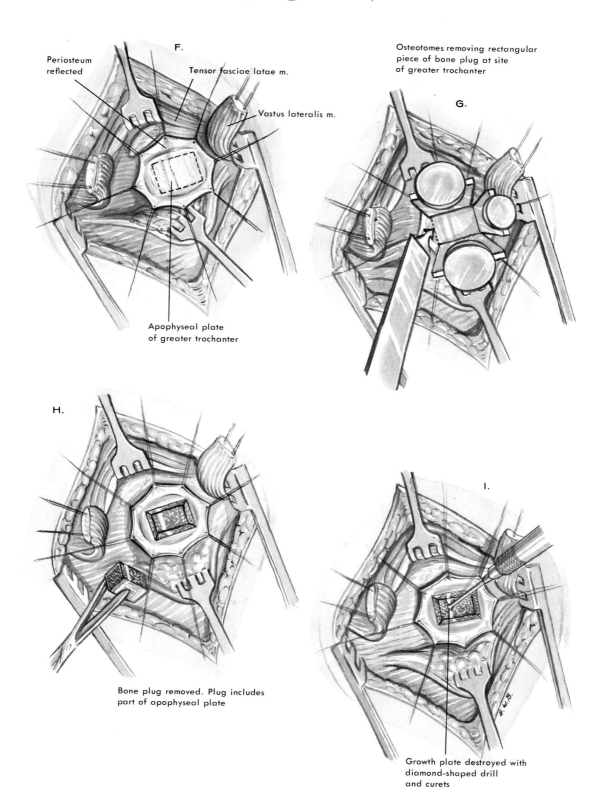

F.

Periosteum reflected

Tensor fasciae latae m.

Vastus lateralis m.

Apophyseal plate of greater trochanter

Osteotomes removing rectangular piece of bone plug at site of greater trochanter

G.

H.

Bone plug removed. Plug includes part of apophyseal plate

I.

Growth plate destroyed with diamond-shaped drill and curets

447

Greater Trochanteric Apophyseodesis (Langenskiöld)
(Continued)

J. With a curved osteotome, cancellous bone is removed from the proximal femoral shaft and packed into the defect at the site of the growth plate.

K and **L.** The bone plug is rotated 180 degrees, replaced in the defect in the greater trochanter, and with an impactor and mallet, is securely seated.

M. The muscles are resutured to their insertion sites, and the vastus lateralis is attached to gluteus medius-minimus tendons at their insertion after closure of the periosteum. The fascia lata is closed with interrupted sutures, and the wound is closed with interrupted and subcuticular skin sutures. It is not necessary to immobilize the hip in any cast.

POSTOPERATIVE CARE

The patient is allowed to be up and around the first day postoperatively, as soon as he is comfortable. He is discharged home within a few days, protecting the limb that was operated on with a three-point crutch gait for three to four weeks.

Plate 20. Greater Trochanteric Apophyseodesis
(Langenskiöld)

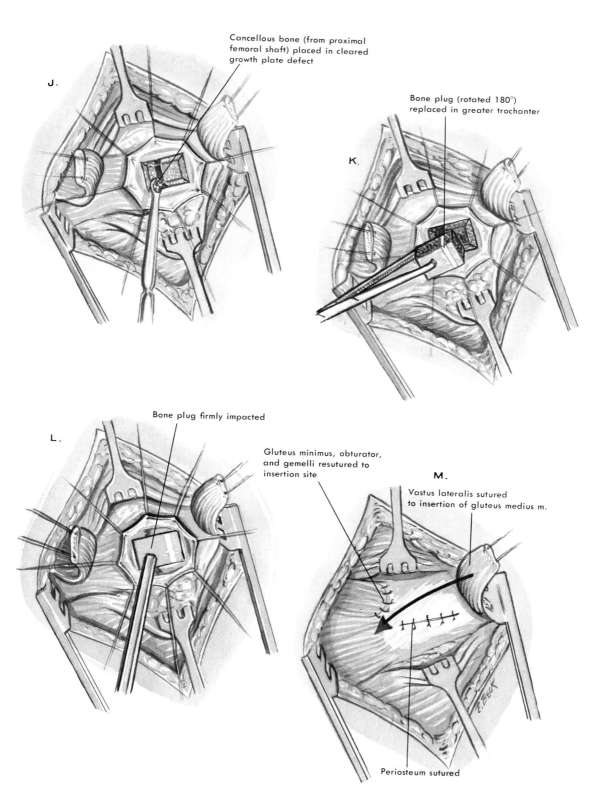

J.

Cancellous bone (from proximal femoral shaft) placed in cleared growth plate defect

K.

Bone plug (rotated 180°) replaced in greater trochanter

L.

Bone plug firmly impacted

M.

Gluteus minimus, obturator, and gemelli resutured to insertion site

Vastus lateralis sutured to insertion of gluteus medius m.

Periosteum sutured

Distal and Lateral Transfer of the Greater Trochanter

The patient's blood should be typed and cross-matched preoperatively for two units of blood.

OPERATIVE TECHNIQUE

A and **B.** The patient is placed on the fracture table with the affected hip in neutral position as to adduction-abduction and in 20 to 30 degrees of medial rotation to bring the greater trochanter forward to facilitate exposure. The opposite hip is placed in 40 degrees of abduction. Image intensifier anteroposterior fluoroscopy is used to show the femoral head and neck, the greater trochanter, and the upper femoral shaft. The hip should be rotated medially so that the greater trochanter is seen in profile and not superimposed over the femoral neck. It is crucial to visualize the trochanteric fossa. The affected hip and upper two thirds of the thigh are prepared and draped in the usual manner.

A straight lateral longitudinal incision is made from the tip of the greater trochanter and extending distally for 10 cm. The subcutaneous tissue is divided in line with the skin incision.

C. The fascia lata is split longitudinally in the direction of its fibers.

D and **E.** The vastus lateralis is detached proximally from the abductor tubercle by a proximally based horseshoe-shaped incision and elevated subperiosteally from the femoral shaft for 5 to 7 cm. Be sure that the vastus lateralis is elevated in its entire width.

Plate 21. Distal and Lateral Transfer of the Greater Trochanter

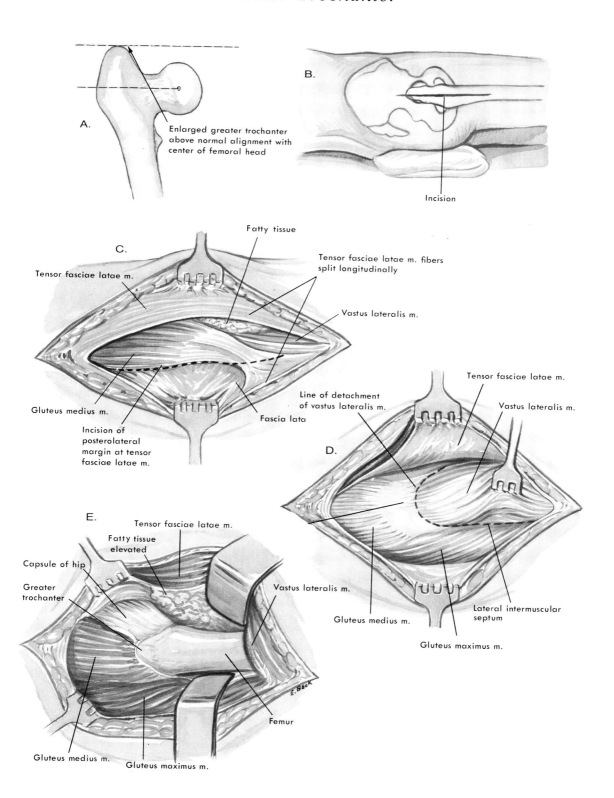

A. Enlarged greater trochanter above normal alignment with center of femoral head

B. Incision

C.
- Fatty tissue
- Tensor fasciae latae m. fibers split longitudinally
- Tensor fasciae latae m.
- Vastus lateralis m.
- Gluteus medius m.
- Fascia lata
- Incision of posterolateral margin at tensor fasciae latae m.

D.
- Line of detachment of vastus lateralis m.
- Tensor fasciae latae m.
- Vastus lateralis m.
- Gluteus medius m.
- Lateral intermuscular septum
- Gluteus maximus m.

E.
- Tensor fasciae latae m.
- Fatty tissue elevated
- Capsule of hip
- Greater trochanter
- Vastus lateralis m.
- Gluteus medius m.
- Gluteus maximus m.
- Femur

Z. BECK

451

Distal and Lateral Transfer of the Greater Trochanter
(Continued)

F. The anterior border of the gluteus medius is identified, and a blunt elevator-retractor is introduced beneath its deep surface, pointing in the direction of the trochanteric fossa.

G. At this time, to orient the plane of the trochanteric osteotomy properly, a smooth Kirschner wire is inserted at the level of the abductor tubercle, pointing to the trochanteric fossa along a line continuous with the upper cortex of the femoral neck. Radiography with image intensification will verify the proper level and depth of the guide wire. The point of the Kirschner wire must not protrude through the medial cortex into the trochanteric fossa.

H. A blunt flat retractor is placed beneath the posterior border of the greater trochanter to protect the soft tissues. The previously applied anterior retractor protects the soft tissues ventrally. With a 2- to 3-cm.-wide reciprocating saw the greater trochanter is divided in the anteroposterior direction, following the proximal border of the Kirschner wire. Care is taken to stop the cut 3 cm. short of the medial cortex of the trochanteric fossa. Injury to the vessels in the trochanteric fossa must be avoided in order to prevent necrosis of the femoral head.

I. Then a 3-mm.-wide flat osteotome is driven through the osteotomy cleft, and the osteotomy site is wedged open by moving the handle of the osteotome craniad. By leverage with the osteotome in the cleft, a greenstick fracture of the medial cortex is produced.

Plate 21. Distal and Lateral Transfer of the Greater Trochanter

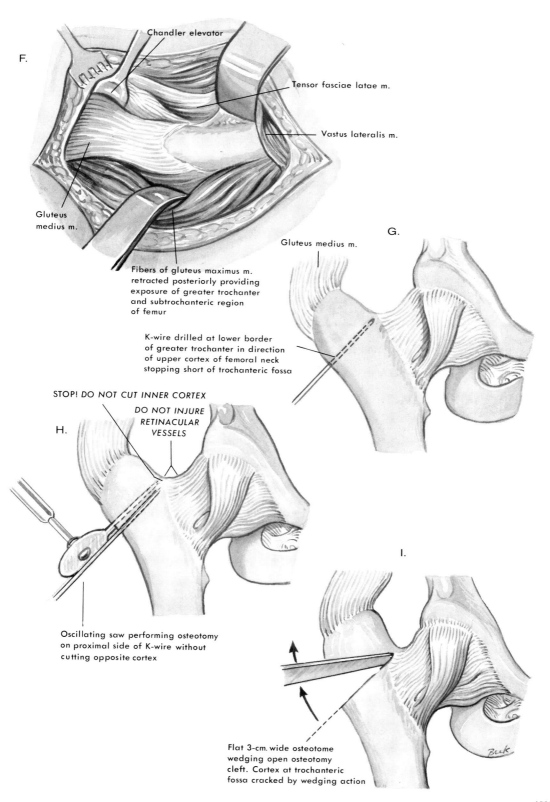

F.

Chandler elevator

Tensor fasciae latae m.

Vastus lateralis m.

Gluteus medius m.

Fibers of gluteus maximus m. retracted posteriorly providing exposure of greater trochanter and subtrochanteric region of femur

G.

Gluteus medius m.

K-wire drilled at lower border of greater trochanter in direction of upper cortex of femoral neck stopping short of trochanteric fossa

STOP! *DO NOT CUT INNER CORTEX*
DO NOT INJURE RETINACULAR VESSELS

H.

Oscillating saw performing osteotomy on proximal side of K-wire without cutting opposite cortex

I.

Flat 3-cm. wide osteotome wedging open osteotomy cleft. Cortex at trochanteric fossa cracked by wedging action

Distal and Lateral Transfer of the Greater Trochanter
(Continued)

J. A large periosteal elevator is placed deep into the osteotomy cleft, opening it up medially by gently levering the handle up and down. The trochanteric fragment is lifted superolaterally with a Lewin bone clamp, and adhesions between the joint capsule and the medial aspect of the greater trochanter are released. This must be done very carefully in order not to injure retinacular blood vessels in the capsule. Do not fracture the greater trochanter! Mobilization is sufficient when, upon lateral and distal traction on the greater trochanter, the muscle response is elastic; if there is still muscle resistance, it means that further adhesions are present that must be freed.

K. After sufficient mobilization of the greater trochanter, the recipient site on the lateral surface of the upper femoral shaft is prepared with a curved osteotome to create a flattened surface. Do not remove too much bone laterally. Next, the greater trochanter is displaced distally and laterally; in excessive femoral antetorsion it may be moved slightly forward. If additional distal advancement is desired, the hip may be abducted on the fracture table.

L and M. The trochanter is held in the desired position and temporarily fixed to the femur with two threaded Kirschner wires of adequate size that are drilled upward and medially. At this point the accuracy of the position of the greater trochanter is verified by image intensifier radiography. As stated previously, the tip of the greater trochanter should be level with the center of the femoral head and at a distance from it of two to two and a half times the radius of the femoral head. If there are problems with proper visualization, a long Kirschner wire is placed horizontally and parallel to both anterior superior iliac spines, crossing the center of the femoral head; then the position of the tip of the greater trochanter is checked.

Plate 21. Distal and Lateral Transfer of the Greater Trochanter

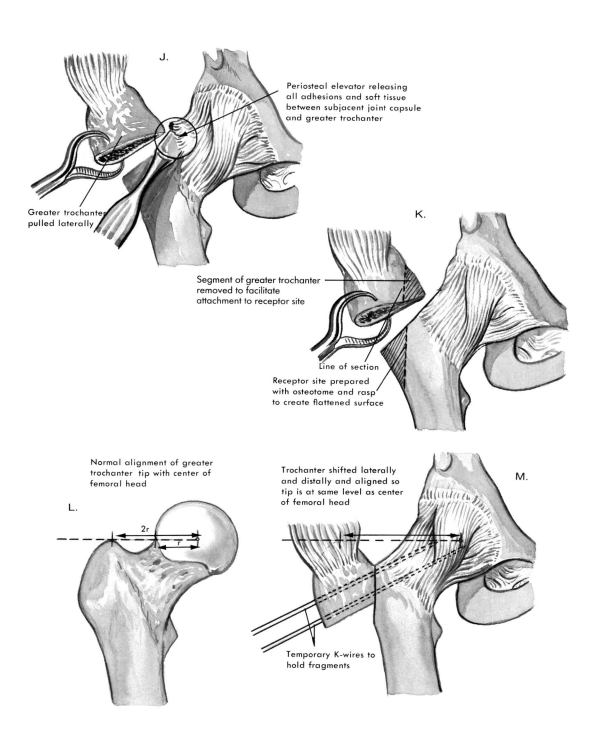

J.

Periosteal elevator releasing all adhesions and soft tissue between subjacent joint capsule and greater trochanter

Greater trochanter pulled laterally

K.

Segment of greater trochanter removed to facilitate attachment to receptor site

Line of section

Receptor site prepared with osteotome and rasp to create flattened surface

Normal alignment of greater trochanter tip with center of femoral head

L.

2r

r

Trochanter shifted laterally and distally and aligned so tip is at same level as center of femoral head

M.

Temporary K-wires to hold fragments

Distal and Lateral Transfer of the Greater Trochanter
(Continued)

N. Prior to osteosynthesis the gluteal muscle is split in the direction of the fibers to expose the bone and to avoid muscle necrosis. The greater trochanter is fixed to the lateral surface of the upper femur with two lag screws (each equipped with a washer), which are directed medially and distally at a 45-degree angle to counteract the pull of the hip abductors. For large trochanters 6.5-mm. cancellous screws with drill bits of appropriate size are used; with smaller trochanters 3.2-mm. screws are used. The outer cortex of the greater trochanter may be overdrilled. Taping of the outer cortex is optional. The washers increase the surface area, avoid cutting through the cortex, ensure more secure fixation, and allow early motion. After both screws are inserted the initial Kirschner wires are removed.

O. An alternative method of fixation is the use of two heavy threaded Kirschner wires directed medially and upward. The resultant pull of the hip abductors through the direction of the wires provides force that will compress the greater trochanter against the lateral surface of the femur. This author does not recommend internal fixation by this method because screw fixation is more stable. However, in an obese or uncooperative patient, threaded Kirschner wires may be used in addition to screw fixation; or a tension wire band may be used as described in lateral advancement of the greater trochanter (Plate 22).

P. Final intraoperative radiographs are made to ensure that the trochanter has been advanced to the desired site. Next, the detached origin of the vastus lateralis is firmly sutured to the tendinous insertion of the gluteus medius and minimus muscles. This tension-band suture absorbs the pull of the hip abductors and reinforces the internal fixation of the greater trochanter. A suction drain is inserted, and the remainder of the wound is closed in routine fashion. The skin closure is subcuticular.

POSTOPERATIVE CARE

The patient is placed in split Russell's traction with each hip in 35 to 40 degrees of abduction. Active assisted exercises are begun as soon as the patient is comfortable, usually the third postoperative day. Adduction and excessive flexion of the hip should be avoided. Hip abduction exercises are performed supine, which eliminates the effect of gravity. Sitting is not permitted for three weeks because, with 60 to 90 degrees of hip flexion, the posterior fibers of the gluteus medius muscle exert a strong lateral rotatory force on the greater trochanter and may loosen its fixation.

The patient is allowed to be out of bed on the third postoperative day on crutches and instructed to walk, a three-point gait with partial weight-bearing protecting the limb that was operated on. The patient is discharged to home as soon as he is independent and secure on crutches. Three weeks after surgery, side-lying hip abduction exercises are started, and the child is allowed to sit and to return to school. At six weeks bony consolidation is usually adequate to begin use of one crutch on the opposite side (to protect the hip that was operated on) and to perform standing Trendelenburg exercises. One-crutch protection should be continued until hip abductor muscles are normal or good in motor strength and Trendelenburg's sign is negative.

The screws are removed three to six months postoperatively. During the screw removal, one should be very cautious not to damage the gluteus medius and minimus muscle fibers. After removal of the screws, the hip is protected by three-point partial weight-bearing on crutches for two to three weeks, and exercises consisting of side-lying hip abduction and standing Trendelenburg exercises are performed to regain the motor strength of the hip abductor muscles.

Plate 21. Distal and Lateral Transfer of the Greater Trochanter

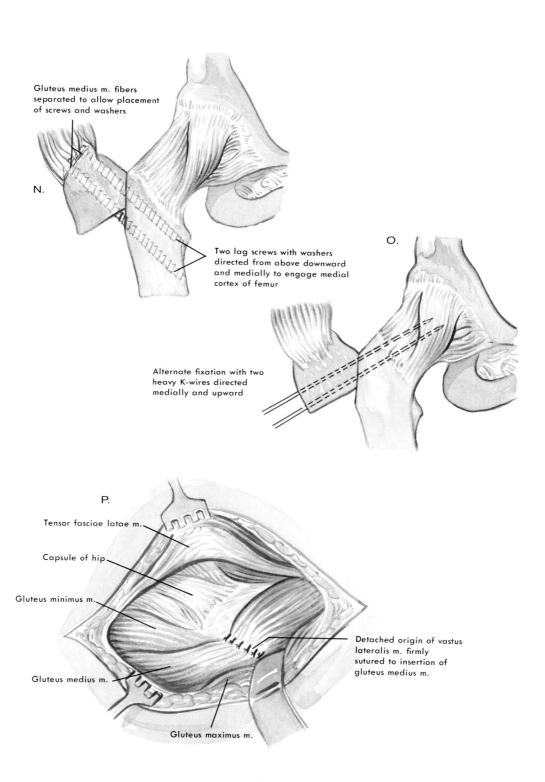

Gluteus medius m. fibers separated to allow placement of screws and washers

N.

Two lag screws with washers directed from above downward and medially to engage medial cortex of femur

O.

Alternate fixation with two heavy K-wires directed medially and upward

P.

Tensor fasciae latae m.

Capsule of hip

Gluteus minimus m.

Gluteus medius m.

Gluteus maximus m.

Detached origin of vastus lateralis m. firmly sutured to insertion of gluteus medius m.

Lateral Advancement of the Greater Trochanter

OPERATIVE TECHNIQUE

A. The surgical exposure of the greater trochanter and upper femoral shaft is similar to that for distal and lateral transfer of the greater trochanter (see Plate 21, Steps **A** to **K**).

B. The tip of the greater trochanter is at its normal level, so it is not necessary to advance it distally. It is kept horizontally level with the center of the femoral head, and its position is maintained by two wide-threaded positional cancellous screws. Insert the screws horizontally perpendicular to the osteotomized lateral surface of the upper femur. The threads of these "positioning" screws grip the trochanter as well as the intertrochanteric region of the femur without compression. The cleft between the greater trochanter and femur is filled with autogenous cancellous iliac bone, taken through a separate incision over the iliac apophysis.

C. Internal fixation is augmented by a taut tension band of heavy wire suture that extends from the neck of each trochanteric screw to a small unicortical screw, anchored 6 cm. distally in the femur. This wire tension band counteracts the pull of the hip abductors.

D. The detached vastus lateralis is then sutured to the insertion of the gluteus medius. The subcutaneous tissue and the skin are closed in the usual manner.

POSTOPERATIVE CARE

Postoperative care is similar to that following distal and lateral transfer of the greater trochanter (see Plate 21).

Plate 22. *Lateral Advancement of the Greater Trochanter*

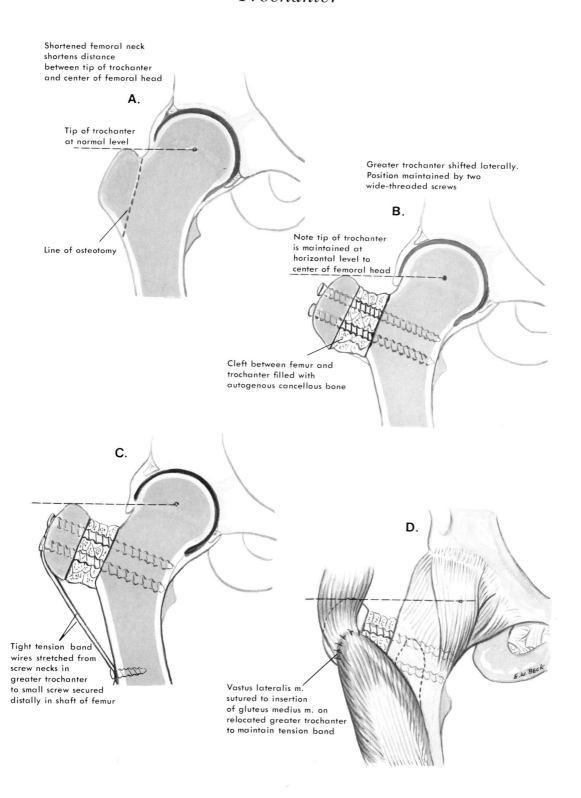

Shortened femoral neck shortens distance between tip of trochanter and center of femoral head

A.

Tip of trochanter at normal level

Line of osteotomy

Greater trochanter shifted laterally. Position maintained by two wide-threaded screws

B.

Note tip of trochanter is maintained at horizontal level to center of femoral head

Cleft between femur and trochanter filled with autogenous cancellous bone

C.

Tight tension band wires stretched from screw necks in greater trochanter to small screw secured distally in shaft of femur

D.

Vastus lateralis m. sutured to insertion of gluteus medius m. on relocated greater trochanter to maintain tension band

E.W. BECK

Wagner's Intertrochanteric Double Osteotomy

The first step of the operation is a soft-tissue release of the hip adductors and iliopsoas muscle through a separate medial incision. Compressive forces between the femoral head and acetabulum should be relieved, since elongation of the femoral neck will increase intra-articular pressure. The objectives are to elongate the femoral neck, restore the neck-shaft angle to normal, and displace the greater trochanter laterally and distally.

The bony procedure consists of two horizontal osteotomies: the first at the base of the greater trochanter at the level of the upper border of the femoral neck; and the second through the upper end of the femoral shaft (above the lesser trochanter), level with the lower margin of the femoral neck. The double osteotomy creates three fragments that can be moved and redirected independently of each other.

OPERATIVE TECHNIQUE

A. The proximal part of the femur is exposed through a lateral longitudinal approach, as described for distal and lateral transfer (see Plate 21, Steps **A** through **K**).

First, a heavy threaded Steinmann pin is inserted in the center of the axis of the femoral head. The pin should stop short of the capital femoral physis. The level of the two horizontal osteotomies is determined under image intensifier. The first should be at the base of the greater trochanter and the second at the upper end of the femoral shaft immediately distal to the base of the femoral neck. These levels are marked by inserting smooth Kirschner wires into bone.

B. A heavy threaded Steinmann pin is inserted in the midportion of the greater trochanter, stopping short of its medial cortex. Next, the two horizontal osteotomies are performed under image intensifier roentgenographic control. It is vital to avoid injury to the vessels in the trochanteric fossa and the retinacular vessels. The deep ends of the osteotomies should stop short of the medial cortex, in which a greenstick fracture is made. First the greater trochanter is pulled cephalad to facilitate exposure. Next, the femoral neck fragment is pushed downward and medially into the desired position; then the distal femoral fragment is pulled laterally so that the medial cortex of the upper end of the femoral shaft serves as a buttress to the inferomedial corner of the femoral neck. This maneuver elongates the femoral neck.

C. When the femoral head and neck and the femoral shaft have been brought into the corrected position, three smooth Kirschner wires are used to transfix and temporarily hold the fragments. Next the greater trochanter is transferred distally and laterally and fixed to the femoral neck with the threaded pin previously inserted in its midportion. Radiographs are made to check the realignment of the three fragments and the correction achieved.

D. Osteosynthesis is performed by a molded semitubular plate, which is prepared as follows: With a powerful wire cutter a vertical slot is cut out from the plate's upper end to the first screw hole. The bifurcated limbs are trimmed at their tips to sharp points and bent inward to form hooks. The semitubular plate is reshaped to fit the superolateral surface of the upper femur. The hooks are inserted in the tip of the greater trochanter, deep into cancellous bone for firm anchorage. The diagonally inserted Kirschner wires transfix the neck and shaft and prevent medial shifting of the femoral neck on the buttress provided by the upper medial cortex of the femoral shaft. All the screws are inserted, and the spaces between the fragments are packed with autogenous cancellous bone obtained from the ilium through a separate incision.

Some surgeons may prefer to use other methods of internal fixation such as a 90- or 130-degree AO right-angle plate and stabilization of the fragments with multiple screws.

POSTOPERATIVE CARE

Osteosynthesis is secure, permitting active assisted exercises three or four days postoperatively. The patient is kept in bilateral split Russell's traction for three weeks, until the hip develops functional range of motion. Then partial weight-bearing is permitted with three-point crutch gait protection. Bone healing is usually solid in three months, at which time full weight-bearing is allowed.

Plate 23. Wagner's Intertrochanteric Double Osteotomy

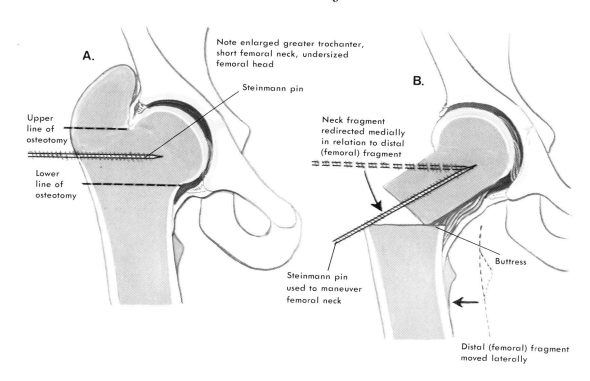

A.

Note enlarged greater trochanter, short femoral neck, undersized femoral head

Steinmann pin

Upper line of osteotomy

Lower line of osteotomy

B.

Neck fragment redirected medially in relation to distal (femoral) fragment

Buttress

Steinmann pin used to maneuver femoral neck

Distal (femoral) fragment moved laterally

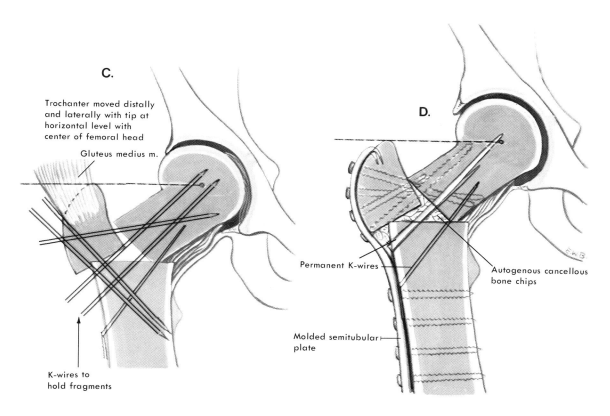

C.

Trochanter moved distally and laterally with tip at horizontal level with center of femoral head

Gluteus medius m.

K-wires to hold fragments

D.

Permanent K-wires

Autogenous cancellous bone chips

Molded semitubular plate

Lateral-Based Closing Wedge Valgization Osteotomy of Proximal Femur With Distal-Lateral Advancement of Greater Trochanter

The greater trochanter and the upper femoral shaft are exposed according to the technique described in Plate 21, Steps **A** through **K**. If the hip adductors are taut they are released through a separate medial incision.

OPERATIVE TECHNIQUE

A and **B.** First the greater trochanter is osteotomized following the technique described for distal and lateral advancement. Then two threaded Steinmann pins are inserted to serve as guides for the level and angle of osteotomy. The apex of the osteotomy stops 1 cm. short of the medial cortex. The length of the base of the wedge depends on the degree of correction of coxa vara required. The wedge of bone is resected with an oscillating saw.

C. With a straight osteotome and the leverage of the pins anchored in the femur, a greenstick fracture is produced in the medial cortex, converting the osteotomy to a short-stemmed Y.

Plate 24. *Lateral-Based Closing Wedge Valgization Osteotomy of Proximal Femur With Distal-Lateral Advancement of Greater Trochanter*

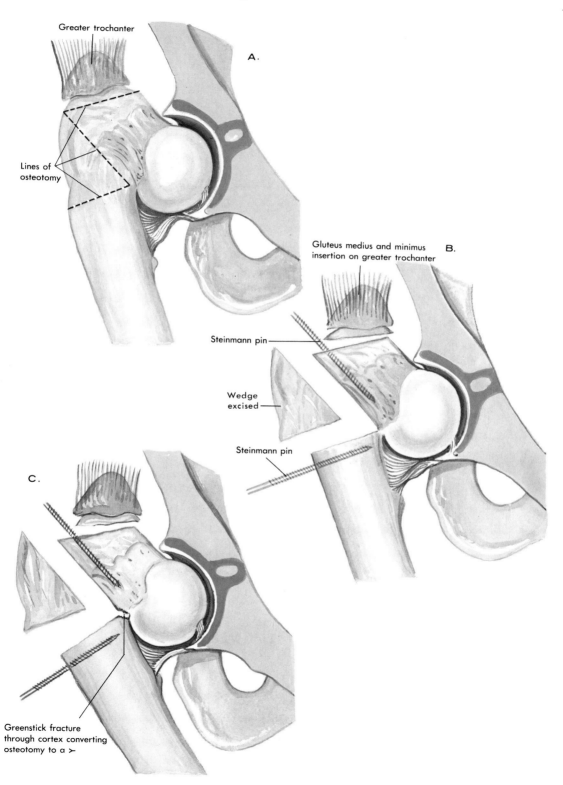

Greater trochanter

A.

Lines of osteotomy

Gluteus medius and minimus insertion on greater trochanter

B.

Steinmann pin

Wedge excised

Steinmann pin

C.

Greenstick fracture through cortex converting osteotomy to a ⊁

Lateral-Based Closing Wedge Valgization Osteotomy
of Proximal Femur With Distal-Lateral Advancement
of Greater Trochanter (Continued)

D. The osteotomy gap is closed by bringing the two Steinmann pins together and by aligning the neck shaft and greater trochanter at a preoperatively determined angle.

E. The greater trochanter is transfixed with a threaded Steinmann pin driven into the neck of the femur.

F. The three fragments are then fixed with a prebent trochanteric hook plate and screws.

POSTOPERATIVE CARE

Care following this operation is similar to that after Wagner's intertrochanteric double osteotomy.

Plate 24. Lateral-Based Closing Wedge Valgization Osteotomy of Proximal Femur With Distal-Lateral Advancement of Greater Trochanter

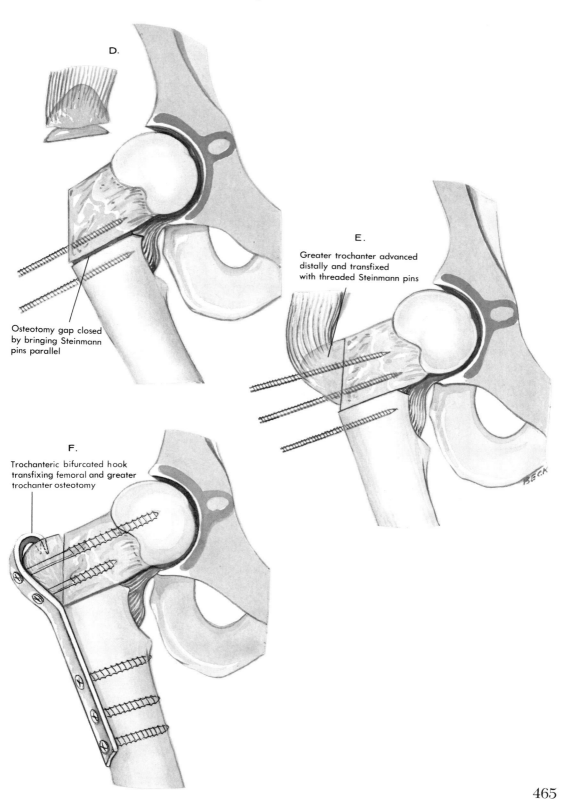

D.

Osteotomy gap closed by bringing Steinmann pins parallel

E.

Greater trochanter advanced distally and transfixed with threaded Steinmann pins

F.

Trochanteric bifurcated hook transfixing femoral and greater trochanter osteotomy

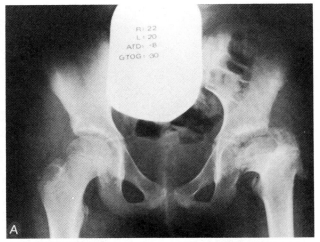

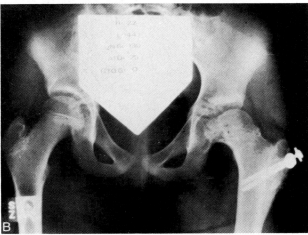

FIGURE 2–206. Avascular necrosis of the left femoral head with resultant coxa breva and relative overgrowth of the greater trochanter treated by distal and lateral advancement of the greater trochanter.

A. Preoperative anteroposterior radiogram of both hips showing the short femoral neck, coxa vara, and relative overgrowth of the greater trochanter. The patient has marked gluteus medius lurch and 4 cm. shortening of the femur. **B.** Postoperative anteroposterior radiogram of the hips showing a closing. (From Kelikian, A. S., and Tachdjian, M. O.:Greater trochanteric advancement. *In* The Hip Society Award Papers. St. Louis, C. V. Mosby, 1983. Reprinted by permission.)

greater trochanter; the hip joint should be congruous and have functional range of motion. The procedure, described and illustrated in Plate 22, lengthens the lever arm of the hip abductors.

Intertrochanteric Double Osteotomy

Wagner has described an intertrochanteric double osteotomy for the correction of the marked overgrowth of the greater trochanter when its tip abuts the lateral wall of the ilium, the femoral neck is very short, the femoral neck-shaft angle is decreased from normal to 100 to 110 degrees, and the hip joint is somewhat congruous. There should be good range of hip motion. The procedure is relatively complicated and technically difficult. An important prerequisite is the technical capability of the surgeon. The operative technique is described and illustrated in Plate 23. An illustrative case is shown in Figure 2–207.

Lateral Based Closing Wedge Valgization Osteotomy of the Proximal Femur with Distal-Lateral Advancement of the Greater Trochanter

Coxa vara with trochanteric overgrowth may also be corrected by a lateral closing wedge osteotomy of the proximal femur combined with greater trochanteric advancement. This procedure is technically simpler than the one just described. A lateral closing wedge osteotomy is made. The apex of this wedge corresponds to the medial neck-shaft junction. The greater trochanter is osteotomized at its base, and the wedge of bone is removed. The osteotomy site is closed by aligning the two Kirschner wires. The neck-shaft and greater trochanteric fragments are aligned as determined preoperatively. Fixation is accomplished by a prebent trochanteric hook plate. Two of this author's patients underwent this procedure. The opera-

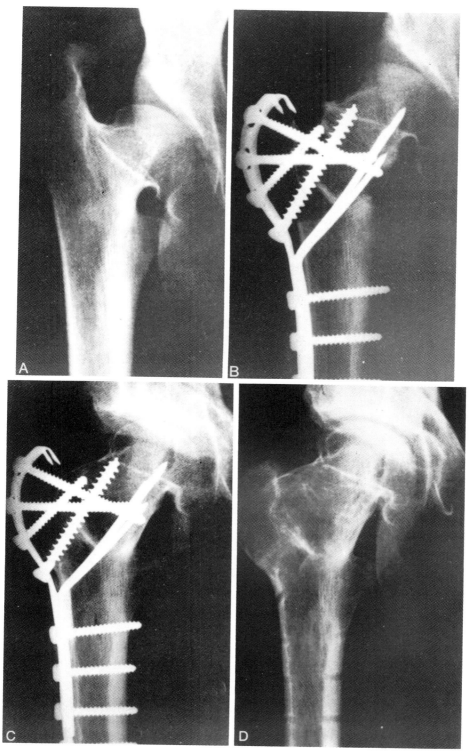

FIGURE 2–207. *Wagner double intertrochanteric osteotomy.*

A. Preoperative anteroposterior radiogram showing the short femoral neck and severe relative overgrowth of the greater trochanter. **B.** Immediate postoperative radiogram showing correction of deformity with elongation of the femoral neck. **C.** One year postoperative radiogram. **D.** Following removal of fixation device. (From Wagner, H.: Femoral osteotomies for congenital hip dislocation. *In* Weil, U. H. (ed): Progress in Orthopedic Surgery. No. 2, Acetabular Dysplasia and Skeletal Dysplasia in Childhood. Heidelberg, Springer-Verlag, 1978. Reprinted by permission.)

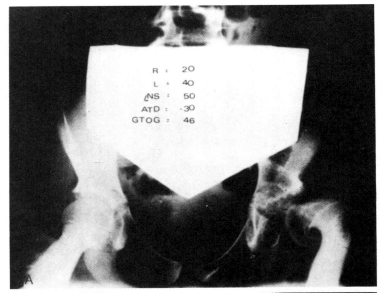

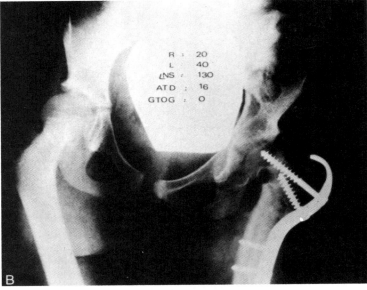

FIGURE 2–208. Modified Pauwel's osteotomy.

A. A 4-cm. leg length of discrepancy caused a severe gluteus medius lurch. **B.** Closing lateral wedge osteotomy of the proximal femur was combined with greater trochanteric advancement. (From Kelikian, A. S., and Tachdjian, M. O.: Greater trochanteric advancement. *In* The Hip Society Award Papers. St. Louis, C. V. Mosby, 1983. Reprinted by permission.)

tive technique is described and illustrated in Plate 24, and an example is shown in Figure 2–208.

HIP DYSPLASIA IN THE ADOLESCENT

By definition, hip dysplasia denotes a deranged articular relationship between an abnormal acetabulum and a deformed upper end of the femur. The acetabulum is maldirected, facing forward and upward owing to excessive antetorsion (Fig. 2–209). It is shallow because of a decrease in its depth, and steep because of a decrease in the width of its roof (Fig. 2–210).

The walls of the acetabulum are deficient superoanteriorly and occasionally also posteriorly. The acetabular fossa is thickened because pressure is reduced owing to the nonconcentricity of the femoral head in the dysplastic acetabulum.

In the dysplastic hip, the upper end of the femur is also deformed. Normally the degree of femoral antetorsion is about 15 degrees, the femoral neck-shaft angle is about 130 degrees, and the tip of the greater trochanter is at, or immediately distal to, the center of the femoral head and laterally displaced about two to two and a half times the radius of the femoral head. In congenital hip dysplasia there is excessive femoral antetorsion, and the femoral head may

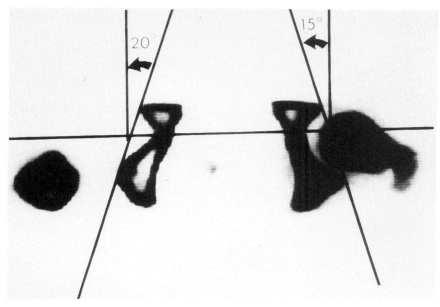

FIGURE 2–209. *Acetabulum is maldirected owing to excessive antetorsion.*

Note that the acetabular antetorsion on the side of the dysplasia is 20 degrees, whereas the normal side is 15 degrees.

be spherical or flattened posteromedially (Fig. 2–211).

Congenital dysplasia of the hip in the adolescent may be complicated by aseptic necrosis of the femoral head due to immobilization in extreme positions after reduction, as in frog-leg, marked abduction, or medial rotation, or after reduction without preliminary traction or open reduction without femoral shortening. In such hips, the biomechanics of the hip are disrupted because of the relative overgrowth of the greater trochanter and the short femoral neck.

Asymmetrical growth arrest of the capital femoral physis, with the lateral part closed and the medial part open, will tilt the femoral head out of the acetabulum. In total necrosis of the femoral head, the femoral neck will be short.

The objective of treatment of hip dysplasia is to prevent osteoarthritis. The successive stages in the evolution of degenerative arthritis secondary to congenital hip subluxation are as follows:

The first and earliest sign is the appearance of the triangle of subchondral bone density in

FIGURE 2–210. *Anteroposterior radiogram of both hips; congenital dysplasia of the right hip.*

Note that the dysplastic acetabulum is shallow and steep, and Shenton's line is disturbed.

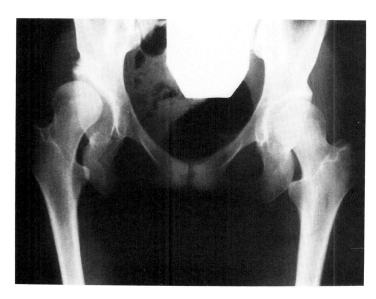

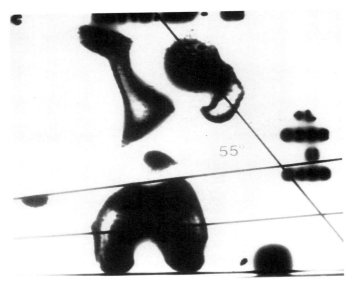

FIGURE 2–211. Torsional study by CT scan of the upper end of the femur in congenital dysplasia of the hip.

Note the excessive antetorsion of 55 degrees.

the acetabular roof. The articular cartilage space is not thinned (Fig. 2–212 A).

In the second stage, the triangular bony condensation in the acetabular roof (sourcil) is steeper and increased in height, and the articular cartilage space is definitely thinned at the rim of the acetabulum (Fig. 2–212 B).

The third stage is characterized by the development of the cyst in the femoral head and the formation of osteophytes medially. The joint space is thinner (Fig. 2–212 C).

The fourth stage consists of extensive cystic changes in both the femoral head and acetabulum, and marked narrowing of the articular cartilage space (Fig. 2–212 D).

Surgical intervention should be carried out in the first, and preferably, no later than the second stage to prevent development of osteoarthritis—before the osteoarthritis has progressed from its incipient to its established stage. When one sees a radiogram such as that shown in Figure 2–213, it is too late to prevent osteoarthritis.

The magnitude of joint pressure and the stress are related to the degree of compressive force and the extent of the area transmitting the load. Reduction of weight-bearing surface will result in an increase in joint pressure. In the dysplastic subluxated hip, the extent of weight-bearing surface is reduced with proportional increase in the magnitude of stress across the joint (Fig. 2–214). The principles of treatment of congenital hip dysplasia are: (1) to create a normal upper end of the femur, (2) to establish normal biomechanics of the hip, and

(3) to provide adequate acetabular coverage of the femoral head.

Indications for Surgical Treatment

The first indication for surgical treatment is hip instability, especially if it is progressive. Instability of the hip is determined by the Trendelenburg test, which should be performed with the tested hip in extension and by flexing only the knee. If the Trendelenburg test is positive, it means that the hip joint is unstable. The delayed Trendelenburg test, as described by Mitchell, is an important way to determine whether the instability is progressive. If you note that the contralateral side of the pelvis drops at the count of 15, and two months later drops at the count of 10, and soon after that at the count of 5, this demonstrates progressive clinical instability of the hip joint, and surgical intervention is indicated.[643] Radiographic determination of hip instability is by weight-bearing views of both hips made with the patient standing first on both feet and then on the affected limb only. An increasing break in Shenton's line indicates progressive instability of the hip joint.

The second indication for surgical intervention is the development of abnormal bone condensation in the roof of the acetabulum. In the normal hip, the outline of the acetabular roof is an even, smooth curve (sourcil). In the subluxated and dysplastic hip, the bony condensation in the roof becomes triangular and migrates laterally toward the acetabular rim.

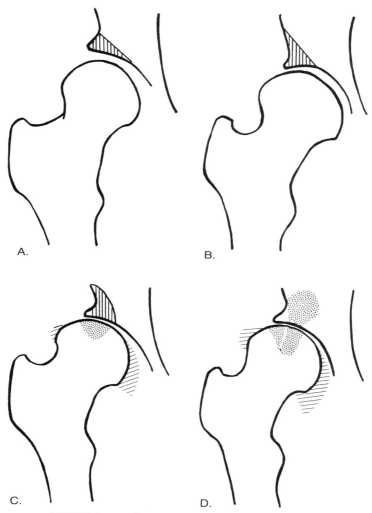

FIGURE 2–212. *The four different stages of osteoarthritis of the hip.*

(Redrawn after Pauwels, Biomechanics of the Normal and Diseased Hip. New York, Springer Verlag, 1976.)

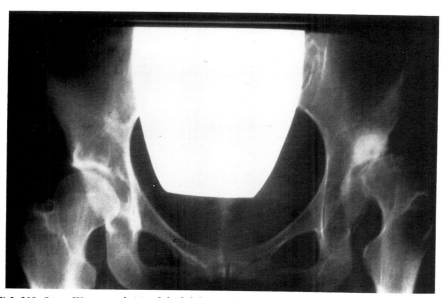

FIGURE 2–213. *Stage IV osteoarthritis of the left hip with congenital hip dysplasia and subluxation of the hip.*

471

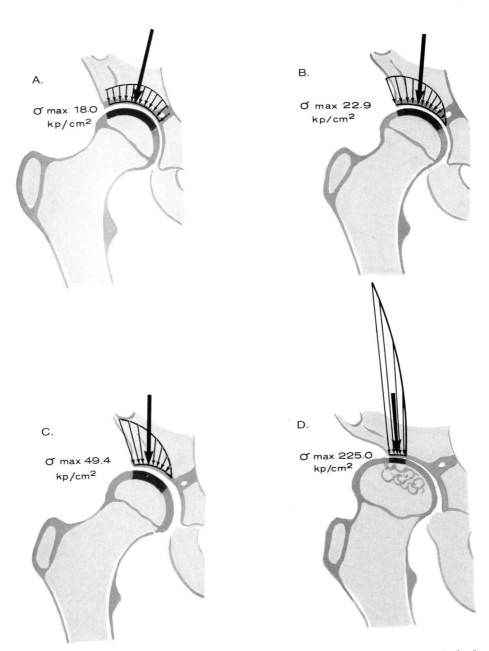

FIGURE 2–214. *Magnitude of joint pressure in relation to the extent of area transmitting the load.*

Drawings show the gradual increase in articular pressure with progressive subluxation of the hip. **A** Normal hip. **B** to **D.** Gradual subluxation. Note the increase of pressure across the joint.

Figure 2–215 A shows a normal sourcil; in Figure 2–215 B you can see that the sourcil is thickened and lateral. Abnormal subchondral bony condensation in the roof of the acetabulum indicates incipient osteoarthritis. It is a biologic response before the onset of pain.

There is controversy about the indications for surgical treatment when a patient is developing a thickened sourcil and instability of the hip joint, but has no pain. Should one operate or should one wait for pain to develop? It is difficult to convince parents that they should put their youngster through a number of operations to prevent osteoarthritis of the hip if the child has no pain and is participating in normal physical activities. This author takes a strong posture that the definition of orthopedics is prevention first and then treatment. Pain does not have to be a prerequisite for reconstruction of a dysplastic hip. A patient who is not physically active and who has no pain should be put through a stress activity test, such as running or a game of tennis, to see whether pain develops. In other words, just as we do a stress test for coronary circulation, we should do a stress test for the hip joint to see whether it is pain-free or painful. If a patient has pain at rest or after minimal physical activity, there should be no question about the need for surgical intervention.

Preoperative Assessment

Prior to surgery, it is crucial to delineate the pathologic changes. A CT scan will determine the exact degree of femoral and acetabular antetorsion; it will show the deficiency of the acetabulum, whether it is anterior or posterior; and it will also assess concentricity of reduction.

Derotation osteotomy of the proximal femur is commonly performed in the treatment of congenital dislocation of the hip. One of the most common problems of the procedure is the creation of femoral retrotorsion owing to over-zealous lateral rotation of the distal segment of the femur. As a result, the femoral head is displaced posteriorly out of the acetabulum. It is crucial that a deformity of the upper end of the femur not be created in an attempt to provide stable reduction of the hip. With a CT scan, it is simple to determine the exact degree of femoral antetorsion by assessing the relationship of the transcondylar axis of the femur to the longitudinal axis of the neck of the femur. In the weight-bearing anteroposterior radiogram of both hips shown in Figure 2–216 A, note that the left femoral head is subluxated and uncovered. When the hip is abducted 40 degrees and medially rotated 30 degrees, Shenton's line can be restored and the femoral head can be contained in the acetabulum, as shown in Figure 2–216 B. If one performs an intertrochanteric varus rotation osteotomy, however, the femoral neck-shaft angle will be 90 degrees and the tip of the greater trochanter will be elevated above the joint line. The result will be a lower limb length discrepancy with a short-leg limp and a gluteus medius lurch. In such cases, it is crucial that concentric reduction of the hip joint be achieved by operations to treat both aspects of the problem; that is, a varus derotation osteotomy of the proximal femur should be combined with a pelvic osteotomy. To repeat, avoid overcorrection; do not create a deformity of the upper end of the femur.

In the preoperative assessment one must study the biomechanics of the hip, keeping in mind that in planning surgical reconstruction one must consider function. Bone is a biologic tissue that will respond to stress. Restoration of normal function is important. If the greater trochanter is elevated owing to relative overgrowth and the patient walks with a gluteus medius lurch, then a distal and lateral transfer of the greater trochanter should be performed. When the biomechanics of the hip joint are restored to normal in a concentrically reduced hip, the acetabulum may respond to function, obviating the need for an innominate osteotomy.

FIGURE 2–215. Subchondral bone condensation in the acetabular roof.

A. In the normal hip the sourcil is smooth. **B.** In the dysplastic hip, the sourcil is thickened and has migrated laterally.

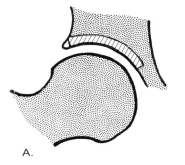
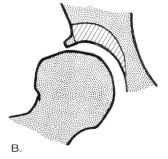

A.   B.

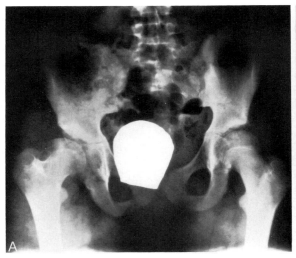

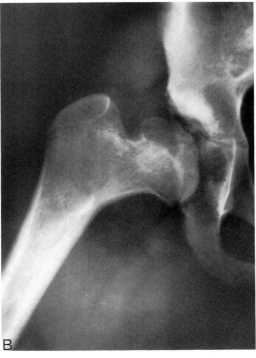

FIGURE 2–216. Congenital dysplasia of the left hip.

A. In weight-bearing position. **B.** With the hip abducted and medially rotated. Note that the femoral head can be contained in the acetabulum by marked abduction of the hip, but that the tip of the greater trochanter is elevated above the joint line.

Classification

Congenital dysplasia of the hip in the adolescent may be classified as: Grade I, stable and congruous but dysplastic; Grade II, unstable and subluxating; Grade III, subluxated, congruous or slightly incongruous, and reducible or irreducible; and Grade IV, subluxated with marked incongruity.

Treatment

Treatment varies according to the type of hip dysplasia and the stability and congruity of the hip joint. If the hip is stable and congruous, one should simply observe the patient with periodic clinical and radiographic assessment. A dysplastic hip does not require surgery unless there is evidence of instability of the hip. If the hip is unstable, as shown by the Trendelenburg test and the break in Shenton's line in the standing radiogram of the hips, surgical intervention may be indicated. As stated earlier, the surgery consists of realignment osteotomy of the proximal femur, an innominate osteotomy, or both. Concentricity of reduction is a prerequisite. If the hip is subluxated, congruous or only slightly incongruous, but concentrically reducible, osteotomy of the proximal femur or of the innominate bone, or both, is performed. If it is irreducible by simple abduction, flexion,

and medial rotation of the hip, an open reduction of the hip joint should be performed first. If the hip is subluxated and markedly incongruous, Chiari's innominate osteotomy is the best operation in the adolescent. Prior to performing a Chiari procedure, one should correct the deformity of the upper end of the femur (especially marked antetorsion). Sometimes a shelf procedure may be performed instead of a Chiari osteotomy, or the two may be combined.

SURGICAL PROCEDURES

Salter's Innominate Osteotomy. The objective of Salter's innominate osteotomy is to derotate a maldirected acetabulum with excessive antetorsion. It is simple to determine the degree of acetabular antetorsion with a CT scan. If this is the problem, Salter's innominate osteotomy is the procedure of choice.

Prerequisites and contraindications have been described previously. The technique is described and illustrated in Plate 18.

Sutherland's Double Innominate Osteotomy. This operation consists of a Salter innominate osteotomy and an osteotomy through the pubis in the interval between the symphysis pubis and the obturator foramen.[911] The operative technique is described and illustrated in Plate 25. In 1966 Hopf described a technique of double innominate osteotomy in which the second osteotomy was performed laterally through the thin isthmus between the acetabulum and the obturator foramen.[423] Hopf's double innominate osteotomy is periacetabular; owing to its proximity to the hip joint it permits greater versatility of correction. Technically it is difficult and risks compromising the blood supply to the hip and entering the hip joint and damaging the articular cartilage. In the Sutherland double innominate osteotomy, the second cut is medial, away from the hip joint, permitting an adequate degree of rotation of the acetabular segment. The Sutherland technique has the definite *advantages* that: (1) the articular cartilage is not endangered, (2) the growth of the triradiate cartilage is not disturbed, (3) the blood supply to the femoral head is not jeopardized, and (4) the design of the operation achieves medial displacement of the hip. The *drawbacks* of the Sutherland procedure are: (1) the orthopedic surgeon's unfamiliarity with the complex anatomy of the symphysis pubis region, especially of the urogenital diaphragm; (2) the danger of injury to the pudendal vessels and nerves; and (3) the necessity for internal fixation of the pubic osteotomy with one threaded Steinmann pin. In the initial stages of familiarizing himself with the surgical technique, the surgeon may find the assistance of a urologist desirable to obviate any problems of surgical exposure. The use of image intensifier radiographic control will avoid the pitfalls of selecting an improper site for the pubic osteotomy, penetration of iliac pins into the hip joint, and injury to neurovascular structures by the pubic pin. Excessive anterior displacement of the hip joint should be avoided. The procedure is biomechanically sound, as it does displace the hip joint medially and provides adequate coverage of the femoral head (Fig. 2–217). The indications and requisites for the procedure are the same as those of triple innominate osteotomy.

Triple Innominate Osteotomy. There are certain limitations to the rotation of the acetabulum that can be obtained by a single osteotomy of the innominate bone; also, in the older patient the inflexibility of the symphysis pubis does not allow sufficient mobility for effective rotation and tilting of the acetabular segment. In their efforts to overcome these problems, LeCoeur, Hopf, and Steel independently described a triple innominate osteotomy in which three cuts are made, the first through the ilium (similar to the Salter procedure), the second through the ramus of the pubis, and the third through the ischium.[422, 423, 538, 539, 897] The additional cuts through the ischium and pubis allow free mobility of the acetabular segment, which is di-

rected to the desired position, fully covering the femoral head by normal articular cartilage and providing stability to the hip in weight-bearing position.

The primary *indication* for triple innominate osteotomy is a dysplastic hip in an adolescent that requires more than 25 degrees of abduction to contain the femoral head concentrically in the acetabulum. If less than 20 degrees of abduction is required for corrective containment, Salter's innominate osteotomy should be performed first; in borderline cases, if adequate containment is not achieved in weight-bearing position, one can proceed to perform the pubic and ischial cuts to mobilize the acetabular segment fully. Another factor to consider is bilaterality of involvement; in the adolescent in whom the symphysis pubis is inflexible, Salter's innominate osteotomy of one hip will aggravate the dysplasia of the opposite hip. Triple innominate osteotomy is therefore the procedure of choice when *both* hips are dysplastic in the adolescent. Other indications are hip joint instability and pain.

The *prerequisites* for triple innominate osteotomy are (1) a congruous hip that can be concentrically reduced, (2) a hip with adequate articular cartilage space, and (3) functional range of hip motion. There is no upper age limit.

Triple innominate osteotomy is *contraindicated* when the hip is stiff, is incongruous, and has lost its articular cartilage space with degenerative arthritis. The hip joint capacity is not enlarged by triple innominate osteotomy; therefore when the femoral head is flattened, enlarged, and uncovered, rotating the acetabulum to cover the anterior and lateral parts of the femoral head will uncover its posterior part. Posterior instability of the hip is undesirable biomechanically and troublesome when total joint replacement is indicated later on in adult life. In paralytic hip subluxation, such as in myelomeningocele or cerebral palsy, the results of triple innominate osteotomy have been poor; in such cases it should be performed with great caution, if ever; shelf acetabular augmentation with or without Chiari's pelvic medial displacement osteotomy is more effective in treatment of paralytic hip subluxation.

There are several surgical approaches to the ischium and pubis for triple innominate osteotomy, namely, the inferior (Steel), posterior (Tönnis), and subinguinal-adductor (Tachdjian and Edelstein).[897, 920, 942] The Steel technique for triple innominate osteotomy is described in Plate 26. There are disadvantages in the Steel technique. (1) In the inferior approach to the

Text continued on page 493

Double Innominate Osteotomy (Sutherland)

The operation is performed with the patient in supine position on a radiolucent table. It is vital that image intensifier fluoroscopy and radiographic control be utilized. The bladder is emptied at the time of surgery by inserting a Foley catheter, which will remain in place for two days. Skin preparation and draping, which should include to the contralateral hip, is carried out. Salter's innominate osteotomy is performed first as illustrated in Plate 18.

OPERATIVE TECHNIQUE

A. A transverse suprapubic incision 7 to 10 cm. long is centered over the symphysis pubis.

B. The subcutaneous tissue and suprapubic fat are divided in line with the skin incision, and the wound edges are retracted. The spermatic cords in the male or the round ligaments in the female are retracted laterally. The aponeurosis of the external abdominal oblique muscle is identified.

C. By dull dissection the attachments of the rectus abdominus and pyramidalis muscles are identified and sharply sectioned from their attachment on the upper border of the pubis. Do not injure the spermatic cords or the round ligaments.

D. Next, the tendons of the adductor longus and gracilis muscles are identified at their origin, freed, and elevated with a periosteal elevator from the anterior surface of the pubis.

Plate 25. Double Innominate Osteotomy (Sutherland)

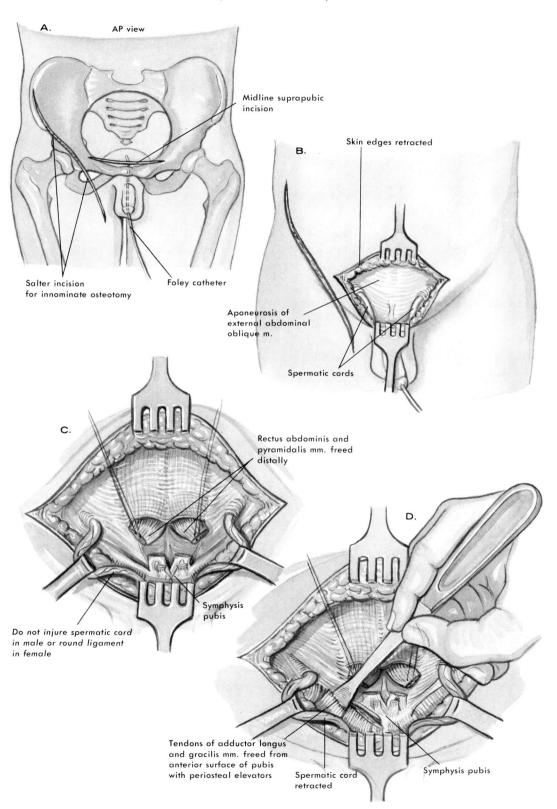

A. AP view

Midline suprapubic incision

Salter incision for innominate osteotomy

Foley catheter

B. Skin edges retracted

Aponeurosis of external abdominal oblique m.

Spermatic cords

C. Rectus abdominis and pyramidalis mm. freed distally

Symphysis pubis

Do not injure spermatic cord in male or round ligament in female

D.

Tendons of adductor longus and gracilis mm. freed from anterior surface of pubis with periosteal elevators

Spermatic cord retracted

Symphysis pubis

477

Double Innominate Osteotomy (Sutherland) (Continued)

E. A Keith hypodermic needle is inserted in the cartilage of the symphysis pubis, and its position is confirmed with an anteroposterior radiogram of the pelvis. Next the periosteum of the symphysis pubis is sectioned transversely and elevated anteriorly and posteriorly, and Chandler retractors are passed around the pubic bone to protect soft tissues during surgery. The internal pudendal artery curves around the medial margin of the inferior ramus of the pubis; the subperiosteal dissection should be gentle and cautious to prevent inadvertent injury to this vessel. The level of osteotomy is marked by drilling a Kirschner wire vertically immediately lateral to the symphysis pubis and medial to the obturator foramen. Again, location of the osteotomy site is visualized by image intensifier radiography.

F. The urogenic diaphragm attaches at the inferior margin of the pubis. The deep dorsal nerve and vessels of the penis pierce the urogenic diaphragm very close to the arcuate ligaments of the penis in the midline. These vital structures are away from the surgical approach, but their proximity and position in the midline should be remembered. With a small rongeur, a wedge of bone 0.7 to 1.3 cm. wide is removed from the pubic bone. The obturator foramen should not be entered.

G and **H.** The lateral pubic segment is elevated with a towel clip, and the attachments of the lower part of the periosteum of the urogenic diaphragm are freed from the inferior margin of the pubis. The stripping of the urogenic diaphragm should extend 2 to 3 cm. laterally.

Plate 25. Double Innominate Osteotomy
(Sutherland)

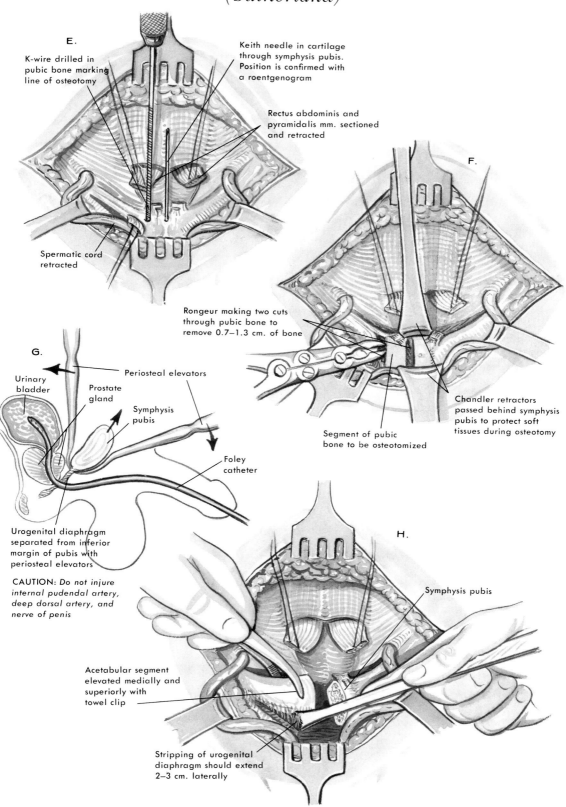

E.

K-wire drilled in pubic bone marking line of osteotomy

Keith needle in cartilage through symphysis pubis. Position is confirmed with a roentgenogram

Rectus abdominis and pyramidalis mm. sectioned and retracted

Spermatic cord retracted

F.

Rongeur making two cuts through pubic bone to remove 0.7–1.3 cm. of bone

Chandler retractors passed behind symphysis pubis to protect soft tissues during osteotomy

Segment of pubic bone to be osteotomized

G.

Urinary bladder

Prostate gland

Symphysis pubis

Periosteal elevators

Foley catheter

Urogenital diaphragm separated from inferior margin of pubis with periosteal elevators

CAUTION: *Do not injure internal pudendal artery, deep dorsal artery, and nerve of penis*

H.

Symphysis pubis

Acetabular segment elevated medially and superiorly with towel clip

Stripping of urogenital diaphragm should extend 2–3 cm. laterally

Double Innominate Osteotomy (Sutherland) (Continued)

I and **J.** A laminar spreader is used at the site of Salter's iliac osteotomy to mobilize the lateral segment. (Do not use a laminar spreader to effect acetabular rotation.) With a towel clip, the lateral acetabular segment is pulled downward and forward, and the medial end of the acetabular segment is pulled upward and medially. The acetabular segment should be displaced superiorly at the site of the pubic osteotomy. By this maneuver, the acetabulum is rotated anteriorly and laterally, and the hip joint is displaced medially.

K. One or two medium-sized threaded Steinmann pins are used to transfix the pubic osteotomy. Do not direct the Steinmann pins in a posterior or inferior direction.

L and **M.** The osteotomized iliac segments of the Salter's osteotomy are fixed with two heavy threaded Kirschner wires transfixing the graft; in the distal fragment they should be posterior and medial to the acetabulum. Closed-suction drainage tubes are inserted, and the wound is closed, and a one and one half hip spica cast is applied.

POSTOPERATIVE CARE

At six weeks in children and eight weeks in adolescents and adults the cast is removed, and radiograms are made to determine the healing of the osteotomy. The pins are removed, and gradually the hip is mobilized. The hip that was operated on is protected with a three-point crutch gait until its functional strength is restored and the Trendelenburg test is negative.

Plate 25. Double Innominate Osteotomy
(Sutherland)

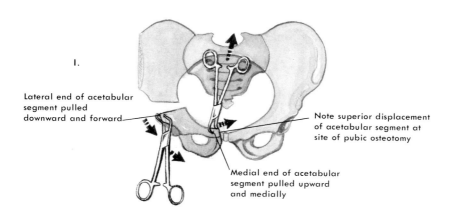

I.

Lateral end of acetabular segment pulled downward and forward

Note superior displacement of acetabular segment at site of pubic osteotomy

Medial end of acetabular segment pulled upward and medially

Arrows show directions of pull to produce anterior and lateral rotation of acetabulum and medial shift of hip joint

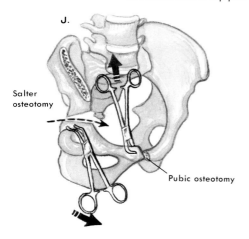

J.

Salter osteotomy

Pubic osteotomy

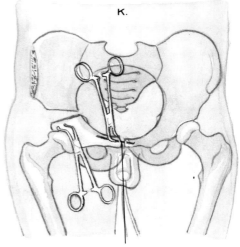

K.

Position of acetabular segment maintained while pubic osteotomy is secured with one or two medium-sized Steinmann pins

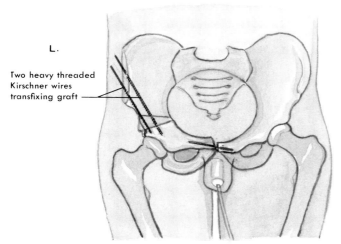

L.

Two heavy threaded Kirschner wires transfixing graft

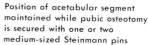

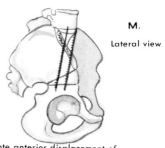

M.

Lateral view

Note anterior displacement of acetabulum and anterior rotation of acetabular segment at site of Salter osteotomy

Steel's Triple Innominate Osteotomy

OPERATIVE TECHNIQUE

A and **B.** In this operation the acetabulum is freed and mobilized by osteotomies of the ischium, superior ramus of the pubis, and ilium from the greater sciatic notch posteriorly to an area between the anterior superior and anterior inferior iliac spines anteriorly. The acetabular segment is rotated to cover the femoral head anteriorly and laterally; the iliac osteotomy is stabilized by a wedge of iliac bone and internal fixation with threaded Steinmann pins or screws.

C. The patient is placed supine on a radiolucent operating table, and the affected hemipelvis, abdomen, lower part of the chest, and entire lower limb are prepared sterile and draped. Preparation of the buttock inferiorly and appropriate shielding of the perineum are important. The draping should allow free motion of the hip and knee during the operation. A nerve stimulator should be available. The osteotomy of the ischium is performed first. The hip and knee of the limb to be operated on are flexed at 90 degrees. (In the drawing both hips are shown in the lithotomy position; it should be emphasized that on the operating table only the hip on the affected side is flexed.) An assistant holds the limb with the hip in neutral position with respect to rotation and adduction-abduction. The ischial tuberosity, which is readily palpated, is marked with indelible ink. A 7- to 9-cm. long transverse incision is made 1 cm. proximal to the subnatal crease and centered over the ischial tuberosity. The subcutaneous tissue and deep fascia are incised in line with the skin incision.

Plate 26. Steel's Triple Innominate Osteotomy

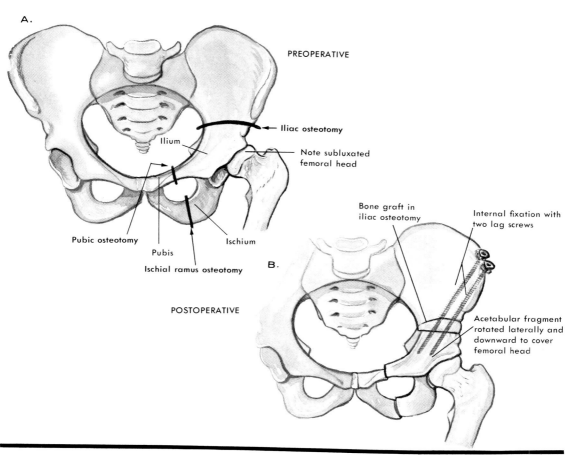

A.

PREOPERATIVE

Iliac osteotomy

Ilium

Note subluxated
femoral head

Pubic osteotomy

Pubis

Ischial ramus osteotomy

Ischium

Bone graft in
iliac osteotomy

Internal fixation with
two lag screws

B.

POSTOPERATIVE

Acetabular fragment
rotated laterally and
downward to cover
femoral head

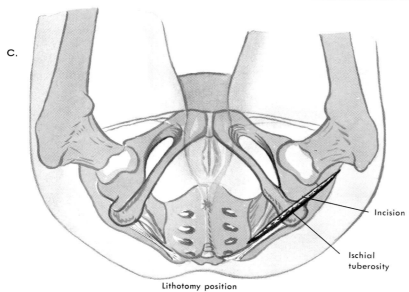

C.

Incision

Ischial
tuberosity

Lithotomy position

Steel's Triple Innominate Osteotomy (Continued)

D. The inferior border of the gluteus maximus is delineated and retracted laterally. The sciatic nerve lies immediately deep to the medial and inferior fibers of the gluteus maximus. Watch for the sciatic nerve and be cautious. It is not necessary to expose the nerve, but its visualization helps to protect it from inadvertent injury during surgery. The ischial bursa, which is superficial to the ischial tuberosity, is identified. The three hamstring muscles take origin from the ischial tuberosity: the biceps femoris is the most superficial, the semitendinosus (which is membranous at its origin) is lateral to the biceps femoris, and the semimembranosus (which is tendinous near its origin) is immediately proximal and lateral to the semitendinosus. The sciatic nerve and semimembranosus muscle look alike; they should not be mistaken for each other. After its exit from the greater sciatic notch, the sciatic nerve courses posterior to the ramus of the ischium and down the limb parallel and lateral to the semimembranosus. It lies far enough laterally to stay out of harm's way. If in doubt use a nerve stimulator. (The leg will jump! Be sure the patient's foot does not hit the assistant's head, contaminating the field.)

E and F. This author detaches the origins of the biceps femoris, the semitendinosus, and the semimembranosus and tags them with sutures for later reattachment. The periosteum over the ischial ramus and tuberosity is incised.

Plate 26. Steel's Triple Innominate Osteotomy

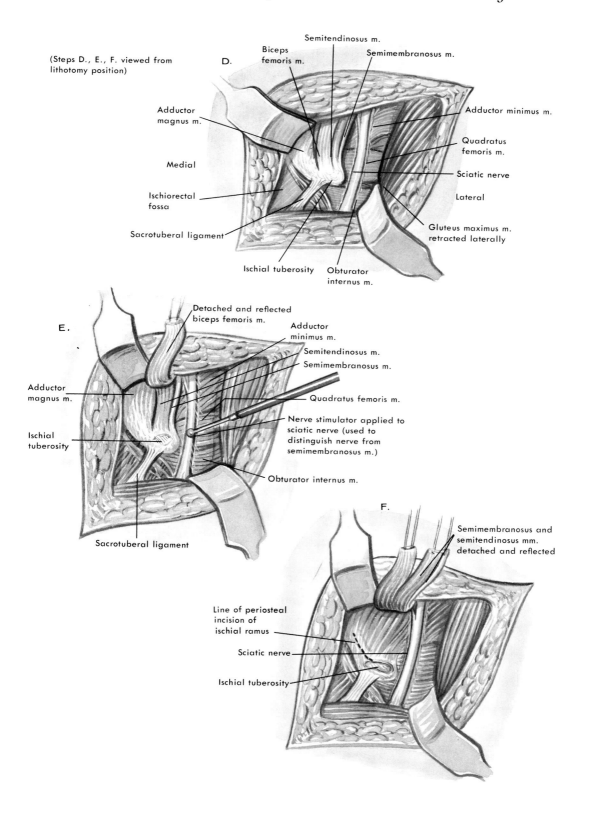

(Steps D., E., F. viewed from lithotomy position)

D.

Biceps femoris m.

Semitendinosus m.

Semimembranosus m.

Adductor magnus m.

Adductor minimus m.

Quadratus femoris m.

Medial

Sciatic nerve

Ischiorectal fossa

Lateral

Sacrotuberal ligament

Gluteus maximus m. retracted laterally

Ischial tuberosity

Obturator internus m.

E.

Detached and reflected biceps femoris m.

Adductor minimus m.

Semitendinosus m.

Semimembranosus m.

Adductor magnus m.

Quadratus femoris m.

Nerve stimulator applied to sciatic nerve (used to distinguish nerve from semimembranosus m.)

Ischial tuberosity

Obturator internus m.

Sacrotuberal ligament

F.

Semimembranosus and semitendinosus mm. detached and reflected

Line of periosteal incision of ischial ramus

Sciatic nerve

Ischial tuberosity

Steel's Triple Innominate Osteotomy (Continued)

G. A curved kidney pedicle forceps is passed subperiosteally superior to the ischial tuberosity, around the ischial ramus, and into the obturator foramen. The importance of staying beneath the periosteum cannot be overemphasized. The internal pudendal vessels and nerves should be protected; they run in Alcock's canal, enclosed in the obturator internus fascia, and emerge from the pelvis to innervate and supply blood to the external genitalia. The site and level of osteotomy is verified by image intensifier fluoroscopy. The lower part of the ischial ramus is sectioned obliquely with an osteotome directed lateromedially.

H. The detached hamstring muscles are resutured to their origin. Hemostasis is obtained; blood loss is usually minimal. Catheters are inserted for closed suction.

I. The edge of the gluteus maximus is sutured to the fascial envelope, and the wound is closed in the usual fashion. Because this phase of the operation is performed in close proximity to the perineum it is advisable to change instruments, gown, and gloves. Appropriate redraping is recommended for the anterior approach.

Plate 26. Steel's Triple Innominate Osteotomy

Patient in lithotomy position

G.

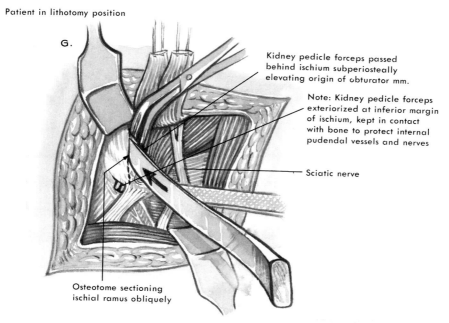

Kidney pedicle forceps passed behind ischium subperiosteally elevating origin of obturator mm.

Note: Kidney pedicle forceps exteriorized at inferior margin of ischium, kept in contact with bone to protect internal pudendal vessels and nerves

Sciatic nerve

Osteotome sectioning ischial ramus obliquely

H.

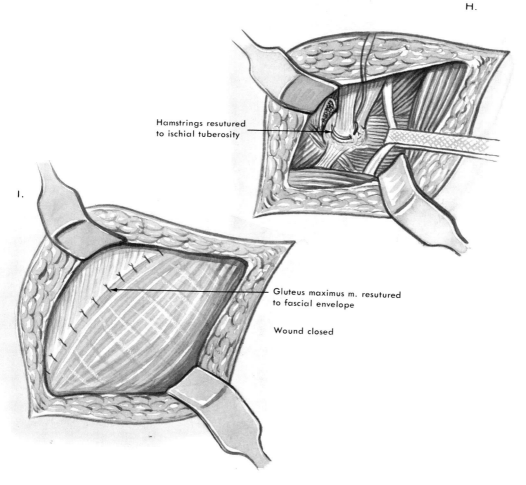

Hamstrings resutured to ischial tuberosity

I.

Gluteus maximus m. resutured to fascial envelope

Wound closed

Steel's Triple Innominate Osteotomy (Continued)

J and **K.** The second surgical approach is the standard iliofemoral one employed for other innominate osteotomies. The cartilaginous iliac apophysis is split; the gluteal and iliac muscles are elevated subperiosteally from lateral and medial walls of the ilium. The sartorius is sectioned at its origin and reflected distally, and the lateral attachments of the inguinal ligament are detached and reflected medially. Both heads of the rectus femoris are divided, elevated, and reflected distally. Keeping the dissection subperiosteal and deep to the iliacus and psoas muscles protects the femoral nerve and vessels. Exposure of the superior ramus of the pubis is facilitated by flexing the hip. The ramus is subperiosteally exposed circumferentially 1 cm. medial to the iliopectineal prominence. There is a tendency to perform the osteotomy too far laterally—in the medial wall of the acetabulum; verify the site radiographically. A curved kidney pedicle forceps is introduced subperiosteally from the upper border of the ramus into the obturator foramen. Injury to obturator vessels and nerves should be avoided. If the pubic bone is very thick, a second forceps may be introduced subperiosteally below and pushed superiorly to meet the upper forceps. The pubic bone is osteotomized with a sharp osteotome directed posteromedially—15 degrees medial from the perpendicular.

Plate 26. Steel's Triple Innominate Osteotomy

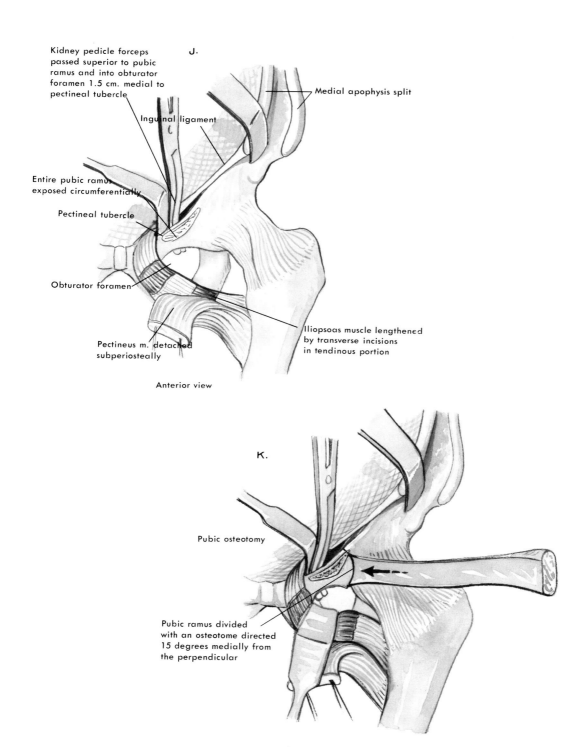

J.

Kidney pedicle forceps passed superior to pubic ramus and into obturator foramen 1.5 cm. medial to pectineal tubercle

Medial apophysis split

Inguinal ligament

Entire pubic ramus exposed circumferentially

Pectineal tubercle

Obturator foramen

Iliopsoas muscle lengthened by transverse incisions in tendinous portion

Pectineus m. detached subperiosteally

Anterior view

K.

Pubic osteotomy

Pubic ramus divided with an osteotome directed 15 degrees medially from the perpendicular

Steel's Triple Innominate Osteotomy (Continued)

L. The iliac bone is divided with a Gigli saw, utilizing the technique described for Salter's innominate osteotomy.

M. After sectioning of the iliac bone, the acetabular segment is mobilized with a laminar spreader and periosteal elevator. When free, the acetabular segment is manipulated into the desired position to cover the femoral head. Lateralization of the acetabulum should be avoided; the medially directed oblique cuts of the ischium and pubis will facilitate its medial shift. With the acetabulum in the proper position, a triangular fragment of bone is removed from the superior margin of the ilium.

N. The iliac segments and the graft are transfixed with two threaded Steinmann pins. The pins may be introduced from below and directed superiorly into the upper iliac segment, or from above down. They should not penetrate the hip joint. This author prefers fixation with two cancellous screws or two pronged tubular plates as in the Wagner technique. He does not find immobilization of the hip in a hip spica cast necessary. (Steel and Coleman apply a one–and–one half hip spica cast.)[153, 155–159, 897–899]

POSTOPERATIVE CARE

This author recommends placing the patient in bilateral split Russell's traction. Gluteus medius and minimus, gluteus maximus, quadriceps femoris, and triceps surae exercises are begun as soon as possible. The patient is allowed to be up and around, walking with three-point toe-touch crutch gait for 10 to 12 weeks.

Steel and Coleman retain the hip spica cast for eight to ten weeks. When the triple osteotomies show healing, partial weight-bearing with crutches is allowed. Full weight-bearing is allowed six months postoperatively, at which time the internal fixation device is removed.

Plate 26. Steel's Triple Innominate Osteotomy

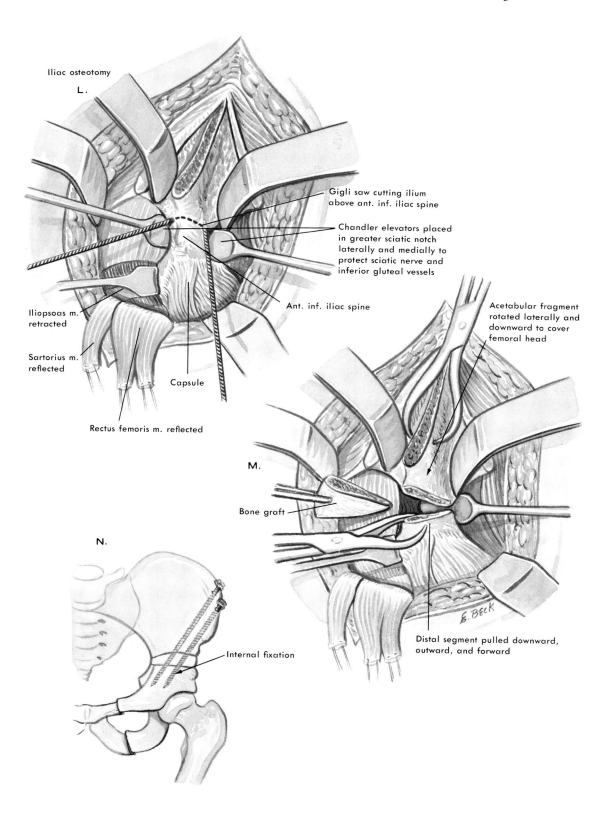

Iliac osteotomy

L.

Gigli saw cutting ilium above ant. inf. iliac spine

Chandler elevators placed in greater sciatic notch laterally and medially to protect sciatic nerve and inferior gluteal vessels

Iliopsoas m. retracted

Sartorius m. reflected

Ant. inf. iliac spine

Capsule

Rectus femoris m. reflected

N.

M.

Acetabular fragment rotated laterally and downward to cover femoral head

Bone graft

E. BECK

Internal fixation

Distal segment pulled downward, outward, and forward

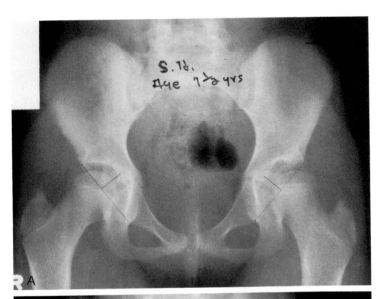

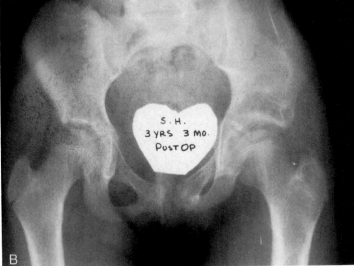

FIGURE 2–217. Sutherland's double innominate osteotomy.

A. Preoperative radiogram. **B.** Postoperative radiogram. (Courtesy of D. Sutherland.)

ischium the surgical wound is close to the rectum and there is always danger of contamination. (2) The dissection and ischial osteotomy are near the sciatic nerve; the nerve should be protected during the procedure. (3) The ischial cut is in the weight-bearing sitting position of the ischium and is not periacetabular. The further away from the hip joint it is, the more limited is the degree of correction that can be obtained. (4) Lateralization of the acetabulum is a definite problem; because a wedge of bone from the ischium is not resected in the Steel procedure, the acetabulum often becomes displaced and rotates laterally despite efforts to move the hip joint medially by directing the pubic and ischial cuts medially. (5) It is difficult to make the pubic cut because its approach is lateral to the iliopsoas tendon; approach to the pubic bone medial to the iliopsoas tendon is technically much easier and lessens the danger of inadvertently entering the hip joint with the osteotomy line. The advantage of Steel's technique is that the ischial tuberosity, especially in the thin patient, is readily palpable, and surgical approach to the ischium is relatively easy.

In the Tönnis technique for triple osteotomy the ischium is sectioned through a posterior approach.[942] First, the patient is placed in prone position, and an oblique incision is made, centered over the ischial tuberosity, in the direction of the gluteus maximus muscle fibers. The subcutaneous tissue and deep fascia are divided in line with the skin incision. Next, with a blunt instrument, the fibers of the gluteus maximus are gently spread, exposing the ischial tuberosity and the sacrotuberous ligament. Care must be taken not to spread the gluteus maximus fibers too far proximally in order to avoid inadvertent injury to the inferior gluteal nerve and vessels. The obturator internus and gemelli are divided transversely immediately above the ischial tuberosity and gently elevated, exposing the ischial ramus to the greater sciatic notch. Next, with a blunt retractor inserted into the sciatic notch, the sciatic nerve is retracted superolaterally and the gluteal nerve and vessels upward. Then two retractors are inserted in the obturator foramen—one lateral to the ischial ramus and the other medial to the ischium (the medial retractor is medial to the sacrotuberous ligament). It is vital to preserve and maintain integrity of the sacrotuberous and sacrospinal ligaments, as they provide stability to the spine. The level and direction of osteotomy are determined under image intensifier radiographic control. With an osteotome, the ischial ramus

is cut from the lateral to the medial side; the plane of osteotomy is frontal to enable rotation of the acetabular segment. The osteotomy should be complete; it is best to double-check its thoroughness with a radiogram. The ischial wound is closed, and the patient is turned to supine posture and reprepared and redraped.

The pubic osteotomy is performed through a separate small transverse incision over the pubic ramus, medial to the psoas muscle. The femoral vessels and nerves with the iliopsoas are retracted laterally, and the pubic cut is made parallel to the hip joint, close to the acetabulum. The iliac osteotomy is performed through an anterior incision similar to Salter's, but instead of a transverse osteotomy of the ilium, Tönnis recommends a curvilinear cut in the superolateral to inferomedial direction.[942] The change of position of the patient from prone to supine is a definite disadvantage of the Tönnis technique because it adds 30 minutes to the operation time. Another problem with the Tönnis technique is injury to the nerve supply of the gluteus maximus, which has occurred in 3 per cent of cases. A technical problem is lateralization of the acetabulum; efforts to move the acetabulum medially are not always successful.

This author has developed a medial-adductor approach to the ischium and pubis for periacetabular triple innominate osteotomy (Plate 27). The advantages of this technique are, first, the exposure of the ischium and pubis through a single transverse medial-adductor incision, which is cosmetically very pleasing. Second, the triple osteotomy is periacetabular; being close to the hip joint it permits a greater degree of correction. Third, taking a wedge of bone from the upper ramus of the ischium, based anteriorly and laterally, allows medial relocation of the hip joint. An illustrative case is shown in Figure 2–218.

Periacetabular Innominate Osteotomy. Wagner and Eppright independently developed a technique of osteotomy to cover the femoral head when the hip joint is congruous and the hyaline cartilage surface of the acetabulum is sufficiently large.[263, 979] In the Wagner Type I osteotomy, a hemispheric section of the cartilaginous osseous acetabulum is cut out of the pelvic isthmus with a special chisel and then turned outward anterolaterally until the femoral head is completely covered. The acetabulum is cut parallel to its articular surface, and the line of osteotomy is guided by image intensifier radiographic control. With spreaders, the acetabulum is loosened and pulled down over the femoral head. The pivot point of the hip is

Text continued on page 503

Periacetabular Triple Innominate Osteotomy Through Subinguinal Adductor Approach

This approach allows performance of a triple innominate osteotomy close to the hip joint and avoids turning the patient from prone to supine and repreparing and redraping (as in the Tönnis gluteal approach).

OPERATIVE TECHNIQUE

A. The patient is placed in completely supine position on a radiolucent operating table so that a C-arm image intensifier can be used. The abdomen, affected side of the pelvis, perineal area, and entire lower limb are prepared and draped to allow free motion of the hip. Adequate shielding, preparing, and draping of the perineum is crucial. Two separate skin incisions are used: first, an oblique iliac incision for the usual Salter innominate osteotomy; and second, a transverse adductor incision such as is used for routine adductor myotomy.

B to **D.** The subcutaneous tissue and fascia are divided. The adductor longus, gracilis, and adductor brevis muscles are detached at their origins, tagged, and retracted distally. Injury to the obturator nerves and vessels should be avoided.

Plate 27. Periacetabular Triple Innominate Osteotomy Through Subinguinal Adductor Approach

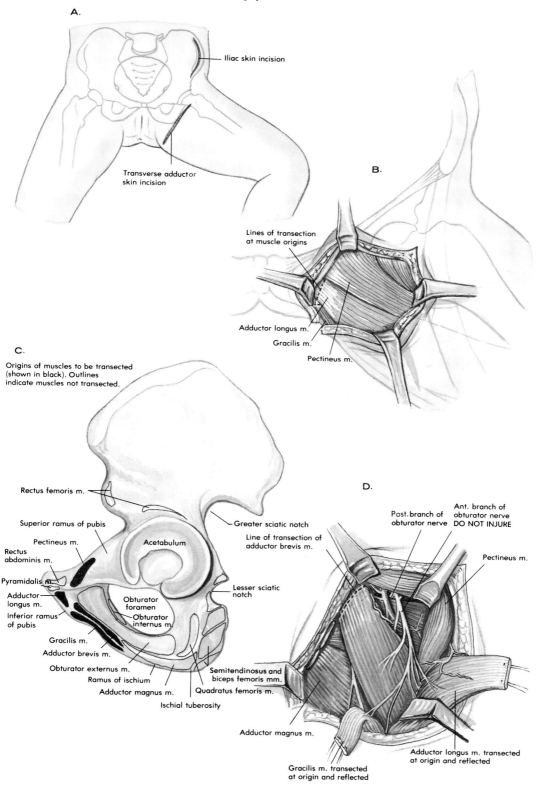

A.

Iliac skin incision

Transverse adductor skin incision

B.

Lines of transection at muscle origins

Adductor longus m.

Gracilis m.

Pectineus m.

C.

Origins of muscles to be transected (shown in black). Outlines indicate muscles not transected.

Rectus femoris m.

Superior ramus of pubis

Pectineus m.

Rectus abdominis m.

Pyramidalis m.

Adductor longus m.

Inferior ramus of pubis

Gracilis m.

Adductor brevis m.

Obturator externus m.

Ramus of ischium

Adductor magnus m.

Ischial tuberosity

Acetabulum

Obturator foramen

Obturator internus m.

Greater sciatic notch

Line of transection of adductor brevis m.

Lesser sciatic notch

Semitendinosus and biceps femoris mm.

Quadratus femoris m.

D.

Post. branch of obturator nerve

Ant. branch of obturator nerve DO NOT INJURE

Pectineus m.

Adductor magnus m.

Gracilis m. transected at origin and reflected

Adductor longus m. transected at origin and reflected

495

Periacetabular Triple Innominate Osteotomy Through Subinguinal Adductor Approach (Continued)

E. The iliopsoas muscle is lengthened at its musculotendinous junction.

F. The avascular plane between the abductor magnus and obturator externus muscles is developed by blunt dissection. The ramus of the ischium is identified and verified by the image intensifier. Tissue in the interval between the adductor magnus and obturator externus is divided with electrocautery, and the ischial ramus is exposed subperiosteally. Two Chandler elevator retractors are placed completely around the ischial ramus.

G. A broad flat osteotome is used to resect a wedge of the ischium, based laterally and anteriorly, about 1.5 to 2.0 cm. inferior to the acetabulum. The osteotome is directed from the lateral to the medial side. The osteotomy should be complete. Taking a wedge of bone prevents lateral displacement of the acetabular segment and allows rotation and medialization of the acetabulum.

H. Next, the superior ramus of the pubis is identified by palpation and verification under image intensifier; it is relatively subcutaneous at this level. The iliopsoas muscle is retracted laterally and the pectineus muscle is elevated. The site of osteotomy of the superior ramus of the pubis is 1.5 cm. medial to the acetabulum, which is verified by image intensifier radiography. The pubic bone is subperiosteally exposed, and two Chandler elevator retractors are inserted behind the pubic ramus.

Plate 27. Periacetabular Triple Innominate Osteotomy Through Subinguinal Adductor Approach

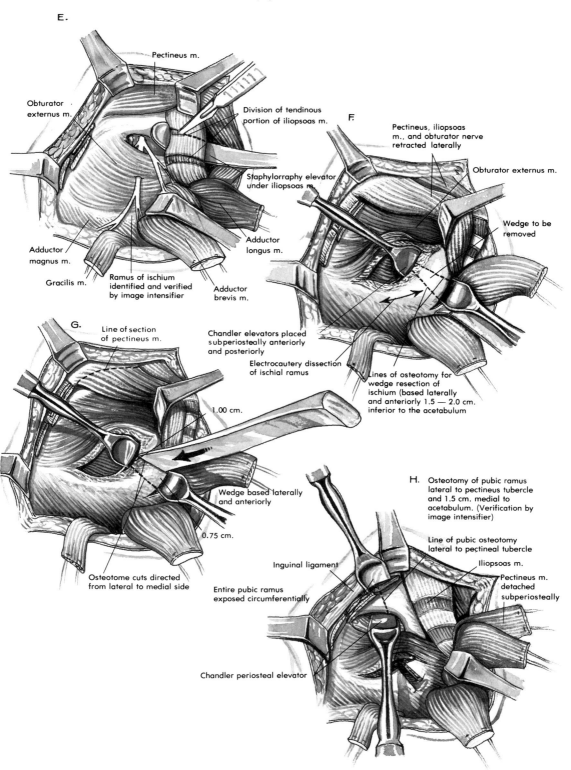

E.

Pectineus m.

Obturator externus m.

Division of tendinous portion of iliopsoas m.

Staphylorraphy elevator under iliopsoas m.

Adductor longus m.

Adductor magnus m.

Gracilis m.

Ramus of ischium identified and verified by image intensifier

Adductor brevis m.

F.

Pectineus, iliopsoas m., and obturator nerve retracted laterally

Obturator externus m.

Wedge to be removed

Chandler elevators placed subperiosteally anteriorly and posteriorly

Electrocautery dissection of ischial ramus

Lines of osteotomy for wedge resection of ischium (based laterally and anteriorly 1.5 — 2.0 cm. inferior to the acetabulum

G.

Line of section of pectineus m.

1.00 cm.

Wedge based laterally and anteriorly

0.75 cm.

Osteotome cuts directed from lateral to medial side

H. Osteotomy of pubic ramus lateral to pectineus tubercle and 1.5 cm. medial to acetabulum. (Verification by image intensifier)

Line of pubic osteotomy lateral to pectineal tubercle

Iliopsoas m.

Pectineus m. detached subperiosteally

Inguinal ligament

Entire pubic ramus exposed circumferentially

Chandler periosteal elevator

497

Periacetabular Triple Innominate Osteotomy Through Subinguinal Adductor Approach (Continued)

I. Pubic osteotomy is performed with the osteotome directed medially and upward.
J and **K.** The iliac osteotomy is performed as described by Salter.

Plate 27. Periacetabular Triple Innominate Osteotomy Through Subinguinal Adductor Approach

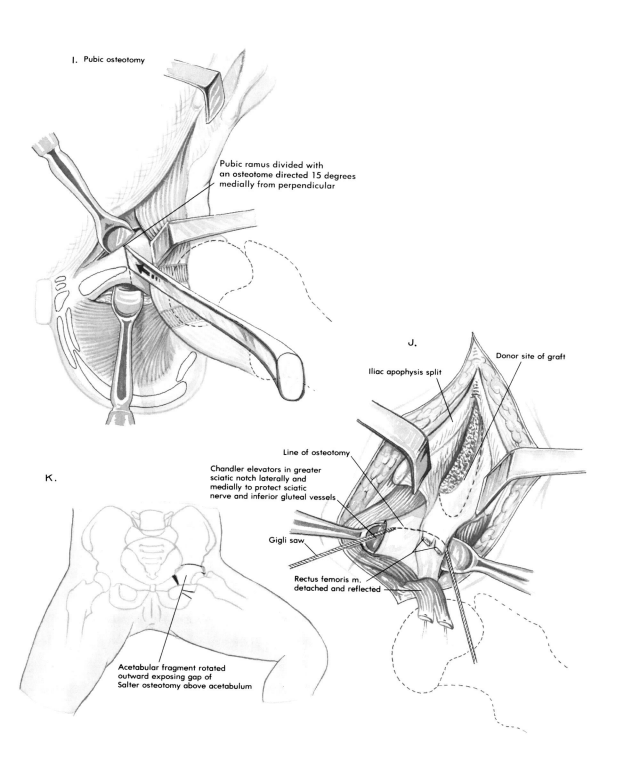

I. Pubic osteotomy

Pubic ramus divided with an osteotome directed 15 degrees medially from perpendicular

J.

Iliac apophysis split

Donor site of graft

Line of osteotomy

Chandler elevators in greater sciatic notch laterally and medially to protect sciatic nerve and inferior gluteal vessels

Gigli saw

Rectus femoris m. detached and reflected

K.

Acetabular fragment rotated outward exposing gap of Salter osteotomy above acetabulum

Periacetabular Triple Innominate Osteotomy Through Subinguinal Adductor Approach (Continued)

L. By rotating the acetabular fragment and manipulating the lower limb, excellent anterior and lateral coverage is provided.

M and **N.** A wedge of bone taken from the ilium is inserted at the iliac osteotomy site and fixed by two threaded Steinmann pins, which may be inserted either superoinferiorly and medially or retrograde inferosuperiorly.

O. Additional fixation by one semitubular plate is recommended. The inferior holes of the semitubular plates are cut with a large pin cutter to create prongs. The sharp prongs are impacted into the rotated acetabulum; cortical screws are inserted from the lateral to the medial surface of the ilium, transfixing the plates. The pubic and ischial osteotomies do not require fixation, but the former may be grafted with a wedge of bone taken from the ischium or ilium.

Final roentgenograms are made for a permanent record. The tendons of the adductor longus, adductor brevis, and gracilis are resutured to their origins. Closed suction tubes are used for 48 hours. The wound is closed in routine fashion. A hip spica cast is not needed unless a concurrent varus femoral osteotomy is performed.

POSTOPERATIVE CARE

The patient is placed in bilateral split Russell's traction. Active assisted and gentle passive exercises are commenced the second day postoperatively. In about seven to ten days postoperatively the patient is allowed to be up and around with a three-point crutch gait protecting the limb that was operated on. Full weight-bearing is delayed until the osteotomies are solidly healed, about two to three months. Internal fixation devices are removed four to six months postoperatively.

Plate 27. Periacetabular Triple Innominate Osteotomy Through Subinguinal Adductor Approach

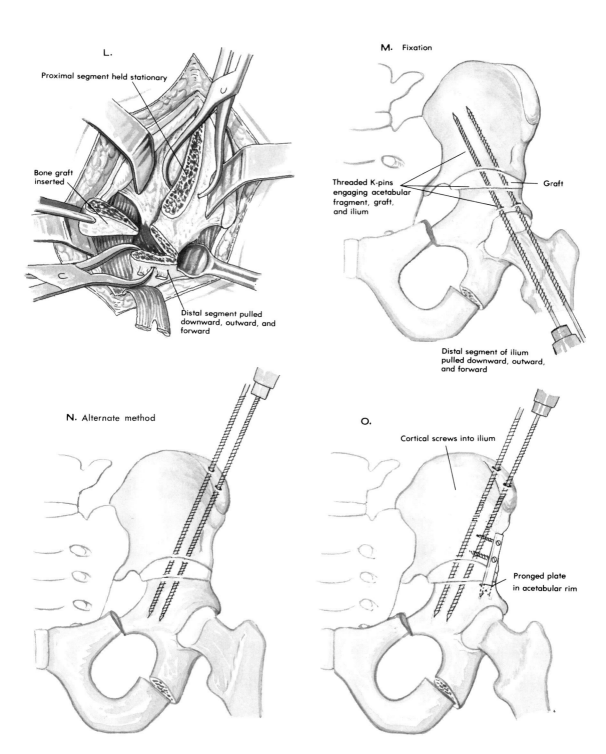

L.

Proximal segment held stationary

Bone graft inserted

Distal segment pulled downward, outward, and forward

M. Fixation

Threaded K-pins engaging acetabular fragment, graft, and ilium

Graft

Distal segment of ilium pulled downward, outward, and forward

N. Alternate method

O.

Cortical screws into ilium

Pronged plate in acetabular rim

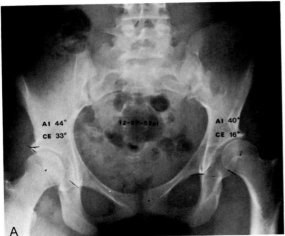

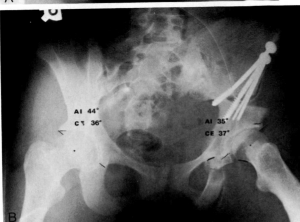

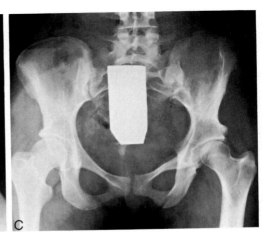

FIGURE 2–218. Dysplasia of the acetabulum treated by triple innominate osteotomy through the inguinal adductor approach.

A. Preoperative radiogram. B. Immediate postoperative radiogram. C. Three years postoperatively.

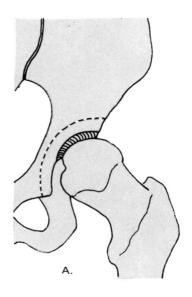

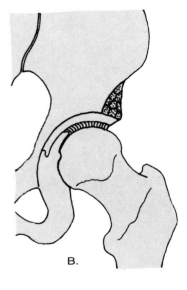

FIGURE 2–219. Wagner Type I periacetabular osteotomy.

A. Line of osteotomy. B. The acetabulum is redirected to cover the femoral head.

A.　　　　　　　B.

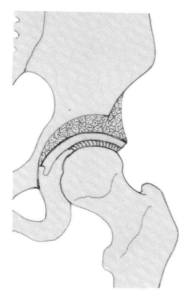

FIGURE 2–220. Wagner Type II periacetabular osteotomy.

In this operation the affected limb is lengthened by insertion of a graft at the osteotomy site.

unchanged. The osteotomy is fixed in the corrected position by means of two hooked plates on the lateral wall of the ilium. The plates are fixed with screws; cortical cancellous bone chips are taken from the iliac crest to fill the space at the osteotomy site (Fig. 2–219).

Wagner has also developed another technique (Type II) to cover the femoral head when the affected lower limb is short. In this technique, a bone graft is inserted at the osteotomy site to lengthen the lower limb (Fig. 2–220).

A third type of Wagner acetabular osteotomy combines the hemispherical osteotomy cut around the dysplastic acetabulum with a transverse osteotomy of the isthmus of the ilium, utilizing Chiari's principle. The distal segment of the ilium is displaced medially, and the bone fragments are fixed with Kirschner wires that are made into staples and are held together by a pronged semitubular plate and cortical screws (Fig. 2–221).

Eppright's dial periacetabular osteotomy is very similar to Wagner's Type I. The only differences are the technique by which the cuts are made and the method of fixation. Eppright utilizes two Steinmann pins with the added support of a hip spica cast for a period of three to four weeks.

The advantage of periacetabular osteotomy is the great degree of coverage of the femoral head that can be provided by being so close to the deformity. Its disadvantages are that technically it is difficult to execute and there is always the danger of the osteotomy entering the hip joint and causing chondrolysis. Aseptic necrosis of the acetabular fragment is another complication. This author prefers triple innominate osteotomy over periacetabular innominate osteotomy.

Chiari's Medial Displacement Pelvic Osteotomy. In 1955 Chiari described a procedure in which the innominate bone is osteotomized between the anterior inferior iliac spine and the greater sciatic notch, immediately above the origin of the capsule of the hip joint, and the inferior segment of the innominate bone is displaced medially. The upper fragment becomes the shelf, and the capsule is interposed between the femoral head and the shelf. The operation is a form of capsular arthroplasty; the interposed thickened capsule converts into fi-

FIGURE 2–221. Wagner Type III periacetabular osteotomy.

The spherical osteotomy cut around the dysplastic acetabulum is combined with a transverse osteotomy of the ilium. After redirection of the acetabulum, the hip joint is shifted medially, following the Chiari principle.

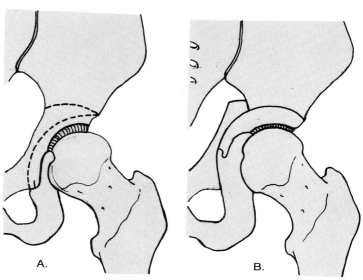

A.   B.

brocartilage.[126] Chiari's pelvic osteotomy is a salvage, not a reconstructive, procedure. Coverage of the femoral head is provided by fibrocartilage and not by hyaline cartilage. Under the stresses of weight-bearing and loading, fibrocartilage is less durable than hyaline cartilage, decreasing the longevity of the hip joint and increasing the likelihood of further development of osteoarthritis. Whenever possible the femoral head should be covered by hyaline cartilage.

Another disadvantage of the Chiari operation is the postoperative narrowing of the pelvis, which is inevitable. The patient and her parents should be forewarned that the narrowed pelvic outlet may obstruct full-term vaginal delivery, and Caesarean section may be necessary; there are, however, numerous reports of successful vaginal delivery after the operation.

The angle of displacement is medial and also slightly upward (15 degrees); therefore some minor degree of shortening of the lower limb may result. The greater the degree of upward displacement, the greater will be the amount of limb shortening.

Sciatic nerve paresis is a calculated risk of the procedure because the nerve is angulated at the osteotomy site and also may be injured by bone splintering at the sciatic notch. The importance of using a Gigli saw or very sharp, thin AO osteotomes to cut the cortex of the sciatic notch cannot be overemphasized. Surgical scarring around the sciatic nerve by prior pelvic osteotomy increases the chance of nerve damage.

The advantages of Chiari's osteotomy are that it enlarges the capacity of the newly formed acetabulum. When the femoral head is flattened, large, extruded more than 30 per cent, and incongruous, an acetabular enlargement innominate osteotomy is indicated. It increases the load-bearing surface on the femoral head and thereby decreases the pressure per square unit on cartilage and bone. Curving the cut in the back toward the ischium near the sciatic notch provides posterior coverage to the enlarged femoral head. Provided the osteotomy line is not too close, the hip joint and the articular cartilage space are not violated and the range of hip motion is maintained. The procedure is extra-articular and does not interfere with the acetabular roof. Medial displacement of the fulcrum of the hip joint shortens the medial arm of the hip abductor lever system, improves the hip mechanics, and diminishes the load on the femoral head (Fig. 2–222). This is a definite advantage of the Chiari operation over the other shelf procedures; the others do

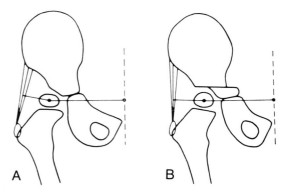

FIGURE 2–222. Medial displacement of fulcrum of hip joint in Chiari's osteotomy.

A and **B.** Diagrams illustrate that the Chiari osteotomy medially displaces the fulcrum of the hip joint and consequently shortens the medial arm of the hip abductor lever system and decreases the load on the femoral head. (From Colton, C. L.: Chiari osteotomy for acetabular dysplasia in young subjects. J. Bone Joint Surg., 54-B:578, 1972. Reprinted by permission.)

not shift the hip joint medially. Medial relocation of the upper femur with the greater trochanter changes the direction of the hip abductors to a more vertical line. This functionally lengthens the lateral arm of the hip abductor lever system (Fig. 2–223). Another advantage of the Chiari pelvic osteotomy over the shelf operation is the immediate formation of a strong live roof that is not absorbed like the grafts of a shelf. Provision of a deep solid acetabular roof will facilitate total hip replacement in the future if necessary.

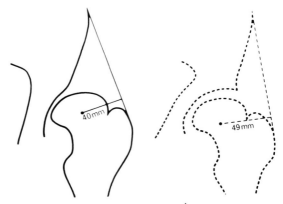

FIGURE 2–223. Medial displacement of femoral head in Chiari's osteotomy.

In Chiari's osteotomy, medial displacement of the femoral head produces a more vertical line of action of the hip abductors; this effectively lengthens the lateral arm of the hip abductor lever system. (From Colton, C. L.: Chiari osteotomy for acetabular dysplasia in young subjects. J. Bone Joint Surg., 54-B:578, 1972. Reprinted by permission.)

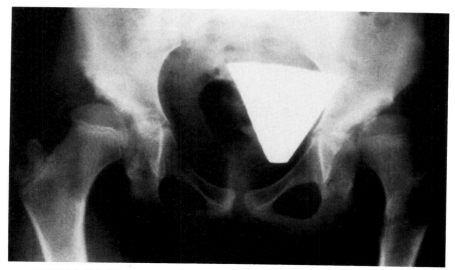

FIGURE 2–224. *Bilateral superolateral subluxation of both hips in a 15-year-old girl.*

Left hip is irreducible.

Indications. Chiari's pelvic osteotomy is indicated for (1) an irreducible laterally subluxated hip with moderate incongruity of the joint in an adolescent or young adult (Fig. 2–224). The procedure relocates the femoral head medially and provides roof coverage. (2) Pain, especially increasing pain, due to beginning osteoarthritis of the hip is alleviated by Chiari's pelvic osteotomy, which increases the acetabular capacity and relieves abnormal joint pressure. (3) Progressive instability in a dysplastic hip in an adolescent with moderate or severe

incongruity of the joint and coxa magna is corrected (Fig. 2–225). Incongruity of the joint precludes the Salter or triple innominate osteotomy, which covers the femoral head by hyaline cartilage; the enlarged femoral head requires an acetabular enlargement operation. (The Salter and triple innominate osteotomies do not increase the capacity of the acetabulum; by tilting the acetabulum anteriorly and laterally, they will uncover the posterior part of the hip joint.)

Progressive instability of the hip joint is de-

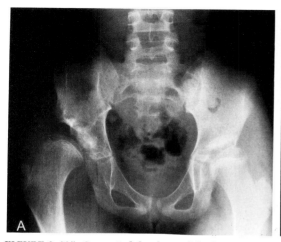
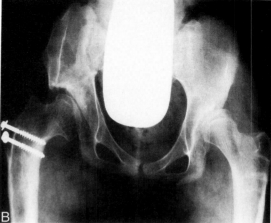

FIGURE 2–225. *Congenital dysplasia of the hip in an adolescent with severe incongruity of the hip joint, coxa magna, and lack of coverage of the femoral head.*

Previously this patient was treated by open reduction and a very poorly performed innominate osteotomy. **A.** Preoperative radiograms. **B.** Postoperative radiogram after Chiari's pelvic osteotomy and distal and lateral transfer of the greater trochanter.

termined clinically by the Trendelenburg test and in standing anteroposterior radiograms of the hip. If there is marked degree of femoral antetorsion or valgus inclination it should be corrected before Chiari's osteotomy is performed.

Contraindications. Chiari's pelvic osteotomy is contraindicated in the presence of severe osteoarthritis of the hip with marked degeneration of articular cartilage and loss of joint motion. Functional range of hip motion is a vital prerequisite. If the joint has been destroyed it cannot be salvaged. A total joint replacement or hip arthrodesis should be considered in these patients. In reducible subluxations with congruity of the hip joint, Chiari's osteotomy should not be performed; a triple or Salter's innominate osteotomy is indicated in these patients.

The technique of Chiari's pelvic osteotomy is described and illustrated in Plate 28. Illustrative cases are shown in Figures 2–226 and 2–227.

If the degree of displacement is more than 50 per cent the osteotomy site is filled with an autogenous bone graft from the ilium.

Complications. *Sciatic nerve palsy* occurs in about 1 per cent of cases. It is vital to protect the nerve by retractors in the sciatic notch and prevent posterior displacement of the osteotomized segments; bone splintering should be avoided by using a Gigli saw to cut the cortex at the sciatic notch. Stay in the subperiosteal plane during surgical exposure, and expose the medial and lateral walls of the ilium. The patient and parents should be forewarned of the possibility of sciatic nerve palsy. Almost always the stretched nerve will recover function; it may, however, require 6 to 12 months for maximal recovery.

Stiff hip may result from cutting the osteotomy too close to the femoral head, entering the joint, and damaging articular cartilage. The use of image intensifier radiographic control is crucial for determining the proper level of osteotomy. Too low a level will fail to provide a sufficient interval between the femoral head and the ilium to accommodate the capsule and will prevent the development of a satisfactory hip joint space.

In the dysplastic hip with a shallow acetabulum the osteotomy line may extend into the sacroiliac joint and cause painful sacroiliac arthritis. When the acetabulum is very shallow it is best to perform a shelf operation.

An ugly prominence of the anterior superior iliac spine and a flexion deformity of the hip are caused by posterior slipping of the distal segment. It may be avoided by curving the osteotomy line into a dome shape, keeping a retractor posterior to the distal fragment once the osteotomy is completed, and using secure internal fixation. The range of hip flexion will be limited postoperatively for quite some time; it is best to forewarn the patient.

Penetration of screws or threaded Steinmann pins into the hip joint should be avoided by appropriate radiographic control.

Kawamura's Dome-shaped Medial Displacement Innominate Osteotomy Through Transtrochanteric Approach. The patient is placed on the table in straight lateral position with the hip that is to be operated on upward. The skin incision extends inferoposteriorly from the anterior superior iliac spine to the greater trochanter and then curves posteriorly to terminate at a point corresponding to the greater sciatic notch. (This author prefers to begin the skin incision at the middle third of the iliac crest to facilitate exposure of the inner wall of the ilium by splitting the iliac apophysis— similar to Salter's technique, except that the lateral wall of the ilium is not exposed superiorly.) The subcutaneous tissue and deep fascia are divided in line with the skin incision. The interval between the gluteus medius posteriorly and the tensor fasciae femoris anteriorly is developed by blunt dissection. Next, the vastus lateralis is detached from the *abductor* tubercle by a horseshoe-shaped incision based proximally and is subperiosteally elevated in its entire width from the femoral shaft for a distance of 5 cm. A blunt elevator retractor is inserted beneath the deep surface of the gluteus medius muscle, passing from its anterior to its posterior margin. The proper level of trochanter osteotomy is determined with a smooth Kirschner wire and image intensifier radiography. The greater trochanter is osteotomized with a reciprocal oscillating electric saw, following the details of technique described for distal-lateral transfer of the greater trochanter (see Plate 21). Be sure the saw stops short of the medial cortex of the trochanteric fossa and that vessels are not cut inadvertently. The greater trochanter with its attached muscles is then reflected superiorly, exposing the superior aspect of the capsule of the hip joint and the adjacent iliac bone. The acetabular origin of the rectus femoris is detached and excised; the direct head of the muscle is sectioned from the anterior inferior iliac spine and reflected distally. The periosteum along the acetabular rim is sharply divided with a scalpel and is elevated from the outer table of the ilium for about 1 cm. The direct

Text continued on page 518

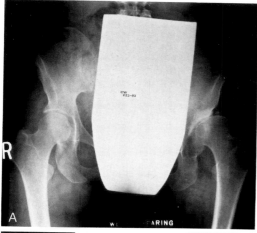

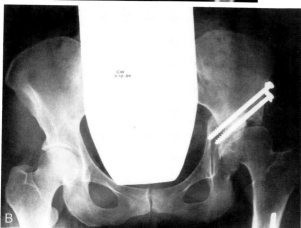

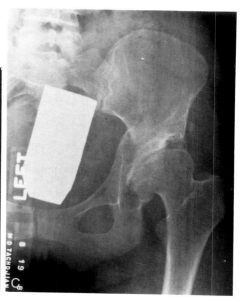

FIGURE 2–226. Chiari's osteotomy for congenital dysplasia of the hip with osteoarthritis.

A. Preoperative radiogram. **B.** Following Chiari's medial displacement osteotomy. **C.** Result 18 months later showing full coverage of the femoral head. Patient had total relief of her symptoms.

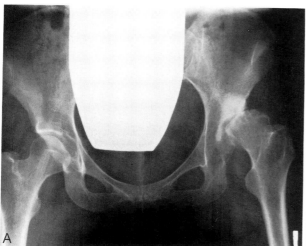

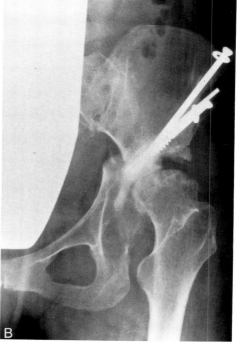

FIGURE 2–227. Chiari's osteotomy for congenital dysplasia of the hip with osteoarthritis.

A. Preoperative radiogram. **B.** Postoperative radiogram.

Chiari's Innominate Osteotomy

The patient is placed supine on a radiolucent operating table. Image intensifier fluoroscopy and radiographic control are vital to control the level, direction, and degree of medial displacement of the osteotomy accurately. Some surgeons prefer to perform the operation on a fracture table with the feet secured to the traction plate; this facilitates the application of a hip spica cast. This author fixes the iliac osteotomy internally with cancellous screws and does not apply a spica cast; therefore, the fracture table, which is cumbersome (especially the perineal post), is unnecessary.

The skin of the affected side of the lower part of the chest, abdomen, pelvis, and entire lower limb is prepared and draped to allow free motion of the hip as it is being operated on.

OPERATIVE TECHNIQUE

A and **B.** The medial and lateral walls of the ilium are exposed by an anterolateral approach similar to that described for Salter's innominate osteotomy (Plate 18). Adequate posterior exposure to visualize the sciatic notch is vital. Also it is imperative to stay in the subperiosteal plane in order to avoid injury to the sciatic nerve and gluteal vessels and nerves. Distal exposure is important. The sartorius muscle must be detached from the anterior superior iliac spine, its free end marked with unabsorbable suture (2-0 Mersilene or Tycron) for later reattachment, and reflected inferiorly and medially.

C. In adolescent hip dysplasia the capsule is thickened and often adherent to the lateral wall of the ilium; the capsule is dissected and elevated off the ilium to the rim of the acetabulum. Occasionally one may have to make a small opening in the hip joint capsule anterosuperiorly to ascertain the correct level of osteotomy.

Plate 28. Chiari's Innominate Osteotomy

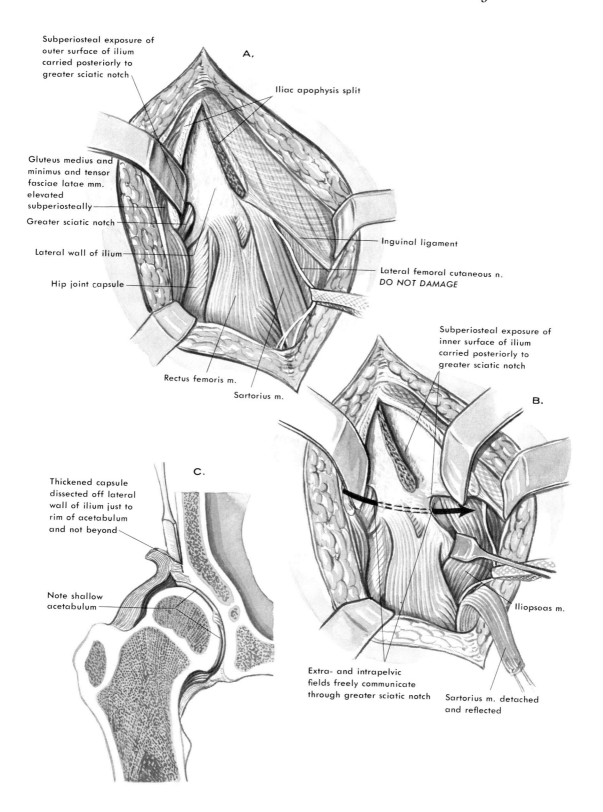

Subperiosteal exposure of outer surface of ilium carried posteriorly to greater sciatic notch

A.

Iliac apophysis split

Gluteus medius and minimus and tensor fasciae latae mm. elevated subperiosteally

Greater sciatic notch

Lateral wall of ilium

Hip joint capsule

Inguinal ligament

Lateral femoral cutaneous n. *DO NOT DAMAGE*

Rectus femoris m.

Sartorius m.

Subperiosteal exposure of inner surface of ilium carried posteriorly to greater sciatic notch

B.

C.

Thickened capsule dissected off lateral wall of ilium just to rim of acetabulum and not beyond

Note shallow acetabulum

Iliopsoas m.

Extra- and intrapelvic fields freely communicate through greater sciatic notch

Sartorius m. detached and reflected

Chiari's Innominate Osteotomy (Continued)

D. Next, the reflected head of the rectus femoris is elevated and detached from the superior margin of the acetabulum. In the older patient the capsule and the reflected head of the rectus femoris may not be separately identifiable. The direct head of the rectus femoris is detached from its origin at the anterior inferior iliac spine; both heads are reflected distally. The hip joint capsule should not be damaged. The taut iliopsoas muscle is lengthened by two transverse incisions of its tendinous fibers only; the underlying muscle fibers are left intact. If there is no hip flexion deformity, routine iliopsoas lengthening is not recommended because, postoperatively, temporary weakness of hip flexion is a problem.

E to G. The ideal level of osteotomy is just above the capsular attachment between the capsule and the reflected head of the rectus femoris. Too low a level will damage the interposed capsule, and too high a level will not provide adequate coverage. The ilium is cut at an angle directed 10 to 15 degrees upward and medially. The osteotomy angle is the angle between the plane of the pelvic osteotomy and the horizontal. If it is directed more than 15 to 20 degrees superiorly, the osteotomy may violate the sacroiliac joint. The danger of entering the joint is great if the acetabulum is shallow. The roof angle is the angle formed between the horizontal and a line joining the original outer acetabular lip to the new acetabular lip. With remodeling of the osteotomy, the "step" region fills in and the roof angle represents the increased acetabular overhang. The CE angle of Wiberg does not accurately express the adequacy of femoral head coverage, because innominate osteotomies at different levels and angles can give the same CE angle but widely varying degrees of acetabular improvement.

Plate 28. Chiari's Innominate Osteotomy

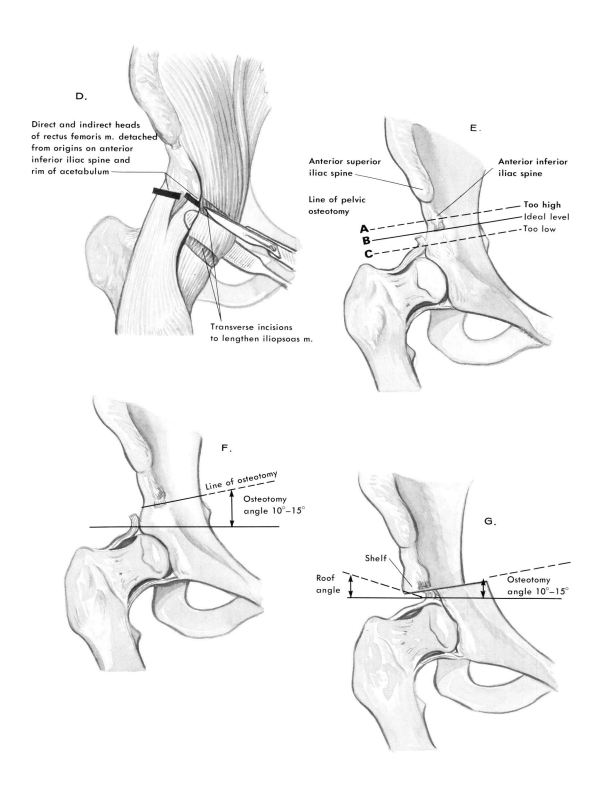

D.

Direct and indirect heads of rectus femoris m. detached from origins on anterior inferior iliac spine and rim of acetabulum

Transverse incisions to lengthen iliopsoas m.

E.

Anterior superior iliac spine

Anterior inferior iliac spine

Line of pelvic osteotomy

Too high
Ideal level
Too low

A
B
C

F.

Line of osteotomy

Osteotomy angle 10°–15°

G.

Shelf

Roof angle

Osteotomy angle 10°–15°

Chiari's Innominate Osteotomy (Continued)

H to J. A smooth Kirschner wire or Steinmann pin is inserted as a guide at the middle of the superior acetabular rim at the proposed level and angle. The exact position and direction of the angle of the pin is determined by image intensifier fluoroscopy and radiograms. The angle should be 10 to 15 degrees medial and upward. The line of osteotomy, which may be marked by multiple drill holes, should be curved, terminating inferior to the anterior inferior iliac spine anteriorly and to the lower part of the greater sciatic notch posteriorly. The curved osteotomy should correspond to the shape of the femoral head.

Plate 28. Chiari's Innominate Osteotomy

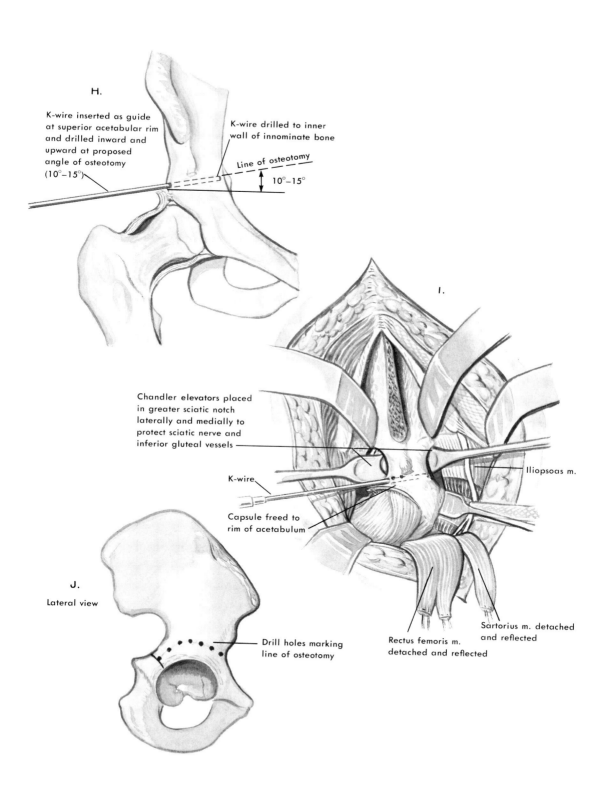

H.

K-wire inserted as guide at superior acetabular rim and drilled inward and upward at proposed angle of osteotomy (10°–15°)

K-wire drilled to inner wall of innominate bone

Line of osteotomy

10°–15°

I.

Chandler elevators placed in greater sciatic notch laterally and medially to protect sciatic nerve and inferior gluteal vessels

K-wire

Capsule freed to rim of acetabulum

Iliopsoas m.

Rectus femoris m. detached and reflected

Sartorius m. detached and reflected

J.

Lateral view

Drill holes marking line of osteotomy

513

Chiari's Innominate Osteotomy (Continued)

K. Straight-line osteotomy may cause posterior displacement of the distal segment that will produce an ugly prominence of the anterior superior iliac spine and a flexion deformity of the hip.

L. Posterior displacement of the distal segment may also cause angulation and kinking of the sciatic nerve and neurapraxia.

M. The osteotomy is performed with ½- or ⅜-inch-wide osteotomes, which should be thin and sharp. Splintering and greenstick fracture of the inner wall of the ilium should be avoided. The position and the direction of the angle of the osteotomes should be double checked by image intensifier fluoroscopy. Several osteotomes are used side by side and advanced together. Osteotomy cuts are first made anteriorly around the capsule and then posteriorly. Narrower osteotomes ensure an adequate curve. An assistant will indicate when the osteotomes penetrate the medial wall of the ilium. An alternate method is to execute the entire cut of the ilium with a Gigli saw.

Plate 28. Chiari's Innominate Osteotomy

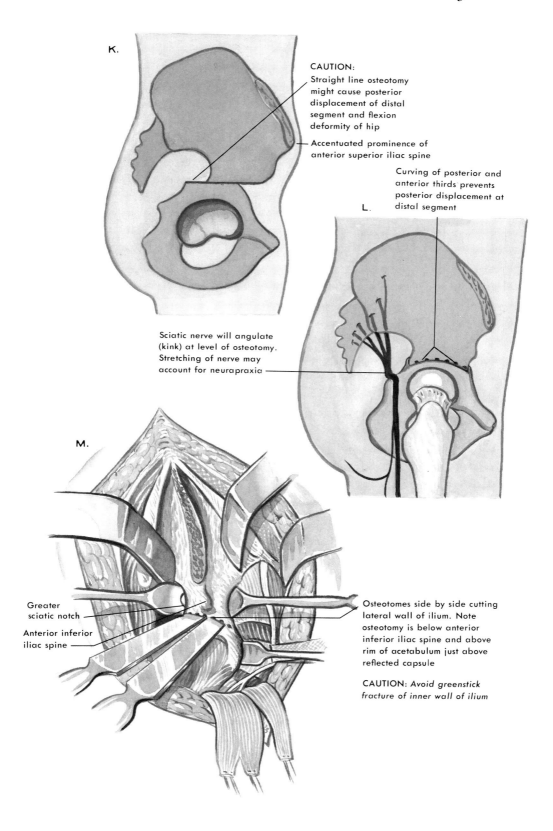

K.

CAUTION:
Straight line osteotomy might cause posterior displacement of distal segment and flexion deformity of hip

Accentuated prominence of anterior superior iliac spine

Curving of posterior and anterior thirds prevents posterior displacement at distal segment

L.

Sciatic nerve will angulate (kink) at level of osteotomy. Stretching of nerve may account for neurapraxia

M.

Greater sciatic notch

Anterior inferior iliac spine

Osteotomes side by side cutting lateral wall of ilium. Note osteotomy is below anterior inferior iliac spine and above rim of acetabulum just above reflected capsule

CAUTION: Avoid greenstick fracture of inner wall of ilium

515

Chiari's Innominate Osteotomy (Continued)

N. The last posterior 1 or 2 cm. of the ilium are cut with a Gigli saw. A Midas Rex saw may be used, but it may not always be available. This author prefers to section the entire ilium with a Gigli saw because the cut is smooth and bone splintering is prevented.

O and **P.** Upon completion of the osteotomy, the cut is opened first by wide osteotomes, periosteal elevators, and then gently by a laminar spreader. The iliac fragments should be fully mobilized. The hip is widely abducted, and the femoral head is displaced medially by the surgeon as an assistant holds the anterior iliac crest firmly. The Chandler retractors (or interlocking small-bladed cobra retractors) should be kept in the greater sciatic notch to prevent posterior displacement and sciatic nerve injury. The hip joint capsule should disappear under the new roof of cancellous bone of the inferior surface of the proximal iliac fragment. The medial displacement or shift is expressed as a percentage of the thickness of the ilium at the level of osteotomy. A common pitfall is medial shifting of the distal iliac fragment due to hinging at the greater sciatic notch, i.e., the distal pelvic segment has rotated inward. The "hinged" osteotomy may give the pseudoappearance of excellent head coverage. Oblique roentgenograms, however, will show the curve at the greater sciatic notch to be unbroken. The medial wall of the iliac wing is a reliable bench mark to assess the degree of medial displacement. It should be remembered that with 50 per cent medial displacement approximately 1.5 cm. of femoral head coverage is provided. Complete separation of the iliac fragments is not desirable and must be avoided. If greater coverage and cupping of the femoral head is required, the Chiari osteotomy is combined with a shelf procedure. Corticocancellous strips of bone ½ inch wide are taken from the ilium and wedged into a slot in the distal iliac segment. The bone grafts are angled a few degrees cephalad and interposed between the capsule and the proximal iliac segment.

Q. One or two threaded Steinmann pins are used to transfix the iliac fragments obliquely. An anteroposterior radiogram is made to determine the degree of femoral head coverage provided. Two cancellous screws with washers are used to transfix the iliac fragments obliquely. It is best to drill from the outer wall of the proximal iliac segment, as it will provide greater stability. The threaded Steinmann pin and cancellous screws should not penetrate the hip joint. The split iliac apophysis is sutured, the sartorius muscle reattached to its origin, and the wound closed in routine fashion. A hip spica cast is not necessary.

POSTOPERATIVE CARE

The patient is placed in bilateral split Russell's traction. Active assisted and gentle passive exercises are begun as soon as the patient is comfortable. On the second to the third postoperative day he is allowed to be up and around with a three-point crutch gait protecting the limb by toe-touch. When the patient is not walking, counterpoised traction is replaced until painless functional range of motion of the hip is achieved and maintained. Crutch protection is continued until complete bony healing has taken place, usually in about six to eight weeks. The threaded Steinmann pins and screws are removed three to four months postoperatively.

Plate 28. Chiari's Innominate Osteotomy

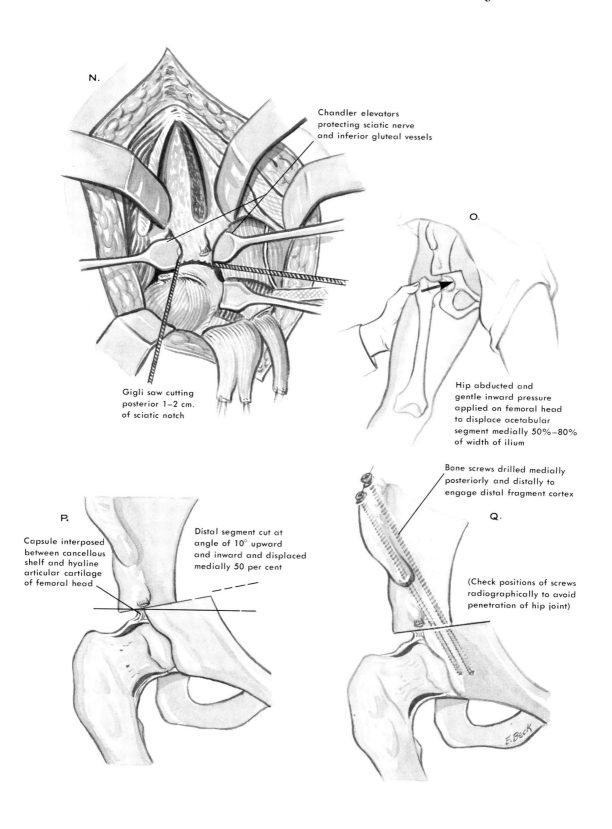

N.

Chandler elevators protecting sciatic nerve and inferior gluteal vessels

Gigli saw cutting posterior 1–2 cm. of sciatic notch

O.

Hip abducted and gentle inward pressure applied on femoral head to displace acetabular segment medially 50%–80% of width of ilium

P.

Capsule interposed between cancellous shelf and hyaline articular cartilage of femoral head

Distal segment cut at angle of 10° upward and inward and displaced medially 50 per cent

Q.

Bone screws drilled medially posteriorly and distally to engage distal fragment cortex

(Check positions of screws radiographically to avoid penetration of hip joint)

E. Beck

lateral approach with osteotomy and elevation of the greater trochanter provides clear visualization of the posterior aspect of the acetabulum and the sciatic notch; inadvertent injury to the sciatic nerve and gluteal vessels is thereby obviated. The transtrochanteric lateral approach also permits clear vision of the upper and anterior aspects of the hip joint, making the execution of a dome osteotomy relatively simple.

Next, the periosteum from the inner wall of the ilium is elevated thoroughly. The use of the Salter iliac apophyseal split technique makes it easy, and it is done under direct vision. The periosteum on the anterior edge of the ilium is incised and elevated, beginning at the anterosuperior iliac spine and extending to the iliopectineal eminence. Then the periosteum on the inner wall of the ilium is completely detached and elevated from the greater sciatic notch to the anterior inferior iliac spine. Kawamura incises and elevates the periosteum from front to back (to the arcuate line) and then posteroanteriorly from the sciatic notch to the arcuate line. This author prefers to elevate the periosteum superoinferiorly as in Salter's innominate osteotomy. The important technical point is complete detachment of the periosteum above the osteotomy line to permit medial shift of the acetabulum. Kawamura recommends the width of the elevated periosteum to be 3 to 5 cm. when it is performed front to back and inferosuperiorly.

Two medium-sized Chandler elevator retractors are then placed subperiosteally in the sciatic notch, one introduced from the lateral and the other from the medial side of the ilium; these retractors keep the sciatic nerve and

gluteal vessels out of harm's way. A Cobra retractor may be placed subperiosteally from the anterior end of the ilium to protect the intrapelvic contents.

Next, a Kirschner wire is drilled into the ilium at the point of insertion of the capsule and its exact position verified by image intensifier radiography. The level of osteotomy should never be too low or too high. It should be immediately above the hypertrophied joint capsule. Multiple drill holes are then made, outlining the dome osteotomy line. Making the osteotomy initially dome-shaped instead of rectangular hastens remodeling. The drill holes are pointed upward 15 degrees in a lateromedial direction. If there is too much capsular hypertrophy, some of the capsule may be sliced off. (The thickness of the capsule is determined by a small incision made in its superior portion.)

The curvature of the dome parallels that of the femoral head (Fig. 2–228). (Formerly Kawamura performed the pelvic osteotomy primarily in a trapezoid shape.) With a thin small osteotome, the osteotomy is completed in the line of the drill holes. Be cautious and do not splinter bone, especially at the sciatic notch. Kawamura utilizes a specially devised drill-type saw to perform the osteotomy.

Next the two segments of the osteotomized pelvis are shifted; the distal segment is displaced medially by abducting the hips and pushing the femoral head inward, while the proximal segment is pulled outward with a large bone hook and periosteal elevator to bring it completely over the femoral head. The fragments hinge at the symphysis pubis and the sacroiliac joint, mostly the former.

The space between the femoral head and the

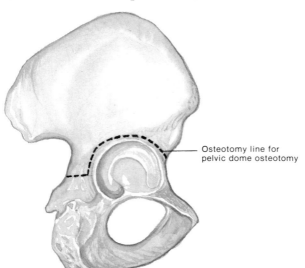

Osteotomy line for pelvic dome osteotomy

FIGURE 2–228. Diagram showing osteotomy line in Kawamura's dome pelvic osteotomy.

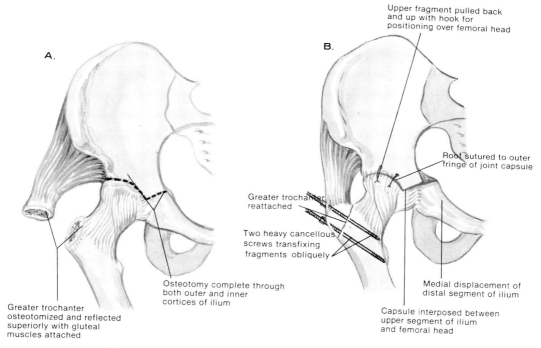

FIGURE 2–229. Kawamura's medial displacement dome pelvic osteotomy.

A. The inclination of the osteotomy. **B.** After displacement and internal fixation. The greater trochanter is reattached.

newly formed acetabular roof is widened by pulling the femur distally, and the ragged inferior surface of the new roof is smoothed with a rasp and reshaped into an even dome. An uneven and rough, ragged acetabular roof should be avoided as it predisposes to osteoarthritis. The two pelvic fragments are transfixed with two threaded Steinmann pins, and radiograms are made to determine the adequacy and completeness of femoral head coverage. This author prefers to fix the pelvic osteotomy with two AO cancellous screws. The edge of the new roof may be sutured to the outer fringe of the joint capsule with several mattress sutures.

The greater trochanter is reattached at the desired level on the proximal femoral shaft with two AO screws (Fig. 2–229). The tip of the greater trochanter should be level with the center of the femoral head; also, it should be lateral from the center of the femoral head, two and one half times the radius of the femoral head. A definite advantage of the Kawamura technique is that it is dome-shaped and that it restores normal biomechanics of the hip. The wounds are closed in the usual fashion. Internal fixation with AO screws obviates the necessity for application of a hip spica cast. The postoperative care is similar to that of Chiari's pelvic osteotomy.

This author recommends Kawamura's lateral transtrochanteric approach when simultaneous transfer of the greater trochanter is to be performed. Often the two procedures are staged by this author; first Chiari's osteotomy is performed, and later on (three to six months) the greater trochanter is transferred distally and laterally. Postoperatively the patients do much better, and disability is minimal, as immobilization in a hip spica cast is not required. This author has had no experience with the posterior approach of Bertrand or with the inferior approach of Klisic.[52, 497] The direct lateral approach originally described by Chiari, in which the fibers of the gluteus medius are split vertically, the gluteus minimus is retracted posteriorly, and the ilium is sectioned under image intensifier radiographic control, should not be used. Both surfaces of the ilium should be fully visualized in order to perform the pelvic osteotomy with accuracy and avoid injury to the sciatic nerves and vessels.

The Shelf Operation. The shelf operation includes a number of procedures in which the bony roof of the acetabulum is extended outward (laterally, posteriorly, and anteriorly) by the addition of bone grafts either within or directly over the capsule of the uncovered femoral head. The source of the bony roof is either the immediately adjacent corticocancellous bone of the ilium, which is reflected downward, or free bone grafts (tibial, rib, or allograft).

The shelf operation increases the capacity of a deficient acetabulum. It stabilizes the hip and prevents superolateral migration of the femoral head. The weight-bearing area of the hip is increased, and the pressure forces across the joints are decreased. The procedure is safe; there is no disturbance of the viability of articular cartilage or the circulation to the femoral head. The operation is extra-articular; there is no danger of progressive stiffness of the hip joint. The anatomy and integrity of the pelvic ring are not disturbed. The danger of sciatic nerve palsy is minimal.

The disadvantage of the shelf procedure is that raw bone fits over the fibrocapsule, which converts into fibrocartilage, which is less durable than hyaline cartilage. A properly executed shelf may, however, stand up to reasonable use for many years; and if later on in adult life total hip joint replacement is required because of painful degenerative joint disease, it can be performed much more easily.[511, 1030–1032] Another disadvantage of the shelf operation is that it does not medially displace the acetabulum. The position of the acetabulum is unchanged; therefore the center of gravity across the hip remains lateral, which is a definite biomechanical drawback.

The shelf operation is one of the oldest of the hip stabilizing procedures. It was very popular in the past, but enthusiasm waned because of the poor results; the shelf was absorbed because it was placed too high and was too small. During the past two decades the recently developed techniques of innominate osteotomy have replaced the older shelf operation. In general this author prefers the Chiari medial displacement innominate osteotomy when coverage of an incongruous, painful, dysplastic hip is indicated; Chiari's osteotomy may be combined with the shelf procedure if additional lateral or posterior coverage is required. If the acetabulum is very shallow, however, Chiari's osteotomy will violate the sacroiliac joint; in such an instance a shelf operation should be performed. Likewise, the shelf operation is probably indicated for a hip that has had multiple operations with scarring around the sciatic notch or that is associated with congenital anomalies of the lumbosacral spine; in such cases there is increased risk of kinking of the sciatic nerve and nerve palsy. In paralytic hip dysplasia and subluxation, the shelf operation is more effective than Chiari's osteotomy. The surgeon may prefer the shelf to a Chiari osteotomy because in their experience

it is a simple and safe procedure, providing adequate support to the subluxated femoral head.

The shelf operation should not be performed in the presence of frank dislocation. If the hip is laterally subluxated and incongruous, the outcome may be unsatisfactory; medial displacement of the acetabulum by the Chiari procedure is much better biomechanically. Preferably, when performing the shelf operation the CE angle should not be less than 0 degrees. Excessive femoral antetorsion should be corrected simultaneously with or prior to the shelf procedure.

It is mandatory to place the shelf precisely at the weight-bearing level of the acetabulum. A high shelf will not respond to loading in weight-bearing and will undergo atrophy and gradually disappear. Thinning of the thickened capsule by partial capsulectomy is a vital part of the procedure; it is the fibrocapsule that will be connected to fibrocartilage. In the literature many varieties of the shelf operation have been described; this author has had personal experience with the technique described by Wilson and the slotted acetabular augmentation technique of Staheli.[887, 1032] Of the two methods, he prefers the Staheli operation because it provides a dome coverage over the femoral head, it can be executed accurately, and internal fixation with Steinmann pins and skeletal traction are unnecessary. For success it is mandatory to pay meticulous attention to the details of technique.

The *Wilson technique* of the shelf operation is as follows: With the patient in supine position and a small sandbag under the hip to be operated on, the hip joint is exposed through an anterior iliofemoral incision (Fig. 2–230 A). The medial and lateral walls of the ilium are exposed subperiosteally. Next the straight head of the rectus femoris is detached and reflected distally. The thickened capsule of the hip is widely exposed in its anterior, superior, and posterior aspects. The capsule, which will be adherent on the lateral wall of the ilium, is released and elevated distally as far as the lateral rim of the acetabulum, which is identified by a small aperture in the capsule (Fig. 2–230 B). The thickened capsule is thinned to ⅛ inch by partial capsulectomy (Fig. 2–230 C). A 2.5- to 3-cm. area on the lateral wall of the ilium immediately superior and slightly anterior to the femoral head is marked with drill holes (Fig. 2–230 D). This area is levered with a ½-inch-wide thin osteotome and turned down as the first layer of the shelf (Fig. 2–230 E). The lateral border of this layer is sutured to the capsule with one or two chromic catgut sutures (Fig. 2–230 F). Next

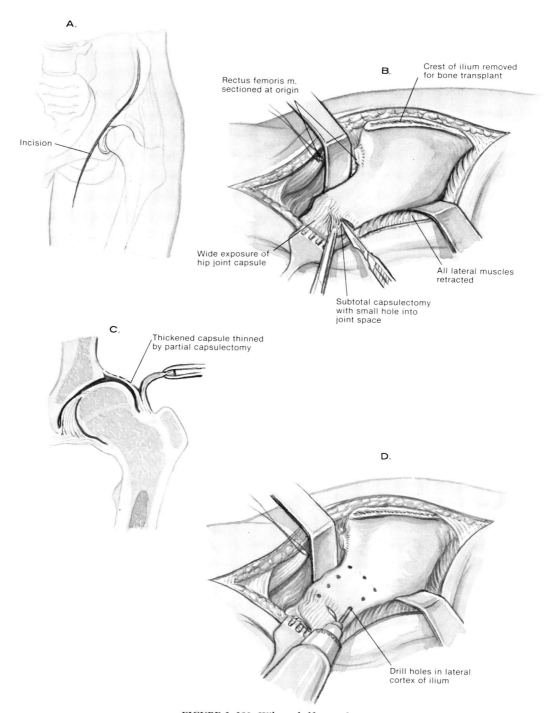

FIGURE 2–230. Wilson shelf procedure.

A, Incision and exposure of the hip joint through an anterior iliofemoral approach. **B.** Sectioning of the straight head of the rectus femoris at its origin and wide exposure of the hip joint capsule. **C.** Thinning of the thickened capsule by partial capsulectomy; only ⅛ inch of capsule covering the femoral head is left. A small aperture in the capsule assists in accurate determination of the lateral margin of the acetabulum. **D.** Small drill holes mark the area of the ilium to be turned downward over the femoral head.

Illustration continued on following page

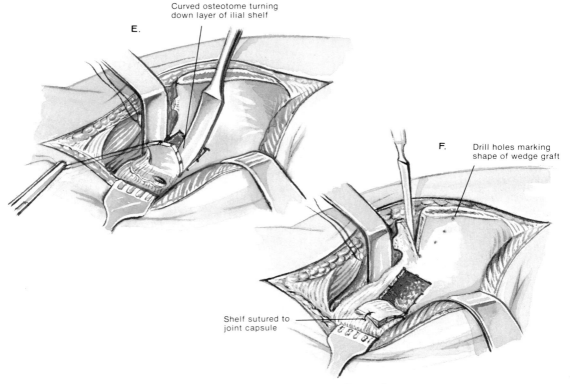

E.

Curved osteotome turning
down layer of ilial shelf

F.

Drill holes marking
shape of wedge graft

Shelf sutured to
joint capsule

FIGURE 2–230 Continued. Wilson shelf procedure.

E. With a sharp curved ½ inch osteotome the first layer of the shelf is elevated and turned down. F. The first layer of the shelf is sutured to the capsule. Drill holes mark the outline of a wedge-shaped graft in the region of the anterosuperior iliac spine.

a defect is made in the lateral wall of the ilium; into this cut a triangular piece of bone taken from the region of the anterosuperior iliac spine is driven (Fig. 2–230 G and H). The graft is fixed to the inner wall of the ilium with one Steinmann pin. Additional grafts are placed on each side of the large graft. The wound is closed, and the child is placed in bilateral skeletal traction. At four weeks the traction is discontinued and a one and one half hip spica cast is applied. The immobilization in the cast is for eight weeks, after which the hip is protected with partial weight-bearing with crutches for an additional six weeks.

Slotted acetabular augmentation, developed by Staheli, is a type of shelf procedure.[887] It provides a congruous acetabular extension in which the size and position of the augmentation are controlled with great ease and accuracy. Precise placement of the slot at the acetabular margin assures a congruous extension of the existing acetabulum. The problem of improper placement of the graft (too high or too low) is obviated. The bone graft consists of thin autogenous cancellous strips of ilium; being flexible,

the grafts do not create focal areas of impingement. No internal fixation with pins is required. The segmented acetabular augmentation may be used as a supplement to redirectional pelvic osteotomy.

According to Staheli, the indication for slotted acetabular augmentation is an extremely deficient acetabulum or an acetabulum with aspherical congruity in which the surgeon prefers the procedure because of its safety, simplicity, and adaptability.

The operative technique of slotted acetabular augmentation is as follows: Small patients are operated on a standard radiolucent operating table, and the involved side is raised 15 degrees on a pad. Heavy patients are best operated on a fracture table, and the affected lower limb is draped free. The hip is exposed via a routine iliofemoral approach through a "bikini" incision made 2 to 3 cm. below and parallel to the iliac crest. The tendon of the reflected head of the rectus femoris is sectioned anteriorly and elevated and retracted posteriorly (later this tendon will be reattached· to stabilize the graft). The capsule of the hip joint is exposed ante-

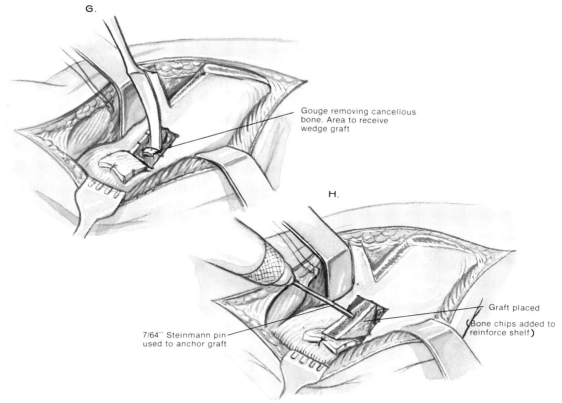

Figure 2–230 Continued. Wilson shelf procedure.

G. With a gouge a defect is made through the cancellous bone of the ilium to the inner cortex. The defect will receive the wedge-shaped graft from the anterosuperior iliac spine. **H.** The triangular piece of graft is anchored in place with a 7/64-inch Steinmann pin. Additional chip grafts from the ilium are used to reinforce the shelf. (Redrawn after Wilson, J. C., Jr.: Surgical treatment of dysplastic acetabulum in adolescents. Clin. Orthop. 98:137, 1974.)

riorly, superiorly, and posteriorly (Fig. 2–231 A). The capsule, thickened and adherent to the lateral wall of the ilium, is elevated from the wall with a periosteal elevator and reflected distally to the acetabular rim. It is best to identify the joint line by image intensifier radiography. Some surgeons prefer to make a small aperture in the capsule to determine the level of the femoral head.

Next a slot is made *exactly* at the margin of the acetabulum. At the selected site a smooth Kirschner wire is inserted and the correct position of the proposed site of the slot is confirmed by an anteroposterior radiogram. The slot is 1 cm. deep and 5 mm. wide; its floor is the articular cartilage of the acetabulum with very little cancellous bone, and its roof is cancellous bone. The slot is made by drilling holes with a 5/32 inch bit (Fig. 2–231 B). The extent of coverage required determines the length of the slot. When there is excessive femoral antetorsion, the slot extends anteriorly; when the acetabulum is deficient posteriorly, it extends

backward. The drilled holes are joined with a rongeur.

The next step is to determine the width of the augmentation and the total length of the graft. This is done on a preoperative standing anteroposterior radiogram of the hips. The actual center edge (CE) angle and the desired normal CE angle of 35 degrees are drawn on the film (Fig. 2–231 C). The extra width necessary to extend the existing socket to obtain the normal CE angle is measured—this is the width of augmentation *(wa)*. The graft length *(gl)* is the sum of the width of augmentation and the slot depth.

Next thin strips of cortical and cancellous bone are taken from the lateral wall of the ilium (Fig. 2–231 D). The inner table of the ilium is left intact. The bone graft strips should extend from the iliac crest to the upper border of the slot—this shallow decortication assures rapid fusion of the graft to the ilium.

Augmentation is carried out in layers. The *first layer* consists of thin strips (1 mm.) of

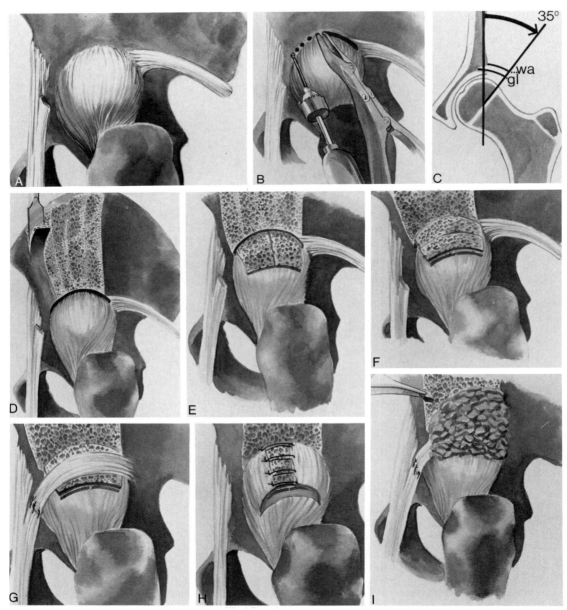

FIGURE 2–231. *Slotted acetabular augmentation*

A. The reflected head of the rectus femoris is sectioned in its anterior part, elevated, and reflected posteriorly. Note the exposure of the thickened capsule of the hip joint in its anterior, superior, and posterior aspects. **B.** The site of the slot is exactly at the margin of the acetabulum. It is made by multiple drill holes that are joined with a narrow rongeur. The slot is 5 mm. wide and 10 mm. deep; its length varies depending on the amount of coverage required. **C.** Method of determining the width of the augmentation (wa) and bone graft length (gl) (See text). **D.** Harvesting of thin strips of cortical and cancellous bone graft from the lateral wall of the ilium. The graft strips are long, extending from the iliac crest to the upper margin of the slot. The inner wall of the ilium is left intact. **E.** First layer of augmentation. The thin strips of bone graft are placed radially into the slot with the concave side downward. **F.** The second layer of augmentation is perpendicular to the first layer, parallel to the acetabular margin. **G.** The first and second layers of bone graft are held in place by reattaching the tendon of the reflected head of the rectus femoris. A capsular flap may be used as an additional measure, if necessary. **H** and **I.** The third layer of the bone graft consists of small pieces of bone, which are packed above the reflected head of the rectus femoris. It is held in place by reattaching the hip abductor to the iliac crest. (From Staheli, L. T.: Slotted acetabular augmentation. J. Pediatr. Orthop., *1*:321, 1981. Reprinted by permission.)

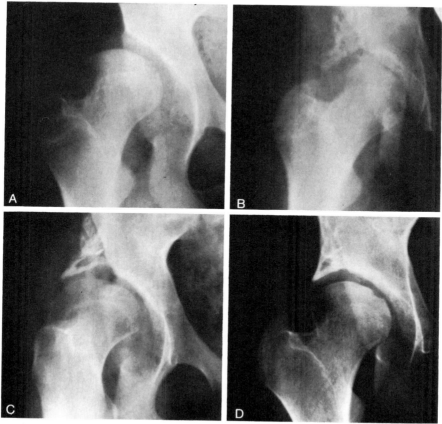

FIGURE 2–232. *Congenital hip dysplasia in a 15-year-old girl treated by the Staheli acetabular augmentation.*

A. Preoperative radiogram. **B.** Immediately postoperative radiogram. **C** and **D.** One and one half years after surgery. Note the excellent coverage of the femoral head. (From Staheli, L. T.: Slotted acetabular augmentation. J. Pediatr. Orthop., *1*:321, 1981. Reprinted by permission.)

cancellous bone that are cut into rectangles about 1 cm. wide and of the appropriate length determined on the preoperative radiograms. The strips of bone graft are placed radially from the "slot" with the concave side down, providing a congruous extension on the femoral head (Fig. 2–231 E). The *second layer* of augmentation is made of thicker bone graft strips (about 2 mm.) with their length equal to that of the extension. They are placed parallel to the acetabulum, at right angles to the first layer of extension (Fig. 2–231 F). The most lateral strip should be thick to provide the extension with a well-defined border. Avoid extending the augmentation too far anteriorly, as it will block hip flexion. Next the detached reflected head of the rectus femoris is pulled forward over the grafts and sutured to its original site. A capsular flap, made by slicing the thickened capsule, may be

sutured over the grafts to secure them to the ilium (Fig. 2–231 G).

The remaining bone grafts are cut into small pieces, packed above the first two layers, and held in place by reattaching the gluteal muscles onto the iliac crest. The *third layer* of augmentation should not protrude beyond the initial two layers (Fig. 2–231 H and I).

The position and width of the augmentation is verified by an anteroposterior radiogram of the hip. The wound is closed in the routine fashion, and a single hip spica cast is applied with the hip in 15 degrees of abduction and 20 degrees of flexion and internal rotation.

Postoperative Care. Immobilization in the cast is for six weeks. The cast is then removed, and three-point crutch-walking gait is permitted with partial weight-bearing on the affected limb until the graft is radiographically shown to be incorporated, usually about three to four months. An illustrative case is shown in Figure 2–232.

References

1. Aarskog, D., Stoa, K. F., and Thorsen, T.: Urinary oestrogen excretion in newborn infants with congenital dysplasia of the hip joint. Acta Paediatr. Scand., 55:394, 1966.
2. Albee, F. H.: The bone graft wedge. Its use in the treatment of relapsing, acquired, and congenital dislocation of hip. N.Y. Med. J., 102:433, 1915.
3. Allen, R. P.: Ischemic necrosis following treatment of hip "dysplasia." J. A. M. A., 180:497, 1962.
4. Almby, B., and Onnerholm, T.: Hip joint instability after the neonatal period. Diagnosis and treatment of 20 consecutive cases. Acta Orthop. Scand., 49:371, 1978.
5. Almby, B., and Rehnberg, L.: Neonatal hip instability. Incidence, diagnosis and treatment at the University Hospital, Uppsala, 1960–1964 and 1970–1974. Acta Orthop. Scand., 48:642, 1977.
6. Almby, B., Hjelmstedt, A., and Lonnerholm, T.: Neonatal hip instability. Reason for failure of early abduction treatment. Acta Orthop. Scand., 50:315, 1979.
7. Anders, G.: Behandlung der Hüftgelenksdysplasie und Hüftluxation mit dem Hanausek-Apparat. 63. Kongress der Deutschen Gesellschaft fur Orthopädie und Traumatologie. Sept., 1976. Z. Orthop., 115:645, 1977.
8. Anderson, M. E., and Bickel, W. H.: Shelf operation for congenital subluxation and dislocation of the hip. J. Bone Joint Surg., 33-A:87, 1951.
9. Anderson, M., Green, W. T., and Messner, M. B.: Growth and predictions of growth in the lower extremities. J. Bone Joint Surg., 45-A:1, 1963.
10. Andren, L.: Instability of the pubic symphysis and congenital dislocation of the hip in newborns. Acta Radiol., 54:123, 1960.
11. Andren, L.: Aetiology and diagnosis of congenital dislocation of the hip in newborns. Radiology, 1:89, 1961.
12. Andren, L.: Frequency and sex distribution of congenital dislocation of the hip among breech presentations. Acta Orthop. Scand., 31:152, 1961.
13. Andren, L.: Pelvic instability in newborns with special reference to congenital dislocation of the hip and hormonal factors. A roentgenologic study. Acta Radiol., Suppl. 212, 1962.
14. Andren, L., and Borglin, N. E.: A disorder of oestrogen metabolism as a causal factor of congenital dislocation of the hip. Acta Orthop. Scand., 30:169, 1961.
15. Andren, L., and Borglin, N. E.: Disturbed urinary excretion pattern of oestrogens in newborns with congenital dislocation of the hip. Acta Endocrinol., 37:423, 1961.
16. Andren, L., and Borglin, N. E.: Disturbed urinary excretion pattern of oestrogens in newborns with congenital dislocation of the hip. II. The excretion of exogenous oestradiol-17B. Acta Endocrinol., 37:427, 1961.
17. Andren, L., and Palmen, K.: Seasonal variation of birth dates of infants with congenital dislocation of the hip. Acta Orthop. Scand., 33:127, 1963.
18. Andren, L., and Rosen, S. von: The diagnosis of dislocation of the hip in newborns and the primary result of immediate treatment. Acta Radiol., 49:89, 1958.
19. Appleton, A. B.: Postural deformities and bone growth. Lancet, 1:451, 1937.
20. Arnold, W. D., Freiberger, R., Robin, D., and Barnett, C.: Observations on congenital hip disease in the Navajo. J. Bone Joint Surg., 46-A:1139, 1964.
21. Artz, T. D., Levine, D. B., Lim, W. N., Salvata, E. A., and Wilson, P. D.: neonatal diagnosis, treatment and related factors of congenital dislocation of the hip. Clin. Orthop., 110:112, 1975.
22. Arzimanoglu, A.: Treatment of congenital hip dislocation by muscle release, skeletal traction and closed reduction in older children. Clin. Orthop., 119:70, 1976.
23. Asher, M. A.: Orthopedic screening: Especially congenital dislocation of the hip and spinal deformity. Pediatr. Clin. North Am., 24:713, 1977.
24. Ashley, R. K., Larsen, L. T., and James, P. M.: Reduction of dislocation of the hip in older children. J. Bone Joint Surg., 54-A:545, 1972.
25. Asplund, S., and Hjelmstedt, A.: Experimentally induced hip dislocation in vitro and in vivo. A study in newborn rabbits. Acta Orthop. Scand. (Suppl.) 199, 1983.
26. Astley, R.: Arthrography in congenital dislocation of the hip. Clin. Radiol., 18:253, 1967.
27. d'Aubigne, R. M.: Traitement Chirurgicale des Malformations Luxantes de la Hanche chez l'Adulte. Paris, Masson, 1962.
28. Bachman, K.-D.: Über die Diagnose der sogangeborenen Hüftgelenksverrenkung in der Neugeborenen-Periode. Geburtshilfe Frauenheillkd., 23:696, 1963.
29. Badgley, C. E.: Correlation of clinical and anatomical facts leading to a conception of the etiology of congenital hip dysplasias. J. Bone Joint Surg., 25:503, 1943.
30. Badgley, C. E.: Etiology of congenital dislocation of the hip. J. Bone Joint Surg., 31-A:341, 1949.
31. Bado, J. L.: Le deviazioni dalls normal nella embriogenesi del muscolo e nella patogenesi di alcune malformazioni congenite. Arch. Putti Chir. Organi Mov., 18:37, 1963.
32. Ball, R. M., and Ryder, C. T.: Flowcharts in orthopaedic surgery. A program for the primary treatment of congenital dislocation of the hip. Orthop. Rev., 5:61, 1976.
33. Barlow, T. G.: Early diagnosis and treatment of congenital dislocation of the hip. J. Bone Joint Surg., 44-B:292, 1962.
34. Barlow, T. G.: Early diagnosis and treatment of congenital dislocation of the hip in the newborn. Proc. R. Soc. Med., 59:1103, 1966.
35. Barlow, T. G.: Neonatal hip dysplasia—treatment results and complications (abridged). Proc. R. Soc. Med., 68:475, 1975.
36. Barta, O.: Über die Spontanheilung der angeborenen Hüftverrenkung. Zentralbl. Chir., 89:164, 1964.
37. Barta, O.: kombienierte funktionelle Behandlung der angeborenen Hüftverrenkung in Alter von über einem Jahre. Z. Orthop., 101:219, 1966.
38. Barta, O.: Prophylaxe und funktionelle Fruhbehandlung der Luxationshüfte mit dem Riemenbugel nach Pavlik. Beitr. Orthop. Traumatol., 24:262, 1977.
39. Bartolomaeus, R., Erfuth, C., Jaster, D., and Tieth, H.: Erfahrungen bei der konservativen Behandlung der Luxationshüfte. Beitr. Orthop. Traumatol., 18:515, 1971.
40. Baubinas, P., and Urmonas, W.: Funktionelle Methoden der Reposition und Therapie der angeborenen Hüftluxation bei Kindern alteren Alters und ihre Resultate. Beitr. Orthop. Traumatol., 17:160, 1970.
41. Bauer, R.: Shortening-adduction osteotomy of the femur. Arch. Orthop. Unfallchir., 67:155, 1969.
42. Beau, Prevot, Guillamot: Principes généraux du traitement actuel de la malformation luxante de la hanche chez l'enfant. Resultats de leur application. Ann. Med. Nancy, 2:194, 1973.

43. Becker, F.: Über die Wandlungen in Auffbessung und Behandlung der kongenitalen Hüftluxation. Dtsch. Med. Wochenschr., *89*:1149, 1956.

44. Becker, F.: Die konservative Behandlung der Hüftdysplasie und Hüftverrenkung. Z. Orthop., *106*:173, 1969.

45. Beddow, F. H.: Facial paralysis complicating splintage for congenital dislocation of the hip in the newborn. J. Bone Joint Surg., *51-B*:714, 1969.

46. Benson, M. K. D., and Jameson Evans, D. C.: The pelvic osteotomy of Chiari: An anatomical study of the hazards and misleading radiographic appearances. J. Bone Joint Surg., *58-B*:164, 1976.

47. Berenyi, P., Szentpetery, J., and Rigo, J.: Festhalten der Fragmente durch Diafixation nach Derotationsosteotomie des oberen Femurendes. Z. Orthop., *101*:374, 1966.

48. Berkley, M. F., Dickson, J. H., Cain, T. E., and Donovan, M. M.: Surgical therapy for congenital dislocation of the hip in patients who are 12 to 36 months old. J. Bone Joint Surg., *66-A*:412, 1984.

49. Bernbeck, R.: Zur Pathologie der Luxatio coxae congenita. Virchow's Arch. Pathol. Anat., *320*:238, 1951.

50. Berquist, T. H.: Magnetic resonance imaging: Preliminary experience in orthopedic radiology. Magnetic Resonance Imaging, *2*:41, 1984.

51. Bertol, P., Macnicol, M. F., and Mitchell, G. P.: Radiographic feature of neonatal congenital dislocation of the hip. J. Bone Joint Surg., *64-B*:176, 1982.

52. Bertrand, P., Benard, H.-M., and Chassagne, A.: Perspectives de l'ostéotomie pelvienne dans la luxation du grand enfant et de l'adulte. Rev. Chir. Orthop., *51*:249, 1965.

53. Beyer, G.: Das Problem des operativen Zungangs zum Hüftgelenk. Brun's Beitr. Klin. Chir., *194*:44, 1957.

54. Bickel, W. H., and Breivis, J. S.: Shelf operation for congenital subluxation and dislocation of the hip. Clin. Orthop., *106*:27, 1975.

55. Bjerkreim, I.: Congenital dislocation of the hip joint in Norway. Part I. Late diagnosis CDH. Acta Orthop. Scand., *157*:1, 1974.

56. Bjerkreim, I.: Congenital dislocation of the hip joint in Norway. Part II: Detection of late cases. Acta Orthop. Scand., *157*:21, 1974.

57. Bjerkreim, I.: Congenital dislocation of the hip joint in Norway. Part III: Neonatal CDH. Acta Orthop. Scand., *157*:47, 1974.

58. Bjerkreim, I.: Congenital dislocation of the hip joint in Norway. Part IV: The incidence in southeast Norway. Acta Orthop. Scand., *157*:75, 1974.

59. Bjerkreim, I.: Congenital dislocation of the hip joint in Norway. A clinical epidemiological study. J. Oslo City Hosp., *26*:79, 1976.

60. Bjerkreim, I., Arseth, P. H.: Congenital dislocation of the hip in Norway. Acta Paediatr. Scand., *67*:329, 1978.

61. Bjerkreim, I., and Van Der Hagen, C. B.: Congenital dislocation of the hip joint in Norway. Part V: Evaluation of genetic and environmental factors. Clin. Genet., *5*:433, 1974.

62. Blavier, L., and Blavier, J.: Traitement de la subluxation de la hanche. Rev. Chir. Orthop., *48*:208, 1962.

63. Blix, M.: Die Länge und die Spannung des Muskels. Skand. Arch. Physiol., *3*:295, 1881.

64. Blockey, N. J.: Congenital dislocation of the hip. *In* Children's Orthopaedics—Practical Problems. London, Butterworth, 1976, pp. 71–112.

65. Blockey, N. J.: Congenital dislocation of the hip. (Editorial.) J. Bone Joint Surg., *64-B*:152, 1982.

66. Blockey, N. J.: Derotation osteotomy in the management of congenital dislocation of the hip. J. Bone Joint Surg., *66-B*:485, 1984.

67. Bohr, H., Baadsgaard, K., and Sager, P. H.: On the development of the epiphysis of the femoral head following dislocation of the hip joint in young rabbits. Acta Orthop. Scand., *39*:280, 1968.

67a. Boal, D. K., and Schwenkter, E. P.: The infant hip: Assessment with real-time US1. Radiology, *157*:667, 1985.

68. Bolton-Maggs, B. G., and Crabtree, S. D.: The opposite hip in congenital dislocation of the hip. J. Bone Joint Surg., *65-B*:279, 1983.

69. Bonitz, K.-H. von: Zur Technik der Beckenosteotomie nach Salter. Osteosynthese mit dem Gabelnagel. Z. Orthop., *104*:175, 1967.

70. Bosch, J.: Die Kontrastfüllung bei der angeborenen Hüftluxation. Z. Orthop., *102*:243, 1966.

71. Bossley, C. J.: The neonatal diagnosis and treatment of congenital dislocation of the hip. J. Bone Joint Surg., *60-B*:286, 1978.

72. Bost, F. C., Hagey, H., Schottstaedt, E. R., and Larsen, L. J.: The results of treatment of congenital dislocation of the hip in infancy. J. Bone Joint Surg., *30-A*:454, 1948.

73. Bosworth, D. M., Ishizuke, T., and Eke, R.: Hip shelf operation in adults. J. Bone Joint Surg., *43-A*:93, 1961.

74. Bosworth, D. M., Fielding, J. W., Liebler, W. A., Ishizuka, T., and Cohen, P.: Hip shelves in children. J. Bone Joint Surg., *42-A*:1223, 1960.

75. Bradford, E. H.: Congenital dislocation of the hip. Am. J. Orthop. Surg., *7*:57, 1909.

76. Brashear, H. R.: Epiphyseal avascular necrosis and its relation to longitudinal bone growth. J. Bone Joint Surg., *45-A*:1423, 1963.

77. Brattstrom, H.: Two sources of error in measurement of the anteversion angle of the femur. Acta Orthop. Scand., *32*:252, 1962.

78. Braun, F. H. T., Jones, K. L., and Smith, D. W.: Breech presentation as an indicator of fetal abnormality. J. Pediatr., *86*:419, 1975.

79. Brizard, J.: Le devenir des hanches luxables ou des luxations découvertes à la naissance. Rev. Rhum., *35*:603, 1968.

80. Brookes, M.: The Blood Supply of Bone. An Approach to Bone Biology. New York, Appleton-Century-Crofts, 1971.

81. Browne, D.: Congenital deformities of mechanical origin. Proc. R. Soc. Med., *29*:1409, 1936.

82. Browne, D.: Treatment of congenital dislocation of the hip. Proc. R. Soc. Med., *41*:388, 1948.

83. Browne, D.: Congenital deformities of mechanical origin. Arch. Dis. Child., *30*:37, 1955.

84. Browne, R. S.: The management of late diagnosed congenital dislocation and subluxation of the hip—with special reference to femoral shortening. J. Bone Joint Surg., *61-B*:7, 1979.

85. Browning, W. H., Rosenkrantz, H., and Tarquinio, T.: Computed tomography in congenital hip dislocation. The role of acetabular anteversion. J. Bone Joint Surg., *64-A*:27, 1982.

86. Brussatis, F.: Ergebnisse der Beckenosteotomie nach Chiari in Abhängichkeit von der Operationstechnik. Verh. Dtsch. Orthop. Ges., *54*:373, 1967.

87. Buchanan, J., Greer, R., and Cotler, J.: Management strategy for prevention of avascular necrosis during treatment of congenital dislocation of the hip. J. Bone Joint Surg., *63-A*:140, 1981.

88. Bucholz, R. W., and Ogden, J. A.: Patterns of ischemic necrosis of the proximal femur in nonoperatively treated congenital hip disease. *In* Proceedings of the Sixth Open Scientific Meeting of the Hip Society. St. Louis, Mosby, 1978, pp. 43–63.

89. Buehler, C. E., and Coleman, S. S.: Colonna arthroplasty for dislocation of the hip in the older child. J. Bone Joint Surg., *54-A*:1799, 1972.

90. Burch, H. B.: Die Becken-Osteotomie von Chiari, theoretische Grundlagen, Hinweis auf erlebte Kom-

plikationen und deren Verhütung. *In* Chapchal, G. (ed.): Beckenosteotomie—Pfannandachplastik. Stuttgart, Thieme, 1965.

91. Burman, M. S., and Clark, H. C.: A roentgenologic study of the hip joint of the infant in the first twelve months of life. A. J. R., *44*:37, 1940.

92. Busse, J., Gasteiger, W., and Tönnis, D.: Eine neue Methode zur röntgenologischer Beurteilung eines Hüftgelenkes—Der Hüftwert. Arch. Orthop. Unfallchir., *72*:1, 1972.

93. Butel, J., Contamin, G., and François, M.: 100 luxations congénitales de la hanche. Resultats lointains du Somerville. Ann. Chir. Infant. (Paris), *13*:159, 1972.

94. Butel, J., Pointu, J., and François, M.: Complementarité des ostéotomies fémorale et pelvienne. Leur indications dans la luxation congénitale de la hanche traitée selon la methode dite de Somerville. Rev. Chir. Orthop. *58*:103, 1972.

95. Butel, J., François, M., Charignon, G., Garrel, J. F., and Faure, C.: Effets de la résection du limbus sur le développement ulterieur du toit cotyloidien. Acta Orthop. Belg., *39*:598, 1973.

96. Buxton, R. A., and McCullough, C. J.: Healing of osteochondritis dissecans following congenital dislocation of the hip: Report of a case. Clin. Orthop., *147*:157, 1980.

97. Cabanac, J., Butel, J., and Contamin, G.: Traitement de la luxation congénitale de la hanche avant 5 ans suivant les principes de Somerville. Ann. Chir. Infant. (Paris), *6*:329, 1963.

98. Caffey, J., Ames, R., Silverman, W. A., Ryder, C. T., and Hough, G.: Contradiction of the congenital dysplasia-predislocation hypothesis of congenital dislocation of the hip through a study of the normal variation in acetabular angles at successive periods in infancy. Pediatrics, *17*:632, 1956.

99. Calandriello, B., and Stellini, L.: La displasia congenita dell'anca nell'eta pediatrica. Anatomia patologica. LVII Congresso della Societa Italiana di Ortopedia e Traumatologia, Bologna, Oct. 1972. Padova, La Garangola, 1972.

100. Campos da Paz, A., Jr., and Kalil, R. K.: Congenital dislocation of the hip in the newborn. A correction of clinical, roentgenographic and anatomical findings. Ital. J. Orthop. Traumatol., *2*:261, 1976.

101. Canale, S. T., and Holand, R. W.: Coventry screw fixation of osteotomies about the pediatric hip. J. Pediatr. Orthop., *3*:592, 1983.

102. Carlioz, H., and Filipe, G.: The natural history of the limbus in congenital dislocation of the Hip: An arthrographic study. *In* Tachdjian, M. O. (ed.): Congenital Dislocation of the Hip. New York, Churchill-Livingstone, 1982, pp. 247–262.

103. Carnochan, J. M.: Etiology, Pathology and Treatment of Congenital Dislocation of the Femur. New York, Wood, 1850.

104. Carter, C. O.: Genetic factors in congenital dislocation of the hip. Proc. R. Soc. Med., *56*:803, 1963.

105. Carter, C. O.: Congenital dislocation of the hip. *In* Sosby, A. (ed.): Clinical Genetics: The Skeletal System. London, Butterworth, 1973, pp. 197–200.

106. Carter, C. O., and Wilkinson, J. A.: Congenital dislocation of the hip. J. Bone Joint Surg., *42-B*:669, 1960.

107. Carter, C. O., and Wilkinson, J. A.: Genetic and environmental factors in the etiology of congenital dislocation of the hip. Clin. Orthop., *33*:119, 1964.

108. Carter, C. O., and Wilkinson, J. A.: Persistent joint laxity and congenital dislocation of the hip. J. Bone Joint Surg., *46-B*:40, 1964.

109. Catterall, A.: Pelvic osteotomy. *In* Rob, C., and Smith, R. (eds.): Operative Surgery. Part II. London, Butterworth, 1979, pp. 632–640.

110. Catterall, A.: Acetabular dysplasia. *In* Tachdjian, M.

111. Catterall, A.: What is congenital dislocation of the hip? (Editorial.) J. Bone Joint Surg., *66-B*:491, 1984.

112. Cedric, C., and Wilkinson, J.: Permanent joint laxity and congenital dislocation of the hip. J. Bone Joint Surg., *46-B*:40, 1964.

113. Chakirgil, G. S.: Radical reduction procedure for treatment of congenital dislocation of the hip in older children. Isr. J. Med. Sci., *16*:344, 1980.

114. Chandler, F. A.: Congenital dislocation of the hip in male infant 11 days old. J. Bone Joint Surg., *11*:546, 1929.

115. Chapchal, G.: Beckenosteotomie—Pfannendachplastik. Stuttgart, Thieme, 1965.

116. Chapchal, G.: Die Behandlung der kongenitalen Hüftdysplasie. Paediatr. Prax., *4*:111, 1965.

117. Chapchal, G.: Butée ostéoplastique ou ostéotomie du bassin? Rev. Chir. Orthop., *51*:243, 1965.

118. Chapchal, G.: Diagnostik und Indikationsstellung bei Deformitäten und Erkrankungen der kindlichen Hüfte. Ann. Paediatr., *205*:477, 1965.

119. Chapchal, G.: Orthopädische Chirurgie und Traumatologie der Hüfte. Stuttgart, Enke, 1965, p. 440.

120. Chapchal, G.: Indications for the various types of pelvic osteotomy. Clin. Orthop., *98*:111, 1974.

121. Chapchal, G. J.: The intertrochanteric osteotomy in the treatment of congenital dysplasia of the hip. Clin. Orthop., *119*:54, 1976.

122. Chapple, C. C., and Davidson, T. D.: A study of the relationship between fetal position and certain congenital deformities. J. Pediatr., *18*:483, 1941.

123. Charnley, J.: Low-Friction Arthroplasty of the Hip. Berlin, Springer, 1979, pp. 332–333.

124. Charnley, J., and Feagin, J. A.: Low-friction arthroplasty in congenital subluxation of the hip. Clin. Orthop., *91*:98, 1973.

125. Chen, R., Weissman, S. L., Salama, R., and Klinberg, M. A.: Congenital dislocation of the hip (CDH) and seasonality: The gestational age of vulnerability to some seasonal factor. Am. J. Epidemiol., *92*:287, 1970.

126. Chiari, K.: Ergebnisse mit der Beckenosteotomie als Pfannendachplastik. Z. Orthop., *87*:14, 1955.

127. Chiari, K.: Die operative Behandlung am Hüftgelenk bei der angeborenen Hüftgelenksverrenkung. Wien. Med. Wochenschr., *107*:1020, 1957.

128. Chiari, K.: *In* proceedings of Societé Internationale de Chirurgie Orthopédique et de Traumatologie. Neuvième congres, Vienna, 1–7 Septembre, 1963–1964.

129. Chiari, K.: Die Beckenosteotomie in der Coxarthrose. Beitr. Orthop., *15*:163, 1968.

130. Chiari, K.: Pelvic osteotomy for hip subluxation. J. Bone Joint Surg., *52-B*:174, 1970.

131. Chiari, K.: Spätergebnisse nach Beckenosteotomie—Verhütung der Präarthrose. Z. Orthop., *112*:603, 1974.

132. Chiari, K.: Medial displacement osteotomy of the pelvis. Clin. Orthop., *98*:55, 1974.

133. Chiari, K.: Bericht über die Beckenosteotomie als Pfannendachplastik nach eigener Methode. *In* Chapchal, G. (ed.): Beckenosteotomie–Pfannendachplastik. Stuttgart, Thieme, 1975, pp. 70–75.

134. Chigot, P. L., and Labbe, G.: Allongement cervicaux après section du grand trochanter chez l'enfant. Rev. Chir. Orthop., *48*:199, 1962.

135. Chigot, P. L., and Vialas, M.: Les resultats tardifs de l'intervention de Colonna. Ann. Chir., *20*:1446, 1966.

136. Chirls, M., Litchman, H., and Robbins, H.: A traction device. J. Bone Joint Surg., *45-A*:1098, 1963.

137. Chrispin, A. R., Harris, H., and Lloyd Roberts, G. C.: A method for calculating acetabular anteversion in children. Pediatr. Radiol., *7*:155, 1978.

138. Chuinard, E. G.: Early weight bearing and correction of anteversion in the treatment of congenital dislocation of the hip. J. Bone Joint Surg., 37-A:229, 1955.

139. Chuinard, E. G.: Femoral osteotomy in the treatment of congenital dysplasia of the hip. Orthop. Clin. North Am., 3:157, 1972.

140. Chuinard, E. G.: Lateral roentgenography in the diagnosis and treatment of dysplasia/dislocation of the hip. Orthopedics, 1:130, 1978.

141. Chuinard, E. G.: Perthes-like changes in congenital dislocation/dysplasia of the hip. Isr. J. Med. Sci., 16:311, 1980.

142. Chuinard, E. G.: Femoral osteotomy in the treatment of congenital dysplasia and dislocation of the hip. In Tachdjian, M. O. (ed.): Congenital Dislocation of the Hip. New York, Churchill-Livingstone, 1982, pp. 437–478.

143. Chuinard, E. G., and Logan, N. D.: Varus-producing and de-rotational subtrochanteric osteotomy in the treatment of congenital dislocation of the hip. J. Bone Joint Surg., 45-A:1397, 1963.

144. Chung, S. M. K.: The arterial supply of the developing proximal end of the human femur. J. Bone Joint Surg., 58-A:961, 1976.

145. Chung, S. M. K.: Musculoskeletal manifestions of hemophilia. In Chung, S. M. K. (ed.): Hip Disorders in Infants and Children. Philadelphia, Lea & Febiger, 1981, pp. 277–289.

146. Chung, S. M. K., and Scholl, H. W.: The Colonna capsular arthroplasty. A long-term follow-up study of fifty-six patients. J. Bone Joint Surg., 53-A:1511, 1971.

147. Clarke, J. J.: Congenital Dislocation of the Hip. London, Baillière, Tindall & Cox, 1910.

148. Cockshott, W. P.: Congenital dislocation of the hip. Br. Med. J., 1:1427, 1960.

148a. Clarke, N. M. P., Clegg, J., and Al-Chalabi, A.: Ultrasound screening of hips at risk for CDH. Failure to reduce the incidence of late cases. J. Bone Joint Surg., 71B:9, 1989.

148b. Clarke, N. M. P., Harcke, H. T., McHugh, P., Lee, M. S., Borns, P. F., and MacEwen, G. D.: Real-time ultrasound in the diagnosis of congenital dislocation and dysplasia of the hip. J. Bone Joint Surg., 67-B(3):406, 1985.

149. Cohen, J.: Congenital dislocation of the hip. Case report of an unusual complication and unusual treatment. J. Bone Joint Surg., 53-A:1007, 1971.

150. Cole, W. G.: Evaluation of a teaching model for the early diagnosis of congenital dislocation of the hip. J. Pediatr. Orthop., 3:2, 1983.

151. Coleman, C. R., Slager, K. F., and Smith, W. S.: The effect of environmental influence on the acetabular development. Surg. Forum, 9:775, 1959.

152. Coleman, S. S.: Diagnosis of congenital dysplasia of the hip in the newborn infant. J. A. M. A., 6:548, 1956.

153. Coleman, S. S.: Treatment of congenital dislocation of the hip in the infant. J. Bone Joint Surg., 47-A:590, 1965.

154. Coleman, S. S.: Congenital dysplasia of the hip in the Navajo infant. Clin. Orthop., 56:179, 1968.

155. Coleman, S. S.: The incomplete pericapsular (Pemberton) and innominate (Salter) osteotomies. A complete analysis. Clin. Orthop., 98:116, 1974.

156. Coleman, S. S.: Salvage procedures in congenital dislocation of the hip utilizing femoral shortening. In The Hip: Proceedings of the Fourth Meeting of the Hip Society, 1976. St. Louis, Mosby, 1976, pp. 29–39.

157. Coleman, S. S.: Congenital Dysplasia and Dislocation of the Hip. St. Louis, Mosby, 1978.

158. Coleman, S. S.: Management of congenital dysplasia and dislocation of the hip from birth to eighteen months of age. In Tachdjian, M. O. (ed.): Congenital Dislocation of the Hip. New York, Churchill-Livingstone, 1982, pp. 181–203.

159. Coleman, S. S.: Problems and complications of Salter's innominate osteotomy. Paper presented at Pediatric Orthopedic International Seminar, Chicago, 1983.

160. Colonna, P. C.: Congenital dislocation of the hip in older subjects. J. Bone Joint Surg., 14:277, 1932.

161. Colonna, P. C.: An arthroplastic operation for congenital dislocation of the hip—a two stage procedure. Surg. Gynecol. Obstet., 63:777, 1936.

162. Colonna, P. C.: An arthroplastic procedure for congenital dislocation in children. J. Bone Joint Surg., 20:604, 1938.

163. Colonna, P. C.: Arthroplasty of the hip for congenital dislocation in children. J. Bone Joint Surg., 29:711, 1947.

164. Colonna, P. C.: Congenital dislocation of the hip in children and adults. A. A. O. S. Instruct. Course Lect., 8:169, 1951.

165. Colonna, P. C.: Care of the infant with congenital subluxation of the hip. J. A. M. A., 166:715, 1958.

166. Colonna, P. C.: Capsular arthroplasty for congenital dislocation of the hip. J. Bone Joint Surg., 35-A:179, 1963.

167. Colton, C. L.: Chiari osteotomy for acetabular dysplasia in young subjects. J. Bone Joint Surg., 54-B:578, 1972.

168. Compère, E. L., and Phemister, D. B.: The tibial peg shelf in congenital dislocation of the hip. J. Bone Joint Surg., 17:60, 1935.

169. Compere, E. L., Garrison, M., and Fahey, J. J.: Deformities of the femur resulting from arrestment of growth of the capital and greater trochanteric epiphysis. J. Bone Joint Surg., 22:909, 1940.

170. Compère, E. L., and Schnute, W. J.: Treatment of congenital dislocation of the hip. J. Bone Joint Surg., 28:555, 1946.

171. Connolly, J. F.: Early diagnosis and misdiagnosis of congenital dislocated hip. Nebr. Med., 60:471, 1975.

172. Conrad, M. B.: Congenital dislocation of the hip. A. O. S. Instruct. Course Lect., 18:207, 1961.

173. Coon, V., Donato, G., Houser, C., and Bleck, E. E.: Normal ranges of hip motion in infants six weeks, three months and six months of age. Clin. Orthop., 110:256, 1975.

174. Cooperman, D. R., Wallensten, R., and Stulbrey, S. D.: Post reduction avascular necrosis in congenital dislocation of the hip. J. Bone Joint Surg., 62-A:247, 1980.

175. Corkery, P. H.: Congenital hip dislocation. Br. Med. J., 3:371, 1971.

176. Corrigan, C., and Segal, S.: The incidence of congenital dislocation of the hip at Island Lake, Manitoba. Can. Med. Assoc. J., 62:535, 1950.

177. Coventry, M. B.: Total hip arthroplasty in the adult with complete congenital dislocation. In The Hip: Proceedings of the Fourth Meeting of the Hip Society, 1976. St. Louis, Mosby, 1976, pp. 77–87.

178. Coventry, M. B., and Harris, L. E.: Congenital muscular torticollis in infancy. Some observations regarding treatment. J. Bone Joint Surg., 41-A:815, 1959.

179. Coventry, M. B., and Johnson, E. W.: Congenital absence of the fibula. J. Bone Joint Surg., 1:941, 1952.

180. Cozen, L.: Some evils of fixed abduction of the hip. Clin. Orthop., 57:203, 1968.

181. Crasselt, C.: Untersuchungen über die teratologische und sogenannten angeborene Hüftgelenksverrenkung. Beitr. Orthop. Traumatol., 15:104, 1968.

182. Crego, C. H., Jr.: Preliminary skeletal traction in the treatment of congenital dislocation of the hip. South. Med. J., 26:845, 1933.

183. Crego, C. H., Jr.: The use of skeletal traction as a preliminary procedure in the treatment of early congenital dislocation of the hip. J. Bone Joint Surg., 21:353, 1939.

184. Crego, C. H., Jr., and Schwarzman, J. R.: Follow-up study of the early treatment of congenital dislocation of the hip. J. Bone Joint Surg., 30-A:428, 1948.

185. Crelin, E. S.: An experimental study of hip stability in human newborn cadavers. Yale J. Biol. Med., 49:109, 1976.

186. Crelin, R. Q.: Innominate osteotomy for congenital dislocation and subluxation of the hip. A follow-up study. Clin. Orthop., 98:171, 1974.

187. Creyssel, J., and Poilleux, F.: Traitment de la luxation congénitale inveterée de la hanche chez l'adulte. Rev. Chir. Orthop., 37:333, 1951.

188. Crock, H. V.: A revision of the anatomy of the arteries supplying the upper end of the human femur. J. Anat., 100:77, 1965.

189. Crock, H. V.: The Blood Supply of the Lower Limb Bones in Man. Edinburgh, Livingstone, 1967.

190. Crock, H. V., and Boni, V.: The management of orthopaedic problems in hemophiliacs. A review of 21 cases. Br. J. Surg., 48:8, 1960.

191. Crowe, J. F., Mani, V. J., and Ranawat, C.: Total hip replacement in congenital dislocation and dysplasia of the hip. J. Bone Joint Surg., 61-A:15, 1979.

192. Cyvin, K. B.: A follow-up study of children with instability of the hip joint at birth. Clinical and radiological investigations with special reference to the anteversion of the femoral neck. Acta Orthop. Scand. (Suppl.), 166:8, 1977.

193. Cyvin, K. B.: Congenital dislocation of the hip joint. Acta Paediatr. Scand. (Suppl.), 66:262, 1977.

194. Cyvin, K. B.: Unsatisfactory results of early treatment of infants with unstable hips at birth. Acta Orthop. Scand., 48:665, 1977.

195. Czeizel, A., Szentpetery, J., and Kellermann, M.: Incidence of congenital dislocation of the hip in Hungary. Br. J. Soc. Prevent. Med., 28:265, 1974.

196. Czeizel, A., Szentpetery, J., Tusnady, G., and Vizkelety, T.: Two family studies of congenital dislocation of the hip after early orthopaedic screening in Hungary. J. Med. Genet., 12:125, 1975.

197. Czeizel, A., Tusnady, G., Vaczo, G., and Vizkelety, T.: The mechanism of genetic predisposition in congenital dislocation of the hip. J. Med. Genet., 12:121, 1975.

198. Dabadie, J.: Le depistage à la naissance de luxation congénitale de la hanche. Ann. Chir. Infant. (Paris), 7:253, 1966.

199. Dabadie, J.: Resultat de 6 ans le depistage et de traitement préventif de la luxation congénitale de la hanche. Ann. Chir. Infant., 12:147, 1971.

200. Dabadie, J., and Lascombes, P. H.: La prévention de la luxation congénitale de la hanche en milieu obstetrical. Rev. Fr. Gynecol. Obstet., 65:45, 1970.

201. Dall, G.: Congenital dislocation of the hip. Management at the Princess Alice Orthopaedic Hospital. S. Afr. Med. J., 56:954, 1979.

202. Dal Monte, A., Soncini, G., and Valdiserri, L.: Acetabuloplasty by triple pelvic osteotomy: Indications and surgical technique. Ital. J. Orthop. Traumatol., 6:5, 1980.

203. Davies, S. J. M., and Walker, G.: Problems in the early recognition of hip dysplasia. J. Bone Joint Surg., 66-B:479, 1984.

204. Day, R. B.: Congenital dysplasia of the hip in the newborn. A second look. J. Maine Med. Assoc., 66:206, 1975.

205. Debrunner, A. M.: Kongenitale Hüftgelenksluxation. Ther. Umsch., 25:538, 1968.

206. Debrunner, H. U.: Die Früherkennung der sogen-annten angeborenen Hüftgelenkverrenkung bei der gezielten Reihenuntersuchung. Schweiz. Med. Wochenschr., 94:1624, 1964.

207. Dega, W.: Ricerche anatomiche e meccaniche sull'anca fetale rivolte a chiarire l'etologie e la patogenesi della lussazione congenita. Chir. Organi Mov., 18:425, 1933.

208. Dega, W.: Surgical treatment of congenital dislocation of the hip in children. J. Bone Joint Surg., 40-A:725, 1958.

209. Dega, W.: Surgical intervention in the treatment of CDH in the child. International Expert Conference, 9th Congress, S.I.C.O.T., Vienna, 1963.

210. Dega, W.: Die anatomische und funktionelle Restitution des kongenital luxierten Hüftgelenkes durch ein einzeitiges Operationsverfahren. Arch. Orthop. Unfallchir., 60:16, 1966.

211. Dega, W.: Transiliac osteotomy in the treatment of congenital hip dysplasia. Chir. Narzadow Ruchu Ortop. Pol., 39:601, 1974.

212. Dega, W.: Der Megatrochanter in der Behandlung der angeborenen Hüftluxation. Z. Orthop., 115:492, 1977.

213. Dega, W.: Development and clinical importance of the dysplastic acetabulum. Prog. Orthop. Surg., 2:47, 1978.

214. Denton, J. R., and Ryder, C. T.: Radiographic follow-up of Salter innominate osteotomy for congenital dysplasia of the hip. Clin. Orthop., 98:210, 1974.

215. Denuce, M.: Luxation congénitale de la hanche. Opération de Hoffa. Rev. Orthop., 4:108, 1893.

216. Desche, P., Courtois, B., Carlioz, H., and Scott, P. J.: Symposium on an experience in screening dislocatable hips. Ann. Orthop. Ouest, 9, 1977.

217. DeWaal Malefijt, M. C., Hoogland, T., and Nielsen, H. K. L.: Chiari osteotomy in the treatment of congenital dislocation and subluxation of the hip. J. Bone Joint Surg., 64-A:996, 1982.

218. Dickerson, R. C.: Congenital subluxation of the hip. Pediatrics, 41:977, 1968.

219. Dickson, F. D.: The shelf operation in the treatment of congenital dislocation of the hip. Surg. Gynecol. Obstet., 55:81, 1932.

220. Dickson, F. D.: The shelf operation in the treatment of congenital dislocation of the hip. J. Bone Joint Surg., 17:43, 1935.

221. Dimon, J. H., III: Observation of the gluteal fold in hip dysplasia. Clin. Orthop., 103:19, 1974.

222. Dogonadze, M. A.: Zur Atropathogenese angeborener Luxationshüften (Hüftdysplasie). Beitr. Orthop. Traumatol., 20:151, 1973.

223. Dogonadze, M. A., Kandelaki, T. A., and Bolkwadse, T. W.: Der Ostrogenstoffwechsel bei der angeborenen Hüftluxation. Beitr. Orthop., 21:100, 1974.

224. Dooley, B. J.: Osteochondritis in congenital dislocation and subluxation of the hip. J. Bone Joint Surg., 46-B:198, 1964.

225. Dorr, W. M.: Erfahrungen mit dem Riemenbugel nach Pavlik in der Behandlung der sog angeborenen Hüftgelenksluxation und ihre Vorstufen. Z. Orthop., 101:535, 1966.

226. Dorr, W. M.: Zur Frühest- und Frühdiagnose der sogenannten angeborenen Hüftgelenksluxation. Dtsch. Med. Wochenschr., 91:168, 1966.

227. Dorr, W. M.: Zur offenen Reposition nach Ludloff. Verh. Dtsch. Orthop. Ges., 54:370, 1968.

228. Dreyer, J., and Pingel, P.: Unsere Erfahrungen bei der Hüftarthrose mit Beckenosteotomie und Kreuzplatte. Arch. Orthop. Unfallchir., 66:310, 1969.

229. Dubousset, J.: Les ostéotomies du bassin dans le traitement de la luxation congénitale de la hanche chez l'enfant et l'adolescent. Rev. Chir. Orthop. (Suppl. 11), 61:313, 1975.

230. Duda, E., Branik, G., and Huziek, E.: Abduktion-sapparat zur Nachbehandlung der angeborenen Hüftluxation. Z. Orthop., *107*:525, 1970.

231. Dunaj, W.: Microscopic structure of articular capsule, ligamentum teres and articular cartilage of femoral head in congenital dislocation of the hip. Chir. Narzadow Ruchu Ortop. Pol., *35*:459, 1970.

232. Dunaj, W.: The myogenic factor in the development of congenital dislocation of the hip. Chir. Narzadow Ruchu Ortop. Pol., *35*:331, 1970.

233. Dunlap, K., Shands, A. R., Jr., Hollister, L. C., Jr., Gail, J. S., and Streit, H. A.: A new method for the determination of torsion of the femur. J. Bone Joint Surg., *35-A*:289, 1953.

234. Dunn, D. M.: Anteversion of the neck of the femur. J. Bone Joint Surg., *34-B*:181, 1952.

235. Dunn, H. K., and Hess, W. E.: Total hip reconstruction in chronically dislocated hips. J. Bone Joint Surg., *58-A*:838, 1976.

236. Dunn, P. M.: The influence of the intrauterine environment in the causation of congenital postural deformities, with special reference to congenital dislocation of the hip. M.D. Thesis, Gainsborough University, 1967.

237. Dunn, P. M.: Congenital dislocation of the hip (CDH): Necropsy studies at birth. Proc. R. Soc. Med., *62*:1034, 1969.

238. Dunn, P. M.: Congenital dislocation of the hip and congenital renal anomalies. Arch. Dis. Child., *46*:878, 1971.

239. Dunn, P. M.: Congenital postural deformities: Further perinatal associations. Proc. R. Soc. Med., *67*:1174, 1974.

240. Dunn, P. M.: Congenital postural deformities. Br. Med. Bull., *32*:71, 1976.

241. Dunn, P. M.: Perinatal observations on the etiology of congenital dislocation of the hip. Clin. Orthop., *119*:11, 1976.

242. Dunn, P. M.: The anatomy and pathology of congenital dislocation of the hip. Clin. Orthop., *119*:23, 1976.

243. Dupuytren, J.: Memoire sur un déplacement original de la tête des fémurs. Rep. Gen. Anat. Physiol., *2*:151, 1826; Leçons Orales de Clinique Chirurgie Paris, *1*:3, 1833 (as cited by Hass, J.: Congenital Dislocation of the Hip. Springfield, Thomas, 1951).

244. Dykes, R. G.: Congenital dislocation of the hip in Southland. N.Z. Med. J., *81*:467, 1975.

245. Ebach, G.: Bisherige Erfahrungen mit der Beckenosteotomie, nach Chiari. Z. Orthop., *102*:262, 1966.

246. Eberhardt, H.: Eine Methode zur Frühbehandlung der Schenkelhalsfehlstellung bei kongenitalen Hüftluxationen. Arch. Orthop. Unfallchir., *55*:306, 1963.

247. Edelson, J. G., Hirsch, M., Weinberg, H., Attar, D., and Barmier, E.: Congenital dislocation of the hip and computerised axial tomography. J. Bone Joint Surg., *66-B*:472, 1984.

248. Edelstein, J.: Congenital dislocation of the hip in the Bantu. J. Bone Joint Surg., *48-B*:397, 1966.

249. Edgren, W.: Coxa plana. A clinical and radiological investigation with particular reference to the importance of the metaphyseal changes for the final shape of the proximal part of the femur. Acta Orthop. Scand., Suppl. 84, 1965.

250. Editorial: Congenital dislocation of the hip. Br. Med. J., *4*:371, 1967.

251. Edwards, J. H.: Familial predisposition in man. Brit. Med. Bull., *25*:84, 1969.

252. El-Adwar, L. I.: A review of the aetiology of congenital dislocation of the hip. Egypt. Orthop. J., *6*:43, 1971.

253. Elftmann, H.: Biomechanics of muscle with particular application to studies in gait. J. Bone Joint Surg., *48-A*:363, 1966.

254. Ellis, G. V.: An account of an instance of remarkable deformity of the lower limbs. Med. Chir. Trans., *36*:439, 1853.

255. Emneus, H.: Some new aspects of the treatment of congenital dislocation of the hip (CDH) according to Palmen-Von Rosen. Acta Orthop. Scand., *37*:311, 1966.

256. Emneus, H.: A note on the Ortolani-Von Rosen-Palmen treatment of congenital dislocation of the hip. J. Bone Joint Surg., *50-B*:537, 1968.

257. Emneus, H.: Brief contributions to the subject. Acta Orthop. Scand. (Suppl.), *130*:56, 1970.

258. Emneus, H., and Undeland, K.: A 4-year prospective study of two different therapeutic regimens for newborns with CDH. Acta Orthop. Scand., *42*:457, 1971.

259. Ender, A.: Die Behandlung der Hüftdysplasie bzw. Luxationshüfte und ihre Ergebnisse an der Orthopädischen Abteilung der Krankenanstalten Hubertusburg seit ihrem Bestehen. Beitr. Orthop. Traumatol., *17*:135, 1970.

260. Endler, F.: Wirkungsprinzipien und Ergebnisse der Beckenosteotomie bei kongenitaler Hüftluxation. Wien. Med. Wochenschr., *122*:408, 1972.

261. Engler, J.: Vorlaufige Behandlungsergebnisse bei Kindern mit in der ersten Lebenswoche festgestelltem Ortolani-Phänomen. Dtsch. Gesund., *22*:1511, 1967.

262. Endo, M., Iinuma, T. A., Umegaki, Y., Tateno, Y., Tanaka, H., and Tsuchiya, K.: Automated diagnosis of congenital dislocation of the hip. Radiology, *122*:25, 1977.

263. Eppright, R. H.: Dial osteotomy of the acetabulum in the treatment of dysplasia of the hip. J. Bone Joint Surg., *57-A*:1172, 1975.

264. Eriksson, U., James, U., and Wilkstrom, G.: The angle of anteversion and the neckshaft angle in children—a roentgenological and clinical study. Acta Soc. Med. Ups., *75*:229, 1970.

265. Estève, R.: Congenital dislocation of the hip. A review and assessment of results of treatment with special reference to frame reduction as compared with manipulative reduction. J. Bone Joint Surg., *42-B*:253, 1960.

266. Eulert, J.: Repositionstechnik der sog. angeborenen Hüftluxation nach der Methode Hoffmann-Daimler. Z. Orthop., *115*:641, 1977.

267. Ewald, F. C., and Hirohashi, K.: Effect of distal transfer of the greater trochanter in growing animals. J. Bone Joint Surg., *55-A*:1064, 1973.

267a. Exner, G. U.: Ultrasound screening for hip dysplasia in neonates. J. Pediatr. Orthop., *8*:656, 1988.

268. Eyre-Brook, A. L.: Treatment of congenital dislocation or subluxation of the hip in children over the age of three years. J. Bone Joint Surg., *48-B*:682, 1966.

269. Eyre-Brook, A. L.: Some aspects of congenital dysplasia of the hip. Ann. R. Coll. Surg. Eng., *43*:1, 1968.

270. Eyre-Brook, A. L., Jones, D. B., and Harris, F. C.: Pemberton's acetabuloplasty for congenital dislocation or subluxation of the hip. J. Bone Joint Surg., *60-B*:18, 1978.

271. Faber, A.: Erbbiologische Untersuchungen über die Anlage zur "angeborenen" Hüftverrenkung. Z. Orthop., *66*:140, 1937.

272. Faber, U.: Untersuchungen über Spätergebnisse bei totaler angeborener Hüftluxation. Arch. Orthop. Unfallchir., *59*:86, 1966.

273. Fabry, G., MacEwen, G. D., and Shands, A. R.: Torsion of femur. A follow-up study in normal and abnormal conditions. J. Bone Joint Surg., *55-A*:1726, 1973.

274. Fairbank, H. A. T.: Operative treatment of dislocated hips. Proc. R. Soc. Med., *3*:15, 1922.

275. Fairbank, H. A. T.: Late results of treatment of congenital dislocation of the hip. Br. J. Surg., *10*:24, 1922.

276. Fairbank, H. A. T.: Congenital dislocation of the hip with special reference to the anatomy. Br. J. Surg., *17*:380, 1930.

277. Fairbank, H. A. T.: Early diagnosis of congenital dislocation of the hip. Br. Med. J., *1*:607, 1939.

278. Farkas, A.: The mechanics of the formation of the "secondary acetabulum" in congenital dislocation of the hip. J. Bone Joint Surg., *20*:885, 1938.

279. Farmer, A. W., and Laurin, C. A.: Congenital absence of the fibula. J. Bone Joint Surg., *42-A*:1, 1960.

280. Farrell, B. P., and Howorth, M. B.: Open reduction in congenital dislocation of the hip. J. Bone Joint Surg., *17*:35, 1935.

281. Fellander, M.: Introduction. *In* Prevention of congenital dislocation of the hip joint in Sweden. Efficiency of early diagnosis and treatment. Acta Orthop. Scand. (Suppl.), *130*:8, 1970.

282. Fellander, M.: General discussion. *In* Prevention of congenital dislocation of the hip joint in Sweden. Efficiency of early diagnosis and treatment. Acta Orthop. Scand. (Suppl.), *130*:59, 1970.

283. Fellander, M., Gladnikoff, H., and Jacobsson, E.: Instability of the hip in the newborn. Classification for selective treatment, pathogenesis of the dislocation and complications. Acta Orthop. Scand. (Suppl.), *130*:35, 1970.

284. Felts, W. J. L.: The prenatal development of the human femur. Am. J. Anat., *94*:1, 1954.

285. Ferguson, A. B., Jr.: Primary open reduction of congenital dislocation of the hip using a median adductor approach. J. Bone Joint Surg., *55-A*:671, 1973.

286. Ferguson, A. B., Jr.: Primary recognition and treatment of congenital dislocation of the hip. Pediatr. Ann., *5*:222, 1976.

287. Ferguson, A. B., Jr.: Treatment of congenital dislocation of the hip in infancy using the medial approach. *In* Tachdjian, M. O. (ed.): Congenital Dislocation of the Hip. New York, Churchill-Livingstone, 1982, pp. 283–293.

288. Ferguson, A. B., Jr., and Howorth, M. B.: Slipping of the upper femoral epiphysis. A study of seventy cases. J. A. M. A., *97*:1867, 1931.

289. Fernandez, C. I.: La Cirugia del Acetabulo en la Luxacion Congenita de la Cadera. Valencia, Editorial Facta, 1965, pp. 77–87.

290. Ferre, R. L., and Schachter, S.: Congenital dislocation of the hip. Innominate osteotomy. Clin. Orthop., *98*:183, 1974.

291. Ferrer-Torrelles, M., and Ceballos, T.: Embryology of the hip in relation to congenital dislocation. *In* Tachdjian, M. O. (ed.): Congenital Dislocation of the Hip. New York, Churchill-Livingstone, 1982, pp. 1–25.

292. Fettweis, E.: Sitz-Hock-Stellungsgips bei Hüftgelenksdysplasien. Arch. Orthop. Unfallchir., *63*:38, 1968.

293. Fettweis, E.: Über Entstehung und Verhütung pathologischer Valgitaten und Antetorsionen des Schenkelhalses beim Hüftluxationsleiden. Z. Orthop., *102*:221, 1970.

294. Fettweis, E.: Erwiderung auf die Bemerkungen von H. Mau über die Arbeit des Verfassers "Zur Prophylaxe des kindlichen Hüftlusxationsleidens." Z. Orthop., *110*:272, 1972.

295. Fettweis, E.: Das Hüftluxationsleiden bei in Beckenendlage Angeboren Kindern. Zur. Pathogenese Bedeutung fur des Luxationsproblem. Z. Orthop., *111*:168, 1973.

296. Fettweis, E.: Die Behandlung der kongenitalen Hüftgelenksdysplasie mit dem Sitz-Hock-Gips. 63. Kongress der deutschen Gesellschaft fur Orthopädie und Traumatologie. Z. Orthop., *115*:648, 1977.

297. Fevre, M. M.: Resultats de l'enquête sur le depistage et le traitement préventif des luxations congénitales de la hanche dans Le Finistère. Pédiatrie, *21*:849, 1966.

298. Fevre, M. M.: Une prophylaxie de la luxation "congénitale" de la hanche pourrait elle supprimer en France ce veritable fléau? Bull. Acad. Med. (Paris), *150*:87, 1966.

299. Fevre, M. M.: Depistage, prophylaxie et traitement précoce des luxations de la hanche. Bull. Acad. Med. (Paris), *151*:273, 1967.

300. Finley, H. V. L., Mandsley, R. H., Bushfield, P. I.: Dislocatable hip and dislocated hip in the newborn infant. Br. Med. J., *4*:377, 1967.

301. Fisher, R. L., and Cary, J. M.: Avascular necrosis complicating congenital dislocation of the hip. Course, prognosis and orthopedic management. Int. Orthop., *2*:229, 1978.

302. Fisher, R. L., Duncan, A. S., and Bronzino, J. D.: The application of axial transverse tomography to the measurement of femoral anteversion. Clin. Orthop., *86*:6, 1972.

303. Flinchum, D.: Shelf reconstruction for hip dysplasia. South. Med. J., *72*:1512, 1979.

304. Floman, Y., and Niska, M.: Dislocation of the hip joint complicating repeated hemarthrosis in hemophilia. J. Pediatr. Orthop., *3*:1, 1983.

305. Frank, G. R., and Michael, H. R.: Treatment of congenital dislocation of the hip: Results obtained with the Pemberton and Salter osteotomies. South. Med. J., *60*:975, 1967.

306. Frankel, V. H., and Burstein, A. H.: Orthopaedic Biomechanics. Philadelphia, Lea & Febiger, 1970, p. 25.

307. Fredensborg, N.: Congenital dislocation of the hip (M.D. Thesis). Lund, Sweden, Lund University, 1975.

308. Fredensborg, N.: Observations in children with congenital dislocation of the hip. Acta Orthop. Scand., *47*:175, 1976.

309. Fredensborg, N.: Overdiagnosis of congenital dislocation of the hip. Clin. Orthop., *119*:89, 1976.

310. Fredensborg, N.: The CE angle of normal hips. Acta Orthop. Scand., *47*:403, 1976.

311. Fredensborg, N.: The results of early treatment of typical congenital dislocation of the hip in Malmo. J. Bone Joint Surg., *58-B*:272, 1976.

312. Fredensborg, N.: Congenital dislocation of the hip. Results of early diagnosis and treatment in Malmo. Int. Orthop. (S.I.C.O.T.), *1*:101, 1977.

313. Fredensborg, N., and Nilsson, B. E.: The effect of early diagnosis of congenital dislocation of the hip. Acta Paediatr. Scand., *65*:323, 1976.

314. Fredensborg, N., and Nilsson, B. E.: Menarcheal age in girls with congenital dislocation of the hip. Acta Paediatr. Scand., *66*:241, 1977.

315. Frejka, B.: Praventation der angeborenen Hüftgelenksluxation durch das Abduktionspolster. Wien. Med. Wochenschr., *91*:523, 1941.

316. Froelich, R.: Zur Profylaxe der angeborenen Hüftverrenkung. Z. Orthop. Chir., *56*, 1932.

317. Frost, H. M.: A chondral modeling theory. Calcif. Tissue Int., *28*:181, 1979.

318. Fuhrman, H.: Spätergebnisse nach Chiarischer Beckenosteotomie. Z. Orthop., *110*:956, 1972.

319. Gaenslen, F. J.: The Schanz subtrochanteric osteotomy for irreducible dislocation of the hip. J. Bone Joint Surg., *17*:76, 1935.

320. Gage, J. R., and Cary, J. M.: The effects of trochan-

teric epiphyseodesis on growth of the proximal end of the femur following necrosis of the capital femoral epiphysis. J. Bone Joint Surg., 62-A:785, 1980.

321. Gage, J. R., and Winter, R. B.: Avascular necrosis of the capital femoral epiphysis as a complication of closed reduction of congenital dislocation of the hip. J. Bone Joint Surg., 54-A:373, 1972.

322. Gallien, R., Bertin, D., and Lirette, R.: Salter procedure in congenital dislocation of the hip. J. Pediatr. Orthop., 4:427, 1984.

323. Gardner, E.: Prenatal development of the human hip joint, femur and hip bone. A. A. O. S. Instruct. Course Lect., 21:1, 1972.

324. Gardner, E., and Gray, D. J.: Prenatal development of the human hip joint. Am. J. Anat., 87:163, 1950.

325. Geiser, M.: Behandlungsergebnisse bei frühzeitig diagnostizierter typischer kongenitaler Hüftluxation. Z. Orthop., 113:67, 1975.

326. Getz, B.: The hip joint in Lapps. Acta Orthop. Scand., Suppl. 22, 1955.

327. Ghormley, R. K.: Use of the anterior superior spine and crest of ilium in surgery of the hip joint. J. Bone Joint Surg., 13:784, 1931.

328. Gibson, D. A.: Congenital dislocation of the hip. A review of adults treated in childhood. Can. J. Surg., 10:288, 1967.

329. Gibson, P. H., and Benson, M. K. D.: Congenital dislocation of the hip. Review at maturity of 147 hips treated by excision of the limbus and derotation osteotomy. J. Bone Joint Surg., 64-B:169, 1982.

330. Gilbert, R. J.: The Chiari procedure for acetabular insufficiency. J. Bone Joint Surg., 56-A:1538, 1974.

331. Gill, A. B.: Operation for old or irreducible congenital dislocation of the hip. J. Bone Joint Surg., 10:696, 1928.

332. Gill, A. B.: Plastic construction of an acetabulum in congenital dislocation of the hip—the shelf operation. J. Bone Joint Surg., 17:48, 1935.

333. Gill, A. B.: An evaluation of present day methods of dealing with congenital dislocation of the hip. J. Bone Joint Surg., 18:487, 1936.

334. Gill, A. B.: End results of bloodless reduction of congenital dislocation of the hip. J. Bone Joint Surg., 25:1, 1943.

335. Gill, A. B.: The end results of early treatment of congenital dislocation of the hip. With an inquiry into the factors that determine the results. J. Bone Joint Surg., 30-A:442, 1948.

336. Gill, A. B.: Progress in orthopaedic surgery for 1946: Congenital dislocation of the hip. Arch. Surg., 58:236, 1949.

337. Gillespie, R., and Torode, I.: Classification and management of congenital abnormalities of the femur. J. Bone Joint Surg., 65-B:447, 1983.

338. Gilmour, J.: Adolescent deformities of the acetabulum. Br. J. Surg., 26:670, 1938.

339. Gilmour, J.: Relationship of acetabular deformity to spontaneous osteo-arthritis of the hip joint. Br. J. Surg., 26:700, 1939.

340. Glauber, A.: Die Funktion und pathomechanische Rolle des Musculus iliopsoas in der Entwicklung der kongenitalen Hüftgelenkverrenkung. Beitr. Orthop. Traumatol., 15:54, 1968.

341. Glauber, A.: Treatment of the dysplastic hip with Pavlik's bandage. J. Bone Joint Surg., 53-B:152, 1971.

342. Glauber, A., and Vizkelety, T.: Ergebnisse der Behandlung der angeborenen Hüftgelenks-luxation mit dem Riemenbugel nach Pavlik. Z. Orthop., 110:108, 1972.

343. Glauber, A., Vizkelety, T., and Szepesi, K.: Die Rolle des M. iliopsoas im Pathomechanismus der sog. angeborenen Hüftluxation. Arch. Orthop. Unfallchir., 62:291, 1967.

344. Gob, A.: Diagnostik der angeborenen Hüftgelenkluxation. Med. Klin. 62:1041, 1967.

345. Gob, A.: Therapie der angeborenen Hüftgelenkluxation. Med. Klin., 62:1090, 1967.

346. Gofton, J. P.: Studies in osteoarthritis of the hip. Part III. Congenital subluxation and osteoarthritis of the hip. Can. Med. Assoc. J., 104:911, 1971.

347. Gold, R. H., and Amstutz, H.: Surgical procedures for congenital dislocation of the hip. Radiol. Clin. North Am., 13:123, 1975.

348. Golfieri, G., Vianello, A., Buzzi, F., and Aluigi, A.: La displasie congénitale de la hanche dans le nouveau-né: Diagnostique et prophylaxie therapeutique. Clin. Pediatr. (Bologna), 50:136, 1968.

349. Good, C., and Walker, G.: The hip in the molded baby syndrome. J. Bone Joint Surg., 66-B:491, 1984.

350. Goodrich, E.: Routine examination of newborn infants for congenital dislocated hips. J.A.M.A., 226:1119, 1973.

351. Gordon, G. C.: Congenital Deformities. Edinburgh, Livingstone, 1961.

352. Gore, D. R.: Iatrogenic avascular necrosis of the hip in young children. A review of six cases. J. Bone Joint Surg., 56-A:493, 1974.

353. Graf, R.: The diagnosis of congenital hip-joint dislocation by the ultrasonic compound treatment. Arch. Orthop. Trauma. Surg., 97:117, 1980.

354. Graf, R.: New possibilities for the diagnosis of congenital hip joint dislocation by ultrasonography. J. Pediatr. Orthop., 3:354, 1983.

354a. Graf, R.: The ultrasonic image of the acetabular rim in infants. Arch. Orthop. Traumat. Surg., 99:35, 1981.

355. Grech, P.: Video-arthrography in hip dysplasia. Clin. Radiol., 23:202, 1972.

356. Grech, P.: Hip Arthrography. London, Chapman & Bell, 1977.

357. Green, N. E., and Griffin, P. P.: Hip dysplasia associated with abduction contracture of the contralateral hip. J. Bone Joint Surg., 64-A:1273, 1982.

358. Greenwald, A. S., and Hayes, D. W.: Weight-bearing areas in the human hip joint. J. Bone Joint Surg., 54-B:157, 1972.

359. Gregersen, H. S.: Congenital dislocation of the hip. Acta Orthop. Scand., 40:53, 1969.

360. Griffin, P. P.: Pitfalls of early treatment of congenital dislocation of the hip and causes of failure. In Tachdjian, M. O. (ed.): Congenital Dislocation of the Hip. New York, Churchill-Livingstone, 1982, pp. 205–213.

360a. Grissom, L. E., Harcke, H. T., Kumar, S. J., Bassett, G. S., and MacEwen, G. D.: Ultrasound evaluation of hip position in the Pavlik harness. J. Ultrasound Med., 7:1, 1988.

361. Gross, F.: Ergebnisse nach Colonnascher plastik. Z. Orthop., 110:988, 1972.

362. Gruca, A.: Surgical critique of late reconstructive procedures for congenital dislocation of the hip. Chir. Narzadow Ruchu Orthop. Pol., 34:459, 1969.

363. Gualtieri, G., Gualtieri, I., and Capelli, A.: Derotation varicizing osteotomy (in children between 5 and 10 years of age). Ital. J. Orthop. Traumatol., 6:53, 1980.

364. Haas, S. L.: Pin fixation in dislocation at the hip joint. J. Bone Joint Surg., 14:346, 1932.

365. Haas, S. S., Epps, C. H., and Adams, J. P.: Normal range of hip motion in the newborn. Clin. Orthop., 91:114, 1973.

366. Haike, H., Breuckmann, G., and Schultze, H.: Ein Beitrag zur operativen Behandlung der sogenannten kongenitalen Hüftluxation. Arch. Orthop. Unfallchir., 66:277, 1969.

367. Haines, R. W.: Cartilage canals. J. Anat., 68:45, 1933.

368. Hallopeau, P.: Traitement de la luxation congénitale irréducible et douloureuse par une greffe d'os mort. Bull. Mem. Soc. Chir. Paris, 49:1198, 1923.

369. Hamacher, P.: Die Problematik der Beckenosteotomie nach Salter. Z. Orthop., 103:454, 1967.

370. Hansson, G.: Neonatal hip instability in Goteborg, Sweden, between 1961 and 1970 (Thesis). Göteborg, Sweden, University of Göteborg, 1980.

371. Hansson, G., Nachemson, A., and Palmen, K.: Screening of children with congenital dislocation of the hip joint on the maternity wards in Sweden. J. Pediatr. Orthop., 3:271, 1983.

372. Hansson, L. I., Olsson, T. H., Selvik, G., and Sunden, G.: A roentgen stereophotogrammetric investigation of innominate osteotomy (Salter). Acta Orthop. Scand., 49:68, 1978.

373. Harris, L. E., Lipscomb, P. R., and Hodgson, J. R.: Early diagnosis of congenital dislocation of the hip. Value of an abduction test. J.A.M.A., 173:229, 1960.

374. Harris, N. H.: A method of measurement of femoral neck anteversion and a preliminary report on its practical application. J. Bone Joint Surg., 47-B:188, 1965.

375. Harris, N. H.: Acetabular growth potential in congenital dislocation of the hip and some factors upon which it may depend. Clin. Orthop., 119:99, 1976.

376. Harris, N. H., and Wilson, D. W.: Significance of femoral neck anteversion and the neck-shaft angle in the management of congenital dislocation of the hip. J. Bone Joint Surg., 52-B:775, 1970.

377. Harris, N. H., Lloyd-Roberts, G. C., and Gallien, R.: Acetabular development in congenital dislocation of the hip. J. Bone Joint Surg., 57-B:46, 1975.

378. Harris, W. H., Crothers, O. D., and Oh, I.: Autogenous bone grafting using the femoral head to correct severe acetabular deficiency for the total hip replacement. *In* The Hip: Proceedings of the Fourth Open Scientific Meeting of the Hip Society, St. Louis, Mosby, 1976, p. 161.

379. Harrison, T. J.: Development of the acetabulum in the rat. Part I. J. Anat., 95:12, 1961.

380. Harrison, T. J.: Development of the acetabulum in the rat. Part II. J. Anat., 92:483, 1958.

381. Harrison, T. J.: Development of the acetabulum in the rat. Part III. J. Anat., 92:483, 1958.

382. Harrold, A. J.: Problems in congenital dislocation of the hip. Br. Med. J., 1:1071, 1977.

383. Hart, V. L.: Primary genetic dysplasia of the hip with and without classical dislocation. J. Bone Joint Surg., 24:753, 1942.

384. Hart, V. L.: Congenital dislocation of the hip joint: Relationship between subluxation and congenital dislocation. J. Bone Joint Surg., 31-A:357, 1949.

385. Hart, V. L.: Congenital dislocation of the hip in the newborn and in early postnatal life. J.A.M.A., 43:1299, 1950.

386. Hart, V. L.: Congenital Dysplasia of the Hip Joint and Sequelae in the Newborn and Early Postnatal Life. Springfield, Ill., Thomas, 1952.

387. Hass, J.: A subtrochanteric osteotomy for pelvic support. J. Bone Joint Surg., 25:281, 1943.

388. Hass, J.: Congenital Dislocation of the Hip. Springfield, Ill., Thomas, 1951.

389. Hass, J.: Can congenital dislocation of the hip be prevented? N.Y. State J. Med., 58:847, 1958.

390. Hass, J., and Hass, R.: Arthrochalasis multiplex congenita. J. Bone Joint Surg., 50-A:663, 1958.

391. Helms, C. A., Moon, K. L., Jr., Genant, H. K., and Chafetz, N.: Magnetic resonance imaging: Skeletal application. Orthopedics, 7:1429, 1984.

392. Henriksson, L.: Measurement of femoral neck anteversion and inclination. A radiographic study in children. Acta Orthop. Scand. (Suppl.), 186:1, 1980.

393. Hensinger, R. N.: Congenital dislocation of the hip. CIBA Clin. Symp., 31:3, 1979.

394. Hensinger, R. N.: Treatment in early infancy: Birth to two months. *In* Tachdjian, M. O. (ed.): Congenital Dislocation of the Hip. New York, Churchill-Livingstone, 1982, pp. 159–171.

395. Hernandez, R. J.: Evaluation of congenital hip dysplasia and tibial torsion by computed tomography. J. Comput. Tomogr., 7:101, 1983.

396. Hernandez, R. J.: Concentric reduction of the dislocated hip: Computed tomographic evaluation. Radiology, 150:266, 1984.

397. Hernandez, R. J., Tachdjian, M. O., and Dias, L. S.: Hip CT in congenital dislocations: Appearance of tight iliopsoas tendon and pulvinar hypertrophy. A.J.R., 139:335, 1982.

398. Hernandez, R. J., Tachdjian, M. O., Poznanski, A. K., and Dias, L. S.: CT determination of femoral torsion. A.J.R., 137:97, 1981.

399. Herold, H. Z.: Avascular necrosis of the femoral head in children under the age of three. Clin. Orthop., 126:193, 1977.

400. Herold, H. Z.: Avascular necrosis of the femoral head due to malposition in untreated congenital dislocation of the hip. Int. Orthop., 2:293, 1979.

401. Herold, H. Z.: Avascular necrosis of the femoral head in congenital dislocation of the hip. Isr. J. Med. Sci., 16:295, 1980.

402. Herold, H. Z.: Unilateral congenital hip dislocation with contralateral avascular necrosis. Clin. Orthop., 148:196, 1980.

403. Herold, H. Z., and Daniel, D.: Reduction of neglected congenital dislocation of the hip in children over the age of six years. J. Bone Joint Surg., 61-B:1, 1979.

404. Heusner, L.: Über die angeborene Hüftluxation. Z. Orthop. Chir., 10:571, 1902.

405. Hey-Groves, E. W.: Some contributions to the reconstructive surgery of the hip. Br. J. Surg., 14:486, 1927.

406. Hey-Groves, E. W.: The treatment of congenital dislocation of the hip joint. *In* Milford, H. (ed.): The Robert Jones Birthday Volume. London, Oxford University, 1928, p. 73.

407. Heyman, C. H.: Long term results following a bone-shelf operation for congenital and some other dislocations of the hip in children. J. Bone Joint Surg., 45-A:1113, 1963.

408. Hiertonn, T., and James, U.: Congenital dislocation of the hip. J. Bone Joint Surg., 50-B:542, 1968.

409. Hilgenreiner, H.: Zur Frühdiagnose und Frühbehandlung der angeborenen Hüftgelenkverrenkung. Med. Klin., 21:1385, 1925.

410. Hippocrates: The Genuine Works of Hippocrates. (Translated by Adams.) London, Baillière, 1937.

411. Hirsch, C., and Scheller, S.: Results of treatment from birth of unstable hips. A clinical and radiographic 5-year follow-up. Clin. Orthop., 62:162, 1969.

412. Hirsch, C., and Scheller, S.: Results of treatment from birth of unstable hips. A 5-year follow-up. Acta Orthop. Scand. (Suppl.), 130:25, 1970.

413. Hjelmstedt, A., and Asplund, S.: Congenital dislocation of the hip: A biomechanical study in autopsy specimens. J. Pediatr. Orthop., 3:491, 1983.

414. Hjelmstedt, A., Asplund, S., and Rauschning, W.: Cryodissection and cryosectioning in biomechanical studies on congenital dislocation of the hip. Anat. Clin., 4:13, 1982.

415. Hoaglund, F. T., Yau, A. C. M. C., and Wong, W. L.: Orthoarthritis of the hip and other joints in South Chinese in Hong Kong. Incidence and related factors. J. Bone Joint Surg., 55-A:545, 1973.

416. Hoaglund, F. T., Kalamchi, A., Poon, R., Chow, S. P., and Yau, A. C. M. C.: Congenital dislocation hip and dysplasia in South Chinese. Int. Orthop., 4:243, 1981.

417. Hodgson, A. R.: Congenital dislocation of the hip. Br. Med. J., 2:647, 1961.
418. Hoffman, D. V., Simmons, E. H., and Barrington, T. W.: The results of the Chiari osteotomy. Clin. Orthop., 98:162, 1974.
419. Hoffmann-Daimler, S.: Ergebnisse und Konsequenzen der funktionellen Methode zur Behandlung der sogenannten angeborenen Hüftluxation. Z. Orthop., 102:569, 1967.
420. Holland, C.: Zur Technik der varisierenden und derotierenden intertrochanteren Femurosteotomie mit gleitlaschen Fixation bein kindlichen Luxationhüften. Z. Orthop., 100:293, 1965.
421. Hommel, H.-J. von: Zur problematik der teratologischen Hüftluxation. Beitr. Orthop. Traumatol., 13:481, 1966.
422. Hopf, A.: Eine biologische Methode zur Pfannengestaltung bei der Hüftdysplasie der Jugendlichen und Erwachsenen. In Verh. D.G.O.T. 52. Kongress, Stuttgart, 1965. Stuttgart, Enke, 1966, p. 420.
423. Hopf, A.: Hüftpfannenverlagerung durch doppelte Beckenosteotomie zur Behandlung der Hüftgelenksdysplasie und Subluxation bei Jungendlichen und Erwachsenen. Z. Orthop., 101:559, 1966.
424. Hopf, A.: Podiumsdiskussion zur Beckenosteotomie. In Verh. D.G.O.T. 56. Kongress, Wien, 1969. Stuttgart, Enke, 1970, p. 223.
425. Hopkins, J.: Neonatal hip examination screening. J. Bone Joint Surg., 57-B:256, 1975. (Abstr.)
426. Howe, W. W., Jr., Lacey, T., II, and Schwartz, R. P.: A study of the gross anatomy of the arteries supplying the proximal portion of the femur and the acetabulum. J. Bone Joint Surg., 32-A:856, 1950.
427. Howorth, B.: Development of present knowledge of congenital displacement of the hip. Clin. Orthop., 125:58, 1977.
428. Howorth, M. B.: Shelf stabilization of the hip—A report of fifty-three cases with particular emphasis on congenital dislocation. J. Bone Joint Surg., 17:945, 1935.
429. Howorth, M. B.: Congenital dislocation of the hip. Ann. Surg., 125:216, 1947.
430. Howorth, M. B.: Congenital dislocation of the hip. Technic of open reduction. Ann. Surg., 135:308, 1952.
431. Howorth, M. B.: The etiology of congenital dislocation of the hip. Clin. Orthop., 29:164, 1963.
432. Howorth, M. B., and Smith, H. W.: Congenital dislocation of the hip treated by open operation. J. Bone Joint Surg., 14:299, 1932.
433. Hoyt, W. A., Weiner, D. S., and O'Dell, H. W.: Congenital dislocation of the hip: An investigation into the efficacy of pre-manipulative traction. The prevention of aseptic necrosis of the hip. (Proc. Am. Orthop. Assoc., June 1972.) J. Bone Joint Surg., 54-A:1799, 1972. (Abstr.)
434. Hoyt, W. A., Troyer, M. L., Reef, T., and Sheik, S.: The proximal femoral epiphyses: Experimental and correlated clinical observations of their potential (Proc. Am. Acad. Orthop. Surg., January 1966.) J. Bone Joint Surg., 48-A:1026, 1966. (Abstr.)
435. Hubbard, D. D., and Staheli, L. T.: The direct radiographic measurement of femoral torsion using axial tomography. Technic and comparison with indirect radiographic method. Clin. Orthop., 86:16, 1972.
436. Huggler, A.: Beckenosteotomie nach Salter und varisierende Derotationsosteotomie des proximalen Femurendes. Z. Orthop., 100:91, 1965.
437. Hughes, J. R.: The surgical treatment of the dysplastic acetabulum in childhood. Proc. 12th Cong. Int. Soc. Orthop. Surg. Traumatol., Tel Aviv, Oct. 9–12, 1972.
438. Hughes, J. R.: Acetabular dysplasia in congenital dislocation of the hip. Proc. R. Soc. Med., 67:1178, 1974.
439. Hughes, J. R.: Intrinsic obstructive factors in congenital dislocation of the hip: The role of arthrography. In Tachdjian, M. O. (ed.): Congenital Dislocation of the Hip. New York, Churchill-Livingstone, 1982, pp. 227–245.
440. Hughes, J. R.: Acetabular dysplasia and acetabuloplasty. In Tachdjian, M. O. (ed.): Congenital Dislocation of the Hip. New York, Churchill-Livingstone, 1982, pp. 665–693.
441. Hummer, C. D., and MacEwen, G. D.: The coexistence of torticollis and congenital dysplasia of the hip. J. Bone Joint Surg., 54-A:1255, 1972.
442. Hummer, C. D., and MacEwen, G. D.: Torticollis and congenital hip dysplasia. J. Bone Joint Surg., 55-B:665, 1973.
443. Idelberger, K.: Die Erbpathologie der sogenanten angeborenen Hüftverrenkung. Munich, Urban & Schwarzenberg, 1951.
444. Igari, T., and Ujiie, K.: Histopathological study on congenital dislocation of the hip—with special reference to changes of the articular cartilage. J. Jpn. Orthop. Assoc., 36:1037, 1963.
445. Ilfeld, F. W.: The management of congenital dislocation and dysplasia of the hip by means of a special splint. J. Bone Joint Surg., 39-A:99, 1957.
446. Ilfeld, F. W., and Makin, M.: Damage to the capital femoral epiphysis due to Frejka pillow treatment. J. Bone Joint Surg., 59-A:654, 1977.
447. Ilfeld, F. W., O'Hara, J., Robins, G., Westin, G. W., and Williamson, M.: Congenital dislocation of the hip. Prognostic signs and methods of treatment with results. Clin. Orthop., 86:21, 1972.
448. Ingram, A. J., and Farrar, E. L.: Congenital dysplasia of the hips. Recognition and treatment. Pediatr. Clin. North Am., 2:1081, 1955.
449. Inman, V. T.: Functional aspects of the abductor muscles of the hip. J. Bone Joint Surg., 29:607, 1947.
450. Ippolito, E., Ishii, Y., and Ponseti, I. V.: Histologic, histochemical, and ultrastructural studies of the hip joint capsule and ligamentum teres in congenital dislocation of the hip. Clin. Orthop., 146:246, 1980.
451. Ishida, K.: Prevention of the development of the typical dislocation of the hip. Clin. Orthop., 126:167, 1977.
452. Ishii, Y., and Asai, H.: Zur Indikation der dreifachen Beckenosteotomie. Z. Orthop., 116:776, 1978.
453. Ishii, Y., and Ponseti, I. V.: Long-term results of closed reduction of complete congenital dislocation of the hip in children under one year of age. Clin. Orthop., 137:167, 1978.
454. Ishii, Y., Weinstein, S. L., and Ponseti, I. V.: Correlation between arthrograms and operative findings in congenital dislocation of the hip. Clin. Orthop., 153:138, 1980.
455. Iwahara, T., and Ikeda, A.: On the ipsilateral involvement of congenital muscular torticollis and congenital dislocation of the hip. J. Jpn. Orthop. Assoc., 35:1221, 1962.
456. Iwasaki, K.: Treatment of congenital dislocation of the hip by the Pavlik harness: Mechanism of reduction and usage. J. Bone Joint Surg., 65-A:760, 1983.
457. Izadpranah, M.: The importance of the combination of the special x-ray with arthrography in congenital displacement of the hip. (Author's transl.). Z. Orthop., 117:816, 1979.
458. Jacobs, J. E.: Metatarsus varus and hip dysplasia. Clin. Orthop., 16:203, 1960.
459. Jager, M., Fischer, V., and Zenker, H.: Indikation und Ergebnisse von Acetabuloplastik und Beckenosteotomie nach Chiari bei angeborener Hüftgelenkdysplasie. Arch. Orthop. Unfallchir., 73:245,A 1972.
460. Jakobsson, A.: The shelf operation: An evaluation of

results in congenital dysplasia, subluxation, and dislocation of the hip joint. Acta Orthop. Scand. (Suppl.), *15*:1, 1954.

461. James, J. I. P.: Editorial: Congenital dislocation of the hip. J. Bone Joint Surg., *54-B*:1, 1972.

462. James, U., and Sevastikoglou, J. A.: Analysis of the material of congenital dislocation of the hip. *In* Prevention of congenital dislocation of the hip joint in Sweden. Acta Orthop. Scand. (Suppl.), *130*:30, 1970.

463. Jani, L.: Die Entwicklung des Schenkelhalses nach der Trochanterversetzung. Arch. Orthop. Unfall-chir., *66*:127, 1969.

464. Jani, L., and Warner, H.: Spätergebnisse der Bernbeck'schen Drehvarisierungsosteotomie. Arch. Orthop. Unfallchir., *66*:30, 1969.

465. Jani, L., and Warner, H.: Die intertrochantere Derotations-variations-osteotomie bei der congenitalen Hüftluxation. *In* Behandlungsergebnisse bei der congenitalen Hüftluxation. Bern, Huber, 1974.

466. Jani, L., and Warner, H.: Die operative Behandlung der praearthrotischen Deformität der Hüftgelenkspfanne bei der congenitalen Hüftluxation. Z. Orthop., *112*:605, 1974.

467. Jansen, K., and Reimann, I.: Den tidlige diagnose of luxatio coxae congenita. Ugeskr. Laeger, *132*:485, 1970.

468. Jauch, G.: Iliosakralgelenksblockierung und pos. Patricksches Phänomen bei der Dysplasichüfte. Beitr. Orthop. Traumatol., *24*:554, 1977.

469. Jequier, S., and Rosman, M.: The double-headed femur—a complication of treatment of congenital hip dislocation. J. Can. Assoc. Radiol., *30*:125, 1979.

470. Joachimsthal, G.: Die angeborene Hüftverrenkung als Teilerscheinung anderer angeborener Anomalien. Z. Orthop., *22*:31, 1908.

471. Johnston, R. C.: Mechanical considerations of the hip joint. Arch. Surg., *107*:411, 1973.

472. Jones, D. A.: An assessment of the value of examination of the hip in the newborn. J. Bone Joint Surg., *55-B*:318, 1977.

473. Jones, D. A.: Sub-capital coxa valga after varus osteotomy for congenital dislocation of the hip. J. Bone Joint Surg., *59-B*:52, 1977.

474. Joyce, J. J., III, and Harty, M.: The anatomical basis of the hip joint exposures. Clin. Orthop., *98*:27, 1974.

475. Judet, J., Letournel, E., and Roy-Camille, R.: L'opération de "suspension" de la hanche. Presse Med., *72*:1367, 1964.

476. Jungmichel, D.: Zur Pathogenese der angeborenen Hüftluxation. Arch. Orthop. Unfallchir., *55*:476, 1963.

477. Juvara, E.: A propos de la butée iliaque: Nouveau procédé pour la construction d'un appui puissant pour le fémur, à l'aide d'un large greffon rigide, en forme de coin, prélévé sur la partie supérieure de la corticale interne du tibia. Rev. Chir., *51*:743, 1932.

478. Kadkhoda, M., Chung, S. M. K., and Adebonojo, F. O.: Congenital dislocation of the hip. Diagnostic screening and treatment. A comparative study of two populations of infants and children. Clin. Pediatr. (Phil.), *15*:239, 1976.

479. Kaiser, G.: Stand der Behandlung der sog. angeborenen Hüftluxation. Beitr. Orthop. Traumatol., *16*:558, 1969.

480. Kalamchi, A.: Modified Salter osteotomy. J. Bone Joint Surg., *64-A*:183, 1982.

481. Kalamchi, A., and MacEwen, G. D.: Avascular necrosis following treatment of congenital dislocation of the hip. J. Bone Joint Surg., *62-A*:876, 1980.

482. Kalamchi, A., and MacEwen, G. D.: Classification of vascular changes following treatment of congenital

dislocation of the hip. *In* Tachdjian, M. O. (ed.): Congenital Dislocation of the Hip. New York, Churchill-Livingstone, 1982, pp. 705–711.

483. Kalamchi, A., and MacFarlane, R.: The Pavlik harness: Results in patients over three months of age. J. Pediatr. Orthop., *2*:3, 1982.

484. Kalamchi, A., Schmidt, T., and MacEwen, G. D.: Congenital dislocation of the hip: Open reduction by the medial approach. Clin. Orthop., *169*:127, 1982.

485. Karpf, P. M., and Batzner, K.: Causes for femur head necrosis in the treatment of congenital hip dislocation. Fortschr. Med., *96*:1947, 1978.

486. Katz, J. F.: Teratological hip dislocation. Isr. J. Med. Sci., *16*:238, 1980.

487. Katz, M. P., GroAgono, B. J. S., and Soper, K. C.: Aetiology and treatment of congenital dislocation of the knee. J. Bone Joint Surg., *49-B*:112, 1967.

488. Kawamura, B.: The transverse pelvic osteotomy. J. Jpn. Orthop. Soc., *32*:65, 1959.

489. Kawamura, B.: Technical points of reconstructing the acetabular roof for the congenitally displaced hip. Proc. 11th Cong. Int. Soc. Orthop. Surg. Traumatol. Mexico, Oct. 6–10, 1969.

490. Kawamura, B., Hosono, S., and Yokogushi, K.: Dome osteotomy of the pelvis. *In* Tachdjian, M. O. (ed.): Congenital Dislocation of the Hip. New York, Churchill-Livingstone, 1982, pp. 609–623.

491. Kelikian, A. S., Tachdjian, M. O., Askew, M. J., and Jasty, M.: Greater trochanteric advancement of the proximal femur: A clinical and biomechanical study. *In* Hungerford, D. S. (ed.): The Hip: Proceedings of the 11th Open Scientific Meeting of the Hip Society, 1983. St. Louis, Mosby, 1983, pp. 77–105.

492. Keller, M. S., Harbhajan, S., and Chawla, S.: Sonographic delineation of the neonatal acetabular labrum. J. Ultrasound Med., *4*:501, 1985.

492a. Keller, M. S., Harbhajan, S. C., and Weiss, A. A.: Real-time sonography of infant hip dislocation. RadioGraphics, *6*(3):447, 1986.

492b. Keller, M. S., and Weiss, A. A.: Sonographic guidance for infant hip reduction under anesthesia. Pediatr. Radiol. *18*:174, 1988.

492c. Keller, M. S., Weltin, G. G., Rattner, Z., Taylor, K. J. W., and Rosenfield, N. S.: Normal instability of the hip in the neonate: US Standards. Radiology, *169*:733, 1988.

493. Kepley, R. F., and Weiner, D. S.: Treatment of congenital dysplasia-subluxation of the hip in children under one year of age. J. Pediatr. Orthop., *4*:413, 1981.

494. King, H. A., and Coleman, S. S.: Open reduction and femoral shortening in congenital dislocation of the hip. Orthop. Trans., *4*:302, 1980.

495. Kleinberg, S. M., and Lieberman, H. S.: The acetabular index in infants in relation to congenital dislocation of the hip. Arch. Surg., *32*:1049, 1936.

496. Klingberg, M. A., Chen, R., Chemke, J., and Levin, S.: Rising rates of congenital dislocation of the hip? Lancet, *2*:583, 1976.

497. Klisic, P.: Ostéotomie du bassin associé à la réduction de la hanche et la correction de l'orientation de la tête fémorale. *In* Chapchal, G. (ed.): Beckenosteotomie Pfannendachplastik. Stuttgart, Thieme, 1965, p. 97.

498. Klisic, P.: Traitement chirurgical de la luxation congénitale de la hanche par réduction-ostéotomie du bassin. Rev. Chir. Orthop., *53*:317, 1967.

499. Klisic, P.: Open reduction with femoral shortening and pelvic osteotomy. *In* Tachdjian, M. O. (ed.): Congenital Dislocation of the Hip. New York, Churchill-Livingstone, 1982, pp. 417–426.

500. Klisic, P., and Jankovic, L.: Combined procedure of

open reduction and shortening of the femur in treatment of congenital dislocation of the hips in older children. Clin. Orthop., *119*:60, 1976.

501. Klopfer, F. von: Zur problematik der Sofortbehandlung bei angeborener Hüftgelenksdysplasia. Z. Orthop., *79*:1, 1950.

502. Knake, J. E., and Kuhns, L. R.: A device to aid in positioning for the Andren-Von Rosen hip view. Radiology, *117*:735, 1975.

503. Knofler, E. W., Sensse, W., and Ziegert, D.: Revalgisierung nach varisierender Osteotomie. Beitr. Orthop. Traumatol., *17*:421, 1970.

504. Kollmann, K.: Frühergebnisse, Fehler und Gefahren der Beckenosteotomie. Z. Orthop., *102*:262, 1966.

505. Komprda, J.: Diagnostika urozene dysplazie Kycle u novorozencu. Acta Chir. Orthop. Traumatol. Cech., *41*:448, 1974.

506. Konig, F.: Osteoplastische Behandlung der kongenitalen Hüftgelenksluxation (mit Demonstration eines Pareparates). Verh. Dtsch. Ges. Chir., *20*:7, 1891.

507. Kovinski, I. T.: Arteriography of the hip in congenital dislocation of the hip. Ortop. Travmatol. Protez (Mosc.), *8*:55, 1969. (Am. Digest Foreign Orthop. Lit., 3rd Quarter, pp. 50–51, 1970. [Abstr.])

508. Kraus, B. S., and Schwartzman, J. R.: Congenital dislocation of the hip among the Fort Apache Indians. J. Bone Joint Surg., *39-A*:448, 1957.

509. Krida, A.: A new departure in the treatment of congenital dislocation of the hip. J. Bone Joint Surg., *13*:811, 1931.

510. Krida, A.: Analysis of results of early treatment of congenital dislocation of the hip by manipulation and osteoclasis for anterior dislocation. J. Bone Joint Surg., *18*:1018, 1936.

511. Kumar, S. J., and MacEwen, G. D.: Shelf operation. *In* Tachdjian, M. O. (ed.): Congenital Dislocation of the Hip. New York, Churchill-Livingstone, 1982, pp. 695–704.

512. Laage, H., Barnett, J. C., Brady, J. M., Dulingan, P. J., Jr., Fett, N. C., Jr., Galleher, T., and Schneider, B. A.: Horizontal lateral roentgenography of the hip in children. J. Bone Joint Surg., *35-A*:387, 1953.

513. LaGasse, D. J., and Staheli, L. T.: The measurement of femoral anteversion. A comparison of the fluoroscopic and biplane roentgenographic methods of measurement. Clin. Orthop., *86*:13, 1972.

514. LaGrange, J., and Dunoyer, J.: La vascularisation de la tête fémorale de l'enfant. Rev. Chir. Orthop., *48*:123, 1962.

515. LaGrange, J., Rigault, P., and Guyonvarch, G.: La réposition sanglante dans le traitement de la luxation inveterée de la hanche chez l'enfant. Opération de Colonna. Ann. Pediatr. (Paris), *14*:288, 1967.

516. LaGrange, J., Rigault, P., and Guyuonvarch, G.: Arthroplastie de la hanche avec interposition cartilagineuse dans le traitement de la luxation congénitale chez l'enfant. Rev. Chir. Orthop., *55*:55, 1969.

517. Lance, M.: Constitution d'une butée ostéoplastique dans les luxations et subluxations congénitales de la hanche. Presse Med., *33*:945, 1925.

518. Lang, J., and Wachsmuth, W.: Praktische Anatomie. 4. Bein und Statik. 2. Auflage. Berlin, Springer, 1972.

519. Lange, B.: Die unblutige Behandlung der angeborenen Hüftverrenkung. Munch. Med. Wochenschr., *51*:872, 1904.

520. Langenskiöld, A.: Technical aspects of the operative reduction of congenital dislocation of the hip. Acta Orthop. Scand., *20*:8, 1950.

521. Langenskiöld, A.: On the transposition of the iliopsoas muscle in operative reduction of congenital hip dislocation. Acta Orthop. Scand., *22*:295, 1952/1953.

522. Langenskiöld, A.: Growth arrest of the greater trochanter for prevention of acquired coxa vara. *In*

Tachdjian, M. O. (ed.): Congenital Dislocation of the Hip. New York, Churchill-Livingstone, 1982, pp. 713–719.

523. Langenskiöld, A., and Laurent, L. E.: Development of the concepts of pathogenesis and treatment of congenital dislocation of the hip. Clin. Orthop., *44*:41, 1966.

524. Langenskiöld, A., and Paavilainen, T.: The effect of traction treatment on the results of closed or open reduction for congenital dislocation of the hip: A preliminary report. *In* Tachdjian, M. O. (ed.): Congenital Dislocation of the Hip. New York, Churchill-Livingstone, 1982, pp. 365–371.

525. Langenskiöld, A., and Salenius, P.: Epiphyseodesis of the greater trochanter. Acta Orthop. Scand., *38*:199, 1967.

526. Langenskiöld, A., Sarpio, C., and Michelsson, J. E.: Experimental dislocation of the hip in the rabbit. J. Bone Joint Surg., *44-B*:209, 1962.

526a. Langer, R.: Ultrasonic investigation of the hip in newborns in the diagnosis of congenital hip dislocation; classification and results of a screening program. Skeletal Radiol., *16*:275, 1987.

527. Lapeyre, M., and Pous, J.-G.: Les ostéotomies fémorales chez l'enfant dans la maladie luxante. Rev. Chir. Orthop., *52*:501, 1966.

528. Larsen, L. J.: Surgical treatment of congenital dislocation of the hip in the older child. Abbot Lecture, 1975. Abbot Proc., *6*:1, 1975.

529. Lasda, N. A., Levinsohn, E. M., Yuan, H. A., and Bunnell, W. P.: Computerized tomography in disorders of the hip. J. Bone Joint Surg., *60-A*:1099, 1978.

530. Laurenson, R. D.: The acetabular index—a critical review. J. Bone Joint Surg., *41-B*:702, 1959.

531. Laurenson, R. D.: Bilateral anomalous development of the hip joint. Post mortem study of a human fetus, twenty-six weeks old. J. Bone Joint Surg., *46-A*:283, 1964.

532. Laurenson, R. D.: Development of the acetabular roof in the fetal hip. J. Bone Joint Surg., *47-A*:975, 1965.

533. Laurent, L. E.: Congenital dislocation of the hip. Acta Chir. Scand. (Suppl.), *179-A*:133, 1953.

534. Laurent, L. E.: Growth disturbances of the proximal end of the femur in the light of animal experiments. Acta Orthop. Scand., *28*:255, 1959.

535. Laurent, L. E.: Capsular arthroplasty (Colonna's operation) for congenital dislocation of the hip. Results of 102 operations. Acta Orthop. Scand., *34*:66, 1964.

536. Lauritzen, J.: Treatment of the congenital dislocation of the hip in the newborn. Acta Orthop. Scand., *45*:724, 1974.

537. Lauritzen, J.: The arterial supply of the femoral head in children. Acta Orthop. Scand., *45*:724, 1974.

538. LeCoeur, P.: Correction des défauts d'orientation de l'articulation coxofémorale par ostéotomie de l'isthme iliaque. Rev. Chir. Orthop., *51*:211, 1965.

539. LeCoeur, P.: Ostéotomie isthmique de bascule. *In* Chapchal, G. (ed.): Beckenosteotomie—Pfannendachplastik. Stuttgart, Thieme, 1965.

540. LeDamany, P.: Die angeborene Hüftgelenks-verrenkung. Z. Orthop. Chir., *21*:129, 1908.

541. LeDamany, P.: La Luxation Congénitale de la Hanche. Etudes d'anatomie comparée d'anthropogénie normale et pathologique, deductions therapeutique. Paris, Alcan, 1912.

542. LeDamany, P.: Congenital luxation of the hip. Am. J. Orthop. Surg., *11*:541, 1914.

543. Leffman, R.: Congenital dysplasia of the hip. J. Bone Joint Surg., *41-B*:689, 1959.

544. Lehman, W. B., Lubliner, J., Rosen, C., and Grant, A.: The use of computerized axial tomography in

congenital dislocation of the hip. Presented at the Pediatric Orthopedic Club of New York, March 17, 1982.

545. Lehman, W. B., Grant, A. D., Nelson, J., Robbins, H., and Milgram, J.: Hospital for Joint Diseases' traction system for preliminary treatment of congenital dislocation of the hip. J. Pediatr. Orthop., 3:104, 1983.

546. Leitz, G.: Pfannendachplastik bei Hüftdysplasie—eine Modifikation der geraden, einfachen Beckenosteotomie nach Chiari fur Erwachsene. Z. Orthop., 109:47, 1971.

547. Leitz, G.: Voraussetzungen zur Pfannenschwenkoperation nach Hopf. Orthop. Praxis, 10:16, 1974.

548. Leitz, G.: Necessarily disappointing results after triple osteotomy in the dysplastic hip joint. Arch. Orthop. Trauma. Surg., 95:241, 1979.

549. Lemoine, A.: Vascular changes after interference with the blood flow of the femoral head of the rabbit. J. Bone Joint Surg., 39-B:763, 1957.

550. Lenz, G.: Behandlung der kongenitalen Hüftluxation durch Extensions-Reposition und Hanausek-Retention. Sept. 1976. Z. Orthop., 115:646, 1977.

551. Leveuf, J.: Primary congenital subluxation of the hip. J. Bone Joint Surg., 29:149, 1947.

552. Leveuf, J.: Results of open reduction of "true" congenital dislocation of the hip. J. Bone Joint Surg., 30-A:875, 1948.

553. Leveuf, J., and Bertrand, P.: L'arthrographie dans la luxation congénitale de la hanche. Presse Méd., 45:437, 1937.

554. Leveuf, J., and Bertrand, P.: Luxations et Subluxations Congénitales de la Hanche. Leur Traitement Basé sur l'Arthrographie. Paris, Doin, 1946.

555. Lima, C., Esteve, R., and Trueta, J.: Osteochondritis in congenital dislocation of the hip. J. Bone Joint Surg., 30-A:875, 1960.

556. Limopaphayom, M., Bhongsvej, S., and Chitinanda, S. P.: Orthopedic problems in the newborn. J. Med. Assoc. Thai., 58:363, 1975.

557. Lindholm, T. S., Laurent, L. E., Osterman, K., and Snellman, O.: Perthes' disease of a severe type developing after satisfactory closed reduction of congenital dislocation of the hip. A report of three cases. J. Bone Joint Surg., 60-B:15, 1978.

558. Lindstrom, J. R., Ponseti, I. V., and Wenger, D. R.: Acetabular development after reduction in congenital dislocation of the hip. J. Bone Joint Surg., 61-A:112, 1979.

559. Lindstrom, N.: Brief contributions to the subject. Prevention of congenital dislocation of the hip in Sweden. Efficiency of early diagnosis and treatment. Acta Orthop. Scand. (Suppl.), 130:55, 1970.

560. Lloyd-Roberts, G. C., and Swann, M.: Pitfalls in the management of congenital dislocation of the hip. J. Bone Joint Surg., 48-B:666, 1966.

561. Lloyd-Roberts, G. C., Wetherill, M. H., and Fraser, M.: Trochanteric advancement for premature arrest of the femoral capital growth plate. J. Bone Joint Surg., 67-B:21, 1985.

562. Lordkipanidse, E. F. von: Genetische Untersuchung der angeborenen Hüftluxation (Zwillingsanalyse). Beitr. Orthop. Traumatol., 24:13, 1977.

563. Lorenz, A.: Pathologie und Therapie der Angeborenen Hüftverrenkung auf Grundlage von Hundert Operative Behandelten Fallen. Urban Schwarzenberg, 8:428, 1895.

564. Lorenz, A.: Cure of congenital luxation of the hip by bloodless reduction and weighting. Trans. Am. Orthop. Assoc., 9:254, 1896.

565. Lorenz, A.: La riduzione della lussazione congenita dell'anca. Arch. Orthop., 14:1, 1897.

566. Lorenz, A.: Die sogenannte angeborene Hüftverrenkung, ihre Pathologie und Therapie. Stuttgart, Enke, 1920.

567. Lorenz, A.: My Life and Work. New York, Scribner & Sons, 1936.

568. Love, B. R. T., Stevens, P. M., and Williams, P. F.: A long-term review of shelf arthroplasty. J. Bone Joint Surg., 62-B:321, 1980.

569. Low, J., and Allen, B. L., Jr.: The Pavlik harness for congenital dislocated hips. Am. J. Occup. Ther., 29:356, 1975.

570. Lowman, C. L.: The double-leaf shelf operation for congenital dislocation of the hip. J. Bone Joint Surg., 13:511, 1931.

571. Lude, L., and Taillard, W.: Le développement de la congruence articulaire de la hanche chez l'enfant. Rev. Chir. Orthop., 50:757, 1964.

572. Ludloff, K.: Zur Pathogenese und Therapie der angeborenen Hüftverrenkung. Jena, Klin. Jahrb., 10, 1902.

573. Ludloff, K.: The open reduction of the congenital hip dislocation by an anterior incision. Am. J. Orthop. Surg., 10:438, 1913.

574. Ludloff, K.: Die Erfahrungen bei der blutigen Reposition der angeborenen Hüftluxation mit seinem vorderen Schnitt. Zentralbl. Chir., 41:156, 1914.

575. Lust, G., Beilman, W. T., Dueland, D. J., and Farrell, P. W.: Intra-articular volume and hip joint instability in dogs with hip dysplasia. J. Bone Joint Surg., 62-A:576, 1980.

576. MacEwen, G. D., and Ramsey, P. L.: The hip. *In* Lovell, W. W., and Winter, R. B. (eds.): Pediatric Orthopedics. Philadelphia, Lippincott, 1978, pp. 721–804.

577. MacEwen, G. D., and Shands, A. R., Jr.: Oblique trochanteric osteotomy. J. Bone Joint Surg., 49-A:345, 1967.

578. MacKenzie, I. G.: Congenital dislocation of the hip: The development of a regional service. J. Bone Joint Surg., 54-B:18, 1972.

579. MacKenzie, I. G., and Wilson, J. G.: Problems encountered in the early diagnosis and management of congenital dislocation of the hip. J. Bone Joint Surg., 63-B:38, 1981.

580. MacKenzie, I. G., Seddon, H. J., and Trevor, D.: Congenital dislocation of the hip. J. Bone Joint Surg., 42-B:689, 1960.

581. McCarroll, H. R.: Congenital dislocation of the hip after the age of infancy. A.A.O.S. Instr. Course Lect., 12:69, 1955.

582. McCarroll, H. R.: Congenital dysplasia and congenital dislocation of the hip in early infancy. A.A.O.S. Instr. Course Lect., 14:183, 1957.

583. McCarroll, H. R.: Diagnosis and treatment of congenital subluxation (dysplasia) and dislocation of the hip in infancy. J. Bone Joint Surg., 47-A:612, 1965.

584. McCarroll, H. R., and Crego, C. H.: Primary anterior congenital dislocation of the hip. J. Bone Joint Surg., 21:648, 1939.

585. McCarroll, H. R., Jr., and McCarroll, H. R.: Primary anterior dislocation of the hip in infancy. J. Bone Joint Surg., 54-A:1340, 1972.

586. McCauley, R. G., Wunderlich, B. K., and Zimbler, S.: Air embolism as a complication of hip arthrography. Skeletal Radiol., 6:11, 1981.

587. McFarland, B.: Some observations on congenital dislocation of the hip. J. Bone Joint Surg., 30-B:54, 1956.

588. McIntosh, R., Merritt, K. K., Richards, M. R., Samuels, M. H., and Bellows, M. T.: The incidence of congenital malformations: A study of 5,964 pregnancies. Pediatrics, 14:505, 1954.

589. McKay, D. W.: A comparison of the innominate and the pericapsular osteotomy in the treatment of con-

genital dislocation of the hip. Clin. Orthop., 98:124, 1974.

590. McKay, D. W.: Classification of pelvic osteotomies: Principles and experiences. *In* Tachdjian, M. O. (ed.): Congenital Dislocation of the Hip. New York, Churchill-Livingstone, 1982, pp. 501–523.

591. McKay, D. W.: Pemberton's innominate osteotomy: Indications, technique, results, pitfalls, and complications. *In* Tachdjian, M. O. (ed.): Congenital Dislocation of the Hip. New York, Churchill-Livingstone, 1982, pp. 543–554.

592. McKay, D. W., Rising, E., and Keblisch, P.: Comparison of the innominate osteotomy (Salter) with the pericapsular osteotomy (Pemberton). Proc. Am. Acad. Orthop. Surg., 50-A:832, 1968.

593. McKibbin, B.: Anatomical factors in the stability of the hip joint in the newborn. J. Bone Joint Surg., 52-B:148, 1970.

594. McKinnon, B., Bosse, M. J., and Browning, W. H.: Congenital dysplasia of the hip: The lax (subluxatable) newborn hip. J. Pediatr. Orthop., 4:422, 1984.

595. McSweeny, A.: A comment from the periphery on innominate osteotomy. Clin. Orthop., 98:195, 1974.

596. Magilligan, D. J.: Calculation of the angle of anteversion by means of horizontal lateral roentgenography. J. Bone Joint Surg., 38-A:1231, 1956.

597. Magnant, J.-S., and Maurin, X.: L'ostéotomie pelvienne. J. Chir. (Paris), 99:275, 1970.

598. Magnant, J.-S., and Maurin, X.: L'arthroacétabuloplastie de Salter. Sa technique, ses indications, et ses resultats. J. Chir. (Paris), 102:53, 1971.

599. Makin, M.: Closure of the epiphysis of the femoral head and of the triradiate cartilage of the acetabulum following surgery for congenital hip dislocation. Isr. J. Med. Sci., 16:307, 1980.

600. Maquet, P.: Réduction de la pression articulaire de la hanche par latéralisation chirurgicale du grand trochanter. Acta Orthop. Belg., 42:266, 1976.

601. Marafioti, R. L., and Westin, G. L.: Factors influencing results of acetabuloplasty in children. J. Bone Joint Surg., 62-A:765, 1980.

602. Marchetti, P. G.: Classification and treatment of hip subluxation in childhood and adolescence. *In* Tachdjian, M. O. (ed.): Congenital Dislocation of the Hip. New York, Churchill-Livingstone, 1982, pp. 321–337.

603. Marchetti, P. G.: Open reduction of congenital dislocation of the hip: 384 consecutive cases. *In* Tachdjian, M. O. (ed.): Congenital Dislocation of the Hip. New York, Churchill-Livingstone, 1982, pp. 401–415.

604. Marchetti, P. G., Faldini, A., and Mar Mau, H.: Bemerkungen zu E. Fettweiss, "Dur Prophylaxes der kindlichen Hüftluxations-keidens." Z. Orthop., 119:207, 1972.

605. Marino, D., and Gabriele, P. P.: Su di un caso de lussazione congenita dell'anca in un feto prematuro. Chir. Organi Mov. (Bologna), 62:71, 1975.

606. Martin, H. E.: Geometrical-anatomical factors and their significance in the early x-ray diagnosis of the hip joint disease in children. Radiology, 56:842, 1951.

607. Martz, C. D., and Taylor, C. C.: The 45-degree angle roentgenographic study of the pelvis in congenital dislocation of the hip. J. Bone Joint Surg., 36-A:528, 1954.

608. Marx, V. O.: New observations in congenital dislocation of the hip in the newborn. J. Bone Joint Surg., 20:1095, 1938.

609. Masse, P., and Guepin, F.: Les conséquences psychologiques du traitement des luxations congénitales de la hanche. Rev. Chir. Orthop., 50:213, 1964.

610. Massie, W. K.: Vascular epiphyseal changes in congenital dislocation of the hip. Results in adults compared with results in coxa plana and in congenital

611. Massie, W. K.: Congenital dislocation of the hip—its causes and effects. Clin. Orthop., 8:103, 1956.

612. Massie, W. K., and Howorth, M. B.: Congenital dislocation of the hip. Part I. Method of grading results. J. Bone Joint Surg., 32-A:519, 1950.

613. Massie, W. K., and Howorth, M. B.: Congenital dislocation of the hip. Part II. Results of open reduction as seen in early adult period. J. Bone Joint Surg., 33-A:171, 1951.

614. Massie, W. K., and Howorth, M. B.: Congenital dislocation of the hip. Part III. Pathogenesis. J. Bone Joint Surg., 33-A:190, 1951.

615. Massie, W. K., and Howorth, M. B.: Vascular epiphysial changes in congenital dislocation of the hip. J. Bone Joint Surg., 33-A:284, 1951.

616. Matles, A. L.: Alterations in the roentgenograms of the newborn hip as a result of position. Clin. Orthop., 38:100, 1965.

617. Matles, A. L.: A microscopic study of the newborn fibrocartilaginous acetabular labrum. Clin. Orthop., 54:197, 1967.

618. Matsoukas, J., Papadimitriou, D., and Euthymidu, C.: Etude histologique des muscles pelvi-fémoraux chez les enfants porteurs d'une luxation congénitale de la hanche. Helv. Paediatr. Acta, 24:201, 1962.

619. Matzen, P. F.: Zur Technik der intertrochanteren varisierenden und detorquierenden Osteotomie. Zentralbl. Chir., 89:1735, 1964.

620. Mau, H.: Die Trochanterresektion als physiologische Behandlung der Coxa vara. Z. Orthop., 85:48, 1955.

621. Mau, H.: Spontaneous straightening of the femoral neck following adduction osteotomy in congenital dysplasia of the hip. J. Bone Joint Surg., 43-A:285, 1961.

622. Mau, H.: Form- und Funktionsprobleme bei der frühkindlichen operativen Behandlung der sogenannten angeborenen Hüftluxation. Langenbecks Arch. Klin. Chir., 306:174, 1964.

623. Mau, H.: Subtrochantarer Ermüdungsbruch bei alter hochstehender Hüftluxation. Z. Orthop., 103:537, 1967.

624. Mau, H.: Bemerkungen zu E. Fettweis "Zur Prophylaxe des kindlichen Hüftluxations-keidens." Z. Orthop., 119:207, 1972.

625. Mau, H., Dorr, W. M., Henkel, L., and Lutsche, J.: Open reduction of congenital dislocation of the hip by Ludloff's method. J. Bone Joint Surg., 53-A:1281, 1971.

626. Mears, D. C., and Fredensborg, N.: Treatment of congenital dislocation of the hip. Lancet, 2:780, 1974.

627. Medalie, J. H., Makin, H. M., Alkalay, E., Yofe, J., Cochair, Z., and Ehrlich, D.: Congenital dislocation of the hip. A clinical-epidemiological study. Jerusalem 1954–1960. I. Retrospective incidence study. Isr. J. Med. Sci., 2:212, 1966.

628. Medbo, I.: Follow-up study of hip joint dysplasia treated from the newborn stage. Acta Orthop. Scand., 35:338, 1965.

629. Mendes, D. G.: A splint for congenital dislocation of the hip. J. Bone Joint Surg., 52-A:588, 1970.

630. Metaizeau, J. P., and Prevot, J.: Le retentissement des ostéotomies innominées sur le cotyle controlateral. Rev. Chir. Orthop., 66:453, 1980.

631. Metaizeau, J. P., Prevot, J., and Piechoki, M.: Pemberton's pelvic osteotomy in the management of residual dysplasias of the socket. Chir. Pediatr., 21:225, 1980.

632. Michelsson, J.-E., and Langenskiöld, A.: Dislocation or subluxation of the hip. Regular sequels of immobilization of the knee in extension in young rabbits. J. Bone Joint Surg., 54-A:1177, 1972.

633. Milgram, J. E.: Viewpoints in treatment of congenital

dislocation of the hip in infancy. J. Bone Joint Surg., 40-A:731, 1958.

634. Milgram, J. E.: Congenital dislocation of the hip in infancy, methods of minimizing aseptic necrosis. Manitoba Med. Rev., 42:426, 1962.

635. Milgram, J. E.: Prevention and treatment of aseptic necrosis in congenital dislocation of the hip. J. Bone Joint Surg., 48-B:48, 1966.

636. Milgram, J. W.: Morphology of untreated bilateral congenital dislocation of the hips in a seventy-four-year-old man. Clin. Orthop., 119:112, 1976.

637. Milgram, J. W., and Tachdjian, M. O.: Pathology of the limbus in untreated teratologic congenital dislocation of the hip. A case report of a ten-month-old infant. Clin. Orthop., 119:107, 1976.

638. Millis, M. B., and Hall, J. E.: Transiliac lengthening of the lower extremity. A modified innominate osteotomy for the treatment of postural imbalance. J. Bone Joint Surg., 61-A:1182, 1979.

639. Misasi, N., and Vallario, V.: Present status of the surgical treatment of congenital dislocation of the hip. Bull. Hosp. Joint Dis., 33:30, 1971.

640. Mitchell, G. P.: Arthrography in congenital displacement of the hip. J. Bone Joint Surg., 45-B:88, 1963.

641. Mitchell, G. P.: Congenital dislocation of the hip. Scot. Med. J., 15:468, 1970.

642. Mitchell, G. P.: Problems in the early diagnosis and management of congenital dislocation of the hip. J. Bone Joint Surg., 54-B:4, 1972.

643. Mitchell, G. P.: The delayed Trendelenburg hip test. Int. Congress Series, No. 291, S.I.C.O.T., 1972.

644. Mitchell, G. P.: Chiari medial displacement osteotomy. Clin. Orthop., 98:146, 1974.

645. Mitchell, G. P.: Congenital dislocation of the hip. J. R. Coll. Surg. Edin., 22:81, 1977.

646. Mitchell, G. P.: Complications of early treatment of congenital dislocation of the hip. *In* Tachdjian, M. O. (ed.): Congenital Dislocation of the Hip. New York, Churchill-Livingstone, 1982, pp. 215–226.

647. Mitchell, G. P.: The subluxating hip following treatment for congenital dislocation. *In* Tachdjian, M. O. (ed.): Congenital Dislocation of the Hip. New York, Churchill-Livingstone, 1982, pp. 305–319.

648. Mittelmeier, H.: Zur Kombination von intertrochanterer Femurosteotomie und Pfannendachplastik (unter Verwendung des Osteotomie-keiles). Beitr. Orthop. Traumatol., 11:9, 1964.

649. Mittelmeier, H.: Simultane Kombination der intertrochanteren Femurosteotomie mit der Pfannendachplastik nach Lance unter Verwendung des Osteotomiekeiles. *In* Int. Symp. Bopfd. Plastik. Stuttgart, G. Thieme, 1965, p. 54.

650. Mohing, W.: The development of the hip joint after intertrochanteric osteotomy. Proc. 8th Cong. Int. Soc. Orthop. Surg. Traumatol., New York, Sept. 4–9, 1960.

651. Monticelli, G.: Intertrochanteric femoral osteotomy with concentric reduction of the femoral head in treatment of residual congenital acetabular dysplasia. Clin. Orthop., 119:48, 1976.

652. Monticelli, G., and Milella, P.: Indications for treatment of congenital dislocation of the hip by the surgical medial approach. *In* Tachdjian, M. O. (ed.): Congenital Dislocation of the Hip. New York, Churchill-Livingstone, 1982, pp. 385–399.

653. Monticelli, G., Mollica, Q., and Milella, P. P.: La displasia congenita dell'anca nell'eta pediatrica—L'osteotomia di centramento. Relazione 57th Congresso Soc. Ital. Ortop. Traum., 1, 1972.

654. Moon, K. L., Genant, H. K., Davis, P. L., Chafetz, N. I., Helms, C. A., Morris, J. M., Rodrigo, J. J., Jergesen, H. E., Brasch, R. C., and Bovill, E. G.: Nuclear magnetic resonance imaging in orthopedics: Principles and applications. J. Orthop. Res., 1:101, 1983.

655. Moore, F. H.: Screening for congenital dislocation of the hip. J. Irish Med. Assoc., 67:104, 1974.

656. Morel, G.: L'ostéotomie de Salter dans le traitement de la malformation luxante de la hanche après l'age de la marche. Rev. Chir. Orthop., 57:175, 1971.

657. Morel, G.: The treatment of congenital dislocation and subluxation of the hip in the older child. Acta Orthop. Scand., 46:364, 1975.

658. Morel, G., and Briard, J. L.: Progressive gradual reduction of the dislocated hip in the child after walking age. *In* Tachdjian, M. O. (ed.): Congenital Dislocation of the Hip. New York, Churchill-Livingstone, 1982, pp. 373–383.

659. Morgan, J. D., and Somerville, E. W.: Normal and abnormal growth of the upper end of the femur. J. Bone Joint Surg., 42-B:264, 1969.

660. Morin, C., Harcke, H. T., and MacEwen, G. D.: The infant hip: Real-time US assessment of acetabular development. Radiology, 157:673, 1985.

661. Morscher, E.: Our experience with Salter's innominate osteotomy in the treatment of hip dysplasia. *In* Weil, U. H. (ed.): Progress in Orthopedic Surgery, Vol. 2. Berlin, Springer, 1978, p. 107.

662. Morville, P.: On the anatomy and pathology of the hip joint. Acta Orthop. Scand., 7:107, 1936.

663. Muller, G. M., and Seddon, H. J.: Late results of treatment of congenital dislocation of the hip. J. Bone Joint Surg., 35-B:342, 1953.

664. Nagura, S.: Zur Ätiologie der angeborenen Hüftverrenkung. Zentralbl. Chir., 80:1933, 1955.

665. Naito, K.: Congenital dislocation of the hip. J. Jpn. Orthop. Assoc., 13:1086, 1968.

666. Nakamura, K.: Arthrographic study of congenital dislocation of the hip joint. J. Jpn. Orthop. Assoc., 42:491, 1968.

667. Nelson, M. A.: Early diagnosis of congenital dislocation of the hip. J. Bone Joint Surg., 48-B:388, 1966.

668. Netter, R.: Technique opératoire. Note sur un procédé clinique de mésure de l'anteversion du col fémoral. Rev. Orthop., 26:374, 1939.

669. Nichols, E. H., and Bradford, E. H.: The surgical anatomy of congenital dislocation of the hip joint. Am. J. Med. Sci., 119:629, 1900.

670. Nicholson, J. T., Kopell, H. P., and Mattei, F. A.: Regional stress angiography of the hip. J. Bone Joint Surg., 36-A:503, 1954.

671. Niclasen, S. D.: Family studies of relation between Perthes disease and congenital dislocation of the hip. J. Med. Genet., 15:296, 1978.

672. Nicod, L.: Ostéotomies du bassin selon Chiari. *In* Chapchal, G. (ed.): Beckenosteotomie—Pfannendachplastik. Stuttgart, Thieme, 1965, p. 120.

673. Nishimura, H.: Incidence of malformations in abortions. *In* Fraser, C., and McKusick, V. A. (eds.): Congenital Malformations. Amsterdam, Excerpta Medica, 1970, p. 275.

673a. Novick, G., Ghelman, B., and Schneider, M.: Sonography of the neonatal and infant hip. AJR, 141:639, 1983.

674. Ogden, J. A.: Anatomic and histologic study of factors affecting development and evolution of avascular necrosis in congenital hip dislocation. *In* The Hip. Proceedings of the Second Annual Meeting of the Hip Society. St. Louis, Mosby, 1974, pp. 125–153.

675. Ogden, J. A.: Changing patterns of proximal femoral vascularity. J. Bone Joint Surg., 56-A:941, 1974.

676. Ogden, J. A.: Treatment positions for congenital dysplasia of the hip. J. Pediatr., 86:732, 1975.

677. Ogden, J. A.: Dynamic pathobiology of congenital

hip dysplasia. *In* Tachdjian, M. O. (ed.): Congenital Dislocation of the Hip. New York, Churchill-Livingstone, 1982, pp. 93–144.

678. Ogden, J. A.: Normal and abnormal circulation. *In* Tachdjian, M. O. (ed.): Congenital Dislocation of the Hip. New York, Churchill-Livingstone, 1982, pp. 59–92.

679. Ogden, J. A., and Jensen, P. S.: Roentgenography of congenital dislocation of the hip. Radiology, *119*:189, 1976.

680. Ogden, J. A., and Moss, H. L.: Pathologic anatomy of congenital hip disease. *In* Progress in Orthopedic Surgery, Vol. 2. Heidelberg, Springer, 1978, p. 3.

681. Ogden, J. A., and Southwick, W. O.: A possible cause of avascular necrosis complicating the treatment of congenital dislocation of the hip. J. Bone Joint Surg., 55-A:1770, 1973.

682. Ogden, J. A., and Southwick, W. O.: Cartilage canals and epiphyseal osteogenesis. Trans. Orthop. Reg. Soc., *1*:85, 1975.

683. Oh, W. H.: Dislocation of the hip in birth defects. Orthop. Clin. North Am., 7:315, 1976.

684. Ohl, E., and Nicod, L.: Röntgenologische Hinweiszeichen auf schwere Kopfumbau Storungen bei der Behandlung kongenitaler Hüftluxationen. Z. Orthop., *114*:960, 1976.

685. Oki, T., Terashim, Y., Murachi, S., and Nogami, H.: Clinical features and treatment of joint dislocations in Larsen's syndrome. Report of three cases in one family. Clin. Orthop., *119*:206, 1976.

686. Olah, J.: Eine neue diagnostische Methode der angeborenen Hüftluxation. Z. Orthop., *106*:422, 1969.

687. O'Malley, A. G.: Congenital dislocation of the hip. J. Bone Joint Surg., *47-B*:188, 1965.

688. Ombredanne, L.: Precis Clinique et Opératoire de Chirurgie Infantile. Paris, Masson, 1932.

689. O'Rahilly, R., and Gardner, E.: The embryology of moveable joints. *In* Sokoloff, L. (ed.): The Joints and Synovial Fluid I. New York, Academic, 1978, p. 82.

690. Ortolani, M.: Un segno poco noto e sue importanza per la diagnosi precoce di preussasione congenita dell'anca. Pediatria, *45*:129, 1937.

691. Ortolani, M.: La lussazione congenital dell'anca. Bologna, Cappelli, 1948.

692. Ortolani, M.: Mezzi divaricatori vecchi e nuovi nella profilasso-correzione della lussazione congenita dell'anca. Chir. Organi Mov., *38*:154, 1953.

693. Ortolani, M.: Le diagnostic clinique, fait par la recherche du signe du ressaut, est le seul moyen permettant le traitement vraiment précoce et total de la luxation congénitale de la hanche. Bull Acad. Nat. Med. (Paris), *141*:188, 1957.

694. Ortolani, M.: La lussazione congenita dell'anca-nuovi criteri diagnostici e profilatico-correttivi. Bologna, Cappelli, 1976.

695. Ortolani, M.: The classic: Congenital hip dysplasia in the light of early and very early diagnosis. Clin. Orthop., *119*:6, 1976.

696. Ortolani, M., and Ortolani, M.: Dysplasia of the hip and pre- and postnatal posture. Clin. Orthop., *26*:219, 1975–1976.

697. Owen, R.: Early diagnosis of the congenitally unstable hip. J. Bone Joint Surg., *50-B*:453, 1968.

698. Owen, R., and Corkery, P. H.: Congenital hip dislocation. Br. Med. J., 3:370, 1971.

699. Ozonoff, M. B.: Controlled arthrography of the hip: A technic of fluoroscopic monitoring and recording. Clin. Orthop., *93*:260, 1973.

700. Paavilainen, T.: Vetohoidon vaikutus synnynnaisen lonkkakuksaation hoitotuloksiin (with English summary: The effect of traction treatment on the results of treatment for congenital dislocation of the hip). Helsinki, Helsinki University, 1980.

701. Packer, J. W., Lefkowitz, L. A., and Ryder, C. T.: Habitual dislocation of the hip treated by innominate osteotomy. Clin. Orthop., *83*:184, 1972.

702. Padovani, J. P.: La réorientation du cotyle par triple ostéotomie du bassin. Technique de Pol Le Coeur. Nouv. Presse Med., 5:921, 1976.

703. Padovani, J. P., Faure, F., Devred, P., Jacquemier, M., and Sarrat, P.: Intérêt et indications de la tomodensitométrie dans le bilan des luxations congénitales de la hanche. Ann. Radiol. (Paris), *22*:188, 1979.

704. Padovani, J. P., and Rigault, P.: Triple ostéotomie pelvienne de Pol Le Coeur. Indications chez l'enfant. Rev. Chir. Orthop., *63*:25, 1977.

705. Palmen, K.: Preluxation of the hip joint: Diagnosis and treatment in the newborn and the diagnosis of the hip joint in Sweden during the years 1948–1960. Acta Pediatr. (Suppl.), *129*:50, 1961.

706. Palmen, K.: Examination of the newborn for congenital dislocation of the hip. Dev. Med. Child Neurol., 5:45, 1963.

707. Palmen, K.: Preluxation of the hip in the newborn. The diagnostic work in Sweden during the years 1953–1966. Acta Orthop. Scand., *130*:8, 1970.

708. Palmen, K.: Late-diagnosis congenital dislocation of the hip joint (CDH). Lakartidningen, 77:2786, 1980.

709. Palmen, K., and Von Rosen, S.: Late diagnosis dislocation of the hip joint in children. Acta Orthop. Scand., *46*:90, 1975.

710. Papadopulos, J. S., Agnantis, J., and Popp, W.: Luxationsperthes—Gibt es röntgenologische Moglichkeiten fur die Voraussage und der Frühdiagnose? Z. Orthop., *115*:752, 1977.

711. Papavasiliou, V. A., and Piggott, H.: Acetabular floor thickening and femoral head enlargement in congenital dislocation of the hip: Lateral displacement of femoral head. J. Pediatr. Orthop., 3:22, 1983.

712. Parisel, F.: Le depistage précoce de la luxation de la hanche. Bruxelles Med., *49*:341, 1969.

713. Parkin, D. M.: The efficiency of notification of congenital dislocation of the hip. Public Health, *94*:68, 1980.

714. Parkkulainen, K. V., and Solomon, K. A.: The influence of early treatment on the prognosis of congenital dislocation of the hip joint. Ann. Paediatr., 5:290, 1959.

715. Paterson, D. C.: Innominate osteotomy. Its role in treatment of congenital dislocation and subluxation of the hip joint. Clin. Orthop., *98*:198, 1974.

716. Paterson, D. C.: The early diagnosis and treatment of congenital dislocation of the hip. Clin. Orthop., *119*:28, 1976.

717. Paterson, D. C.: The early diagnosis and screening of congenital dislocation of the hip. *In* Tachdjian, M. O. (ed.): Congenital Dislocation of the Hip. New York, Churchill-Livingstone, 1982, pp. 145–157.

718. Pauwels, F.: Gesommelte Abhandlungen zur Funktionellen Anatomie des Bewegungsapparates. New York, Springer, 1965.

719. Pavlik, A.: Die funktionelle Behandlungsmethode mittels Reimenbugel als Prinzip der konservativen Therapie bei angeborenen Hüftgelenksverrenkungen der Sauglinge. Z. Orthop., *89*:341, 1957.

720. Peic, S.: Verhalten der Beinlänge bei "angeborener" Hüftverrenkung. Z. Orthop., *119*:435, 1972.

721. Pemberton, P. A.: Osteotomy of the ilium with rotation of the acetabular roof for congenital dislocation of the hip. J. Bone Joint Surg., *40-A*:724, 1958.

722. Pemberton, P. A.: Pericapsular osteotomy of the ilium for congenital subluxation and dislocation of the hip. J. Bone Joint Surg., 47-A:65, 1965.

723. Pemberton, P. A.: Pericapsular osteotomy of the ilium for the treatment of congenitally dislocated hips. Clin. Orthop., *98*:41, 1974.

724. Perkins, G.: Signs by which to diagnose congenital dislocation of the hip. Lancet, 1:648, 1928.

725. Perlik, P. C., Westin, G. W., and Marafioti, R. L.: Combination pelvic osteotomy for acetabular dysplasia in children. J. Bone Joint Surg., 67-A:842, 1985.

726. Peterson, H. A., Klassen, R. A., McLeod, R. A., and Hoffman, A. D.: The use of computed tomography in dislocation of the hip and femoral neck antetorsion in children. J. Bone Joint Surg., 63-B:198, 1981.

727. Petit, P., Queneau, P., and Borde, J.: Traitement des luxations et subluxations congénitales de la hanche dans la première enfance. Rev. Chir. Orthop., 48:148, 1962.

728. Petit, P., Queneau, P., Carioz, H., Dubousset, J., Lebard, J. P., and Mechin, J. F.: Monographie des Annales de Chirurgie. Paris, L'Expansion Scientifique, 1974.

729. Petrie, J. G.: Congenital dislocation of the hip in infancy. J. Bone Joint Surg., 47-A:607, 1965.

730. Place, M. J., Parkin, D. M., and Fritton, J. M.: Effectiveness of neonatal screening for congenital dislocation of the hip. Lancet, 2:249, 1978.

731. Platou, E.: Luxatio coxae congenita. A follow-up study of four hundred and six cases of closed reduction. J. Bone Joint Surg., 35-A:843, 1953.

732. Platou, E.: Rotation osteotomy in the treatment of congenital dislocation of the hip. J. Bone Joint Surg., 35-A:48, 1953.

733. Platt, H.: Congenital dislocation of the hip (editorial). J. Bone Joint Surg., 35-B:339, 1953.

734. Platt, H.: Congenital dislocation of the hip: Its early recognition and treatment. Br. J. Surg., 45:438, 1958.

735. Poggi, A.: Contribution to the radical treatment of congenital unilateral coxo-femoral dislocation. Clin. Orthop., 98:5, 1974.

736. Pointu, J., François, M., and Butel, J.: Notre pratique de l'intervention de Salter dans le traitement des luxations et subluxations congénitales de la hanche. Rev. Chir. Orthop., 58:65, 1972.

737. Ponseti, I. V.: Causes of failure of the treatment of congenital dislocation of the hip. J. Bone Joint Surg., 26:775, 1944.

738. Ponseti, I. V.: Pathomechanics of the hip after the shelf operation. J. Bone Joint Surg., 28:229, 1946.

739. Ponseti, I. V.: Congenital dislocation of the hip in the infant. A.A.O.S. Instruct. Course Lect., 10:161, 1953.

740. Ponseti, I. V.: Non-surgical treatment of congenital dislocation of the hip. J. Bone Joint Surg., 48:1392, 1966.

741. Ponseti, I. V.: Growth and development of the acetabulum in the normal child. Anatomical, histological, and roentgenographic studies. J. Bone Joint Surg., 60-A:575, 1978.

742. Ponseti, I. V.: Morphology of the acetabulum in congenital dislocation of the hip. Gross, histological and roentgenographic studies. J. Bone Joint Surg., 60-A:586, 1978.

743. Ponseti, I. V., and Becker, J. R.: Congenital metatarsus adductus: The results of treatment. J. Bone Joint Surg., 48:702, 1966.

744. Ponseti, I. V., and Frigerio, E. R.: Results of treatment of congenital dislocation of the hip. J. Bone Joint Surg., 41-A:823, 1959.

745. Potter, E. L.: Bilateral renal agenesis. J. Pediat., 29:68, 1946.

746. Potter, E. L.: Bilateral absence of ureters and kidneys. A report of 50 cases. Obstet. Gynecol., 25:3, 1965.

747. Pous, J. G., Dimeglio, A., and Daoud, A.: Is treatment of CDH by progressive reduction by traction still advisable? (Author's transl.) Rev. Chir. Orthop., 65:327, 1979.

748. Pouliquen, L., and Denis, P.: Le depistage radiologique précoce de la luxation congénitale de la hanche. J. Radiol., 46:572, 1965.

749. Purath, W.: Observation of the so-called "anti-Chiari effect": subsequent to osteotomy of the pelvis in children. (Author's transl.) Z. Orthop., 117:301, 1979.

750. Putti, V.: Congenital dislocation of the hip. Surg. Gynecol. Obstet., 42:449, 1926.

751. Putti, V.: Per la cura precoce della lussazione congenital dell'anca. Arch. Ital. Chir., 18:653, 1927.

752. Putti, V.: Early treatment of congenital dislocation of the hip. J. Bone Joint Surg., 11:798, 1929.

753. Putti, V.: Treatment of congenital absence of tibia or fibula. Chir. Organi Mov., 7:513, 1929.

754. Putti, V.: Early treatment of congenital dislocation of the hip. J. Bone Joint Surg., 15:16, 1933.

755. Putti, V.: Anatomia Della Lussazione Congenita Dell'Anca. Bologna, Cappelli, 1935.

756. Putti, V.: Die Anatomie der angeborenen Hüftverrenkung. Stuttgart, F. Enke, 1937.

757. Putti, V.: Early treatment of congenital dislocation of the hip. J. Bone Joint Surg., 47:602, 1965.

758. Putti, V., and Zanoli, R.: Tecnica dell'artrotomia per la riduzione della lussazione congenita dell'anca. Chir. Organi Mov., 16:1, 1931.

759. Rab, G. T.: Biomechanical aspects of the Salter osteotomy. In The Hip: Proceedings of the Fourth Meeting of the Hip Society, 1976. St. Louis, Mosby, 1976, pp. 67–74.

760. Rab, G. T.: Biomechanical aspects of Salter osteotomy. Clin. Orthop., 132:82, 1978.

761. Rab, G. T.: Preoperative roentgenographic evaluation for osteotomies about the hip in children. J. Bone Joint Surg., 63-A:306, 1981.

762. Rabin, D. L., Barnett, C. R., Arnold, W. D., Freiberger, R. H., and Brooks, G.: Untreated congenital hip disease: A study of the epidemiology, natural history and social aspect of the disease in a Navajo population. Am. J. Publ. Health, 55:1, 1965.

763. Race, C., and Herring, J. A.: Congenital dislocation of the hip: An evaluation of closed reduction. J. Pediatr. Orthop., 3:166, 1983.

764. Radin, E. L., and Paul, I. L.: The biomechanics of congenital dislocated hips and their treatment. Clin. Orthop., 98:32, 1974.

765. Raine, G. E.: Acute traumatic dislocation of a congenitally dysplastic hip. Report of a case. J. Bone Joint Surg., 55-B:640, 1973.

766. Ralis, Z., and McKibbin, B.: Changes in the shape of the human hip joint during its development and their relation to its stability. J. Bone Joint Surg., 55-B:780, 1973.

767. Ramsey, P. L.: Congenital hip dislocation before and after walking age. Postgrad. Med., 60:114, 1976.

768. Ramsey, P. L., and Hensinger, R. N.: Congenital dislocation of the hip associated with central core disease. J. Bone Joint Surg., 57-A:648, 1975.

769. Ramsey, P. L., Lasser, S., and MacEwen, G. D.: Congenital dislocation of the hip: Use of the Pavlik harness in the child during the first 6 months of life. J. Bone Joint Surg., 58-A:1000, 1976.

770. Ranft, G., and Pissarek, H.: Pädiatrisch-orthopädische Zusammenarbeit bei der Früherkennung und Behandlung der Luxationshüfte. Pädiatr. Grenzgeb., 9:251, 1970.

771. Record, R. G., and Edwards, J. H.: Environmental influences related to the etiology of congenital dislocation of the hip. Br. J. Prevent. Soc. Med., 12:8, 1958.

772. Reiter, R.: Erfahrungen mit dem Riemenzugel nach Pavlik. Z. Orthop., 95:220, 1961.

773. Rengeval, J. P., Normand, X., Laidi, A., Queneau, P., and Seringe, R.: Congenital dislocation of the hip treated by the Somerville technique at the age of

walking. A long term review. Rev. Chir. Orthop., 66:83, 1980.

774. Renoirte, P., and Saussez, M.: L'ostéotomie de Chiari dans les dysplasies coxofémorales acquises de la seconde enfance. Acta Orthop. Belg., 36:209, 1970.

775. Renshaw, R. S.: Inadequate reduction of congenital dislocation of the hip. J. Bone Joint Surg., 63:1114, 1981.

776. Ridlon, J.: Congenital dislocation of the hip. R.I. Med. J., 16:135, 1933.

777. Riedl, K.: Die Anwendung der Pavlik-Bandage bei der Behandlung der sog. angeborenen Hüftluxation. Z. Orthop., 115:639, 1977.

778. Rigault, J.-P.: Le depistage des hanches luxable en maternité. Rev. Fr. Gynecol. Obstet., 66:427, 1971.

779. Ring, P. A.: The treatment of unreduced congenital dislocation of the hip in adults. J. Bone Joint Surg., 41-B:299, 1959.

780. Ringrose, C. A. D.: Congenital dislocation of the hip as a cause of malpresentation during labor. Am. J. Obstet. Gynecol., 123:916, 1975.

781. Ritter, M. A.: Congenital dislocation of the hip in the newborn. Am. J. Dis. Child., 125:30, 1973.

782. Ritter, M. A., and Wilson, P. D., Jr.: Colonna capsular arthroplasty. A long-term follow-up of forty hips. J. Bone Joint Surg., 50-A:1305, 1968.

783. Robin, D. L., Barnett, C. R., Arnold, M. D., Freiberger, R. H., and Brooks, G.: Untreated congenital hip disease. A study of the epidemiology, natural history and social aspects of the disease in a Navajo population. Am. J. Publ. Health, 55:1, 1965.

784. Robinson, G. W.: Birth characteristics of children with congenital dislocation of the hip. Am. J. Epidemiol., 87:276, 1968.

785. Roper, A.: Hip dysplasia in the African Bantu. J. Bone Joint Surg., 58-B:155, 1976.

786. Roose, P. E., Chingren, G. L., Klaaren, H. E., and Broock, G.: Open reduction for congenital dislocation of the hip using the Ferguson procedure. A review of twenty-six cases. J. Bone Joint Surg., 61-A:915, 1979.

787. Rosen, S. von: Early diagnosis and treatment of congenital dislocation of the hip joint. Acta Orthop. Scand., 26:136, 1956.

788. Rosen, S. von: Diagnosis and treatment of congenital dislocation of the hip joint in the newborn. J. Bone Joint Surg., 44-B:284, 1962.

789. Rosen, S. von: Further experience with congenital dislocation of the hip in the newborn. J. Bone Joint Surg., 50-B:538, 1968.

790. Rosen, S. von: Instability of the hip in the newborn. Fifteen years' experiences in Malmo. Acta Orthop. Scand., 130:13, 1970.

791. Rosman, M. A.: Congenital hip dislocation diagnosed after walking age: Results of treatment. Can. J. Surg., 19:169, 1976.

792. Roth, A., Gibson, D. A., and Hall, J. E.: The experience of five orthopedic surgeons with innominate osteotomy in the treatment of congenital dislocation and subluxation of the hip. Clin. Orthop., 98:178, 1974.

793. Rott, Z.: Röntgenologische Untersuchung von Familien mit Vockommen von angeborener Hüftverrenkung. Z. Orthop., 104:181, 1967.

794. Ruby, L., Mital, M. A., O'Connor, J., and Patel, U.: Anteversion of the femoral neck. Comparison of methods of measurement in patients. J. Bone Joint Surg., 61-A:46, 1979.

795. Ryder, C. T., and Crane, L.: Measuring femoral anteversion: The problem and a method. J. Bone Joint Surg., 35-A:321, 1953.

796. Ryder, C. T., and Mellin, G. W.: A prospective epidemiological study of the clinical and roentgeno-

graphic characteristics of the hip joint in the first year of life—From the foetal life study. J. Bone Joint Surg., 48-A:1024, 1966.

797. Ryder, C. T., Mellin, G. W., and Caffey, J.: The infant's hip—normal or dysplastic. Clin. Orthop., 22:7, 1962.

798. Ryerson, E. W.: An improved shelf operation at the hip. J. Bone Joint Surg., 23:782, 1941.

799. Sainton, R.: De l'anatomie de l'articulation de la hanche chez l'enfant et de la luxation congénitale de cette articulation (étude pathogénique). Thèse de Paris, No. 226, 12, 1892–1893.

800. Saito, T.: Photo-elastic studies on technic of Colonna's hip arthroplasty (Japanese). Sapporo Med. J., 30:120, 1966.

801. Sakaguchi, R.: The treatment of congenital dislocation of the hip. Rinsho Seikeigeka (Tokyo), 2:597, 1967. (Abstract in Am. Dig. Foreign Orthop. Lit., 3rd Quarter, 1971, pp. 8–11.)

802. Salenius, P., and Videman, T.: Growth disturbances of the proximal end of the femur. An experimental study with tetracycline. Acta Orthop. Scand., 41:199, 1970.

803. Sallis, J. G., and Smith, R. G.: A study of the development of the acetabular roof in congenital dislocation of the hip. Br. J. Surg., 52:44, 1965.

804. Salter, R. B.: Innominate osteotomy in the treatment of congenital dislocation and subluxation of the hip. J. Bone Joint Surg., 43-B:518, 1961.

805. Salter, R. B.: Role of innominate osteotomy in the treatment of congenital dislocation and subluxation of the hip in the older child. J. Bone Joint Surg., 48-A:1413, 1966.

806. Salter, R. B.: The principle and technique of innominate osteotomy (motion picture with sound track). Chicago, Film Library, American Academy of Orthopedic Surgeons, 1966.

807. Salter, R. B.: Congenital dislocation of the hip. *In* Graham, W. D. (ed.): Modern Trends in Orthopedics, No. 5. London, Butterworth, 1967, p. 140.

808. Salter, R. B.: Etiology, pathology, pathogenesis and possible prevention of congenital dislocation of the hip. Can. Med. Assoc. J., 98:933, 1968.

809. Salter, R. B.: An operative treatment for congenital dislocation and subluxation of the hip in the older child. *In* Apley, A. G. (ed.): Recent Advances in Orthopaedics. London, Churchill, 1969, p. 325.

810. Salter, R. B.: Textbook of Disorders and Injuries of the Musculoskeletal System. Baltimore, Williams & Wilkins, 1970, p. 98.

811. Salter, R. B.: Specific guidelines in the application of the principle of innominate osteotomy. Orthop. Clin. North Am., 3:149, 1972.

812. Salter, R. B.: Innominate osteotomy. *In* The Hip: Proceedings of the Fourth Meeting of the Hip Society, 1976. St. Louis, Mosby, 1976, p. 40.

813. Salter, R. B., and Dubos, J.-P.: The first fifteen years' personal experience with innominate osteotomy in the treatment of congenital dislocation and subluxation of the hip. Clin. Orthop., 98:72, 1974.

814. Salter, R. B., and Field, P.: The effects of continuous compression on living articular cartilage. J. Bone Joint Surg., 42-A:31, 1960.

815. Salter, R. B., and Thompson, G. H.: The role of innominate osteotomy in young adults. *In* The Hip: Proceedings of the Seventh Open Scientific Meeting of the Hip Society, 1979. St. Louis, Mosby, 1979, p. 278.

816. Salter, R. B., Kostiuk, S., and Dallas, S.: Avascular necrosis of the femoral head as a complication of treatment for congenital dislocation of the hip in young children: A clinical and experimental investigation. Can. J. Surg., 12:44, 1969.

817. Salter, R. B., Kostiuk, J., and Schatzker, J.: Exper-

imental dysplasia of the hip and its reversibility in newborn pigs. J. Bone Joint Surg., 45-A:1781, 1963.

818. Salvati, E. A., and Wilson, P. D.: Treatment of irreducible hip subluxation by Chiari. Clin. Orthop., 98:151, 1974.

819. Salzer, M., and Zuckriegl, H.: Die Operationstechnik der offenen Hüftgelenkreposition nach Ludloff. Z. Orthop., 103:409, 1967.

820. Samuelson, K. M., Nixon, G. W., and Morrow, R. E.: Tomography for evaluation of congenital dislocation of the hip while in a spica cast. J. Bone Joint Surg., 56-A:844, 1974.

821. Sayle-Creer, W., and Barlow, T. G.: Congenital dislocation of the hip. Br. Med. J., 1:1427, 1960.

822. Scaglietti, O., and Calandriello, B.: Open reduction of congenital dislocation of the hip. J. Bone Joint Surg., 44-B:257, 1962.

823. Scammon, R. E., and Calkins, L. A.: The development and growth of the external dimensions of the human body in the fetal period. Minneapolis, University of Minnesota, 1929, p. 48.

824. Scapinelli, R., and Ortolani, M.: La displasia congenita dell'anca nell'eta pediatrica. Diganosi e trattamento precoci e ultraprecoci. LVII Congresso della Societa Italiana di Ortopedia e Traumatologia, Bologna, October 1972. Padova, La Garangola, 1972.

825. Schanz, A.: Zur Behandlung der veralteten angeborenen Hüftverrenkung. Munch. Med. Wochenschr., 69:930, 1922.

826. Schede, F.: Zur pathologischen Anatomie der kongenitalen Hüftverrenkung. Z. Orthop. Chir., 32:427, 1913.

827. Schede, F.: Ergebnisse unserer Behandlung der angeborenen Hüftverrenkung. Z. Orthop., 71:3, 1941.

828. Schede, F.: Die Ergebnisse der Luxationsbehandlung. Z. Orthop., 82:1, 1952.

829. Schneider, P. G.: Zur offenen Reposition der angeborenen Hüftverrenkung. Z. Orthop., 100:201, 1965.

830. Schneider, P. G.: Eine einfache, verstelbare Luxationsschiene. Z. Orthop., 98:201, 1964.

831. Schneider, P. G., and Grueter, H.: Röntgenologische und histologische Reaktionen nach dosierter Trochanterversetzung und intertrochanterer Osteotomie bei Luxationshüften. Z. Orthop., 98:145, 1964.

832. Schneider, P. G., and Thull-Emden, J.: Ligamentum capitis femoris und operative Reposition kindlicher Luxationshüften. Z. Orthop., 109:365, 1971.

833. Schoenecker, P. L., Bitz, D. M., and Whiteside, L. A.: The acute effect of position of immobilization on capital femoral epiphyseal blood flow. J. Bone Joint Surg., 60-A:899, 1978.

834. Schoenecker, P. L., and Strecker, W. B.: Congenital dislocation of the hip in children. Comparison of the effects of femoral shortening and of skeletal traction in treatment. J. Bone Joint Surg., 66-A:21, 1984.

835. Scholder-Hegi, P.: Mathematische Betrachtungen über die schräge Varisations- und Derotationsosteotomie nach Bernbeck. Z. Orthop., 96:298, 1962.

836. Schottstaedt, E. R.: Treatment of congenital dislocation of the hip in infancy. J. Bone Joint Surg., 47:602, 1965.

837. Schreiber, A., and Meyer, H. R.: Spätresultate konservative behandelter kongenitaler Hüftluxationen. Z. Orthop., 100:265, 1965.

838. Schulitz, K.-P.: Die Retrotorsion des Femur nach Derotations-Varisierungosteotomien im Kindesalter. Z. Orthop., 107:241, 1970.

839. Schulze, H., and Kramer, J.: Ergebnisse der Beckenosteotomie nach Chiari. Z. Orthop., 113:891, 1975.

840. Schuster, W.: Röntgenologische Beurteilung der dysplastischen Hüftpfanne. Orthopäde, 2:219, 1973.

841. Schuster, W.: Radiologic interpretation of dysplasia of the acetabulum. *In* Progress in Orthopedic Surgery, Vol 2. Heidelberg, Springer, 1978, p. 73.

842. Schwartz, A., and Goldberg, M.: Hip arthrography in children. Skeletal Radiol., 3:155, 1978.

843. Schwartz, D. R.: Acetabular development after reduction of congenital dislocation of the hip. J. Bone Joint Surg., 47-A:705, 1965.

844. Scott, J. C.: Frame reduction in congenital dislocation of the hip. J. Bone Joint Surg., 35-B:372, 1953.

845. Seddon, H. J.: Dislocation of the hip. J. Bone Joint Surg., 44-B:255, 1962.

846. Seewald, K.: Eine Modifikation der perikapsularen Darmbeinosteotomie nach Pemberton. Wien. Med. Wochenschr., 117:690, 1967.

847. Serre, H., Izran, P., Simon, L., and Rogues, J. M.: Les attients de la hanche au cours de l'hémophile. Marseille Med., 106:483, 1969.

848. Severin, E.: Arthrography in congenital dislocation of the hip. J. Bone Joint Surg., 21:304, 1939.

849. Severin, E.: Arthrograms of hip joints of children. Surg. Gynecol. Obstet., 72:601, 1941.

850. Severin, E.: Contribution to the knowledge of congenital dislocation of the hip joint. Late results of closed reduction and arthrographic studies of recent cases. Acta Chir. Scand., Suppl. 63, 1941.

851. Severin, E.: Arthrography in sequelae to acute infectious arthritis of hips of young children. Acta Chir. Scand., 93:389, 1946.

852. Severin, E.: Congenital dislocation of the hip. Development of the joint after closed reduction. J. Bone Joint Surg., 32-A:507, 1950.

853. Severin, E.: Frekvensen av luxatio coxae congenita och pes equino-varus congenitus i Sverige. Nord Med., 55:221, 1956.

854. Seyfarth, H.: Beitrag zur Beckenosteotomie in der Behandlung der Luxationshüfte. Beitr. Orthop. Traumatol., 12:462, 1965.

855. Seyfarth, H.: Aktuelle Gesichtspunkte zur operativen Behandlung der Luxationshüfte. Beitr. Orthop. Traumatol., 13:677, 1966.

856. Shands, A. R., and Steele, M. K.: Torsion of the femur. J. Bone Joint Surg., 40-A:803, 1958.

857. Sharp, I. K.: Acetabular dysplasia. The acetabular angle. J. Bone Joint Surg., 43-B:268, 1971.

858. Sharrard, W. J.: Neonatal diagnosis of congenital dislocation of the hip. Dev. Med. Child Neurol., 20:389, 1978.

859. Sharrard, W. J.: Paediatric Orthopedics and Fractures. 2nd Ed. Oxford, Blackwell, 1979, pp. 318–427.

860. Shih, J. S., Chen, H. T., and Liu, H. C.: Interim follow-up studies of innominate osteotomy for congenital dislocation of the hip. Clin. Orthop., 152:261, 1980.

861. Shino, K.: Über der Hüftpläne. Z. Morphol. Anthropol., 17:325, 1915.

862. Shulze, H., and Kraemer, J.: Ergebnisse der Beckenosteotomie nach Chiari. Z. Orthop., 113:891, 1975.

863. Siffert, R. S., Ehrlich, M. G., and Katz, J. F.: Management of congenital dislocation of the hip. Clin. Orthop., 86:28, 1972.

864. Sijbrandjii, S.: Dislocation of the hip in young rats produced experimentally by prolonged extension. J. Bone Joint Surg., 47-B:792, 1965.

865. Simons, G. W.: A comparative evaluation of the current methods for open reduction of the congenitally displaced hip. Orthop. Clin. North Am., 11:161, 1980.

866. Sinios, A.: Die Präluxation am Hüftgelenk des Neugeborenen. Monatsschr. Kinderheilkd., 111:281, 1963.

867. Smaill, G. B.: Congenital dislocation of the hip in the newborn. J. Bone Joint Surg., 50-B:525, 1968.

868. Smith, D. W.: Recognizable Patterns of Human Deformation. Philadelphia, Saunders, 1981, pp. 19–22.

869. Smith, M. G. H.: The results of neonatal treatment of congenital hip dislocation: A personal series. J. Pediatr. Orthop., 4:311, 1984.

870. Smith, P. B., and Robinson, A. W.: A radiographic jig for the von Rosen view. Radiography, 35:168, 1969.

871. Smith, W. S.: Experimental aspects of so-called congenital dysplasia of the hip. Proc. 8th Cong. Int. Soc. Orthop. Surg. Traumatol., 277, New York, Sept. 4–9, 1960.

872. Smith, W. S., Ireton, R. J., and Coleman, C. R.: Sequelae of experimental dislocation of a weight-bearing ball-and-socket joint in a young growing animal. J. Bone Joint Surg., 40-A:1121, 1958.

873. Smith, W. S., Badgley, C. E., Orwig, J. B., and Harper, J. M.: Correlation of post-reduction roentgenograms and thirty-one year follow-up in congenital dislocation of the hip. J. Bone Joint Surg., 50-A:1081, 1968.

874. Smith, W. S., Coleman, C. R., Olix, M. L., and Slager, R. F.: Etiology of congenital dislocation of the hip. An experimental approach to the problem using young dogs. J. Bone Joint Surg., 45:491, 1963.

875. Solomon, L., and Breighton, P.: Osteoarthritis of the hip and its relationship to pre-existing disorders in an African population. J. Bone Joint Surg., 58-B:389, 1976.

876. Somerville, E. W.: Development of congenital dislocation of the hip. J. Bone Joint Surg., 35-B:568, 1953.

877. Somerville, E. W.: Open reduction in congenital dislocation of the hip. J. Bone Joint Surg., 35-B:363, 1953.

878. Somerville, E. W.: Persistent foetal alignment of the hip. J. Bone Joint Surg., 39-B:106, 1957.

879. Somerville, E. W.: The nature of hip dysplasia. Proc. 8th Cong. Int. Soc. Orthop. Surg. Traumatol., 278, New York, Sept. 4–9, 1960.

880. Somerville, E. W.: Results of treatment of 100 congenitally dislocated hips. J. Bone Joint Surg., 40-B:258, 1967.

881. Somerville, E. W.: The nature of the congenitally dislocated hip. Proc. R. Soc. Med., 67:1169, 1974.

882. Somerville, E. W.: A long-term follow-up of congenital dislocation of the hip. J. Bone Joint Surg., 60-B:25, 1978.

883. Somerville, E. W., and Scott, J. C.: The direct approach to congenital dislocation of the hip. J. Bone Joint Surg., 39-B:623, 1957.

884. Sommer, J.: Atypical hip click in the newborn. Acta Orthop. Scand., 42:353, 1971.

885. Soutter, R., and Lovett, R. W.: Congenital dislocation of the hip: A study of 227 dislocations. J.A.M.A., 82:171, 1924.

886. Specht, E. E.: Congenital dislocation of the hip. Am. Fam. Physician, 988, 1974.

887. Staheli, L. T.: Slotted acetabular augmentation. J. Pediatr. Orthop., 1:321, 1981.

888. Staheli, L. T.: Medial approach open reduction for congenitally dislocated hips: A critical analysis of forty cases. In Tachdjian, M. O. (ed.): Congenital Dislocation of the Hip. New York, Churchill-Livingstone, 1982, pp. 295–303.

889. Staheli, L. T., Dion, M., and Tuell, J. I.: The effect of the inverted limbus on closed management of congenital hip dislocation. Clin. Orthop., 137:163, 1978.

890. Stanisavljevic, S.: Examination of hips in newborn babies and results. Henry Ford Hosp. Med. Bull., 9:214, 1961.

891. Stanisavljevic, S.: Radiologic diagnosis of prenatal congenital hip dislocation and subluxation in the newborn. Radiology, 79:606, 1962.

892. Stanisavljevic, S.: Diagnosis and Treatment of Congenital Hip Pathology in the Newborn. Baltimore, Williams & Wilkins, 1964.

893. Stanisavljevic, S.: Tribute to Marino Ortolani. Clin. Orthop., 119:4, 1976.

894. Stanisavljevic, S.: Anatomical basis as the rationale for the treatment of congenital hip pathology. Presented at the Symposium on Congenital Dislocation of the Hip, October 1979, Jerusalem, Israel.

895. Stanisavljevic, S.: Part I: Etiology of congenital hip pathology. Part II: Anatomy of congenital hip pathology. In Tachdjian, M. O. (ed.): Congenital Dislocation of the Hip. New York, Churchill-Livingstone, 1982, pp. 27–57.

896. Stanisavljevic, S., and Mitchell, C. L.: Congenital dysplasia, subluxation and dislocation of the hip in stillborn and newborn infants. An anatomical-pathological study. J. Bone Joint Surg., 45-A:1147, 1963.

897. Steel, H. H.: Triple osteotomy of the innominate bone. J. Bone Joint Surg., 55-A:343, 1973.

898. Steel, H. H.: Triple osteotomy of the innominate bone. A procedure to accomplish coverage of the dislocated or subluxated femoral head in the older patient. Orthop. Clin., 122:16, 1977.

899. Steel, H. H.: Triple osteotomy of the innominate bone. In Tachdjian, M. O. (ed.): Congenital Dislocation of the Hip. New York, Churchill-Livingstone, 1982, pp. 567–594.

900. Stein, I. F.: Deflexion attitudes in breech presentation. J.A.M.A., 117:1430, 1941.

901. Stojimirovic, I.: Our way of open reduction for congenital dislocation of the hip. Acta Chir. Iugosl., 6:202, 1959.

902. Stojimirovic, I.: A new method to the hip joint in our way of open reduction for congenital dislocation of the hip. Acta Chir. Iugosl., 8:51, 1961.

903. Strange, F. G.: The Hip. Baltimore, Williams & Wilkins, 1965.

904. Straub, H. J.: Chiari pelvic osteotomy for hip dysplasia in patients below the age of 20. In Progress in Orthopedic Surgery, Vol. 2. Heidelberg, Springer, 1978, p. 121.

905. Strauss, H. J.: Chiari pelvic osteotomy for hip dysplasia in patients below the age of 20. Progr. Orthop. Surg., 2, 1978.

906. Strayer, L. M., Jr.: Embryology of the human hip joint. Yale J. Biol. Med., 16:13, 1943.

907. Strayer, L. M., Jr.: Embryology of the human hip joint. Clin. Orthop., 74:221, 1971.

908. Stulberg, S. D., and Harris, W.: Acetabular dysplasia and development of osteoarthritis of the hip. In The Hip. Proceedings of the Second Open Scientific Meeting of the Hip Society. St. Louis, Mosby, 1974, p. 82.

909. Sutherland, D. H.: Double innominate osteotomy in congenital hip dislocation or dysplasia. In Tachdjian, M. O. (ed.): Congenital Dislocation of the Hip. New York, Churchill-Livingstone, 1982, pp. 595–608.

910. Sutherland, D. H., and Greenfield, R.: Medial pubic osteotomy in difficult Salter procedures. (Proc. West. Orthop. Assoc.) J. Bone Joint Surg., 57-A:135, 1975. (Abstr.)

911. Sutherland, D. H., and Greenfield, R.: Double innominate osteotomy. J. Bone Joint Surg., 59-A:1082, 1977.

912. Suzuki, R.: Treatment of congenital dislocation of the hip with Pavlik's bandage. J. West. Pacific Orthop. Assoc., 3:79, 1966.

913. Suzuki, R.: Complications of the treatment of congenital dislocation of the hip by the Pavlik harness. Int. Orthop., 3:77, 1979.

914. Suzuki, R., and Sato, K.: Evaluation of Pavlik's

bandage method for the treatment of congenital hip dislocation. Fukushima J. Med. Sci., *15*:61, 1968.

915. Swiderski, G., Marciniak, W., and Milanowski, Z.: Schräge transiliakale Osteotomie in der Behandlungen der angeborene Hüftgelenksubluxation. Beitr. Orthop. Traumatol., *17*:152, 1975.

915a. Szoke, N., Kuhl, L., and Heinrichs, J.: Ultrasound examination in the diagnosis of congenital hip dysplasia of newborns. J. Pediatr. Orthop., *8*:12, 1988.

916. Szulc, W.: The significance of the hormonal and mechanical factors in the etiology and pathogenesis of the congenital dislocation of the hip. Chir. Narzadow Ruchu Ortop. Pol., *35*:1, 1970.

917. Tachdjian, M. O.: Salter's innominate osteotomy to derotate the maldirected acetabulum. *In* Tachdjian, M. O. (ed.): Congenital Dislocation of the Hip. New York, Churchill-Livingstone, 1982, pp. 525–541.

918. Tachdjian, M. O.: Treatment after walking age. *In* Tachdjian, M. O. (ed.): Congenital Dislocation of the Hip. New York, Churchill-Livingstone, 1982, pp. 339–363.

919. Tachdjian, M. O.: Treatment of hip dysplasia in the older child and adolescent: Factors in decision making. *In* Tachdjian, M. O. (ed.): Congenital Dislocation of the Hip. New York, Churchill-Livingstone, 1982, pp. 625–641.

920. Tachdjian, M. O., and Edelstein, D.: Periacetabular osteotomy through the subinguinal medial adductor approach. Paper presented at the American Orthopedic Association Annual Meeting, 1985, San Diego. Orthop. Trans., *9*:No. 2, Spring, 1985.

921. Tachdjian, M. O., and Kelikian, A. S.: Distal and lateral advancement of the greater trochanter. *In* Tachdjian, M. O. (ed.): Congenital Dislocation of the Hip. New York, Churchill-Livingstone, 1982, pp. 721–739.

922. Tanabe, G., Kotakemori, K., Miyake, Y., and Mohri, M.: Early diagnosis of congenital dislocation of the hip. Acta Orthop. Scand., *43*:511, 1972.

923. Tauber, C., Ganel, A., Horoszowski, H., and Farine, I.: Distal transfer of the greater trochanter in coxa vara. Acta Orthop. Scand., *51*:611, 1980.

924. Thieme, W. T., Wynne-Davies, R., Balir, H. A. F., Bell, E. T., and Lorane, J. A.: Clinical examination and urinary oestrogen assays in newborn children with congenital dislocation of the hip. J. Bone Joint Surg., *50-B*:546, 1968.

925. Thiery, J., and Rigault, P.: Residual femoral anteversion after treatment of dislocating dysplasia of the hip by cushion abduction. Acta Orthop. Belg., *43*:465, 1977.

926. Thomas, C. L., Gage, J. R., and Ogden, J. A.: Treatment concepts for proximal femoral ischemic necrosis complicating congenital hip disease. J. Bone Joint Surg., *64-A*:817, 1982.

927. Thomas, G.: Zur operativen Technik der Pfannendachplastik. *In* Chapchal, G. (ed.): Beckenosteotomie—Pfannendachplastik. Stuttgart, Theime, 1965, pp. 40–41, 125.

928. Thompson, R. C.: A new physical test in dislocation of the hip. J. Bone Joint Surg., *54-A*:1326, 1972.

929. Tikhonenkov, E.: Effect of reconstruction of its roof on acetabular development. Orthop. Travmatol. Protez (Mosc.), *4*:36, 1970.

930. Tönnis, D.: Elektromyographische und histologische Untersuchungen zur Frage der Entstehung der angeborenen Hüftluxation. Z. Orthop., *105*:527, 1969.

931. Tönnis, D.: A modified acetabular roof osteotomy combined with intertrochanteric detorsion-varus osteotomy. Proc. 12th Cong. Int. Soc. Orthop. Surg. Traumatol., 688, Tel Aviv, Oct. 9–12, 1972.

932. Tönnis, D.: An evaluation of conservative and operative methods in the treatment of congenital hip dislocation. Clin. Orthop., *199*:76, 1976.

933. Tönnis, D.: Normal values of the hip joint for the evaluation of x-ray in children and adults. Clin. Orthop., *119*:39, 1976.

934. Tönnis, D.: Zum Aspekt der Hüftdysplasie in Klinik und Röntgenologie. Z. Orthop., *114*:98, 1976.

935. Tönnis, D.: Einleitung. (63. Kongress der Deutschen Gesellschaft fur Orthopädie und Traumatologie, September 1976.) Z. Orthop., *115*:636, 1977.

936. Tönnis, D.: Indikation und Wirksamkeit verschiedener Operationsmethoden bei angeborener Hüftdysplasie. Z. Orthop., *115*:726, 1977.

937. Tönnis, D.: Statistische Auswertungen der Hüftkopfnekroserate bei konservativer und nachträglicher operative Behandlung der angeborenen Hüftluxation. (63. Kongress der Deutschen Gesellschaft fur Orthopädie und Traumatologie, September, 1976.) Z. Orthop., *115*:653, 1977.

938. Tönnis, D.: Zusammenfassung der Podiums-diskussion. (63. Kongress der Deutschen Gesellschaft fur Orthopädie und Traumatologie, September, 1976.) Z. Orthop., *115*:653, 1977.

939. Tönnis, D.: Der Leistenschnitt als Zugang zur Operation Hüftreposition. Z. Orthop., *116*:130, 1978.

940. Tönnis, D.: Eine neue Form der hüftpfannen Schrenkung durch Dreifachosteotomie zur Ermöglichung späterer Hüftprothese. Orthop. Praxis, *15*:1003, 1979.

941. Tönnis, D.: Congenital Hip Dislocation: Avascular Necrosis. New York, Thieme-Stratton, 1982.

942. Tönnis, D.: Triple osteotomy close to the hip joint. *In* Tachdjian, M. O. (ed.): Congenital Dislocation of the Hip. New York, Churchill-Livingstone, 1982, pp. 555–565.

943. Tönnis, D.: Congenital Dysplasia and Dislocation of the Hip in Children and Adults. With collaboration of Helmut Legal and Reinhard Graf. Berlin, Springer-Verlag, 1984.

944. Tönnis, D., and Kuhlmann, G. P.: Untersuchungen über die Haufigkeit von Hüftkopfnekrosen bei Spreizhosenbehandlung und verschiedenen konservativen Behandlungsmethoden der angeborenen Hüftdysplasie und Hüftluxation. Z. Orthop., *106*:651, 1969.

945. Tönnis, D., and Letz, A.: Untersuchungen über das Verhalten des Pfannendach- und des Schenkelhalswinkels nach intertroch. Derotationsvarisierungsosteotomie und die Indikation zur Acetabuloplastik. Arch. Orthop. Unfallchir., *66*:171, 1969.

946. Tönnis, D., and Trede, B.: Untersuchungen über den Einfluss des Spreizhoschens auf den Hüftpfannendachwinkel bei angeborener Hüftdysplasie. Z. Orthop., *107*:263, 1970.

947. Tönnis, D., Behrens, K., and Tscharani, F.: Eine neue Technik der Dreifach-Osteotomie zur Schwenkung dysplastischer Hüftpfannen bei Jugendlichen und Erwachsenen. Z. Orthop., *119*:253, 1981.

948. Tönnis, D., Veigel, B., Groher, W., and Rauterberg, E.: Nachuntersuchungsergebnisse einer Acetabuloplastik kombiniert mit der Derotationsvarisierungsosteotomie unter Gleichzeitiger Verwendung des Osteotomiekeiles. Z. Orthop., *110*:489, 1972.

949. Trager, G. von, and Blankenburg, H.: Ergebnisse der konservativen Behandlung der sogenannten angeborenen Hüftluxation der Subluxation und der Dysplasie. Beitr. Orthop. Traumatol., *15*:700, 1968.

950. Tredwell, S. J., and Bell, H. M.: Efficacy of neonatal hip examination. J. Pediatr. Orthop., *1*:61, 1981.

951. Trevor, D.: Osteotomy in the treatment of congenital dislocation of the hip. Proc. R. Soc. Med., *51*:1045, 1958.

952. Trevor, D.: Treatment of congenital hip dislocation in older children. Proc. R. Soc. Med., *53*:481, 1960.

953. Trevor, D.: The place of the Hey Groves–Colonna operation in the treatment of congenital dislocation of the hip. Ann. R. Coll. Surg. Engl., *48*:241, 1968.

954. Trevor, D.: Congenital dislocation of the hip. Ann. R. Coll. Surg. Engl., *50*:213, 1972.

955. Trevor, D., Johns, D. L., and Fixsen, J. A.: Acetabuloplasty in the treatment of congenital dislocation of the hip. J. Bone Joint Surg., *57-B*:167, 1975.

956. Tronzo, R. G., and Okin, E. M.: Anatomic restoration of the congenital hip dysplasia in adulthood by total hip replacement. Clin. Orthop., *106*:94, 1975.

957. Trueta, J.: The normal vascular anatomy of the human femoral head during growth. J. Bone Joint Surg., *39-B*:358, 1957.

958. Trueta, J., and Amata, V. P.: The vascular contribution to osteogenesis. III. Changes in the growth cartilage caused by experimentally induced ischemia. J. Bone Joint Surg., *42-B*:571, 1960.

959. Tsoukas, S., Aboussouan, G. S., and Gonzalo-Vivar, F.: Considerations sur les arthrodèses de hanche. Rev. Med. Moyen Orient., *31*:414, 1964.

960. Tsuchiya, K., and Yamada, K.: Open reduction of congenital dislocation of the hip in infancy using Ludloff's approach. Int. Orthop., *1*:337, 1978.

961. Tsuyama, N., and Sakaguchi, R.: Treatment of congenital dislocation of the hip with the Pavlik dynamic splint. *In* Tachdjian, M. O. (ed.): Congenital Dislocation of the Hip. New York, Churchill-Livingstone, 1982, pp. 173–180.

962. Tucker, F. R.: Arterial supply of the femoral head and its clinical importance. J. Bone Joint Surg., *31-B*:82, 1949.

963. Tylman, D., and Sotirov, B.: The mechanism of pelvic stabilization following abduction-supportive osteotomies of the femur. Chir. Narzadow Ruchu Ortop. Pol., *34*:83, 1969.

964. Ueda, F., Ueke, T., Okuda, H., Taneka, H., Suda, M., Sujerki, Y., and Ando, Y.: X-ray study of so-called spontaneous healing in congenital dislocation of the hip joint. Nagoya Med. J., *8*:5, 1967.

965. Ueno, R., Funauchi, M., Kura, K., Tamai, A., and Nagatsuru, Y.: Die Behandlung der angeborenen Hüftgelenksluxation durch die Pavlik-Bandage: Ergebnisse von 168 eigenen Fallen. Z. Orthop., *113*:1090, 1975.

966. Ullmann, K.: Zur Frage der röntgenologischen Beurteilung des knochernen Pfannendachs mit weiteren Ergebnissen der Röntgenstammbaumforschung. *In* Verh. Dtsch. Orthop. Ges. 33. Kongress, 1939. Beitr. Orthop., 1939, p. 268.

967. Utterback, T. D., and MacEwen, G. D.: Comparison of pelvic osteotomies for the surgical correction of the congenital hip. Clin. Orthop., *98*:104, 1974.

968. Valerio, V.: Primary surgical treatment of congenital hip dislocation. Clin. Orthop., *26*:148, 1975–1976.

969. Van Meerdervoort, H. F.: Congenital dislocation of the hip in black patients. S. Afr. Med. J., *48*:2436, 1974.

970. Vartan, C. K.: The behaviour of the foetus in utero with special reference to the incidence of breech presentation at term. J. Obstet. Gynaecol. Br. Empire, *52*:471, 1945.

971. Visser, J. D.: Functional Treatment of Congenital Dislocation of the Hip. Groningen, The Netherlands, Drukerij van Denderen B. V., 1984.

972. Voutsinas, S. A., MacEwen, G. D., and Boos, M. L.: Home traction in the management of congenital dislocation of the hip. Arch. Orthop. Trauma. Surg., *102*:135, 1984.

973. Wagner, H.: Korrektur der Hüftgelenksdysplasie durch die sphärische Pfannendachplastik International Symposium. *In* Chapchal, G. (ed.): Beckenosteotomie—Pfannendachplastik. Stuttgart, Thieme, 1965.

974. Wagner, H.: Osteosynthese bei der Beckenosteotomie nach Chiari. *In* Chapchal, G. (ed.): Beckenosteotomie—Pfannendachplastik. Stuttgart, Thieme, 1965, p. 92.

975. Wagner, H.: Erfahrungen mit der Pfannenosteotomie bei der Korrektur der dysplastischen Hüftgelenkpfanne. Orthopäde, *2*:253, 1973.

976. Wagner, H.: Der alloplastische Gelenkflachenersatz am Hüftgelenk. Arch. Orthop. Unfallchir., *82*:101, 1975.

977. Wagner, H.: Osteotomies for congenital hip dislocation. *In* The Hip: Proceedings of the Fourth Meeting of the Hip Society, 1976. St. Louis, Mosby, 1976, pp. 45–66.

978. Wagner, H.: Experiences with spherical acetabular osteotomy for the correction of the dysplastic acetabulum. *In* Weil, U. H. (ed.): Progress in Orthopedic Surgery, Vol. 2. Heidelberg, Springer, 1978, p. 131.

979. Wagner, H.: Femoral osteotomies for congenital hip dislocation. *In* Weil, U. H. (ed.): Progress in Orthopedic Surgery, Vol. 2. Acetabular Dysplasia and Skeletal Dysplasia in Childhood. Heidelberg, Springer, 1978, p. 85.

980. Wagner, H., and Keck, P.: Ergebnisse der operativen Behandlung der Dysplasiarthrose des Hüftgelenkes. Orthopäde, *2*:260, 1973.

981. Waigand, D.: Zur Indikation und Technik der Beckenosteotomie nach Chiari. *In* Chapchal, G. (ed.): Beckenosteotomie—Pfannendachplastik. Stuttgart, Thieme, 1965, pp. 94–96.

982. Waigand, D.: Die Stellung der Röntgenologie bei Diagnostik und Therapie der dysplastischen Hüfte. Ann. Radiol., *11*:315, 1968.

983. Wainwright, D.: The shelf operation for hip dysplasia in adolescence. J. Bone Joint Surg., *58-B*:159, 1976.

984. Walker, G.: Problems in the early recognition of congenital hip dislocation. Br. Med. J., *17*:147, 1971.

985. Walker, J. M.: A preliminary investigation of congenital hip disease in the Island Lake Reserve population, Manitoba. University of Manitoba, Anthropology Papers, No. 7, 1973.

986. Walker, J. M.: Morphologic variants of the human fetal hip joint. Their significance in congenital hip disease. J. Bone Joint Surg., *62-A*:1073, 1980.

987. Walker, J. M.: Histological study of the fetal development of the human acetabulum and labrum: Significance in congenital hip disease. Yale J. Biol. Med., *54*:255, 1981.

988. Walker, J. M.: Comparison of normal and abnormal human fetal hip joints: A quantitative study with significance to congenital hip disease. J. Pediatr. Orthop., *3*:173, 1983.

989. Walker, J. M., and Goldsmith, C.: Morphometric study of the fetal development of the human hip joint: Significance for congenital hip disease. Yale J. Biol. Med., *55*:411, 1982.

990. Walter, R., and Donaldson, J. S.: Ultrasound screening of high-risk newborns: A method to decrease the incidence of late diagnosis congenital dysplasia of the hip. Submitted for publication.

991. Warkany, J.: Congenital Malformations. Chicago, Year Book, 1971, pp. 992–997.

992. Watanabe, B. M., Dallas, T. G., and Westin, G. W.: Skeletal traction versus femoral shortening methods in the treatment of older congenitally dislocated hip patients. Orthop. Trans., *4*:303, 1980.

993. Watanabe, R. S.: Embryology of the human hip. Clin. Orthop., *98*:8, 1974.

994. Weathersby, H. T.: The origin of the artery of the ligamentum teres femoris. J. Bone Joint Surg., *41-A*:261, 1959.

995. Wedge, J. H., and Salter, R. B.: Innominate osteotomy: Its role in the arrest of secondary arthritis of the hip in the adult. Clin. Orthop., *98*:114, 1974.

996. Wedge, J. H., and Wasylenko, M. J.: The natural history of congenital dislocation of the hip. A critical review. Clin. Orthop., *137*:154, 1978.

997. Weickert, H. von: Zur Differenzierung von Femurkopfnekrose und Femurkopfaufbaustörung bei der

Behandlung der Luxationshüfte. Z. Orthop., *107*:440, 1970.

998. Weickert, H. von: Die Acetabuloplastik bei der Behandlung der Luxationshüfte. Beitr. Orthop., *31*:333, 1974.

999. Weickert, H. von, and Lohr, R.: Erfahrungen bei der Behandlung des Luxationsperthes unter besonderer Berucksichtigung der anwendung anaboler Wirkstoff. Z. Orthop., *100*:302, 1965.

1000. Weickert, H. von, and Luther, K.-P.: Ergebnisse der Frühbehandlung der Luxationshüfte mit dem beckerschen Spreizhoschen. Kinderaerztl. Prax., *39*:470, 1971.

1001. Weighill, F. J.: The treatment of developmental coxa vara by abduction. Clin. Orthop., *116*:116, 1976.

1002. Weiner, D. S.: Congenital dislocation of the hip associated with congenital muscular torticollis. Clin. Orthop., *121*:163, 1976.

1003. Weiner, D. S., Cook, A. J., Hoyt, W. A., and Oravec, C. E.: Computed tomography in measurement of femoral anteversion. Orthopedics, *1*:299, 1978.

1004. Weiner, D. S., Hoyt, W. A., and O'Dell, H. W.: Congenital dislocation of the hip—The relationship of pre-manipulation traction and age to avascular necrosis of the femoral head. J. Bone Joint Surg., *59*:306, 1977.

1005. Weinstein, S. L., and Ponseti, I. V.: Congenital dislocation of the hip. J. Bone Joint Surg., *61-A*:119, 1979.

1006. Weintroub, S., Green, I., Terdiman, R., and Weissman, S. L.: Growth and development of congenitally dislocated hips reduced in early infancy. J. Bone Joint Surg., *61-A*:125, 1979.

1007. Weissman, S. L.: Congenital dysplasia of the hip. J. Bone Joint Surg., *36-B*:385, 1954.

1008. Weissman, S. L.: Transplantation of the trochanteric epiphysis into the acetabulum after septic arthritis of the hip. J. Bone Joint Surg., *49-A*:1647, 1967.

1009. Weissman, S. L.: Troubles de croissance de l'extrémité proximale du fémur dans les suites du traitement de la luxation congénitale de la hanche. Rev. Chir. Orthop., *55*:331, 1969.

1010. Weissman, S. L.: Osteochondritis dissecans following congenital dislocation of the hip. J. Bone Joint Surg., *56-B*:454, 1974.

1011. Weissman, S. L., and Salama, R.: Treatment of congenital dislocation of the hip in the newborn infant. J. Bone Joint Surg., *48-A*:1319, 1966.

1012. Westin, G. W.: The stick femur. J. Bone Joint Surg., *52-B*:778, 1970.

1013. Westin, G. W., Ilfeld, F. W., and Provost, J.: Total avascular necrosis of the capital femoral epiphysis in congenital dislocation. Clin. Orthop., *119*:95, 1976.

1014. Westin, G. W., Dallas, T. G., Watanabe, B. M., and Ilfeld, F. W.: Skeletal traction vs. femoral shortening in treatment of older children with congenital hip dislocation. Isr. J. Med. Sci., *16*:318, 1980.

1015. White, R. E., Jr., and Sherman, F. C.: The hip-shelf procedure. A long-term evaluation. J. Bone Joint Surg., *62-A*:928, 1980.

1016. Wiberg, G.: Relation between congenital subluxation of the hip and arthritis deformans (roentgenological study). Acta Orthop. Scand., *10*:351, 1939.

1017. Wiberg, G.: Studies on dysplastic acetabula and congenital subluxation of the hip joint, with special reference to the complications of osteoarthritis. Acta Chir. Scand., *58*:83, 1939.

1018. Wiberg, G.: Studien über das normale Arthrographiebild des Hüftgelenks bei Kleinkindern. Z. Orthop., *72*:35, 1941.

1019. Wiberg, G.: Shelf operation in congenital dysplasia of the acetabulum and in subluxation and dislocation of the hip. J. Bone Joint Surg., *35-A*:65, 1953.

1020. Wiley, G.: Studies on dysplastic acetabular and congenital subluxation of the hip joint. Acta Chir. Scand., Suppl. 58:83, 1939.

1021. Wilkinson, J. A.: Femoral anteversion in the rabbit. J. Bone Joint Surg., *44-B*:386, 1962.

1022. Wilkinson, J. A.: Prime factors in the etiology of congenital dislocation of the hip. J. Bone Joint Surg., *45-B*:268, 1963.

1023. Wilkinson, J. A.: The effects of breech malposition. J. Bone Joint Surg., *46-B*:156, 1964.

1024. Wilkinson, J. A.: Breech malposition and intrauterine dislocations. Proc. R. Soc. Med., *59*:1106, 1966.

1025. Wilkinson, J. A.: A post-natal survey for congenital displacement of the hip. J. Bone Joint Surg., *54-B*:40, 1972.

1026. Wilkinson, J. A.: Failures in the management of congenital hip displacement in the newborn. Proc. R. Soc. Med., *68*:476, 1975.

1027. Wilkinson, J. A., and Carter, C.: Congenital dislocation of the hip. J. Bone Joint Surg., *42-B*:669, 1960.

1028. Williams, P. F.: Basic problems in the management of congenital dislocation of the hip. *In* Tachdjian, M. O. (ed.): Congenital Dislocation of the Hip. New York, Churchill-Livingstone, 1982, pp. 741–744.

1029. Williamson, J.: Difficulties of early diagnosis and treatment of congenital dislocation of the hip in Northern Ireland. J. Bone Joint Surg., *54-B*:13, 1972.

1030. Wilson, D. W.: Congenital dislocation of the hip. J. Bone Joint Surg., *46-B*:163, 1964.

1031. Wilson, J. C., Jr.: Traitement chirurgical de la dysplasie acétabulaire chez l'adolescente. Rev. Chir. Orthop., *58*:320, 1972.

1032. Wilson, J. C., Jr.: Surgical treatment of the dysplastic acetabulum in adolescence. Clin. Orthop., *98*:137, 1974.

1033. Wilson, J. C., Jr.: Congenital dislocation of the hip—then and now. West. J. Med., *124*:56, 1976.

1034. Winkler, W., and Weber, A.: Beckenosteotomie nach Chiari. Z. Orthop., *115*:167, 1977.

1035. Witt, A. N., and Jager, M.: Die Berechtigung und Indikation autoplastischer Spantransplantation in der heitigen Chirurgie. Chir. Plast. Reconstruct., *2*:48, 1966.

1036. Woolf, C. M., Koehn, J., and Coleman, S. S.: Congenital hip disease in Utah: The influence of genetic and non-genetic factors. Am. J. Hum. Genet., *20*:430, 1968.

1037. Wynne-Davies, R.: Acetabular dysplasia and familial joint laxity: Two aetiological factors in congenital dislocation of the hip. A review of 589 patients and their families. J. Bone Joint Surg., *52-B*:704, 1970.

1038. Wynne-Davies, R.: A family study of neonatal and late-diagnosis congenital dislocation of the hip. J. Med. Genet., 7:315, 1970.

1039. Wynne-Davies, R.: The epidemiology of congenital dislocation of the hip. Dev. Med. Child Neurol., *14*:515, 1972.

1040. Wynne-Davies, R.: Heritable Disorders in Orthopaedic Practice. Oxford, Blackwell, 1973.

1041. Wynne-Davies, R.: A review of genetics in orthopaedics. Acta Orthop. Scand., *46*:338, 1975.

1042. Yamada, Y.: Axial-transverse-tomographic study on residual subluxation of the hip. J. Jpn. Orthop. Assoc., *43*:361, 1969. (Abstract in Am. Digest Foreign Orthop. Lit., 1st quarter, 1972, pp. 88–91.)

1043. Yamaguchi, M., and Izumida, S.: Pfannendachbildender Effekt verschiedener operativer Eingriffe in der Behandlung der sogenannten kongenitalen Hüftgelenksluxation. Z. Orthop., *114*:156, 1976.

1044. Yosipovitch, Z.: Hip deformities after successful treatment of congenital dislocation of the hip in infancy. Isr. J. Med. Sci., *16*:314, 1980.

1045. Yousefzadeh, D. K., and Ramilo, J. L.: Normal hip

in children: Correlation of US with anatomic and cryomicrotome sections. Radiology, *165*:647, 1987.

1046. Zanoli, R.: Early diagnosis and late results of the early treatment of congenital dislocation of the hip. *In* Excerpta Medica, International Congress Series, No. 116. Amsterdam, Excerpta Medica, 1966, pp. 33–35.

1047. Zapfe, E.: Reposition mit der Overhead-Extension. (63. Kongress der Deutschen Gesellschaft für Orthopädie und Traumatologie, September, 1976.) Z. Orthop., *115*:642, 1977.

1048. Zieger, M., Hilpert, S., and Schulz, R. D.: Ultrasound of the infant hip. Part 1. Basic principles. Pediatr. Radiol., *16*:483, 1986.

1049. Zieger, M.: Ultrasound of the infant hip. Part 2. Validity of the method. Pediatr. Radiol., *16*:488, 1986.

1050. Zieger, M., and Schulz, R. D.: Ultrasonography of the infant hip. Part III. Clinical application. Pediatr. Radiol., *17*:226, 1987.

1051. Zippel, H.: Ätiologische Probleme der angeborenen Luxationshüfte unter besonderer Berucksichtigung zytogenetscher Untersuchungbefunde. Beitr. Orthop. Traumatol., *18*:541, 1971.

1052. Zsernaviczky, J., and Turk, G.: Two new radiological signs in the early diagnosis of congenital dysplasia of the hip joint. Int. Orthop., *2*:223, 1978.

CONGENITAL ABDUCTION CONTRACTURE OF THE HIP AND PELVIC OBLIQUITY

Congenital abduction contracture of the hip is much more common than congenital dislocation of the hip. It seems to arise from fetal malposition.

When the infant lies prone with the affected hip in abduction, the pelvis is level and at a right angle to the longitudinal axis of the spine, which remains straight (Fig. 2–233 A and B). When the affected limb is brought down into weight-bearing position, i.e., parallel with the vertical axis of the trunk and the opposite lower limb, lateral force is brought to bear on the pelvis, which assumes an oblique position (Fig. 2–233 C and D). The posterior superior iliac spine, the iliac crest, and the anterior superior iliac spine are low on the side of the abduction contracture and high on the opposite

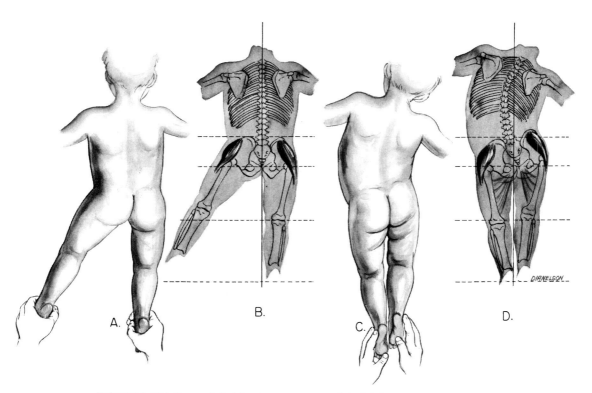

FIGURE 2–233. *Congenital abduction contracture of the left hip and pelvic obliquity.*

A and **B.** When the left hip is maintained in abduction, the pelvis is level and at a right angle to the longitudinal axis of the spine, which remains straight. **C** and **D.** When the left leg is brought down into weight-bearing position, parallel with the vertical axis of the trunk and the opposite extremity, the pelvis assumes an oblique position. Note the low iliac crest on the left, with apparent lengthening of the left lower extremity, the asymmetry of thigh folds and popliteal creases, the scoliosis, and the shortening of the right hip adductors.

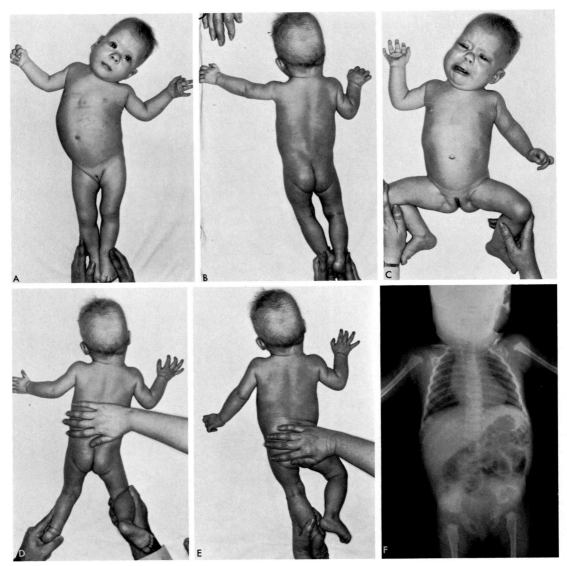

FIGURE 2–234. *Congenital abduction contracture of the right hip and pelvic obliquity in a two-month-old infant.*

A and **B.** Asymmetry of thigh folds and popliteal and gluteal creases with apparent shortening of the left lower extremity. Note the right lumbodorsal scoliosis and the left torticollis in the anteroposterior view. **C.** Limited abduction of left hip. **D.** Limited adduction of right hip. **E.** There is no limitation of adduction of left hip. **F.** Anteroposterior radiogram of whole torso. Note the obliquity of the pelvis and the delay of ossification of the left femoral head. Ortolani's and Barlow's signs were negative for dislocation or instability of the left hip. This patient was treated by passive stretching exercises for abduction contracture of right hip and adduction contracture of left hip.

side. There is asymmetry of the skin folds of the thigh and the popliteal creases, with apparent lengthening of the affected lower extremity (Fig. 2–234). Furthermore, scoliosis of the lumbar spine may result from the pelvic obliquity and the combined lengthening of the lateral trunk muscles on the abduction contracture side and shortening on the opposite side. Often there is associated lateral rotation contracture of the affected hip, and usually there is a varying degree of adduction contracture of the opposite hip. Other associated deformities due to fetal malposition are positional torticollis, valgus deformity of the foot on the abducted side, and pes varus on the adducted side. Ober's test is used to determine the degree of severity of abduction contracture (see Fig. 1–22).

In congenital abduction contracture of the hip, as opposed to congenital dislocation of the hip, Ortolani's and Barlow's signs are negative; the femoral head can be felt in its normal position beneath the femoral artery at the middle of the inguinal ligament, and there is neither piston mobility nor abnormal looseness of the hip. It is essential to differentiate the two conditions.

Radiograms of the hips in both the anteroposterior and 45-degree abduction views are taken. Because of the decreased concentric pressure of the femoral head, ossification of the roof of the acetabulum may be somewhat delayed in the adducted hip (i.e., the side opposite to the abduction contracture). If a severe abduction contracture of the hip is left untreated, subluxation of the opposite hip may occur. Roentgenograms also rule out congenital deformities of the lumbosacral spine, such as hemi-vertebrae and congenital scoliosis, as causes of congenital pelvic obliquity.

Treatment should be started early, preferably in the first two weeks after birth. The mother is taught to stretch the contracted hip abductors passively (Fig. 2–235). If there is contracture of the adductors of the opposite hip, the lateral rotators of the same hip, or the opposite lateral trunk muscles, they also are stretched. The exercises should be performed 20 times slowly in each direction 4 to 6 times a day.

If stretching exercises are begun at a very early age and performed regularly, the contractures will be corrected within four to eight weeks (see Fig. 2–234). Occasionally, when the parents are unequal to the task or the abduction contracture is severe, an infant has to be admitted to the hospital, where the deformity can be corrected by traction and exercises followed by immobilization in a bilateral hip spica cast that holds the affected hip in adduction, extension, and medial rotation, and the opposite hip in 90 degrees of flexion, 60 degrees of lateral rotation, and 50 degrees of abduction. Usually a period of three to four weeks of immobilization in a cast is sufficient to prevent recurrence of the deformity. A hip spica cast is also used in

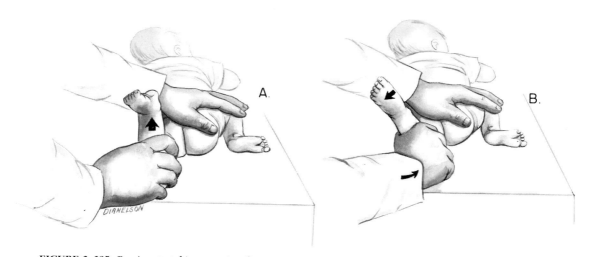

FIGURE 2–235. Passive stretching exercises for correction of congenital abduction contracture of the left hip.

A. The infant is placed prone with the opposite hip and knee flexed in order to get them out of the way and flatten the lumbar spine. The mother steadies the pelvis and opposite thigh with her left hand; with her right hand she grasps the thigh and leg at the knee and maximally extends the affected hip by lifting the thigh toward the ceiling. **B.** Next she adducts the hip by pushing the thigh toward the opposite leg, and rotates the hip medially by twisting the leg out. She keeps the left hip abductors stretched to the count of 10 and then lets go. The exercise is performed 20 times, 4 to 6 times a day.

the rare case in which there is subluxation of the hip opposite to the side of the abduction contracture.

Green and Griffin reported 18 children with unilateral dysplasia of the hip with asymmetrical gluteal folds and apparent lower limb length inequality secondary to pelvic obliquity due to abduction contracture of the contralateral hip. These 18 dysplastic hips were treated by abduction splinting and stretching exercises of the hip with the abduction contracture. In all these cases treatment produced excellent results and normal radiographic appearance.[4]

References

1. Browne, D.: Congenital deformities of mechanical origin. Arch. Dis. Child., 30:37, 1955.
2. Cozen, L.: Some evils of fixed abduction of the hip. Clin. Orthop., 57:203, 1968.
3. Dunn, P. M.: Congenital postural deformities. Br. Med. Bull., 32:71, 1976.
4. Green, N. E., and Griffin, P. P.: Hip dysplasia associ-

Table 2–19. Nine Classes of Congenital

	Class				
	I	II	III	IV	V
Diagram					
Femoral shortening (%)	—	70–90	45–80	40–67	48–85
Femoral-pelvic abnormalities	Femur absent Ischiopubic bone structures underdeveloped and deficient Lack of acetabular development	Femoral head absent Ischiopubic bone structures delayed in ossification	No osseous connection between femoral shaft and head Femoral head ossification delayed Acetabulum may be absent Femoral condyles maldeveloped Infrequent irregular tuft on proximal end of femur	Femoral head and shaft joined by irregular calcification in a fibro-cartilaginous matrix	Femur incompletely ossified, hypoplastic, and irregular Mid-shaft of femur abnormal
Associated abnormalities	Fibula absent	Tibia shortened Fibula, foot, knee-joint, and ankle-joint abnormal	Tibia shortened 0–40% Fibula shortened 5–100% Patella absent or small and high riding Knee-joint instability frequent Foot malformed	Tibia shortened 0–20% Fibula shortened 4–60% Knee-joint instability frequent Foot small with infrequent malformations	Tibia shortened 4–27% Fibula shortened 10–100% Knee-joint instability frequent Severe malformations of the foot frequent
Treatment objectives	Prosthetic management	Pelvic-femoral stability through prosthetic management	Union between femoral shaft and hip for hip stability Prosthetic management	Union between femoral head, neck, and shaft Prosthetic management	Prosthetic management

*From Pappas, A. M.: Congenital abnormalities of the femur. J. Pediatr. Orthop., 3:45, 1983. Reprinted by permission.

ated with abduction contracture of the contralateral hip.
J. Bone Joint Surg., *64-A*:1273, 1982.

CONGENITAL LONGITUDINAL DEFICIENCY OF THE FEMUR

The spectrum of defective development of the femur ranges from simple hypoplasia (congenital short femur) to complete hypoplasia (congenital absence of the femur). Congenital defects of the femur can be subdivided into two main categories—those with and those without an osseous defect. Deficiencies of the femur with an osseous defect of the upper third are generally referred to as proximal focal deficiency. Deficiencies may also occur in its midportion or distally.

The femoral deficiencies without an osseous defect are generally referred to as hypoplasia of the femur or congenital short femur. They are of three types: simple hypoplasia, or congenital short femur in which proportions are normal; hypoplastic femur with coxa vara; and hypoplastic femur with coxa valga.

*Abnormalities of the Femur**

VI	VII	VIII	IX
30–60	10–50	10–41	6–20
Distal femur short, irregular, and hypoplastic	Coxa vara	Coxa valga	Hypoplastic femur
Irregular distal femoral diaphysis	Hypoplastic femur	Hypoplastic femur	
	Proximal femoral diaphysis irregular with thickened cortex	Femoral head and neck smaller	
	Lateral femoral condyle deficiency frequent	Proximal femoral physis horizontal	
	Valgus distal femur	Abnormality of femoral condyles frequent with associated bowing of shaft and valgus of distal femur	
Single bone lower leg	Tibia shortened <10–24%	Tibia shortened 0–36%	Tibia shortened 0–15%
Patella absent	Fibula shortened <10–100%	Fibula shortened 0–100%	Fibula shortened 3–30%
Foot malformed	Lateral and high riding patella frequent	Lateral and high riding patella frequent	Additional ipsilateral and contralateral malformations frequent
		Foot malformed	
Prosthetic management	Extremity length equality	Extremity length equality	Extremity length equality
	Improved alignment of (a) proximal and (b) distal femur	Improved alignment of (a) proximal and (b) distal femur	

Pappas proposed the following comprehensive classification of congenital abnormalities of the femur.

Class I. Congenital absence of the femur

Class II. Proximal femoral and pelvic deficiency

Class III. Proximal femoral deficiency with no osseous connection between femoral shaft and head

Class IV. Proximal femoral deficiency with disorganized fibro-osseous disconnection between femoral shaft and head

Class V. Midfemoral deficiency with hypoplastic proximal and distal development

Class VI. Distal femoral deficiency

Class VII. Hypoplastic femur with coxa vara and sclerosed diaphysis

Class VIII. Hypoplastic femur with coxa valga

Class IX. Hypoplastic femur with normal proportions[85]

He arrived at this classification in a thorough study of 125 children with 139 congenital abnormalities of the femur who were followed for a major portion of their growing years. A comprehensive longitudinal analysis of the data provided the definition of each classification; a forecast of the range of growth discrepancy of the femur and other bones in the lower limb, and the likelihood of associated malformations; and recognition of the clinical factors that must be coordinated with treatment considerations and long-term functional potential. These are summarized in Table 2–19.

PROXIMAL FEMORAL FOCAL DEFICIENCY

The malformation is a congenital defect. Components of the acetabulum and proximal femur develop from a common cartilaginous anlage. The hip joint is created by the formation of a cleft. At nine weeks of fetal life it resembles that of an adult. An outline of the development of the human femur from four weeks to term is given in Table 2–20. During the period of limb bud formation and differentiation, a noxious agent may produce proximal femoral focal deficiency. Experimentally, Duraswami produced this deformity by injecting insulin into the yolk sac on the sixth day of development of chick embryos.[24] Of the numerous teratologic agents— such as irradiation, anoxia, ischemia, bacterial toxins, viral infection, mechanical and thermal injury, toxic chemicals, and hormones—only the drug thalidomide has been demonstrated to be a definite cause in the human.

The limbs develop in a proximodistal direction; the acetabulum and the upper elements of the femur form first, and then the leg and foot follow. Therefore, in the absence of an acetabulum, there is no femoral head and vice versa. If an acetabulum is seen in the radiogram it denotes the presence of a femoral head and neck, though they may not be visualized in the radiogram because they are unossified.

Classification

It is essential to classify proximal femoral focal deficiency and outline a goal-oriented plan of management, which depends on the natural history of its various types and is based on the anticipated growth and development of the defective limb. Various classifications have been proposed by several authors—by Frantz and O'Rahilly; by Hall, Brooks, and Denis; and by King.[30, 41, 54–58] Infantile, or developmental, coxa vara should definitely not be classified under proximal femoral focal deficiency. There is also some controversy as to whether the milder forms of simple hypoplasia of the femur should be included under this classification. This author strongly feels that problems in management of the congenital short femur are different, and it should be regarded as a separate clinical entity.

Gillespie and Torode subdivided congenital longitudinal deficiencies into two major groups: *Group I*, or congenital hypoplastic femur, in which the hip and knee are or can be made functional and lower limb equalization may be possible; and *Group II*, or true proximal femoral focal deficiency, in which the hip is never normal and the ultimate lower limb discrepancy is of such magnitude that these patients need prosthetic management and all surgical procedures are designed to facilitate the fitting of the prosthesis.[34, 107]

Aitken classified proximal femoral focal deficiency into four different types on the basis of the radiographic features; this classification is endorsed by King.[3, 54–58] Radiographic findings depend on the age of the patient. In *Type A* the femur is short with coxa vara and lateral bowing of its upper third; the medial femoral cortex at the site of bowing is thickened. There is always an adequate acetabulum that contains a femoral head (Fig. 2–236 A). During the first year of life the lower two thirds of the femoral shaft are ossified, but the upper third and the femoral head and neck are cartilaginous (Figs. 2–237 A). The acetabulum is present and normal. The upper end of the distal bony shaft is

Table 2–20. *Development of the Human Femur From Four Weeks to Term**

Embryo			
Size (mm)	Age (weeks)	Length of femur (mm)	Development of Femur
5–7	4–5	—	1. Histologically undifferentiated limb bud and apical ectodermal ridge 2. Contiguous to lower spine area
9–12	5–6	2	1. Paddle-shaped limb 2. Mesodermal differentiation starts. Blastema to chondral and myogenic differentiation 3. Pelvis and femur two separate cellular mosaics. Femoral head will develop as part pelvic mosaic 4. Ectodermal changes—preneurogenesis
15–20	6–7	3–4	1. Chondral formation in shaft at least two of five cell phases 2. Fibula and lateral femoral condyle; tibia and medial femoral condyle develop in proximal distal relationship 3. Early zone formation in areas of joint development 4. Outline of femoral head 5. Early neuromyogenesis 6. Peripheral digital outline
20–30	7–8.5	6–8	1. Chondral model complete 2. Acetabulum, femoral head, greater trochanter, and femoral condyles in chondral model 3. Periosteal sleeve 4. Central shaft chondral to osseous transition 5. Vascularization 6. Joint cavitation 7. Evidence of neuromuscular activity in upper extremity
30–40	8.5–10	8–10	1. Center of femur ossified—extension of ossification proximal and distal (more rapid distally) 2. Hip and knee joints formed with evidence of interarticular structures 3. Evidence of neuromuscular activity lower extremity. All muscle groups identifiable 4. Femoral retroversion of approximately 10°
70	12	18	1. Ossification extends to metaphyseal levels—proximal and distal 2. Vascularization of intertrochanteric and condylar regions 3. Intra-articular structures and ligaments—complete 4. Femoral retroversion changes to anteversion of 5 to 10°
100–term	15–40	27–100	1. Extension of vascularization and ossification into femoral neck-head 2. Cavitation of femoral diaphysis 3. Femoral anteversion increases to 30–40° 4. Rapid growth and development of all structures

*From Pappas, A. M.: Congenital abnormalities of the femur and related lower extremity malformations: Classification and treatment. J. Pediatr. Orthop., 3:45, 1983. Reprinted by permission.

TYPE		FEMORAL HEAD	ACETABULUM	FEMORAL SEGMENT	RELATIONSHIP AMONG COMPONENTS OF FEMUR AND ACETABULUM AT SKELETAL MATURITY
A	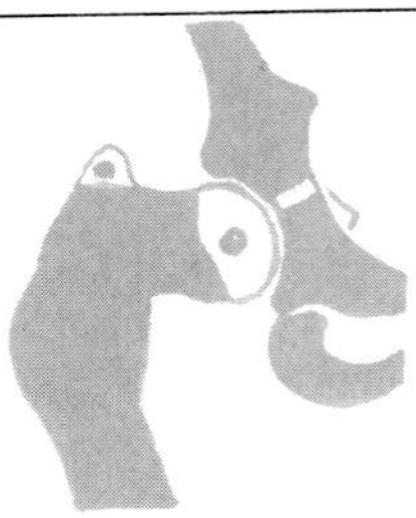	Present	Normal	Short	Bony connection between components of femur Femoral head in acetabulum Subtrochanteric varus angulation, often with pseudarthrosis
B	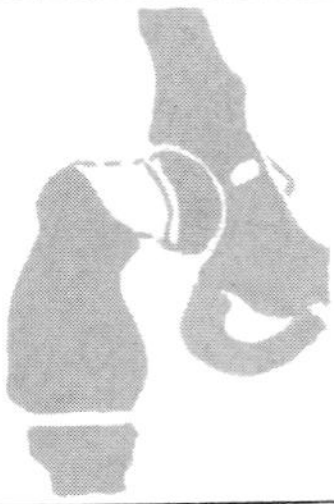	Present	Adequate or moderately dysplastic	Short, usually proximal bony tuft	No osseous connection between head and shaft Femoral head in acetabulum
C	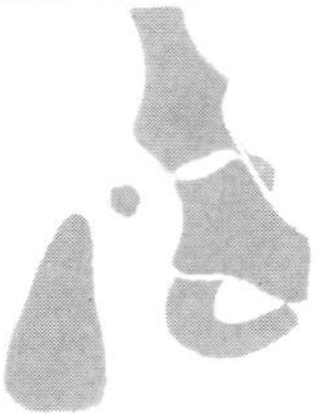	Absent or represented by ossicle	Severely dysplastic	Short, usually proximally tapered	May be osseous connection between shaft and proximal ossicle No articular relation between femur and acetabulum
D	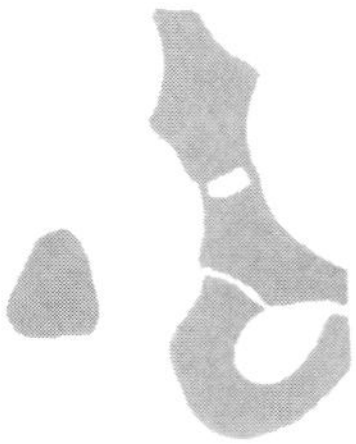	Absent	Absent Obturator foramen enlarged Pelvis squared in bilateral cases	Short, deformed	(none)

FIGURE 2–236. *Aitken classification of proximal femoral focal deficiency.*

A to D. The four types of deficiency. See text for explanation.

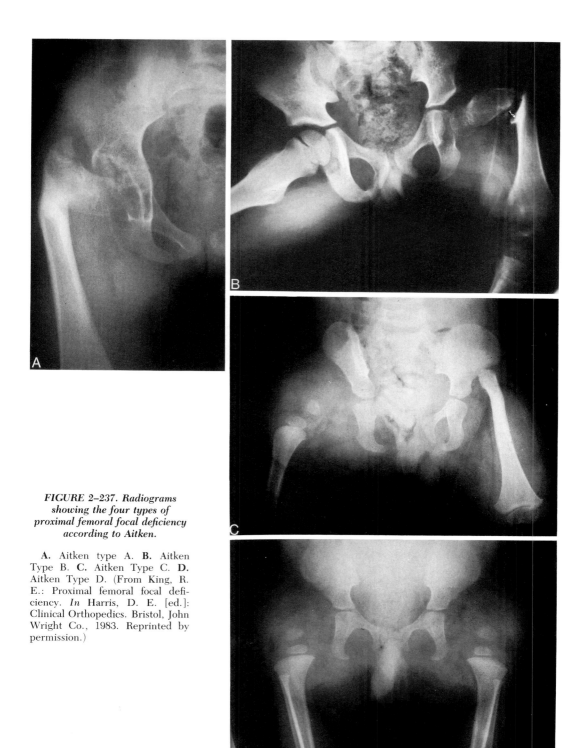

FIGURE 2–237. Radiograms showing the four types of proximal femoral focal deficiency according to Aitken.

A. Aitken type A. **B.** Aitken Type B. **C.** Aitken Type C. **D.** Aitken Type D. (From King, R. E.: Proximal femoral focal deficiency. *In* Harris, D. E. [ed.]: Clinical Orthopedics. Bristol, John Wright Co., 1983. Reprinted by permission.)

usually bulbous rather than spiky, and it is separated from the acetabulum by a considerable gap. The ossified femoral shaft is thinner than normal. The femur is markedly short. By the end of the second year or early in the third year of life, the ossification center of the femoral head develops, and the proximal shaft of the femur gradually ossifies. At the subtrochanteric region a pseudarthrosis develops, and increasing varus deformity of the upper femur ensues with angulation at the site of the pseudarthrosis. This is in contrast to varus angulation in developmental coxa vara (or infantile coxa vara), in which the deformity occurs at the metaphyseal region in the neck of the femur. At skeletal maturity, ossification of the pseudarthrosis will take place in most cases, but the varus angulation at the subtrochanteric region may be very severe (Fig. 2–238). Morphologic findings in an autopsy specimen from one case of Type A proximal femoral focal deficiency has been reported by Epps.[26]

In *Type B* there are always an acetabulum and a femoral head; however, the ossification of the capital femoral epiphysis is delayed, and the acetabulum is mildly dysplastic (Fig. 2–236 B). The upper end of the femoral shaft is displaced laterally and upward, with its proximal end lying above the femoral head. The femoral shaft is short and deformed and has a small bony bulbous tuft at its upper end (Fig. 2–237 B). The junction between the femoral

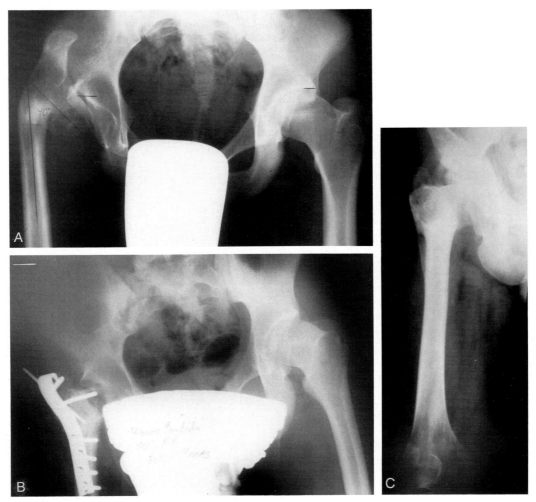

FIGURE 2–238.
Proximal femoral focal deficiency of the right femur with severe coxa vara.

A. The neck-shaft angle is 40 degrees, and the tip of the greater trochanter is markedly elevated. **B.** After subtrochanteric abduction osteotomy with distal transfer of the greater trochanter. **C.** Two years postoperatively, showing the neck-shaft angle to be 110 degrees.

head and shaft is by defective cartilage that fails to ossify at skeletal maturity. The resultant subtrochanteric varus deformity may be extensive.

In *Type C* the acetabulum is markedly dysplastic, and the femoral head never ossifies (Fig. 2–236 C). The femoral shaft is very short, and at its upper end there is a small tuft of dysplastic ossified tissue that tapers sharply to a point. The hip is very unstable; there is no synchronous motion between the femoral shaft and head. The tapered, sclerotic upper end of the femoral shaft appears to move on the lateral wall of the ilium (Figs. 2–237 C and 2–239). It migrates progressively upward.

Type D is the most severe deficiency (Fig. 2–236 D). Both the acetabulum and femoral head are absent. The femoral shaft is very short

with no proximal tufting; the femur appears to be represented by the distal femoral condyles (Fig. 2–237 D).

Definitive classification of proximal femoral focal deficiency during infancy is difficult because of the marked delay of ossification of the cartilaginous portion of the proximal femur. It is important *to assess serial radiograms* during maturation of the skeleton. Differentiation of Type A from Type B is particularly difficult until the femoral head and neck are ossified. The presence of an acetabulum indicates the presence of a femoral head. Arthrography will also demonstrate it, but routine arthrography is not recommended. This author performs it to depict the configuration of the femoral head and neck and to determine the degree of coxa vara, as progressive decrease of the femoral

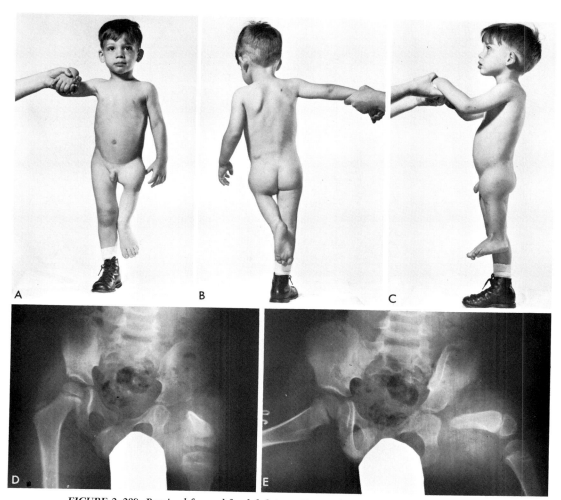

FIGURE 2–239. *Proximal femoral focal deficiency Type C (Aitken) in a three-year-old boy.*

A to **C.** Photographs of patient depicting deformities. **D** and **E.** Anteroposterior and frog-leg lateral radiograms of both hips. Note the presence of an acetabular socket on the left, indicating that there is a cartilaginous femoral head.

Illustration continued on following page

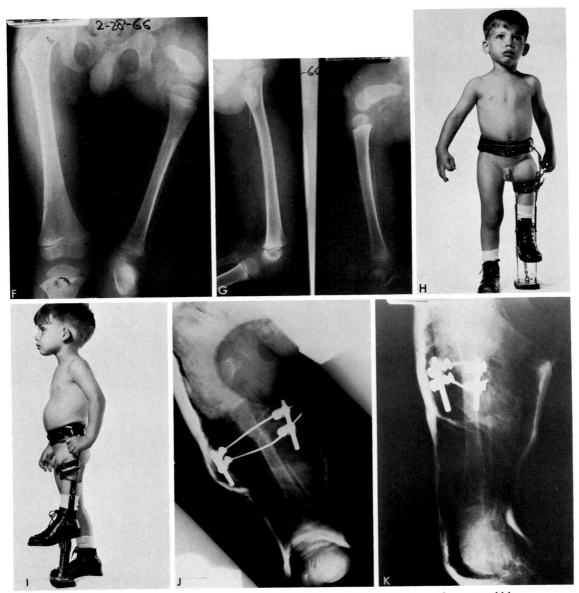

FIGURE 2–239 Continued *Proximal femoral focal deficiency Type C (Aitken) in a three-year-old boy.*

F and **G.** Anteroposterior and lateral radiograms of the entire femur on the right and the lower limb on the left, showing that the left ankle joint is at the same level as the right knee. The left proximal fibula is not ossified. **H** and **I.** Patient demonstrating the above-knee orthosis used for ambulation. A spring traction device is attached on the shoe to hold the limb in neutral position. The pelvic band controls rotation. (At present, the author uses a quadrilateral ischial socket orthosis that extends high on the ilium to prevent hip abduction.) At four years of age a Van Nes rotation-plasty was performed. **J** and **K.** Immediate postoperative radiograms through the hip spica cast, showing the threaded Steinmann pins and Roger Anderson device utilized to hold the osteotomized fragments together firmly.

Illustration continued on following page

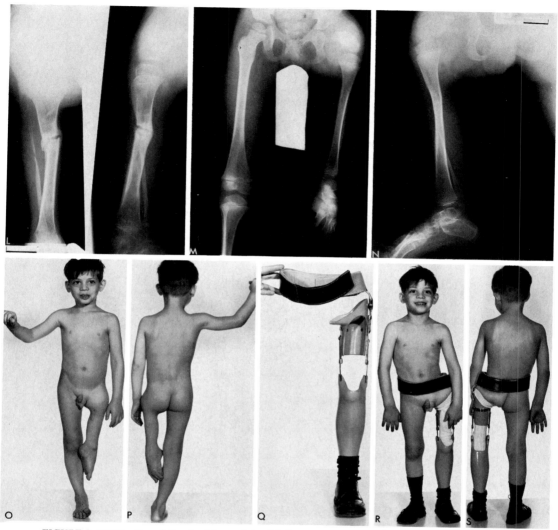

FIGURE 2–239 *Continued Proximal femoral focal deficiency Type C (Aitken) in a three-year-old boy.*

L. Anteroposterior and lateral radiograms of the left tibia, ten months following surgery. The osteotomy is healed. The patient has been fitted with a prosthesis for ambulation. **M** and **N.** Anteroposterior and lateral radiograms one year following rotation-plasty. **O** and **P.** Clinical appearance of patient one year post-rotation-plasty. Note the tendency toward derotation. **Q.** The prosthesis used for walking. The pelvic band attachment is for control of rotation. **R** and **S.** The patient wearing the prosthesis.

shaft-neck angle, especially to 90 degrees or less, is an indication for early valgization osteotomy of the upper end of the femur with or without autogenous bone grafting (Fig. 2–240).

Associated Anomalies

There is a high incidence of associated anomalies: 69 per cent in the series reported by Aitken and 65 per cent of those reported by Koman and associates (Fig. 2–241).[3, 59] This indicates a multifocal teratogenic process that

acts over a period of time. Congenital longitudinal deficiency of the fibula is the most common associated anomaly, its incidence reported as 50 per cent by Nilsonne, 70 per cent by Aitken, and 80 per cent by Amstutz and Wilson.[2–5, 8, 80] In the affected limb there is a varying degree of shortening of the tibia and fibula (if present) due to growth retardation; the patella may be absent or small and high riding; the patellofemoral joint may be laterally subluxated or dislocated, and flexion deformity of the knee and genu valgum are common. The knee joint

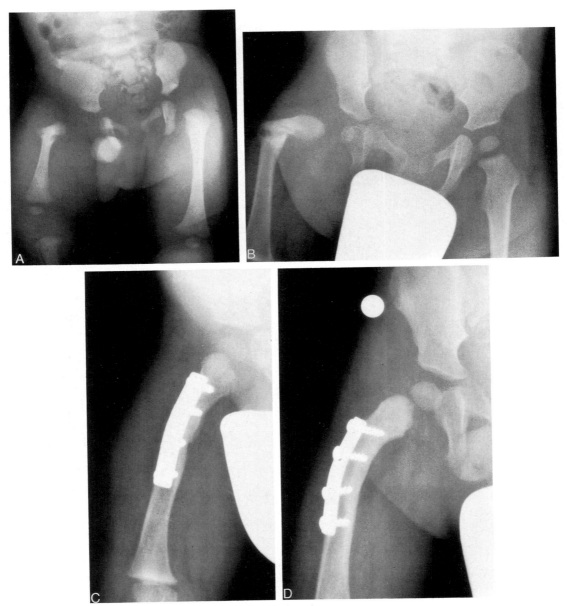

FIGURE 2–240. *Proximal femoral focal deficiency Type A.*

A. Anteroposterior radiogram of one-month-old boy. Note the coxa vara deformity of about 110 degrees, the marked shortening of the femur, and the delay in ossification of the upper end of the femur. **B.** At age 10 months the coxa vara deformity remains uncorrected. **C** and **D.** Anteroposterior and lateral radiograms after valgization osteotomy.

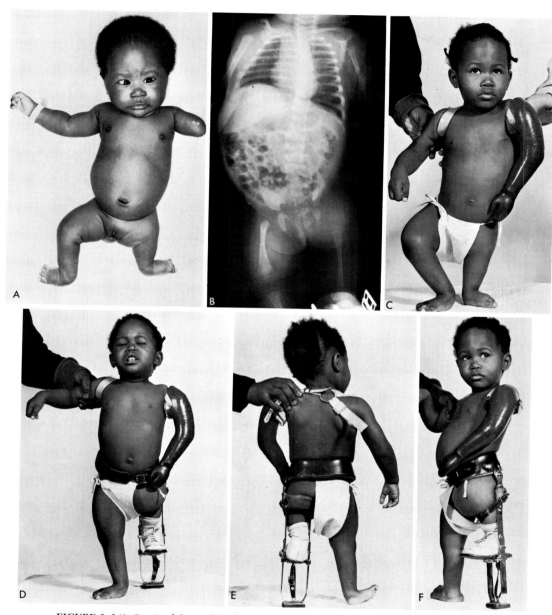

FIGURE 2–241. Proximal femoral focal deficiency Type B (Aitken) with associated anomalies.

Both fibulae are absent, and there is valgus deformity of the ankles. Note the congenital absence of the left forearm and distal half of the arm. **A.** Clinical appearance of infant with multiple deformities. **B.** Anteroposterior radiogram of whole torso and lower limbs. The dysgenetic left femur is cartilaginous. The acetabular socket is very shallow. Note bilateral absence of the fibula. **C.** Same patient at 18 months of age. The opposite knee is flexed to compensate for the marked shortening of the left femur. An artificial mitten hand has been fitted. **D to F.** The child is fitted with a brace. The traction force on the shoe is to prevent increase in the degree of flexion-abduction contracture of the left hip. The ischial ring of the brace, instead of the cartilaginous proximal femur, bears the stresses of body weight. (At present, the author uses an ischial socket.)

Illustration continued on following page

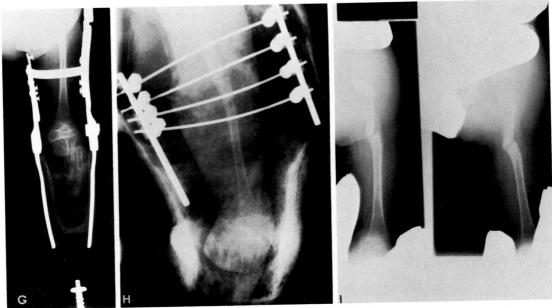

FIGURE 2–241 *Continued Proximal femoral focal deficiency Type B (Aitken) with associated anomalies.*

G. Radiogram of the left lower limb with the orthosis on. A rotation-plasty was performed at three years of age. **H** and **I.** Immediate and three-months-postoperative radiograms.

may be unstable, and associated malformations of the foot range from mild hypoplasia to severe anomalies such as absence of rays and tarsal coalition; talipes equinovarus or vertical talus is rare.

It is vital to assess both the total lower limb and the entire child when outlining the treatment plan. Contralateral lower limb and upper limb deformities may be present. Spine deformities are rare. Occasionally there may be associated congenital heart lesions or cleft palate.

Clinical Picture

The deformity is obvious, with a characteristic appearance at birth. The thigh is bulky and short; the degree of lower limb length disparity varies, depending on the type of proximal femoral focal deficiency. Often the degree of limb length discrepancy is so great that the ankle on the affected side is level with the contralateral knee (Fig. 2–241 A to C). There are flexion, abduction, and lateral rotation contractures of the involved hip, and flexion contracture of the knee. On testing range of motion of the hip, it is often difficult to determine whether the motion is taking place at the femoropelvic junction, the pseudarthrosis of the femur, or the knee joint. The quadriceps femoris is often hypoplastic with a high-riding vestigial patella. The

sartorius muscle is strong and contracts on attempted knee extension—its action being to draw the leg into the "sitting-tailor's position," the hip assumes a position of flexion–abduction–lateral rotation, and the knee is pulled into flexion. Action of the iliopsoas and hamstrings at the site of pseudarthrosis of the upper femoral shaft aggravates the deformity. Passive motion at the hip or pseudarthrosis site is not painful. There is little or no telescoping at the site of nonunion.

The infant should be thoroughly examined to rule out the presence of other associated congenital malformations. In about 50 per cent of cases, the ipsilateral fibula is absent and the tibia is shortened. In complete longitudinal deficiency (complete absence) of the fibula, the lateral malleolus cannot be palpated and the foot is in valgus position. The patella may be absent or hypoplastic and riding high and laterally. Coalition of the tarsal bones and other major malformations of the foot (such as absence of lateral rays) may be present. There may be congenital absence or hypoplasia of other parts of the body, particularly in the upper limb (Fig. 2–241 A).

When the infant begins to stand and take steps, the foot on the involved side is plantar flexed, and the contralateral knee is held in flexion in an attempt to compensate for the marked limb length discrepancy. The patient walks with a short-leg limp. In severe shortening, he may be unable to ambulate unless an extension orthosis is provided. The shortening is progressive; with the relative retardation of growth of the affected side, the knee rides higher and higher. The hip and knee flexion deformities increase, making the limb functionally shorter. A gluteus medius lurch is common.

Treatment

Proximal femoral focal deficiency can involve one or both lower limbs to a varying degree. The problem is complex and is further complicated by the associated deformities such as fibular hemimelia, a markedly malformed foot, or an unstable hip. Each patient must be evaluated individually. Treatment must be based on a thorough assessment of the pathologic anatomy and on the prediction of the natural history according to classification type. The primary objective of treatment is to provide optimal function; improvement of appearance should always be a secondary consideration.

There is no single method of management. Several modalities of treatment are utilized, including surgery and fitting of special prosthetic devices. The psyche of a severely deformed child should not be forgotten. Preventive psychological counseling and total habilitation are essential.

BILATERAL PROXIMAL FEMORAL FOCAL DEFICIENCY

When both femora are involved, the malformation generally tends to be more severe and the stature extremely short (Fig. 2–242). The standing height of the patient is further decreased by flexion deformity of both hips. The center of gravity of the body is lowered toward the ground, however, and the gait, despite being of the waddling type, is very agile and effective. The main problem is one of cosmesis. The primary consideration, however, should be given to function and not to appearance. It is vital that the ability to walk be preserved. These children can be given considerable added height by using bilateral extension prostheses with an augmentation segment below the feet, with or without knee joints. With the extension prostheses the child's height can be increased to normal. The prosthesis employed is a nonstandard above-knee type that is fitted around the feet with the knee joints mounted under the feet. Often these patients will require crutches for ambulation. If the feet and ankles are plantigrade, however, these children walk and run very well; no prostheses can replace the agility they possess with their short lower limbs. Increasing their stature to that of their peers is of no value if they lose mobility and are unable to play or even walk with their

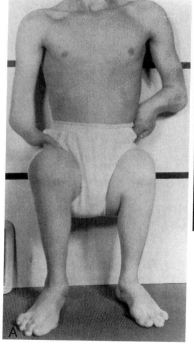
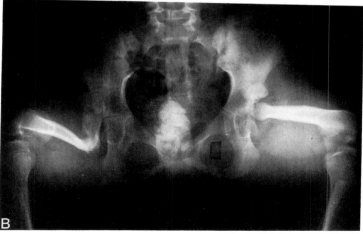

FIGURE 2–242. Bilateral proximal femoral focal deficiency.

A. Clinical appearance. **B.** Radiograms. (Courtesy of Edward Millar, M.D., Chief of Staff, Shriners Hospital, Chicago.)

friends. It is best to leave these children alone. Surgical intervention may improve their appearance but deprive them of function.

In cases in which there are associated distal anomalies, such as absence of the fibula, kyphotic hypoplastic tibiae, and rigid valgus feet, weight-bearing and ambulation may be very difficult or impossible. Only in such an instance should Syme amputation and knee fusion be performed to make prosthetic fitting simpler and to allow functional ambulation.

UNILATERAL INVOLVEMENT

When only one lower limb is affected, the following major deformities require treatment: (1) inequality in lower limb length, (2) pelvifemoral instability, (3) malrotation of the entire lower limb with flexion–abduction–lateral rotation contracture of the hip and flexion contracture of the knee and, (4) inadequacy of the proximal musculature. The severity of these biomechanical deficiencies varies according to the type of proximal femoral focal deficiency; they are discussed according to the age of the child, and a rational plan of treatment is outlined.

Malrotation of the Entire Lower Limb. In the newborn and infant up to 9 to 12 months of age, efforts are directed toward lessening or preventing progression of the flexion, abduction, and lateral rotation contractures of the hip and flexion contracture of the knee. Passive stretching exercises are performed several times a day, pulling the hip into extension, adduction, and medial rotation, and the knee into extension. The direction of passive pull should be in the line of deformity.

In the severe fixed contractural deformity, such as hip flexion of 40 degrees and lateral rotation of 35 degrees, one should apply *bilateral* split Russell skin traction with a medial rotation strap on the affected thigh. After a short period in the hospital—and proper instructions to the parents—the traction is applied at home at night and at nap time.

The sartorius is a deforming force in the pathogenesis of flexion–abduction–lateral rotation contracture of the hip and flexion deformity of the knee.[84] One may recess the origin of the sartorius muscle from the anterior superior iliac spine to the anterior aspect of the upper femoral shaft in the subtrochanteric region. This author recommends transfer of its insertion distally from the medial surface of the upper tibia to the patellar tendon at its insertion. He has found this sartorius transfer to be effective in reinforcing the weak quadriceps femoris muscle, providing active knee extension, and re-

lieving its deforming action at the hip. The operation is performed at three to four years of age.

Pelvifemoral Instability. In proximal femoral focal deficiency, providing a stable anatomic relationship between the proximal femur and the pelvis is crucial for a satisfactory gait. The biomechanical problems are created by progressive coxa vara, persisting instability at the pseudarthrosis site, and failure of development of the hip joint due to deficiencies of the acetabulum and neck-head of the femur.

Progressive coxa vara takes place at the "pseudarthrosis" site in the subtrochanteric region. Arthrography will assist in the accurate determination of the varus deformity. When the two femoral segments are connected by fibrocartilage, a subtrochanteric valgus osteotomy is performed at the site of the pseudarthrosis. The fibrocartilaginous connection may be excised to provide bone-to-bone contact. Bone grafting (from the ilium) is usually not necessary. In severe cases adductor myotomy of the hip is performed first. Internal fixation is by side plate. Injury to the upper femoral physis and the epiphysis of the greater trochanter should be avoided. A one–and–one half hip spica cast is applied for external support. Technical difficulties are minimal. Union occurs readily.

When there is no connection between the two femoral segments, as shown by arthrography and cineradiography, the site of pseudarthrosis is explored, fibrocartilaginous elements are excised, varus deformity is corrected, and internal fixation is provided by nail and plate or a side plate. The pseudarthrosis site is grafted with autogenous bone from the ipsilateral ilium. Union is more difficult to achieve in these cases; re-exploration and regrafting may be necessary in some. One should refrain from violating the hip joint while grafting, in order to prevent limitation of motion of an already compromised hip joint. A stiff hip will make gait training and prosthetic rehabilitation difficult.

When the femoral head-neck and the acetabulum are deficient or absent (Type D proximal femoral focal deficiency), there is gross pelvifemoral instability, for correction of which various surgical procedures have been advocated in the literature. Construction of an acetabulum by means of Chiari's medial displacement iliac osteotomy will provide a roof to which the distal femur is fused, thereby converting the knee to function as a hip (Fig. 2–243). Femoropelvic arthrodesis provides stability but has the definite disadvantage of loss of joint mobility. The ball-and-socket hip joint is converted into a

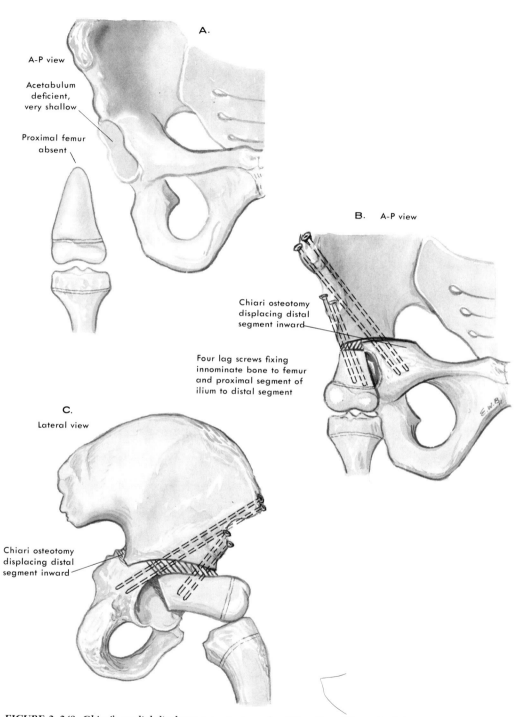

A.

A-P view

Acetabulum
deficient,
very shallow

Proximal femur
absent

B.   A-P view

Chiari osteotomy
displacing distal
segment inward

Four lag screws fixing
innominate bone to femur
and proximal segment of
ilium to distal segment

C.
Lateral view

Chiari osteotomy
displacing distal
segment inward

FIGURE 2–243. Chiari's medial displacement osteotomy for Aitken Type IV proximal femoral focal deficiency.

A. Acetabulum is almost absent, and only the distal femoral shaft is present. **B** and **C.** Postoperative drawing shows the Chiari medial displacement osteotomy and fusion of the distal femoral shaft to the proximal segment of the ilium.

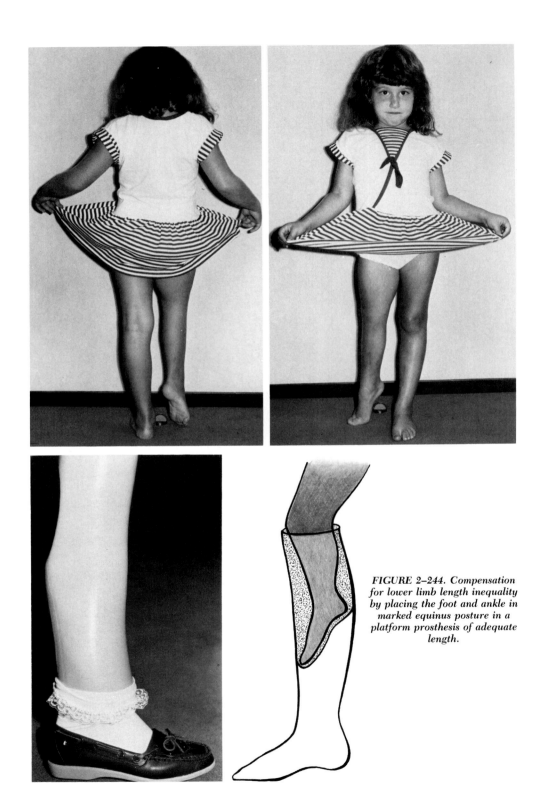

FIGURE 2–244. Compensation for lower limb length inequality by placing the foot and ankle in marked equinus posture in a platform prosthesis of adequate length.

hinge joint with flexion-extension as the only movement. It is perhaps best to ignore the osseous-articular defect and not to perform hip fusion, but instead, to provide stability by increasing motor strength of the hip musculature, which is stimulated by active weight-bearing.

Other surgical attempts to provide pelvifemoral stability in Type D proximal femoral focal deficiency that have been cited in the literature are excision of the femur and placement of the tibia in the acetabulum, excision of the vestigial femoral head-neck and transplantation of the fibula, an allograft hip joint transplant, and an adjustable internal hip joint–proximal femoral replacement prosthesis.[7, 20] This author has had no personal experience with these procedures.

Lower Limb Length Inequality. When the child begins to stand and bear weight, the lower limb discrepancy may not be so great initially; in such a case a patten-bottom extension orthosis will provide adequate weight-bearing and allow the child to walk. The orthosis is best fitted with an ischial socket, relatively high anteriorly and laterally, on the upper thigh; this will act as a buttress and assist in checking progression of the flexion–abduction–lateral rotation deformity of the hip. A well-fitted ischial portion may protect the cartilaginous proximal femur and the pseudarthrosis from the stress of weight-bearing; it is, however, questionable whether it will be effective in preventing cephalad migration of the femoral shaft. A pelvic band with a drop-lock hip joint will control lateral rotation of the hip. It has been conventional to have a traction device on the shoe attached to the patten bottom; this will control posture of the leg in the orthotic device.

When the child is two to three years of age one can quite accurately predict the lower limb length at skeletal maturity.

In proximal femoral focal deficiency the involved femur has constant relative growth inhibition. The percentage of growth inhibition is calculated by the difference between the normal and abnormal lengths divided by the normal length and multiplied by 100. Next, the anticipated normal limb segment length is determined by using serial scanograms and plotting the limb lengths on the Green-Anderson graph according to skeletal age. By transcribing the same spatial relationship of the growth curve to the main growth curve line at maturity, one can predict the normal length. The anticipated normal limb length segment is multiplied by the percentage of growth inhibition, and the length of the involved limb segment at skeletal

maturity can be determined.[7] The use of Moseley charts will expedite this calculation.

Types B, C, and D of proximal femoral focal deficiency require prosthetic restoration to minimize the biomechanical losses and to provide maximal function. This is because there is marked shortening of the affected limb with severe biomechanical problems of hip instability, inadequate proximal musculature, and malrotation. Several important decisions have to be made at this time: first, whether the child should be treated by surgical conversion or extension prosthesis.

When surgical conversion is not allowed by the parents or not chosen by the surgeon, the foot and ankle are placed in full equinus position on a platform, and a prosthesis of adequate length is provided to compensate for the limb length disparity (Fig. 2–244). The length of the prosthesis can be adjusted to accommodate growth. As the shortening increases, the problem may be solved by placing both the knee and the foot within the socket of an extension prosthesis; the hinge of the prosthetic knee is below the child's foot (Fig. 2–245). These types of prostheses are cosmetically unacceptable and

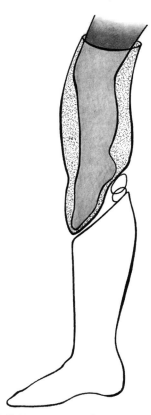

FIGURE 2–245. *Extension prosthesis with the hinge of the prosthetic knee below the child's foot.*

functionally inferior to the conversion prosthetic devices because they cannot provide a normal ratio of thigh to leg length.

Conversion surgery is performed to provide a stump that can be fitted into a conventional prosthesis. The surgeon and the family should make a decision whether to manage the patient as an above-knee or below-knee amputee. An above-knee stump is provided by knee fusion, Syme amputation, and sometimes epiphysiodesis at the distal femur or proximal tibia to level the knees (Fig. 2–246). A below-knee stump is provided by the Van Nes procedure of rotation-plasty (Fig. 2–247). It is best for the child's parents to have the opportunity to see another patient who has had surgical conversion; they should observe the other child walk and play while wearing the prosthesis. If possible, video films are of great value. If the patient is old enough, he should participate in the decision-making process.

Van Nes Rotation-plasty. Borggreve, in 1930, described a turnabout procedure in which the

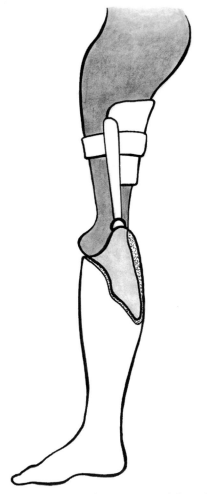

FIGURE 2–247. *Rotation-plasty in proximal femoral deficiency.*

The ankle and foot are turned 180 degrees to activate the knee of the prosthesis.

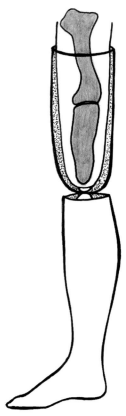

FIGURE 2–246. *Conventional prosthesis used for limb length inequality in proximal femoral focal deficiency.*

The knee is fused, and a Syme amputation is performed.

limb is rotated 180 degrees on a vertical axis, turning the foot posteriorly and using the ankle joint as a knee; thus, dorsiflexion of the foot in the prosthesis would flex the prosthetic knee joint. The patient originally described by Borggreve had lost a large segment of the femur, and the lower segment of his limb was rotated through the gap left by resection of the distal femur.[14] Van Nes popularized the procedure in 1950, reporting the results of rotation-plasty in three patients. He performed rotation through the femur in one case, through the femur and knee in two stages in the second case, and through the knee joint in the third case. Rotating the lower limb through 180 degrees is commonly referred to as the Van Nes rotation-plasty.[109] The original technique of Van Nes was modified later by Kostuik, Gillespie, Hall, and Hubbard, and by Kritter; they rotated the limb by osteotomizing the tibia and fibula.[60, 61] The tibial osteotomy was fixed in a number of ways: fibular strut, plate and screws, multiple Kirschner wires, staples, or intramedullary rods. Bevan-Thomas and Millar reported the results of Van Nes rotation-plasty in three patients.[11] Hall and Bochmann performed the operation in 9 of 19 patients with unilateral proximal femoral focal deficiency.[43]

Prior to performing a Syme amputation and knee fusion and fitting a knee disarticulation type of prosthesis, one should consider the Van Nes rotation-plasty. The turnabout procedure has its distinct advantages and drawbacks; each should be individually evaluated. If possible, it is advisable that both the parents and the child see another patient who has had the procedure done previously or, at least, see the photographs or movies. The child's appearance with the posteriorly rotated foot will be highly unnatural and bizarre without the prosthesis; this objection is not a functional consideration, however, only a cosmetic one. In order to minimize neurovascular compromise, the limb is shortened while being rotated—this markedly diminishes the ambulatory function of the patient without the prosthesis. *The Van Nes rotation-plasty should not be performed in bilateral proximal femoral focal deficiency.* Another drawback of the tibial rotation-plasty is gradual derotation of the leg by the twisted musculature following surgery; this is especially a problem in the child under 12 to 14 years of age. Rerotation may be required every three to five years. Should one wait until completion of skeletal growth before performing turnabout-plasty? The advantage of early functional use of the ankle as a knee joint outweighs the disadvantage of a repeat second or third derotation tibial osteotomy.

The muscles arising proximal to and inserting distal to the line of osteotomy act in a spiral line and exert torque force across the open growing physis. Torode and Gillespie have described an operative technique in which the rotation of the tibia is performed through the knee at the time of knee fusion to the degree permitted by the soft tissues (usually 140 degrees or more) and final rotation through a diaphyseal tibial osteotomy. Fixation is with an intramedullary rod. Their technique eliminates the spiral component of the action of the crural muscles, obviates the necessity for a second operation to achieve knee fusion and rotation,

and permits earlier fitting of a definitive prosthesis.[107] The Torode and Gillespie operative technique of rotation-plasty of the lower limb is illustrated in Plate 29. They performed the procedure in five patients; the wounds and osteotomies healed primarily, and there were no neurovascular complications. The youngest patient was two years old. The operation can be performed in young children without difficulty as long as the proximal tibial epiphyseal ossific nucleus is large enough to allow solid knee fusion. With early surgery, the period in an extension prosthesis is reduced, providing greater mobility of the foot and ankle.

The turnabout procedure has definite advantages over amputation. Position sense is maintained by preserving the foot. There is an added sensory feedback in the below-knee stump versus the above-knee stump. In the modified prosthesis the "knee" (i.e., the 180-degree-turned-about ankle) provides extension of the prosthetic knee when the foot is plantar-flexed and flexion of the prosthetic knee when the foot is dorsiflexed. It gives greater stability and better control of gait in the swing phase (Fig. 2–248). Its principal advantage is the ability to flex the knee in sitting or bicycle riding. Kneeling may still be difficult because the maximum knee flexion that can be obtained is usually less than 90 degrees. An extension prosthesis, while providing an effective gait, does not bend at the knee either during walking or sitting. In a knee-disarticulation type of prosthesis (fitted after Syme amputation and knee fusion) the gait is awkward because knee stability and control are poor.

The requirements for Van Nes rotation-plasty are (1) an ankle joint with normal range of motion and motor power, (2) unilateral involvement, (3) a predicted lower limb inequality that would place the ankle of the deficient limb at the level of the opposite normal knee, and (4) preferably a stable hip.[107, 109]

Should all the toes be amputated after Van Nes rotation-plasty? Removal of the toes will give a rounded contour and better-appearing stump; this benefit is, however, outweighed by the decrease in the power of the stump and the loss of position sense and the child's feeling that he can grip the prosthetic socket with his toes.

The *above-the-knee stump* is achieved by Syme amputation and knee fusion; epiphysiodesis of the distal femur or proximal tibia may be required to level the knees.

Arthrodesis of the knee in extension is performed in Types B and C proximal femoral focal deficiency. The procedure creates a single skel-

Text continued on page 576

Rotation-Plasty of the Lower Limb Through the Knee With Simultaneous Knee Fusion (Torode and Gillespie)

The patient is placed supine on the operating table, and the entire affected lower limb, hip, and pelvis are prepared and draped free. It is vital to be able to palpate the contralateral lower limb through the drapes in order to estimate the amount of shortening required to level the ankle of the deficient limb with the knee of the opposite normal limb.

OPERATIVE TECHNIQUE

A. An anterolateral longitudinal skin incision is made. It begins proximally below the hip. At the knee it curves medially and extends distally along the line of the tibia, terminating 2.5 cm. above the medial malleolus. The subcutaneous tissue is divided in line with the skin incision.

B. Next, the capsule of the knee and the patellar tendon are exposed. The tendon is sectioned and the knee capsule is incised. The patellar and quadriceps muscles are retracted upward, exposing the joint. On the medial aspect of the distal thigh the insertion of the adductor magnus is located, and the adductor hiatus with the neurovascular bundle is identified. In proximal femoral focal deficiency the adductor magnus usually traverses from the pubis at a 70- to 80-degree angle to insert into the femur. The adductor magnus insertion is sectioned distal to the adductor hiatus, facilitating distal exposure of the femoral and popliteal arteries. The sartorius and medial hamstrings are sectioned near their insertions.

C. Next, the lateral aspect of the distal thigh and knee is exposed. Dissection should be careful. If there is associated fibular hemimelia, the peroneal nerve will abut the proximal tibia rather than taking its normal course around the fibular neck. Dissect the peroneal nerve and trace it proximally to its junction with the sciatic nerve.

D. The neurovascular structures both medially and laterally are retracted, and the capsule is divided all around the knee joint. Next, the medial and lateral heads of the gastrocnemius are sectioned, freeing the knee of all muscle and ligamentous attachments. The proximal tibial physis and the distal femoral physis are identified under radiographic control. Next, with an oscillating saw, the hyaline articular cartilage of the proximal tibia and of the distal femoral epiphysis is removed. The level of section of the distal femur is governed by the overall length of the limb and by the length that is required to make the ankle of the affected limb level with the normal knee at skeletal maturity.

Plate 29. Rotation-Plasty of the Lower Limb Through the Knee With Simultaneous Knee Fusion (Torode and Gillespie)

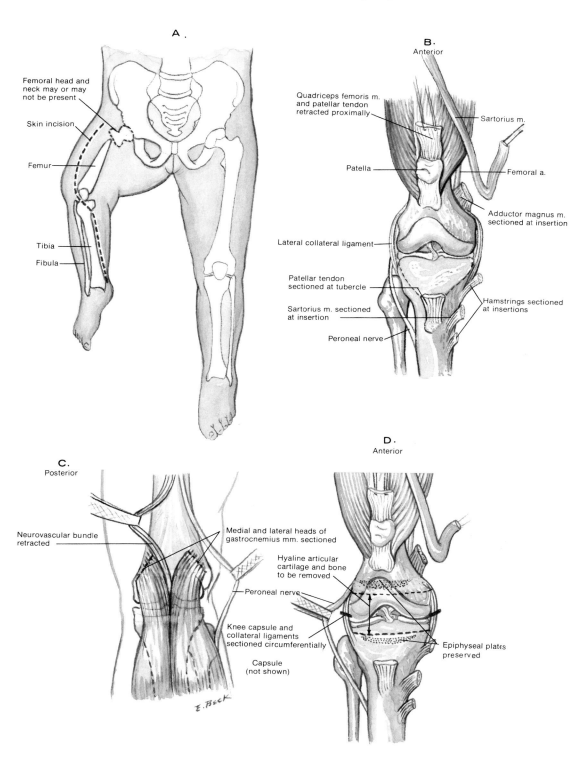

A.

Femoral head and neck may or may not be present

Skin incision

Femur

Tibia

Fibula

B.
Anterior

Quadriceps femoris m. and patellar tendon retracted proximally

Sartorius m.

Patella

Femoral a.

Adductor magnus m. sectioned at insertion

Lateral collateral ligament

Patellar tendon sectioned at tubercle

Hamstrings sectioned at insertions

Sartorius m. sectioned at insertion

Peroneal nerve

C.
Posterior

Neurovascular bundle retracted

Medial and lateral heads of gastrocnemius mm. sectioned

Peroneal nerve

Knee capsule and collateral ligaments sectioned circumferentially

Capsule (not shown)

E. Beck

D.
Anterior

Hyaline articular cartilage and bone to be removed

Epiphyseal plates preserved

573

Rotation-Plasty of the Lower Limb Through the Knee With Simultaneous Knee Fusion (Torode and Gillespie) (Continued)

E. Next insert an intramedullary rod into the distal femur, bring it out through the gluteal region, and hammer it distally into the level of the resected knee. Then rotate the leg laterally at the resected knee level gradually, as much as possible. With care, 120 to 140 degrees of rotation may be possible. At this stage the femoral vessels will slide forward anteromedial to the distal femur.

F. Next, expose the tibia and fibula and subperiosteally perform fasciotomies of all compartments. With an oscillating electric saw, the tibia and fibula are sectioned at the middle of their shafts. Segments of bone may be excised from the tibia and fibula if necessary to elevate the foot to the desired level.

G. The lower segment is rotated so that it points posteriorly and the intramedullary rod is driven across the knee fusion and through the osteotomy site. The rod provides stability both in the sagittal and coronal planes; a hip spica cast incorporating the foot is applied to maintain rotary stability.

If postoperative swelling and vascular embarrassment dictate that the degree of rotation be decreased, the hip spica cast is removed and rotation is reduced. When the swelling subsides the lower segment is rotated to the desired degree. This safety measure is not provided by internal fixation with plate and screws.

POSTOPERATIVE CARE

By six to eight weeks union is obtained at both the knee fusion and tibial osteotomy levels. The cast is removed and the prosthesis is fitted. Physical therapy is instituted to develop motor power of the triceps surae muscle and increase range of plantar flexion of the ankle and foot. The child is instructed in how to move the below-knee section of the modified prosthesis (Fig. 2–248).

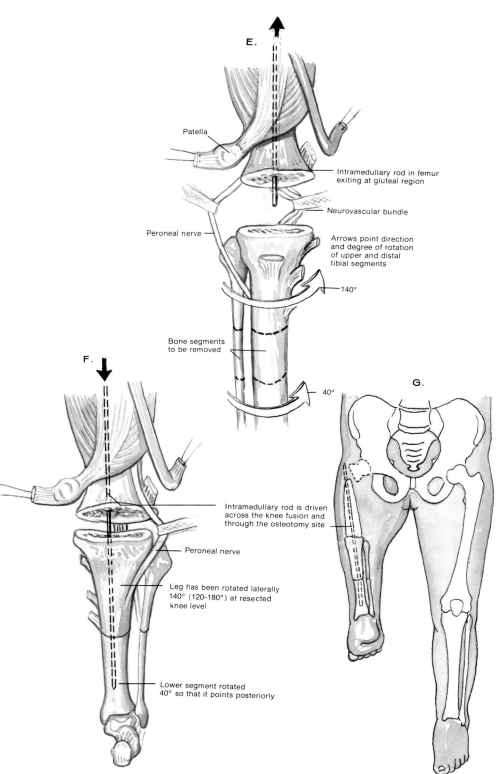

E.

Patella

Intramedullary rod in femur exiting at gluteal region

Neurovascular bundle

Peroneal nerve

Arrows point direction and degree of rotation of upper and distal tibial segments

140°

Bone segments to be removed

40°

F.

G.

Intramedullary rod is driven across the knee fusion and through the osteotomy site

Peroneal nerve

Leg has been rotated laterally 140° (120-180°) at resected knee level

Lower segment rotated 40° so that it points posteriorly

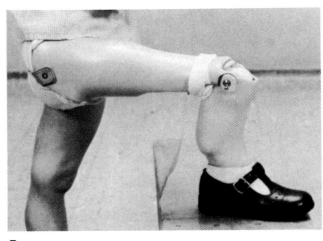

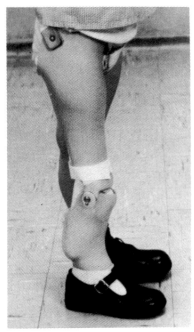

B

A

FIGURE 2–248. *A three-year-old child with right proximal femoral focal deficiency treated by knee fusion and rotation-plasty of the lower limb by the technique described by Torode and Gillespie.*

She is fitted with a modified below-knee prosthesis. Note the flexion and extension of her new "knee" joint powered by the triceps surae muscle. (From Torode, I. P., and Gillespie, R.: Rotation-plasty of the lower limb for congenital defects of the femur. J. Bone Joint Surg., 65-*B*:569, 1983. Reprinted by permission.)

etal lever. Such conversion makes the muscles function more effectively across the hip joint and provides better motor control of the prosthesis. Conversion of the lower limb into a single lever by knee fusion decreases the fixed flexion deformity. King recommends one-stage reconstruction—the arthrodesis of the knee in extension and pelvifemoral stabilization by metaphyseal-epiphyseal synostosis are performed at one operation.[54–58] Articular cartilage is resected from both sides of the knee joint with the ossific nucleus exposed. The growth plates of the distal femur and proximal tibia are not injured. The intramedullary rod (an 8 mm. Küntscher nail) is inserted retrograde from the knee fusion site distally to emerge from the sole of the foot; there it is pushed proximally through the knee joint into the femoral segment. The operative technique is described and illustrated in Plate 30. Central penetration of the distal femoral physis and the proximal tibial physis does not disturb growth. Syme's ankle disarticulation is performed at the time the intramedullary Küntscher nail is removed. In Syme's amputation, the heel pad provides an excellent end-bearing stump, allowing early weight-bearing and fitting of a prosthesis. An illustrative

case is shown in Figure 2–249. Some surgeons prefer to save the calcaneus and fuse it to the distal tibial epiphysis (Boyd amputation), because thereby the heel pad remains centered with no tendency for migration and, being bulbous, assists in suspension of the prosthesis.

There is some controversy about the timing of surgery. Advocates of ablation at an early age recommend it when the infant begins to stand; the advantages of early surgery are that psychologically the amputation is probably a less traumatic experience and the growing child's immediate acceptance of and adaption to a prosthesis are better. Often the parents are the problem.

If the foot of the involved limb is normal and reaches the ground, enabling the child to walk without assistance, amputation should be delayed. With a 5- to 7.5-cm. disparity of limb length, these children can play, swim, and get around quite satisfactorily. With growth the limb length disparity increases; by the age of three to five years (before school age), the shortening of the thigh and leg segments is of such magnitude that ablation of the foot is more readily accepted by the parents.

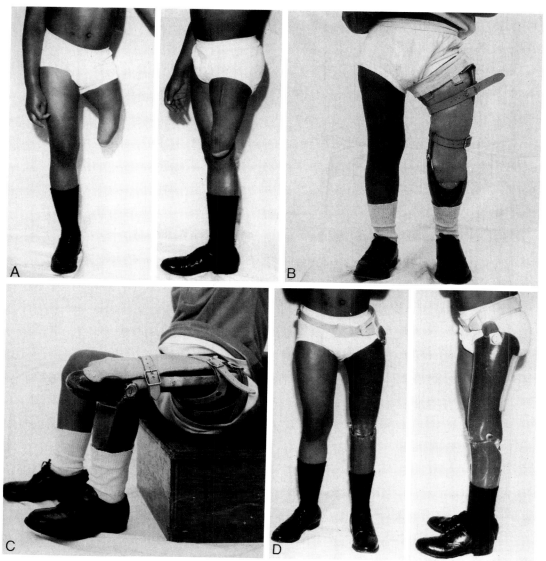

FIGURE 2–249. Proximal femoral focal deficiency treated by King's method.

The knee is fused in extension to create a single skeletal lever, and a Syme amputation is performed to provide an end-bearing stump to be fitted into the prosthesis. **A.** Clinical appearance of the patient without the prosthesis. **B to D.** With the prosthesis.

Knee Fusion for Prosthetic Conversion in Proximal Femoral Focal Deficiency (King)

King's method converts the proximal femoral focal deficient limb into a single skeletal lever arm by arthrodesis of the knee in extension and Syme's ankle disarticulation.

OPERATIVE TECHNIQUE

A. With the patient in supine position, an anterior S-shaped incision is made to expose the anterior aspect of the lower femur and upper tibia. If there is a definite pseudarthrosis in the metaphyseal-diaphyseal subtrochanteric region, King recommends repairing it by excision of its fibrocartilaginous site. Proximally the incision is extended laterally to expose the lateral aspect of the upper femur.

B. The capsule and synovium of the knee joint are opened, and the articular cartilage of the lower end of the femur and the upper end of the tibia is excised with an oscillating electric saw until the ossific nucleus of the epiphysis is seen. Injury to the growth plates should be avoided.

C. Next an 8-mm. Küntscher or similar nail is inserted retrograde. First, it is inserted distally into the tibia, exiting from the sole of the foot.

D. It is then passed proximally into the femur, impacting the lower end of the femur and the upper epiphysis of the tibia in extension. Care is taken to provide proper rotational alignment of the lower limb and ensure that the fused knee is not in flexion. The intramedullary nail should be in the center of the physes of the distal femur and the proximal tibia to avoid growth retardation.

If the pseudarthrosis site is excised, the intramedullary nail is inserted to fix the upper femoral segments internally (not shown in the drawing).

The wound is closed in routine fashion. A one–and–one half hip spica cast is applied for immobilization.

E. Six weeks postoperatively, when the intramedullary nail is removed, a Syme's amputation is performed.

Plate 30. Knee Fusion for Prosthetic Conversion in Proximal Femoral Focal Deficiency (King)

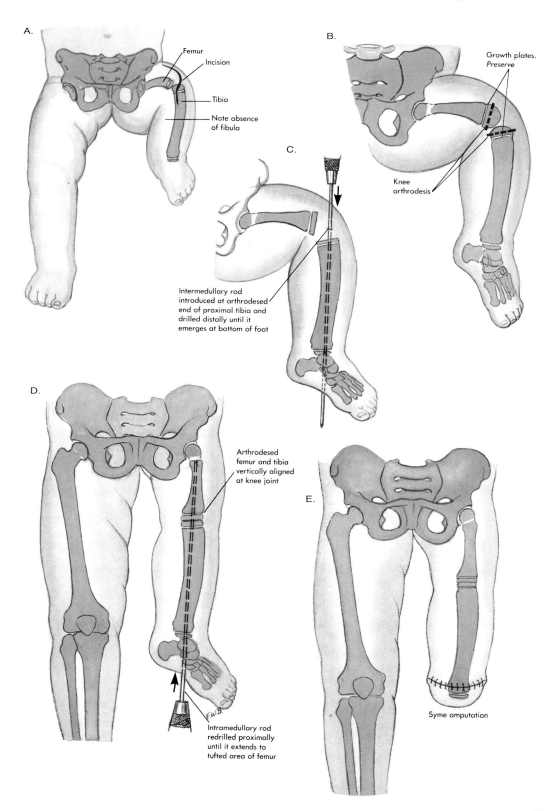

A.

Femur

Incision

Tibia

Note absence of fibula

B.

Growth plates. *Preserve*

Knee arthrodesis

C.

Intermedullary rod introduced at arthrodesed end of proximal tibia and drilled distally until it emerges at bottom of foot

D.

Arthrodesed femur and tibia vertically aligned at knee joint

Intramedullary rod redrilled proximally until it extends to tufted area of femur

E.

Syme amputation

References

1. Acker, R. B.: Congenital absence of femur and fibula—report of two cases. Clin. Orthop., *15*:203, 1959.
2. Aitken, G. T.: Amputation as a treatment for certain lower-extremity congenital abnormalities. J. Bone Joint Surg., *41-A*:1267, 1959.
3. Aitken, G. T.: Proximal femoral focal deficiency—definition, classification and management. *In* Proximal Femoral Focal Deficiency: A Congenital Anomaly. Nat. Acad. Sci., *1734*:1, 1969.
4. Aitken, G. T.: Proximal femoral focal deficiency. *In* Swinyard, C. A. (ed.): Limb Development and Deformity: Problems of Evaluation and Rehabilitation. Springfield, Ill., Thomas, 1969.
5. Aitken, G. T.: Congenital lower limb deficiencies. A.A.O.S. Instruct. Course Lect., *24*:81, 1975.
6. Amstutz, H. C.: Prognosis for growth and development of congenital anomalies of the lower extremities. J. Bone Joint Surg., *49-A*:1011, 1967.
7. Amstutz, H. C.: The morphology, natural history, and treatment of proximal femoral focal deficiency. *In* Aitken, G. T. (ed.): Proximal Femoral Focal Deficiency: A Congenital Anomaly. Nat. Acad. Sci., *1734*:50, 1969.
8. Amstutz, H. C., and Wilson, P. D., Jr.: Dysgenesis of the proximal femur (coxa vara) and its surgical management. J. Bone Joint Surg., *44-A*:1, 1962.
9. Bagg, J. J.: Etiology of certain congenital structural defects. Am. J. Obstet. Gynecol., *8*:131, 1924.
10. Bailey, J. A., II, and Beighton, P.: Bilateral femoral dysgenesis. Clin. Pediatr., *9*:668, 1970.
11. Bevan-Thomas, W. H., and Millar, E. A.: A review of proximal focal femoral deficiencies. J. Bone Joint Surg., *49-A*:1376, 1967.
12. Blauth, W.: Der Congenitale Femurdefekt. Stuttgart, Springer Verlag, 1967.
13. Blencke, A.: Über congenitalen Femurdefekt. Z. Orthop. Chir., *9*:584, 1901.
14. Borggreve: Kniegelenksersatz durch das in der Beinlangsachse um 180 degree gedrehte Fussgelenk. Arch. Orthop. Unfallchir., *28*:175, 1930.
15. Burck, U., Riebel, T., Held, K. R., and Stoeckenius, M.: Bilateral femoral dysgenesis with micrognathia. Cleft palate. Anomalies of the spine and pelvis, and foot deformities. Clinical and radiological findings. Helv. Paediatr. Acta, *36*:473, 1981.
16. Burgess, E.: The surgical means of obtaining hip stability with motion in congenital proximal femoral deficiency. Inter-clin. Inform. Bull., *1*:1, 1961.
17. Chapchal, G., and Van de Kerkhove, W.: Die Umdrehplastik des Sprunggelenkes bei der Behandlung des kongenitalen Femurdefektes. Arch. Orthop. Unfallchir., *41*:109, 1941.
18. Colonna, P. C.: Some common congenital deformities and their orthopedic treatment. N.Y. State J. Med., *28*:713, 1928.
19. Compere, E. L., Garrison, M., and Fahey, J. J.: Deformities of the femur resulting from arrestment of the capital and greater trochanteric epiphyses. J. Bone Joint Surg., *22*:909, 1940.
20. Cristini, J. A.: Surgical management of the proximal femoral focal deficient extremity. J. Bone Joint Surg., *55-A*:424, 1973.
21. Doig, G.: Proximal femoral phocomelia. J. Bone Joint Surg., *52-B*:394, 1970.
22. Drachman, D. B., and Sokoloff, L.: The role of movement in embryonic joint development. Dev. Biol., *14*:401, 1966.
23. Drehmann, G.: Über kongenitalen Femurdefekt. Z. Orthop., *11*:220, 1903.
24. Duraiswami, P. K.: Experimental causation of congenital skeletal defects and its significance in orthopaedic surgery. J. Bone Joint Surg., *34-B*:646, 1952.
25. Ellis, G. V.: An account of an instance of remarkable deformity of the lower limbs. Med. Chir. Trans., *36*:439, 1853.
26. Epps, C. H., Jr.: Proximal femoral focal deficiency: A case report of a necropsy. Inter-Clin. Inform. Bull., *6*:1, 1967.
27. Epps, C. H., Jr.: Proximal femoral focal deficiency. J. Bone Joint Surg., *65-A*:867, 1983.
28. Fixsen, J. A., and Lloyd Roberts, G. C.: The natural history and early treatment of proximal femoral dysplasia. J. Bone Joint Surg., *56-B*:86, 1974.
29. Fock, G., and Sulammaa, M.: Congenital short femur. Acta Orthop. Scand., *36*:294, 1965.
30. Frantz, C. H., and O'Rahilly, R.: Congenital skeletal limb deficiencies. J. Bone Joint Surg., *43-A*:1202, 1961.
31. Freund, E.: Congenital defects of femur, fibula and tibia. Arch. Surg., *33*:349, 1936.
32. Gardner, E. D.: The development and growth of bones and joints. J. Bone Joint Surg., *45-A*:856, 1963.
33. Gardner, E. D.: Prenatal development of the human hip joint, femur, and hip bone. A.A.O.S. Instruct. Course Lect., *21*:138, 1972.
34. Gillespie, R., and Torode, I. P.: Classification and management of congenital abnormalities of the femur. J. Bone Joint Surg., *65-B*:557, 1983.
35. Gilsanz, V.: Distal focal femoral deficiency. Radiology, *147*:104, 1983.
36. Golding, F. C.: Congenital coxa vara and the short femur. Proc. R. Soc. Med., *32*:641, 1939.
37. Goldman, A. B., Schneider, R., and Wilson, P. D., Jr.: Proximal focal femoral deficiency. J. Can. Assoc. Radiol., *29*:101, 1978.
38. Guilleminet, M., and Michel, L.: Un cas d'absence congénitale complète du fémur avec adaption tibio-cotiloidienne progressive. Lyon Chir., *47*:460, 1952.
39. Guilleminet, M., Michel, L., and Michel, C. R.: Aplasie des deux tiers supérieurs de la diaphyse fémorale. Rotation-plastie à 12 ans. Lyon Chir., *58*:418, 1962.
40. Gupta, D. K. S., and Gupta, S. K.: Familial bilateral proximal femoral focal deficiency. Report of a kindred. J. Bone Joint Surg., *66-A*:1470, 1984.
41. Hall, C. B., Brooks, M. B., and Dennis, J. F.: Congenital skeletal deficiencies of the extremities: classification and fundamentals of treatment. J.A.M.A., *181*:590, 1962.
42. Hall, J. E.: Rotation of congenitally hypoplastic lower limbs to use the ankle joint as a knee: A preliminary report. Inter-Clin. Inform. Bull., *6*:3, 1966.
43. Hall, J. E., and Bochmann, D.: The surgical and prosthetic management of proximal femoral focal deficiency. *In* Aitken, G. T. (ed.): Proximal Femoral Focal Deficiency: A Symposium. Washington, D. C.: National Academy of Sciences, Publication 1734, 1969.
44. Hamanishi, C.: Congenital short femur: Clinical, genetic, and epidemiological comparison of the naturally occurring condition with that caused by thalidomide. J. Bone Joint Surg., *62-B*:307, 1980.
45. Haring, O. M., and Lewis, F. J.: The etiology of congenital developmental anomalies. Int. Abstr. Surg., *113*:1, 1961.
46. Henkel, L., and Willert, H. G.: Dysmelia. J. Bone Joint Surg., *51-B*:399, 1969.
47. Holden, C. E.: Congenital shortening of one femur in one identical twin. Postgrad. Med. J., *44*:813, 1968.
48. Ibos, P.: L'absence congénitale du fémur. Thèse de Paris, 1927.
49. Johansson, E., and Aparisi, T.: Missing cruciate ligament in congenital short femur. J. Bone Joint Surg., *65-A*:1109, 1985.

50. Kalamchi, A., Cowell, H. R., and Kim, K. I.: Congenital deficiency of the femur. J. Pediatr. Orthop., 5:129, 1985.

51. Katdare, S. S.: Congenital absence of the shaft of the femur on both sides. Indian Med. Gaz., 80:297, 1945.

52. Kay, H. W.: The proposed international terminology for the classification of congenital limb deficiencies. Dev. Med. Child Neurol., 17(Suppl.):1, 1975.

53. Kelly, T. E.: Familial proximal focal femoral deficiency (PFFD). Birth Defects, Original Art. Series, Vol. 10, No. 12, Excerpta Medica International Congress Series, No. 335, Amsterdam, Excerpta Medica, 1974, p. 195.

54. King, R. E.: Providing a single skeletal lever in PFFD. Inter-Clin. Inform. Bull., 6:23, 1966.

55. King, R. E.: Some concepts of proximal femoral focal deficiency. J. Bone Joint Surg., 49-A:1470, 1967.

56. King, R. E.: Some concepts of proximal femoral focal deficiency. *In* Aitken, G. T. (ed.): Proximal Femoral Focal Deficiency: A Symposium. Washington, D. C., National Academy of Sciences, 1969, pp. 23–49.

57. King, R. E.: Proximal femoral focal deficiencies. *In* Tronzo, R. G. (ed.): Surgery of the Hip Joint. Philadelphia, Lea & Febiger, 1975.

58. King, R. E.: Proximal femoral focal deficiency. *In* Harris, N. (ed.): Clinical Orthopedics. Bristol, Wright, 1983, pp. 184–193.

59. Koman, L. A., Meyer, L. C., and Warren, F. H.: Proximal femoral focal deficiency: Natural history and treatment. Clin. Orthop., 162:135, 1982.

60. Kostuik, J. P., Gillespie, R., Hall, J. E., and Hubbard, S.: Van Nes rotational osteotomy for treatment of proximal femoral focal deficiency and congenital short femur. J. Bone Joint Surg., 57-A:1039, 1975.

61. Kritter, A. E.: Tibial rotation-plasty for proximal femoral focal deficiency. J. Bone Joint Surg., 59-A:927, 1977.

62. Kruger, L. M.: Classification and prosthetic management of limb-deficient children. Inter-Clin. Inform. Bull., 7:1, 1968.

63. Lange, D. R., Schoenecker, P. L., and Baker, C. L.: Proximal femoral focal deficiency: Treatment and classification in forty-two cases. Clin. Orthop., 135:15, 1978.

64. Lange, M.: Die Coxa vara: Ihr klinisches Bild und ihre heutige Behandlung. Munch. Med. Wochenschr., 85:1637, 1938.

65. Langston, H. H.: Congenital defects of the shaft of the femur. Br. J. Surg., 27:162, 1939.

66. Laurenson, R. D.: Development of the acetabular roof in the fetal hip. J. Bone Joint Surg., 47-A:975, 1965.

67. Levinson, E. D., Ozonoff, M. B., and Royen, P. M.: Proximal femoral focal deficiency (PFFD). Radiology, 125:197, 1977.

68. Lewin, P.: Congenital absence or defects of bones of extremities. A.J.R., 4:431, 1917.

69. Lloyd-Roberts, G. C., and Stone, K. H.: Congenital hypoplasia of the upper femur. J. Bone Joint Surg., 45-B:557, 1963.

70. Lutken, P.: The development of the upper end of the femur. J. Bone Joint Surg., 43-A:285, 1961.

71. Maguire, C.: Congenital deformity of femur. Br. Med. J., 1:413, 1914.

72. Maisels, D. O., and Stilwell, J. H.: The Pierre Robin syndrome associated with femoral dysgenesis. Br. J. Plast. Surg., 33:337, 1980.

73. Manohar, K.: Congenital absence of right femur. Br. J. Surg., 27:158, 1939.

74. Meyer, L. M., Friddle, D., and Pratt, R. W.: Problems of treating and fitting the patient with PFFD. Inter-Clin. Inform. Bull., 10:1, 1971.

75. Michel, L.: Deux nouveaux cas d'absence congénitale complète du fémur avec connexion tibiocotyloidienne. Presse Méd., 65:1213, 1957.

76. Mital, M. A., Masalawalla, K. S., and Desai, M. G.: Bilateral congenital aplasia of the femur. J. Bone Joint Surg., 45-B:561, 1963.

77. Morgan, J. D., and Somerville, E. W.: Normal and abnormal growth at the upper end of the femur. J. Bone Joint Surg., 42-B:264, 1960.

78. Mouchet, A., and Ibos, P.: Consideration sur l'absence congénitale du fémur. Rev. Orthop., 35:117, 1928.

79. Murat, J. E., Guilleminet, M., and Descamps, R.: Long-term results of rotation-plasty in two patients with subtotal aplasia of the femur. Am. J. Surg., 113:676, 1967.

80. Nilsonne, H.: Über den kongenitalen Femurdefekt. Arch. Orthop. Unfallchir., 26:138, 1928.

81. Ogden, W., and Meyer, L. C.: Proximal femoral focal deficiency. Presented at the South Carolina Orthopedic Association, Hilton Head Island, September, 1970.

82. Ollerenshaw, R.: Congenital defects of the long bones of the lower limb: A contribution to the study of their causes, effects, and treatment. J. Bone Joint Surg., 7:528, 1925.

83. O'Rahilly, R.: Morphological patterns in limb deficiencies and duplications. Am. J. Anat., 89:135, 1951.

84. Panting, A. L., and Williams, P. F.: Proximal femoral focal deficiency. J. Bone Joint Surg., 60-B:46, 1978.

85. Pappas, A. M.: Congenital abnormalities of the femur and related lower extremity malformations: Classification and treatment. J. Pediatr. Orthop., 3:45, 1983.

86. Pick, J. W., Stack, J. K., and Anson, B. J.: Measurements on the human femur. I. Lengths, diameters and angles. Q. Bull. Northwest. Univ. Med. School, 15:281, 1941.

87. Ramsay, J.: Congenital absence of the right femur. J. Coll. Surg. Australia, 1:247, 1928.

88. Reiner, M.: Ueber den congenitalen Femurdefect. Z. Orthop. Chir., 9:544, 1901.

89. Richardson, E. G., and Rambach, B. E.: Proximal femoral focal deficiency: A clinical appraisal. South. Med. J., 72:166, 1979.

90. Ring, P. A.: Congenital short femur. J. Bone Joint Surg., 41-B:73, 1959.

91. Ring, P. A.: Congenital abnormalities of the femur. Arch. Dis. Child., 36:410, 1961.

92. Rogala, E. J., Wynne-Davies, R., Littlejohn, A., and Gormley, J.: Congenital limb anomalies: Frequency and aetiological factors. Data from the Edinburgh Register of the Newborn (1964–1968). J. Med. Genet., 11:221, 1974.

93. Rossi, T. V., and Kruger, L.: Proximal femoral focal deficiency and its treatment. Orthot. Prosthet., 29:37, 1975.

94. Ryder, C. T., Dick, H. M., and Stinchfield, F. E.: The cartilage angle type of femoral dysgenesis. J. Bone Joint Surg., 49-A:1470, 1967.

95. Schatz, S. L., and Kopits, S. E.: Proximal femoral focal deficiency. A.J.R., 131:389, 1978.

96. Shands, A. R., Jr.: Congenital absence of the femur, patella, tarsal scaphoid and ischium associated with other abnormalities. A.J.R., 19:531, 1928.

97. Shands, A. R., Jr., and MacEwen, G. D.: Congenital abnormalities of the femur. Acta Orthop. Scand., 32:307, 1962.

98. Scheer, G. B.: Treatment of proximal focal femoral deficiency. Clin. Orthop., 85:292, 1972.

99. Siffert, R. S.: Patterns of deformity of the developing hip. Clin. Orthop., 160:14, 1981.

100. Stransky, E., and Abad-Vazquez, L.: On congenital malformations of the femur (first observed case in the Philippines). Ann. Paediatr., 200:31, 1963.

101. Streeter, G. L.: Focal deficiencies in fetal tissues and their relation to intra-uterine amputation. Contrib. Embryol., 22:1, 1930.

102. Swanson, A. B.: A classification for congenital limb malformation. J. Hand Surg., *1*:8, 1976.

103. Tablada, C.: A technique for fitting converted proximal femoral focal deficiencies. Artif. Limbs, *15*:27, 1971.

104. Tleson, D.: Substitution of an ankle for the knee joint of a prosthesis. Adelphi Hosp. Bull., 5:2, 1946.

105. Theobalds, F.: Congenital deformity of femur. Br. Med. J., *1*:532, 1914.

106. Tobin, W. J., and Stewart, T. D.: The upper end of the femur. A.A.O.S. Instruct. Course Lect., 1953. *10*:213, 223, 1953.

107. Torode, I. P., and Gillespie, R.: Rotationplasty of the lower limb for congenital defects of the femur. J. Bone Joint Surg., *65-B*:569, 1983.

108. Tsou, P. M.: Congenital distal femoral focal deficiency: Report of a unique case. Clin. Orthop., *162*:99, 1982.

109. Van Nes, C. P.: Rotation-plasty for congenital defects of the femur. Making use of the ankle of the shortened limb to control the knee joint of a prosthesis. J. Bone Joint Surg., *32-B*:12, 1950.

110. Veitch, V. C.: Imperfect development of the upper end of the femur. Proc. R. Soc. Med., *20*:884, 1926.

111. Vlachos, D.: Contribution à l'étude de l'évolution naturelle des fémurs courts congénitaux. Thèse Médicine, Paris, 1973.

112. Vlachos, D., and Carlioz, H.: Malformations of the femur: their spontaneous development. Rev. Chir. Orthop., *59*:629, 1973.

113. Wagner, H.: Operative lengthening of the femur. Clin. Orthop., *136*:125, 1978.

114. Wagner, H.: Allongement chirurgical du fémur. A propos d'une série de cinquante-huit cas. Ann. Chir., *34*:263, 1980.

115. Warkany, J.: Some factors in the etiology of congenital malformations. Am. J. Ment. Defic., *50*:231, 1945.

116. Warkany, J.: Congenital anomalies. Pediatrics, *7*:607, 1951.

117. Westin, G. W.: Femoral lengthening using a periosteal sleeve. J. Bone Joint Surg., *49-A*:836, 1967.

118. Westin, G. W., and Gunderson, F. O.: Proximal femoral focal deficiency. *In* Aitken, G. T. (ed.): Proximal Femoral Focal Deficiency: A Congenital Anomaly. Washington, D. C., National Academy of Science, 1969, p. 100.

HYPOPLASIA OF THE FEMUR

Hypoplasia of the femur is the most common form of longitudinal deficiency of the femur; there are no other defects; the femur is simply short. The hip joint and femoral neck-shaft angle are normal (Fig. 2–250). The term "miniature femur" is truly descriptive. Involvement is almost always unilateral. In contrast to proximal femoral focal deficiency, congenital short femur is usually not associated with other congenital defects of the skeletal system, but congenital absence of the cruciate ligaments and knee instability are commonly present. There is no predilection for sex; the cases occur sporadically. Congenital shortening of one femur in one of identical twins has been reported by Holder.[1]

Clinically the shortening of the thigh is evident. The Galleazzi test is positive. In the infant

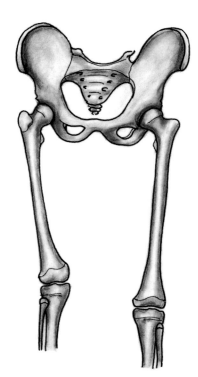

FIGURE 2–250. Diagram showing congenital short femur.

The hip joint and femoral neck-shaft angle are normal.

the involved lower limb tends to assume a posture in lateral rotation, and medial rotation of the hips in extension is limited. Abduction of the hip is not limited. Sometimes the thigh is bowed laterally in its middle third. The Ortolani and Barlow tests are negative for hip dislocation or instability.

Radiograms depict the "miniature" femur, which otherwise is normal. Often there is some delay of ossification of the upper femoral epiphysis, but eventually, with skeletal growth, the femoral head and acetabulum are normal. If there is some lateral bowing of the femoral shaft, it is at its middle third; at the site of the bow the lateral cortex is thickened, but there is no narrowing of the medullary canal.

The percentage of femoral shortening (inhibition) is constant, the two femora keeping a similar relationship in length at skeletal maturity.[3, 4] The percentage of growth inhibition is calculated as follows:

The eventual length of the normal femur at skeletal maturity is determined on the Green-Anderson growth chart or the straight-line graph of Moseley. Then that of the short femur is predicted by multiplying the length of the normal femur by the percentage of femoral shortening. The result can quite accurately forecast the eventual disparity of lower limb length at skeletal maturity. If there is associated hypoplasia of the ipsilateral tibia it should be considered in the calculation.

The congenitally short femur is approximately 10 per cent shorter than the normal one.[4] The total lower limb inequality is rarely greater than 6 cm.

Treatment

A child can easily compensate for some degree of lower limb shortening by tilting the ipsilateral side of the pelvis down without developing any problem with structural scoliosis or fixed pelvic obliquity. In childhood a shoe lift of appropriate height is given to eliminate a short-leg limp and minimize compensatory mechanisms for equalizing leg lengths such as flexing the knee of the long limb in stance or adopting an equinus posture of the short limb in gait. Usually it is unnecessary to compensate for all of the disparity in limb length. If a lift of less than 1 inch is needed, only the heel is raised; if more than 1 inch is needed, the raise should extend to the entire shoe, the prescription reading "sole to balance the heel."

If the predicted lower limb discrepancy is less than 5 cm. at the appropriate skeletal age, lower limb length is equalized by epiphysiodesis of the long distal femur. If it is greater than 2 inches, elongation of the short femur should be considered. The operative techniques of epiphysiodesis and femoral elongation are discussed in Chapter 7.

References

1. Holder, C. E.: Congenital shortening of one femur in one identical twin. Postgrad. Med. J., *44*:813, 1968.
2. Lenz, W., and Feldman, U.: Unilateral and asymmetric limb defects in man: Delineation of the femur-fibula-ulna complex. Birth Defects, *13*:269, 1977.
3. Ring, P. A.: Congenital short femur—simple femoral hypoplasia. J. Bone Joint Surg., *41-B*:73, 1959.
4. Vlachos, D., and Carlioz, H.: Les malformations du fémur. Leur évolution spontanée. Rev. Chir. Orthop., *59*:41, 1973.

APLASIA OF THE FEMUR

In this extremely rare major deficiency there is complete absence of the femur. The upper epiphysis of the tibia tends to articulate with a deficient acetabulum. The opposite lower limb may also be involved with varying degrees of longitudinal deficiency of the femur or the tibia. Treatment is the same as in Type IV proximal femoral focal deficiency.

DEVELOPMENTAL COXA VARA

In this developmental abnormality of the proximal end of the femur there is a primary cartilaginous defect in the femoral neck with abnormal decrease in the femoral neck-shaft angle and shortening of the affected lower limb.

Historically, Fiorani, in 1881, was the first to publish a clinical description of a case of bending of the neck of the femur.[51] The term *coxa vara* was coined by Hofmeister in 1894.[76] Coxa vara's association with other malformations was noted by Kredel in 1896.[95]

There is some controversy in the literature as to the exact term to describe the condition. It has been variously called congenital, developmental, cervical, or infantile. Amstutz, in 1970, reported two patients with coxa vara who had previously had normal radiograms of the hips.[2] Obviously, some patients who develop coxa vara without marked shortening of the femur do not have a clinical or radiographic deformity detectable at birth. By definition a *congenital* deformity should be restricted to defects that are detectable at birth either clinically, radiographically, or chemically. A developmental deformity may not be detectable at birth, but may develop later. The term *developmental coxa vara* was first used by Hoffa in 1905 and later by Duncan.[40, 75] This author agrees with Amstutz and prefers the connotation of the term *developmental coxa vara*, but does not object to the term *infantile* as used by Elmslie, Fairbank, and Pylkkänen.[44, 47–49, 151]

Developmental coxa vara should be distinguished from congenital coxa vara with marked shortening of the femur, the deformity that is present at birth and associated with significant shortening of the femur, is due to growth abnormality of the upper end of the femur, and is classified under proximal femoral focal deficiency (see p. 553). Congenital short femur may exist without coxa vara. Coxa vara may also be a manifestation of a generalized developmental skeletal dysplasia such as Morquio's disease, cleidocranial dysostosis, multiple epiphyseal dysplasia, or metaphyseal dysostosis. Developmental coxa vara should also be distinguished from acquired coxa vara and coxa breva (short femoral neck) due to aseptic necrosis of the upper femoral epiphysis and physis caused by infection or trauma, or as a sequela of Legg-Perthes disease.

Incidence

Developmental coxa vara is rare; its incidence is estimated by Johanning to be 1 in 25,000 live births in the Scandinavian population.[86] Le-Mesurier compared the incidence of developmental coxa vara with that of congenital dislocation of the hip in the same geographic area, noting 1 case of coxa vara to every 13 cases of dislocation. The incidence of congenital dislocation of the hip is 1 per 1000, making that of developmental coxa vara 1 per 13,000 live individuals.[105]

There is no racial predilection. It is equally distributed among males and females. Unilateral involvement is more common than bilateral in the ratio of approximately 2 to 1 (Pylkkänen, 1.9 to 1; Magnusson, 2.2 to 1; and Zimmerman, 3 to 1).[112, 151, 181]

Heredity

That the underlying cause is most likely genetic is supported by the familial incidence of developmental coxa vara and by its occurrence in identical and nonidentical twins.[1, 2, 10, 41, 54, 104, 116, 159]

Early in fetal development, the epiphyseal plate of the proximal femur appears to stretch across the upper end of the bone as a crescentic line of cartilage columns that soon differentiates into cervical epiphyseal and trochanteric apophyseal portions.[123] The medial cervical portion matures early, elongating the femoral neck, and the ossification center of the capital femoral epiphysis appears within the first three to six months of postnatal life. With walking and activity of the hip abductors, the lateral portion of the crescentic preplate becomes organized, and the greater trochanteric apophysis begins to ossify at four years of age. Thus there are two separate areas of development at the proximal end of the femur where rapid growth is taking place. The neck-shaft angle and the length of the upper end of the femur are determined by the relative amount of growth in these two sites. According to Von Lanz and Mayet, the mean angle of the femoral neck and shaft is 148 degrees at one year of age, gradually decreasing to 120 degrees in the adult (Fig. 2–251).[172]

Pathogenesis

Probably the result of a primary defect in enchondral ossification of the medial part of the femoral neck, coxa vara's exact cause is unknown.

Anatomic descriptions of coxa vara were first published by Hoffa in 1905, by Helbing in 1906, and by Schwartz in 1913.[71, 75, 165] Later reports were published by Barr, Camitz, Zimmerman, and Burckhardt.[9, 21, 24, 481] In investigations of fetal femoral head specimens, large amounts of fibrous tissue rather than cancellous bone were found in the medial part of the metaphysis of the femoral neck. Thus the mechanically weak femoral neck could be passively deformed into a varus angulation under the stress of muscle forces and body weight.[2, 136–139]

Biomechanics

In the normal hip the compressive force (R) is perpendicular to the center of the hip joint (Fig. 2–252 A). As a result the physeal cartilage and hyaline cartilage of the acetabulum are stressed by compression (D), which is evenly distributed throughout. Stresses on the medial side of the femoral neck are compressive (D), whereas those on the lateral side are tensile

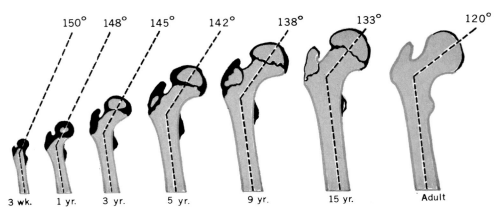

FIGURE 2–251. *Mean angle of the femoral neck-shaft in different age groups.*

(Adapted from von Lanz, T., and Wachsmuth, W.: Praktische Anatomie. Berlin, Julius Springer, 1938, p. 143.)

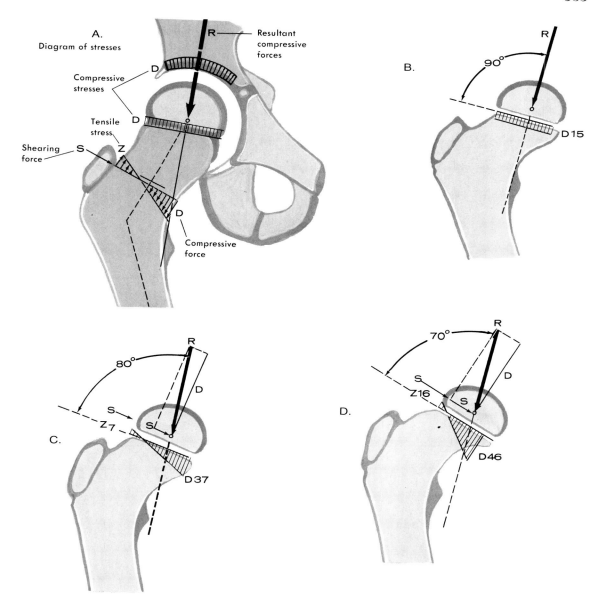

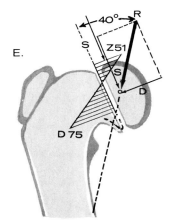

FIGURE 2–252. *Compressive and tensile forces across the hip joint are normal in coxa vara.*

A and **B.** The normal hip. **C** to **E.** Coxa vara. See text for explanation. (Redrawn after Pauwels, F.: Biomechanics of the Normal and Diseased Hip. New York, Springer-Verlag, 1976, pp. 42–44.)

(Z). In Figure 2–252 A, S represents the shearing forces. Normally the physis is perpendicular to the resultant compressive force R (Fig. 2–252 B).

In coxa vara, with progressive decrease in the femoral neck-shaft angle the physis changes its position from horizontal to vertical, and thereby the physis becomes progressively inclined to force R (Fig. 2–252 C to E). The shearing forces (S) across the physis gradually increase. The upper femoral epiphysis tends to tilt and become displaced medially, and the tensile stresses (Z) increase. Growth of the femoral neck is less on the medial side than on the lateral.

The femoral neck-shaft angle affects the direction, position, and magnitude of loading and stressing of the proximal end of the femur (Fig. 2–253). In coxa vara the femoral neck-shaft angle is decreased; consequently the tip of the greater trochanter is elevated, and the position and direction of muscular force M are altered. The point of intersection (X) of muscular force M with the line of action of the partial body weight (K) is lowered. The resultant compressive force R (which connects the point X with

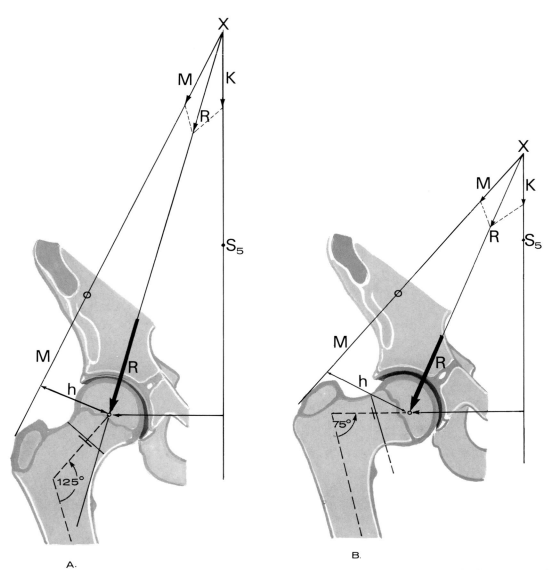

FIGURE 2–253. The effect of the femoral neck-shaft angle on the direction and position of, and the loading stress on the proximal end of the femur.

A. Normal hip. **B.** Coxa vara. See text for explanation. (Redrawn after Pauwels, F.: Biomechanics of the Normal and Diseased Hip. New York, Springer-Verlag, 1976, p. 25.)

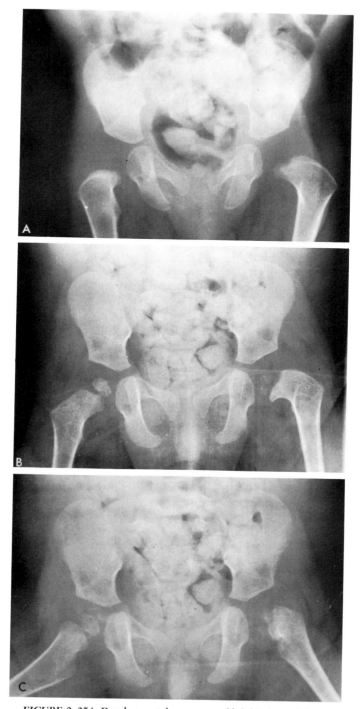

FIGURE 2–254. Developmental coxa vara of left hip in an infant.

A. Anteroposterior radiograms of both hips at three months of age, taken because of limited abduction of left hip and suspicion of congenital hip dislocation. It was interpreted to be normal. **B** and **C.** Radiograms of the hips of same patient at one year of age when he started walking with a painless gluteus medius lurch on the left. Varus deformity of the left hip is evident.

the center of the femoral head) diverges more than normal in coxa vara, and the lever arm (h) of the abductor muscles is lengthened.

Clinical Features

The deformity does not become manifest until after birth and usually not until the age of walking (Figs. 2–254 and 2–255). Clinically, the child presents with a painless, lurching limp.[6, 59, 69, 86, 104, 129, 152, 180] Easy fatigability may be a complaint. Both hips may be affected; the ratio of unilateral to bilateral involvement is 2 to 1. In bilateral coxa vara, the gait may be of a "duck waddle" type, similar to that seen in bilateral dislocation of the hips.

The patients are usually short and sometimes have excessive lumbar lordosis, especially when the deformity is bilateral. The range of abduction and medial rotation of the affected hip is limited. With increasing coxa vara, the tip of the greater trochanter rises in relation to the center of the femoral head, and the origin and insertion of the hip abductors approach each other. The patient develops a gluteus medius lurch, and the Trendelenburg test becomes positive. There is no telescoping, and Ortolani's sign is negative. The affected lower limb is short, the actual amount depending on the extent of the depression of the head and neck of the femur on the femoral shaft.

Radiographic Findings

In addition to a decrease in the shaft-neck angle, radiograms show a triangular piece of bone in the femoral neck close to the head, bounded by two radiolucent bands traversing the neck and forming an inverted V (Fig. 2–256). The inner band is the capital femoral epiphyseal plate; the lateral line is an abnormal area of increased radiolucency marking the site of the faulty maturation of cartilage and irregular ossification. The varus deformity is likely to progress during growth as weight-bearing exerts force on the weakened area. The wider and the more vertical the zone of rarefaction, the greater is the progression of the coxa vara.

In the differential diagnosis, one should rule out causes of acquired coxa vara, such as avascular necrosis of the femoral head (secondary to congenital dislocation of the hip, Legg-Perthes disease, or Gaucher's disease); slipped capital femoral epiphysis; osteomyelitis of the femoral neck; septic arthritis with destruction of the epiphyseal plate of the capital femoral epiphysis

and arrest of its growth; fibrous dysplasia; and severe rickets.

Coxa Breva

The length of the femoral neck affects the magnitude of its mechanical stressing. The length of the lever arm (h) of the muscular force (M) is diminished by shortening of the femoral neck (Fig. 2–257). In response to efforts to preserve equilibrium, the muscle forces and resultant compressive forces (R) increase. Therefore, shortening of the femoral neck increases bending stress.

Treatment

The goals of treatment are: stimulation of ossification and healing of the defective femoral neck, correction of the femoral neck-shaft angle to normal and conversion of the posterior position of the capital femoral physis from nearly vertical to horizontal, and restoration of normal muscle physiology of the hip abductors. These treatment objectives can be achieved only by surgical intervention. Nonoperative measures are futile. Splinting in abduction and medial rotation (recommended by Elmsie) and traction (attempted by Nilsonne and LeMesurier) have proved to be ineffective in correcting the deformity—the "weak gap" in the femoral neck proves stronger than anticipated.[43, 104, 128] Orthotic devices to unload the hip are of no value. The only nonoperative measures employed by this author are passive exercises to stretch the hip adductors and lateral rotators, and a lift in the shoe if the lower limb inequality is significant and decompensates the spine.

Untreated developmental coxa vara tends to be steadily progressive from early infancy to adolescence. Pseudarthrosis may develop within the femoral neck, and the femoral head may be widely separated from the neck. Spontaneous recovery is extremely rare, but occasionally the neck-shaft angle does not increase.[84, 87] In untreated cases secondary dysplastic changes in the acetabulum develop.[62]

Correction of deformity can be achieved only by surgical measures; the problem is to decide the optimal time for surgery and which operative technique to employ. Factors that enter into the decision are the severity of the varus deformity and its interference with function, the age of the patient and the relative amount of remaining growth, and whether the deformity is progressive.

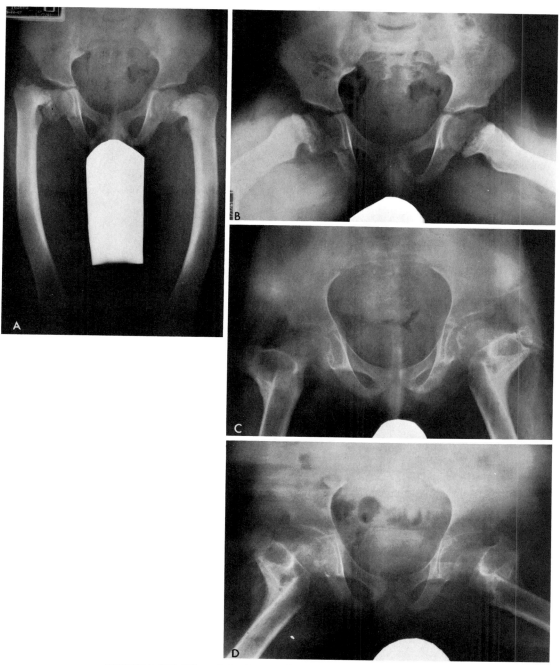

FIGURE 2–255. Bilateral developmental coxa vara in a six-year-old boy.

A and **B.** Anteroposterior and lateral radiograms of both hips. Note the defect in the femoral neck and lateral bowing of the femur. The femoral neck-shaft angle is 90 degrees on the left and 80 degrees on the right. **C** and **D.** Nine-months-postoperative radiograms of both hips. A bilateral abduction osteotomy of the proximal femur was performed.

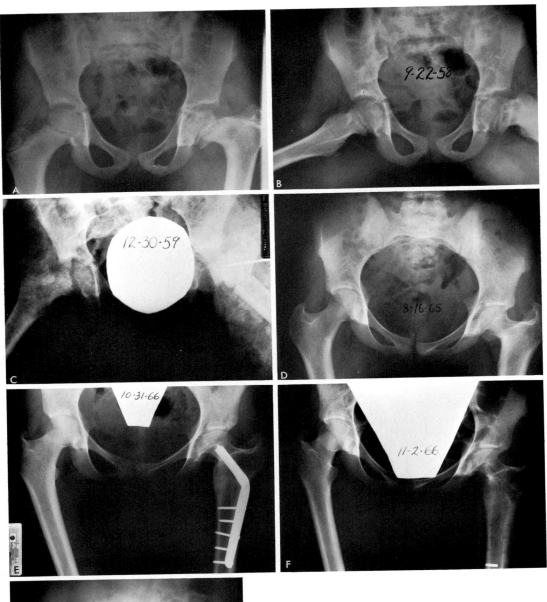

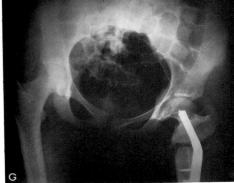

FIGURE 2–256. Developmental coxa vara of left hip.

A and **B.** Anteroposterior and lateral radiograms of both hips at nine years of age. **C.** Radiogram of both hips through the cast, following an abduction osteotomy. **D.** Six-years-postoperative radiogram of the hips at completion of growth. There is some recurrence of varus deformity on the left with approximation of the greater trochanter toward the ilium. Patient had a short-leg gluteus medius limp. **E** to **G.** Postoperative radiograms showing correction of varus deformity by subtrochanteric osteotomy.

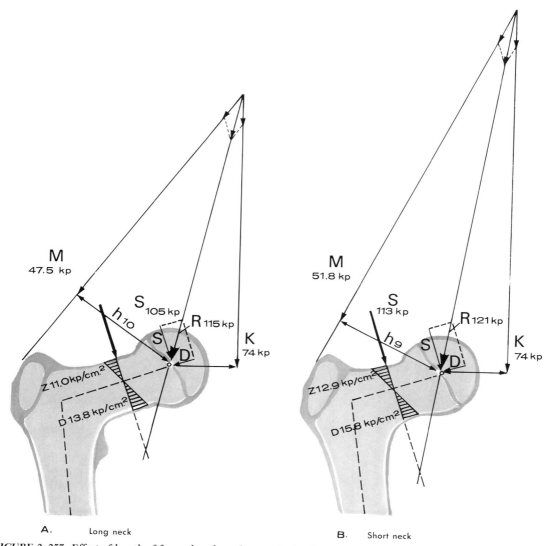

FIGURE 2-257. *Effect of length of femoral neck on the magnitude of mechanical stressing of the upper end of the femur.*

A. Long neck. **B.** Short neck. See text for explanation.

Initially Langenskiöld and Salenius recommended epiphysiodesis of the greater trochanter in an attempt to modify the growth pattern of the upper femur.[99] Mau and Pylkkänen tried growth arrest of the greater trochanter in mild cases of coxa vara.[116, 151] With further experience, Langenskiöld and Salenius concluded that the results of greater trochanteric epiphysiodesis in coxa vara infantum are unreliable.[99] This author does not recommend arrest of the greater trochanteric growth in the developmental form of coxa vara.

Attempts to fix the defect of the femoral neck by pins or bone grafts or both have been described in the literature.[77, 104, 107] The proce-

dure does not, however, correct the varus deformity, and the results are unpredictable and variable as to prevention of progressive deformation of the femoral neck. Le Mesurier, who initially recommended bone grafting of the femoral neck defect, later on found the operation had failed in all three of his cases and, therefore, repudiated the procedure.[104, 105] A further drawback of internal fixation or bone grafting in the femoral neck is growth arrest of the capital femoral physis. Injury and premature closure of the proximal femoral physis will cause progressive shortening of the femur and should be avoided in all operative procedures.

Valgus osteotomy of the upper femur at the

intertrochanteric or subtrochanteric level is the most effective way to correct the varus deformity, to rotate the femoral neck from vertical to horizontal position (relieving shearing stresses on it), and to enhance ossification of the defect.

The osteotomy is indicated when there is a defect in the femoral neck, when the neck-shaft angle is 105 degrees or less, when there is progression of the varus deformity, and when there is a gluteus medius lurch. Of these, the primary indication for surgery is a vertical defect in the femoral neck. Weinstein and associates in a retrospective review of 22 cases of congenital coxa vara introduced the Hilgenreiner epiphyseal (HE) angle as measured on the anteroposterior radiogram of the hips to determine the degree of coxa vara deformity. The HE angle is the angle between Hilgenreiner's line on the horizontal axis and the line through the metaphyseal side of the defect on the femoral neck on the vertical axis (Fig. 2–258). In seven patients in whom the HE angle was greater than 60 degrees, the coxa vara deformity increased. In three cases with HE angles of less than 60 degrees the varus deformity did not increase; in two patients with HE angles of 40 and 49 degrees, the varus deformity improved. These authors concluded that (1) if the HE angle is greater than 60 degrees, progression of coxa vara can be anticipated; (2) if the HE angle is less than 60 degrees and greater than 45 degrees, these hips represented a "gray zone"—they should be observed: HE angles of less than 45 degrees will gradually correct spontaneously without operative intervention. They recommended surgical correction of the HE angle to less than 45 degrees.[180] There is some variance of opinion as to the timing and technique of the operation.

It has been recommended that surgery be postponed until puberty because of the tendency for the deformity to recur after osteotomy. There are, however, definite disadvantages in such a delay, such as secondary dysplastic changes in the acetabulum, pseudarthrosis of the femoral neck, and technical difficulties in achieving correction of the deformity. In a child over eight years of age, the prognosis for providing a normal hip rapidly diminishes. If an operation is indicated, it is best to proceed with the valgus osteotomy as early as possible, as it offers the best opportunity to achieve a fully mobile, painless hip and obviates further varus deformation of the femoral neck. Perhaps the best time for surgery is between one and a half and two years of age. In the occasional instance when varus deformity recurs, the operation is repeated.

In the literature, ever since Keetly performed the first subtrochanteric osteotomy in 1888, many ingenious operative techniques have been described for valgus osteotomy of the upper femur to correct coxa vara, suggesting that no one method has been found to be totally satisfactory in every case.* Also, various methods of internal fixation have been utilized, such as the Blount blade plate, McLaughlin nail spline, and bifurcated blade plate (Wagner, Altdorf), all, of which afford secure fixation of osteotomized fragments, but have the definite disadvantage of requiring a second open operation to remove the internal fixation device.

In a child or adolescent the osseous tissue in the femoral neck is hard, and nails are difficult to introduce. Another drawback of internal fixation devices is the risk of injury to the greater trochanter and capital femoral physis through faulty operative technique or error. Percutaneous fixation with pins, Crow pins and Roger Anderson apparatus, and wire loop and double staples do not fix the fragments securely enough, and loss of correction can occur. Recently, external fixation devices such as Ilizarov and DeBastiani Orthofix have been effective in producing stable fixation of the osteotomy fragments.

Should the site of osteotomy be intertrochanteric or subtrochanteric? At the intertrochanteric level the bone is more cancellous (therefore, more rapid-healing) and the site of correction is closer to the deformity (hence, greater correction can be obtained); the osteotomy is, however, close to the growth plates of the femoral head and greater trochanter, with the potential for injury.

Haas described a technique for correcting coxa vara and simultaneously lengthening the femur. An oblique trochanteric osteotomy is performed, extending medially and distally from the greater to the lesser trochanter but remaining distal to the greater trochanteric growth plate. The limb is placed in traction with a threaded Steinmann pin through the distal femur, pulling the limb into wide abduction. Thus, the varus deformity is corrected and femoral lengthening obtained at the same time. Traction is continued for a period of six to eight weeks, until the osteotomy has united.[66] Roberts has found the procedure to be satisfactory and, because of the advantage of simultaneous femoral lengthening with correction of coxa vara, recommends it in unilateral cases.[153] In the modern era of femoral lengthening and advances in internal fixation, the Haas tech-

*See references 4, 17, 70, 87, 90, 100, 137–139, 141, 150, 152.

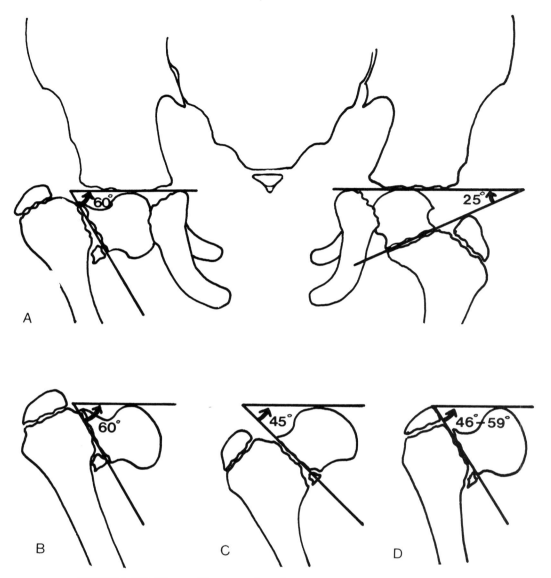

FIGURE 2–258. Diagram illustrating the Hilgenreiner epiphyseal angle (HE angle).

A. The HE angle is 60 degrees on the right with congenital coxa vara, whereas in the left, normal hip it is 25 degrees. **B.** HE angle of greater than 60 degrees is an indication for surgery. **C.** HE angle of 45 degrees or less will have a good prognosis and will tend to correct spontaneously without operative intervention. **D.** HE angle greater than 45 degrees and less than 60 degrees—"gray zone." This hip should be observed.

nique is no longer performed and is not recommended by this author.

In Langenskiöld's technique, the line of osteotomy reaches but does not cross the defect in the femoral neck, thus avoiding the capital femoral physis (Fig. 2–259).[100] The lateral portion of the proximal end of the femoral shaft is roughened and brought against the femoral neck by extreme abduction of the hip. Initially, the fragments were fixed with a wire loop, but fixation was not stable enough, and frequently

the deformity recurred. Therefore, Pylkkänen advocates using a McLaughlin nail for internal fixation.[151] The femoral head is rotated into valgus position by adducting the hip into neutral position. The lower limbs are immobilized in a one–and–one half hip spica cast with the hip that has been operated on in 20 degrees of abduction until firm union of the osteotomy takes place, usually in eight weeks. Technically the Langenskiöld osteotomy is difficult to perform. It does bring normal bone closer to the

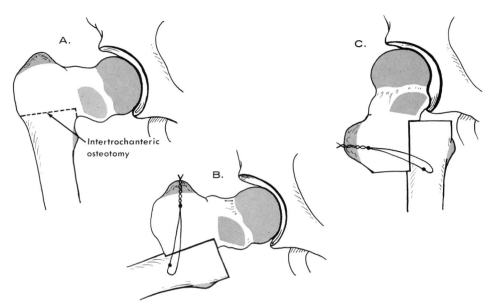

FIGURE 2–259. *Langenskiöld osteotomy for developmental coxa vara.*

Pylkkänen recommends using the McLaughlin nail for internal fixation, as fixation with a wire loop is not stable enough. (Modified from Pylkkänen, P. V.: Acta Orthop. Scand., Suppl. 48, 1960.)

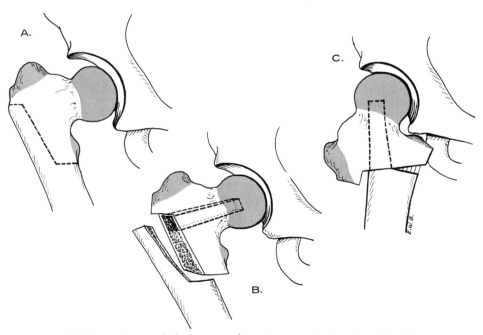

FIGURE 2–260. *Interlocking intertrochanteric osteotomy to correct coxa vara.*

A. A strong spike of lateral cortex is fashioned on the distal fragment, **B,** and mortised into a slot cut in the proximal fragment. **C.** Variations in the length of the lateral spike and depth of the neck mortise depend upon the correction angle and the desirability of crossing the epiphyseal plate with the spike. (Adapted from Amstutz, H. C., and Wilson, P. D., Jr.: J. Bone Joint Surg., *44-A*:16, 1962.)

medial aspect of the femoral neck and achieves excellent correction. Instead of a McLaughlin nail, the bifurcated blade plate of Wagner (and Altdorf) is a better way of fixation in a child. This author's experience with the Langenskiöld technique is very limited.

Amstutz and Wilson recommend an interlocking high intertrochanteric osteotomy in which a strong spike of lateral cortex is fashioned on the distal fragment and mortised into a slot cut in the proximal fragment (Fig. 2–260).[3a] Use of an electric bone cutting saw makes this an easy procedure. They recommend percutaneous pin fixation of both fragments for six weeks if for any reason the correct position is not stable after osteotomy. Also, they stress a minimum of ten weeks of immobilization in a double hip spica cast. The advantages of the Amstutz and Wilson technique are, again, that it brings normal bone closer to the medial aspect of the femoral neck and that recurrence of deformity is less likely. The disadvantages are the technical difficulty and loss of correction due to instability of the fragments even after fixation with pins and incorporation in a hip spica cast.

In unilateral involvement a vital consideration is to avoid further shortening of the limb.

A closing-wedge osteotomy will decrease the already short limb length, whereas an opening-wedge osteotomy will elongate the limb.

Borden, Spencer, and Herndon described a technique of valgus osteotomy in which the trochanteric region and the proximal shaft of the femur are exposed through a lateral longitudinal approach (Fig. 2–261).[17] Under image intensifier radiographic control a guide wire is inserted into the center of the superior half of the femoral neck parallel to its upper border. The guide pin is used as a landmark while the blade of a blade-plate of appropriate size with an angle of 140 degrees is inserted into the neck. The blade should be parallel to the long axis of the femoral neck. Predrilling a slot will facilitate insertion of the blade. Next, an intertrochanteric transverse osteotomy is made under radiographic control. The level of osteotomy should be at a distance of 2 to 2.5 cm. (the diameter of the femoral shaft at that level) distal to the angle of the blade. The lateral surface of the proximal fragment is roughened. The head and neck of the femur are adducted by using the blade as a lever, and the femoral shaft is abducted. Thereby the lateral cortex of the upper fragment is approximated to the upper end of the osteotomized lower fragment. Rota-

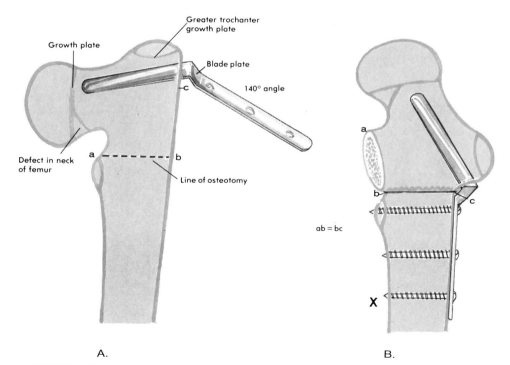

FIGURE 2–261. *Intertrochanteric valgus osteotomy according to Borden, Spencer, and Herndon.*

A. Line of osteotomy and insertion of 140 degree angle–blade parallel to the superior border of the femoral neck. **B.** Varus deformity corrected by adducting femoral head and neck using the blade as a lever. The femoral shaft is abducted. Note that the lateral cortex of the upper fragment is approximated to the upper end of the lower fragment. The plate is secured to the femoral shaft by screws.

tion of the fragments should not be allowed. Adductor myotomy will facilitate correction of the deformity. The plate of the blade-plate is fixed to the shaft with screws. The guide pin is removed. The wound is closed, and a one–and-one half hip spica cast is applied. The cast is removed when the osteotomy is healed. Full weight-bearing is permitted when the defect in the femoral neck is ossified.

MacEwen and Shands employed a technique of oblique trochanteric osteotomy in which coxa vara and associated retroversion of the upper femur are simultaneously corrected.[111] The procedure is a modification of the technique of oblique trochanteric osteotomy in which coxa vara and associated retroversion of the upper femur are simultaneously corrected, originally suggested by J. Warren White in 1946.[179b] Merle d'Aubigne and Descamps previously had investigated the use of oblique osteotomy, and later on, Merle d'Aubigne and Vaillant reported 41 adult cases with degenerative arthritis in whom the oblique osteotomy of the femur was employed to decrease the neck-shaft angle and the increased antetorsion.[118, 119] The procedure is based on the theory that an oblique cut through the bone in a single plane permits a change in both the angulation and rotation of the fragments if the osteotomized surfaces are kept in contact. The relative change in angulation and rotation is determined by the direction and obliquity of the osteotomy. At the trochanteric level of the femur, if an oblique osteotomy running from the anterior surface of the femur distally and posteriorly is performed, adduction of the lower fragment will decrease coxa valga and antetorsion, and abduction of the lower fragment will correct coxa vara and retrotorsion (Fig. 2–262 A to E). The degree of femoral torsion present preoperatively is determined by CT scan. The precise angle of the osteotomy in relation to the long axis of the femur is determined on the graph published by Merle d'Aubigne and Vaillant.[119] The degree of change in the rotation is plotted on the abscissa. The point of intersection of these two lines determines the angle of the cut in relation to the long axis of the femur (Fig. 2–262 F). The more oblique the cut, the less the correction of torsion and the greater the correction of angulation; and the closer the plane of osteotomy to a right angle to the long axis of the femur, the greater the correction of torsion.

The oblique trochanteric osteotomy for correction of coxa vara, as described by MacEwen and Shands, in the older child is preferably performed with the patient on a fracture table with both feet attached to the foot plates.[111] The

hip to be operated on is rotated medially so that the femoral head and neck are aligned with the plane of osteotomy. Through a direct lateral approach, the upper part of the femoral shaft and the greater trochanter are exposed. Next, in order to control the position of the upper fragment, under image intensifier radiographic control, a heavy threaded Steinmann pin is inserted into the neck of the femur along its longitudinal axis. The pin should stop short of the capital femoral physis. Then a second heavy threaded Steinmann pin is inserted into the middle third of the femoral shaft at a predetermined angle of rotation and angulation so that when the lower fragment is abducted the distal pin will be parallel to the proximal pin. The deep end of the distal pin should engage the medial cortex. MacEwen and Shands do not insert a distal pin, but this author finds it will ensure accuracy of the degree of correction obtained. The level of proposed osteotomy is determined under radiographic control. Next, with an electric drill, holes are made along the line of osteotomy, which extends from anterosuperior to posteroinferior at a predetermined angle. The osteotomy is completed with an electric saw. Next, the varus deformity and retrotorsion are corrected by abducting the lower fragment, keeping the osteotomized bony surfaces in close apposition. MacEwen and Shands recommend fixing the bone fragments with a single screw inserted across the osteotomy site and incorporating the proximal Steinmann pin in the hip spica cast. This makes it possible to change the neck-shaft angle after surgery if necessary. This author recommends internal fixation of the osteotomized femoral fragments with a four-hole or preferably six-hole plate. The position of the fragments and the degree of correction obtained are checked by anteroposterior and lateral radiograms. The wounds are closed and a one–and-one half hip spica cast is applied. MacEwen and Shands remove the proximal pin at three weeks. This author recommends removal of the pin immediately after application of the hip spica cast. The cast is removed six to eight weeks postoperatively when the osteotomy is healed. The plate and screws are removed four to six months later by a second open operation.

The operative technique of valgus intertrochanteric osteotomy of the proximal femur for correction of coxa vara and internal fixation with bifurcated blade plate is as follows (see Plate 16, p. 396):

The operation is performed under image intensifier radiographic control and with the patient in supine position.

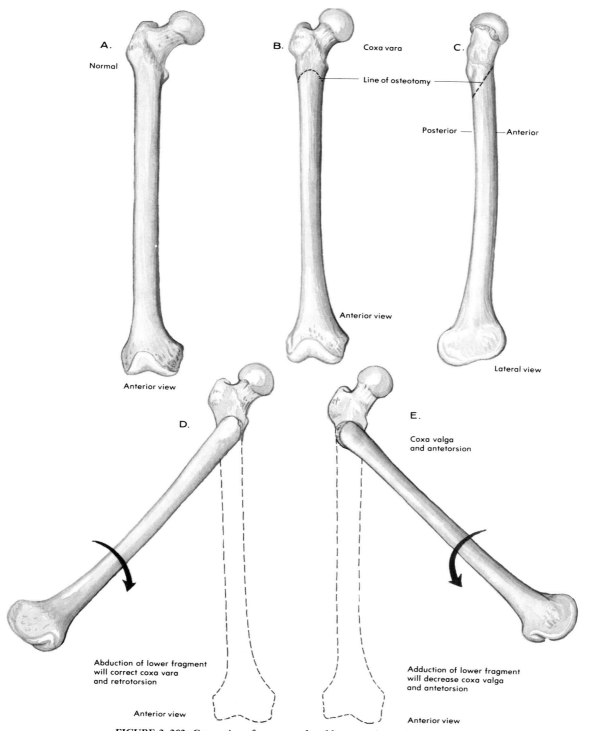

FIGURE 2–262. Correction of coxa vara by oblique trochanteric osteotomy.

A. Normal femur. **B.** Anterior view of the femur with coxa vara. **C.** Lateral view of the femur. In B and C, note the line of oblique osteotomy in the trochanteric area; it runs from the anterior surface of the femur distally and posteriorly. **D.** Coxa vara and retrotorsion are corrected by abduction of the distal fragment. **E.** Adduction of distal fragment will decrease coxa valga and antetorsion. **F.** Merle d'Aubigné and Vaillant graph for determination of the precise angle of the osteotomy in relation to long axis of the femur. See text for explanation.

(From MacEwen, G. D., and Shands, A. R.: Oblique trochanteric osteotomy. J. Bone Joint Surg., *49-A*:345, 1967. Reprinted by permission.)

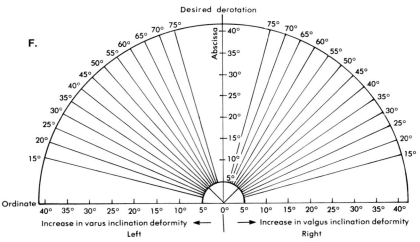

FIGURE 2–262 Continued *Correction of coxa vara by oblique trochanteric osteotomy.*

F. Merle d'Aubigné and Vaillant graph for determination of the precise angle of the osteotomy in relation to long axis of the femur. See text for explanation.

The proximal shaft of the femur and trochanteric region are exposed through a lateral longitudinal approach. First, a threaded Steinmann pin of appropriate diameter is drilled medially through the greater trochanter into the femoral neck in its superior half, along its longitudinal axis, and stopping short of the capital physis. Next, a second threaded Steinmann pin is drilled into the middle half of the femoral shaft, engaging the medial cortex. The relationship of these two pins before and after completion of the osteotomy will measure the degree of correction of varus deformity and retrotorsion.

With an oscillating saw and under image intensifier control, the intertrochanteric osteotomy is performed, terminating medially at a point immediately below the inferomedial corner of the femoral neck. Do not enter and break the medial cortex of the femoral neck. It is also essential to have smooth cut surfaces in order to achieve accurate apposition and stable contact. Avoid using osteotomes and splintering bone.

A wide flat osteotome is inserted between the bone fragments to open up the osteotomy cleft by adducting and rotating the lower limb. Next, with an oscillating saw, a wedge of bone is removed from the upper end of the femoral shaft.

The distal fragment is displaced medially about one third to one half of the diameter of the shaft. By displacing the distal fragment medially and bringing it closer to the center of the hip, compression forces are increased, better bony support is provided, and bone healing is stimulated. Appropriate size and angle of the bifurcated blade-plate are chosen. The bifur-

cated ends of the plate should not penetrate and injure the capital physis. Immediately below the angulation of the blade-plate there is a round hole through which a screw can be inserted into the proximal fragment; this screw should not penetrate the upper femoral physis. The blade-plate is securely held in a special holding instrument, and by careful hammer blows, under image intensifier radiographic control, the bifurcated blade is inserted into the osteotomized surfaces of the proximal fragment parallel to the longitudinal axis of the femoral neck. The site of insertion of the blade will determine the degree of medial displacement. The blade should be placed in the center of the femoral neck, and its bifurcated ends should not protrude from the cortices. The blade is driven proximally into the osteotomized surface and buried almost to the angle of the plate. The holding instrument is removed, and the blade is impacted further with a punch. Its position is checked under image intensifier control in the anteroposterior, lateral, and various oblique projections.

Next, the distal fragment is manipulated, bringing it into the desired degrees of abduction to correct coxa vara and of medial rotation to correct retrotorsion. The osteotomy fragments are firmly fixed together with a bone clamp, and radiograms are made to check the degree of correction of the varus angulation.

Next, a cortical screw of appropriate size is inserted through the most distal hole of the plate first, and then a cancellous screw through the most proximal hole into the femoral neck, and last, a cortical screw through the middle hole. By tightening the screws the bone fragments are compressed and the distal fragment is pulled toward the plate. The wounds are closed in the usual fashion.

In the young child (under six years of age) a one–and–one half hip spica cast is applied. The cast is removed in six to eight weeks when radiograms disclose that the osteotomy is solidly healed. In the older and cooperative child a hip spica cast is not necessary because osteosynthesis with a Wagner bifurcated blade-plate is stable. Active and gentle passive exercises are performed to regain functional range of motion of the hip and knee. Then walking is allowed, first with the protection of crutches, later with three-point gait, and finally with full weight-bearing. Side-lying hip abduction and standing Trendelenburg exercises are performed to develop the motor strength of the gluteus medius. The child is followed, and roentgenograms are

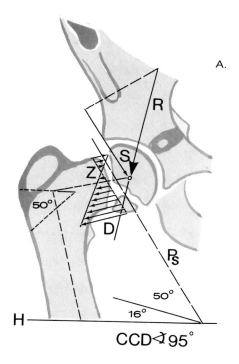

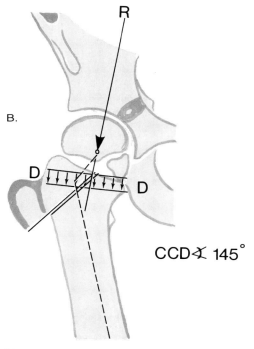

FIGURE 2–263. Objective of Pauwels' osteotomy.

See text for explanation.

taken periodically until maturity. As long as there is a defect in the femoral neck the deformity may recur.

The cuneiform Y-shaped intertrochanteric osteotomy of Pauwel is described in Plate 31.

The objectives of intertrochanteric Y osteotomy are to place the capital femoral physis perpendicular to the resultant compressive force and to decrease the bending stress in the femoral neck. Medial displacement of the upper end of the femoral shaft widens the femoral neck and shifts the compressive force within the core of the cross section of the neck, eliminating the tension stresses caused by bending (Fig. 2–263).

The operation must be executed precisely in order to achieve the objectives. It must be planned on drawings made from radiograms.

Proper choice of radiograms is essential; they must demonstrate clearly the physeal cartilage and the zone of resorption in the femoral neck, must be centered on the femoral head, and exposures must be made at various rotations. Examination with the image intensifier will be of great assistance.

The operation diagram is drawn as shown in Figure 2–264. On a transparent paper placed on the radiogram, draw the hip joint, the physis, and the axis of the shaft of the femur. First, draw a horizontal line H, which transects the axis of the femoral shaft 4 to 6 cm. below the lesser trochanter. Second, draw an interrupted line Ps through the physis and extend it inferiorly until it intersects the horizontal line H. Third, from the point of intersection of the lines H and Ps, draw a line inclined upward 16

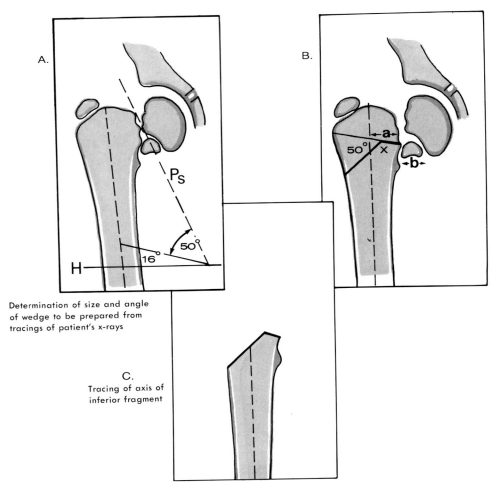

A.

Determination of size and angle
of wedge to be prepared from
tracings of patient's x-rays

B.

C.
Tracing of axis of
inferior fragment

FIGURE 2–264. *Tracings of radiogram to determine the angle of bone wedge to be resected for Pauwels' intertrochanteric osteotomy (see text for explanation).*

Illustration continued on opposite page

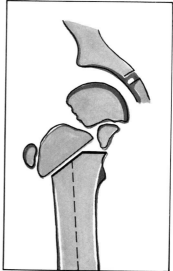

E.
Upper tracing sheet rotated back
and slid upward parallel to
axis of femur until femoral head
lies in socket of original sheet.
Socket is then traced

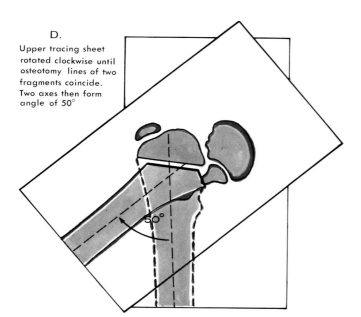

D.
Upper tracing sheet
rotated clockwise until
osteotomy lines of two
fragments coincide.
Two axes then form
angle of 50°

50°

FIGURE 2–264 Continued Tracings of radiogram to determine the angle of bone wedge to be resected for Pauwels'
intertrochanteric osteotomy.

degrees from the horizontal and extend it laterally to intersect the axis of the femoral shaft
(this line is approximately at right angles to the
direction of the resultant compressive force R)
(Fig. 2–264 A). The angle formed between the
third line (inclined upward) and the interrupted
line Ps is the size of the wedge to be resected
(50 degrees in the drawing). Next draw the
upper line of the intertrochanteric osteotomy.
It should extend medially to transect the capital
physis at the zone of resorption in the femoral
neck. Then draw the wedge to be resected with
its apex reaching the upper osteotomy line at
the point X. The part of the upper femoral shaft
vertical to the apex of the wedge (X) must be
equal to the width of the medial part of the
femoral neck separated by the zone of resorption (Fig. 2–264 B).

Superimpose a new sheet of transparent paper on the first and trace the inferior fragment
of the osteotomy with its axis (Fig. 2–264 C).
Rotate the upper tracing sheet clockwise until
the osteotomy lines of the two fragments coincide. Then trace the upper fragment, and the
two axes of the femoral shaft should form an
angle of 50 degrees (Fig. 2–264 D).

Rotate the upper tracing sheet back, slide it
upward parallel to the femoral axis until the
femoral head lies in the acetabular socket of the
original sheet, and trace the acetabulum (Fig.
2–264 E).

References

1. Almond, H. G.: Familial infantile coxa vara. J. Bone
   Joint Surg., 38-B:539, 1956.
2. Amstutz, H. C.: Developmental (infantile) coxa
   vara—a distinct entity. Report of two patients with
   previously normal roentgenograms. Clin. Orthop.,
   72:242, 1970.
3. Amstutz, H. C., and Freiberger, R. H.: Coxa vara in
   children. Clin. Orthop., 22:73, 1962.
3a. Amstutz, H. C., and Wilson, P. J., Jr.: Dysgenesis
    of the proximal femur (coxa vara) and its surgical
    management. J. Bone Joint Surg., 44-A:1, 1962.
4. Armstrong, J. R.: A case of infantile coxa vara, with
   notes on aetiology. Lancet, 1:1498, 1935.
5. Atasu, M., Taysi, K., and Say, B.: Dermatoglyphic
   findings in familial coxa vara with dominant inheritance. Turk. J. Pediatr., 16:15, 1974.
6. Babb, F. S., Ghormley, R. K., and Chatterton, C.
   C.: Congenital coxa vara. J. Bone Joint Surg., 31-
   A:115, 1949.
7. Bade, A.: Zur Abgrenzung der verschiedenen Formen
   von Coxa vara. Z. Orthop. Chir., 59:53, 1933.
8. Barcikowski, W.: Diagnostic difficulties in focal defects

References continued on page 606

Pauwels' Intertrochanteric Y Osteotomy

The patient is placed supine on a radiolucent operating table. The hip and the upper end of the femur should be clearly visualized on the image intensifier. The entire hip and the whole lower limb are prepared and draped to permit free passive motion. The child over six to eight years of age is best operated on on a fracture table. The upper end of the femur and the trochanteric region are exposed through a direct lateral approach.

OPERATIVE TECHNIQUE

A. The angle of the bone wedge to be resected as prepared from tracings of the radiogram (see Fig. 2–264).

B. Under image intensifier radiographic control the lines of osteotomy are determined by drilling Kirschner wires above and below the wedge resection lines. The upper Kirschner wire should stop short of the capital physis and the defect in the neck of the femur, and the tip of the lower Kirschner wire should be just below the upper osteotomy line and terminate medial to the point X, which marks the apex of the bone to be resected.

C. With an oscillating saw, the upper intertrochanteric osteotomy is performed, and the wedge of bone is resected.

D. The wedge of bone is removed with flat osteotomes.

Plate 31. Pauwels' Intertrochanteric Y Osteotomy

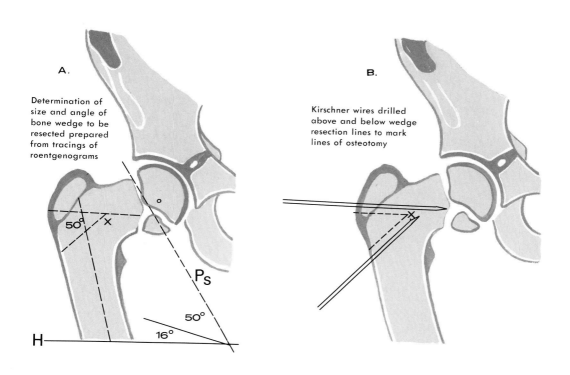

A.

Determination of size and angle of bone wedge to be resected prepared from tracings of roentgenograms

50°

X

o

P_S

50°

16°

H

B.

Kirschner wires drilled above and below wedge resection lines to mark lines of osteotomy

X

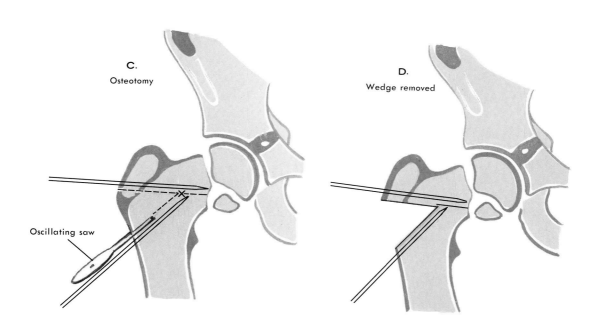

C.
Osteotomy

X

Oscillating saw

D.
Wedge removed

Pauwels' Intertrochanteric Y Osteotomy (Continued)

E. A hook over the greater trochanter is used to pull the upper segment distally, and the two Kirschner wires are made parallel to each other, closing the gap.

F. Pauwels recommends fixing the osteotomy fragments with a metal tension band. First, two holes are made with 2-mm. Kirschner wires parallel to the osteotomy surfaces, the first 1 cm. below and the second 1 cm. above the osteotomy line. These Kirschner wires are directed from the middle of the lateral surface of the shaft to the anterior aspect of the femoral neck. A wire is passed through the two holes and twisted on the lateral aspect of the femur. Pauwels finds that this method of fixation is adequate and maintains the osteotomized surfaces in compression, and he applies a plaster of Paris spica cast for six to eight weeks.

G. This author prefers internal fixation with screws and a band plate hooked over the greater trochanter. In the cooperative child over six years of age, hip spica cast immobilization is not necessary.

Plate 31. Pauwels' Intertrochanteric Y Osteotomy

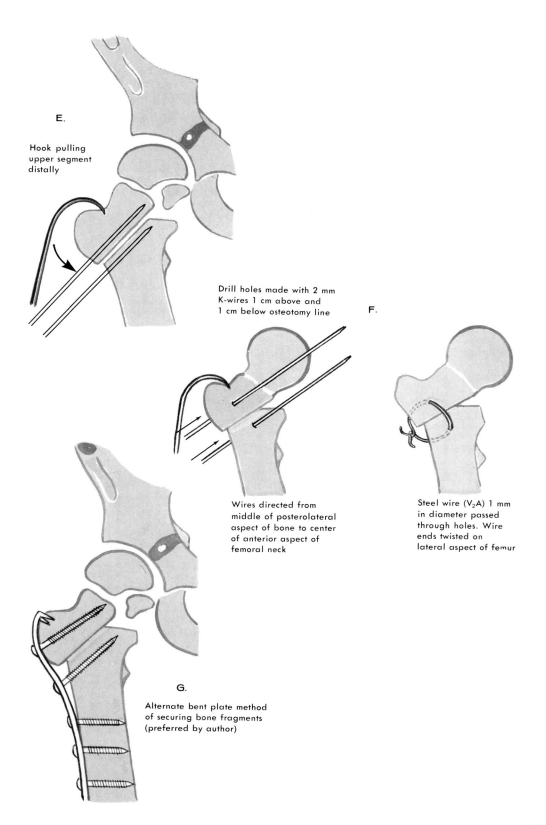

E.

Hook pulling
upper segment
distally

Drill holes made with 2 mm
K-wires 1 cm above and
1 cm below osteotomy line

F.

Wires directed from
middle of posterolateral
aspect of bone to center
of anterior aspect of
femoral neck

Steel wire (V₂A) 1 mm
in diameter passed
through holes. Wire
ends twisted on
lateral aspect of femur

G.

Alternate bent plate method
of securing bone fragments
(preferred by author)

of upper segments of the femoral bone. Wiad. Lek., *18*:1869, 1965.

9. Barr, J. S.: Congenital coxa vara. Arch. Surg., *18*:1909, 1929.

10. Barrington-Ward, L. E.: Double coxa vara with other deformities occurring in brother and sister. Lancet, *1*:157, 1912.

11. Bauer, R.: Ein beitrag zur Coxa vara congenita bzw. sum angeborenen Femurdefekt. Der. Chirurg., *141*:34, 1970.

12. Becton, J. L., and Diamond, L. S.: Persistent limp in congenital coxa vara. South. Med. J., *60*:921, 1967.

13. Bell, M.: Surgical management of coxa vara. Orthop. Trans., *3*:344, 1979.

14. Blauth, W.: Zur Morphologie und Pathogenese der primären Coxa vara congenita und ihren Beziehungen zum sogenannten Femurdefekt. Z. Orthop., *100*:271, 1965.

15. Blockey, N. J.: Observations on infantile coxa vara. J. Bone Joint Surg., *51-B*:106, 1969.

16. Blount, W. P.: Blade-plate internal fixation for high femoral osteotomies. J. Bone Joint Surg., *25*:319, 1943.

17. Borden, J., Spencer, G. E., Jr., and Herndon, C. H.: Treatment of coxa vara in children by means of a modified osteotomy. J. Bone Joint Surg., *48-A*:1106, 1966.

18. Borggreve, J.: Kniegelenksersatz durch das in der Beinlängsache um 180° gedrehte Fussgelenk. Arch. Orthop. Chir., *28*:175, 1930.

19. Brandes, M.: Zur Behandlung der Coxa vara. Z. Orthop., *44*:266, 1924.

20. Brandes, M.: Behandlung der Coxa vara mit Resektion des Trochanter major. Verh. Deutsch. Orthop. Ges., *24*:80, 1929.

21. Burckhardt, E.: Zur klinik und pathologischen Anatomie der Coxa vara infantum. Helv. Chir. Acta, *13*:28, 1946.

22. Cabras, G.: Coxa vara congenita, cosi detta congenita e forme di passagio. La Clinica Orthopedica, Vol. 4, 1952, pp. 145–188.

23. Calhound, J. D., and Pierret, G.: Infantile coxa vara. A.J.R., *115*:561, 1972.

24. Camitz, H.: Etude comparée sur la coxa vara dite congénitale et ostéochondrite coxale juvenile (coxa plana). Acta Chir. Scand., *73*:521, 1934.

25. Capener, N.: The operation of intertrochanteric osteotomy. Proc. R. Soc. Med., *32*:646, 1939.

26. Carter, H. R., and Vitale, C. C.: Developmental coxa vara, a new type of internal fixation for subtrochanteric osteotomies. Can. J. Surg., *3*:324, 1960.

27. Chemke, J., Fishel, E., Zalish, M., and Sagiv, M.: Multiple skeletal anomalies in the '13q −' syndrome. Eur. J. Pediatr., *128*:27, 1978.

28. Chung, S. M.: The arterial supply of the developing proximal end of the human femur. J. Bone Joint Surg., *58-A*:961, 1976.

29. Chung, S. M., and Riser, W. H.: The histological characteristics of congenital coxa vara: A case report of a five year old boy. Clin. Orthop., *132*:71, 1978.

30. Clark, J. M., and Jacobson, G.: Congenital coxa vara. Radiology, *63*:59, 1954.

31. Cleveland, M., Bosworth, D. M., and Della Pietra, A.: Subtrochanteric osteotomy and splint fixation for certain disabilities of the hip joint. A preliminary report. J. Bone Joint Surg., *33-A*:351, 1961.

32. Compere, E. L., Garrison, M., and Fahey, J. S.: Deformities of femur resulting from arrestment of growth of capital or greater trochanteric epiphyses. J. Bone Joint Surg., *22*:909, 1940.

33. Dann, P., Haike, H., and Schulze, H.: Experimental animal studies on the development of static coxa valga and coxa vara. Cosmetologica, *19*:247, 1970.

34. Davis, A.: Infratrochanteric approach to the hip joint (abord de la hanche par voie infratrochantérienne). Acta Orthop. Belg., *39*:658, 1973.

35. Delitala, F.: Sulla coxa vara congenita. Contributo anatomo-patologico. Arch. Ortop., *30*:382, 1913.

36. Delitch, M.: Les troubles du développement du cotyle dans les coxa vara. Rev. Chir. Orthop., *52*:635, 1966.

37. Drehman, G.: Beitrage zur atiologie und therapie der coxa vara. Ver. Dtsch. Orthop. Ges., 8:360, 1909.

38. Drehman, G.: Die coxa vara. Ergebn. Chir. Orthop., 2:453, 1911

39. Dreyfus, J. R.: Sur quelques données nouvelles du traitement opératoire de la coxa-vara. Rev. Chir., 5:378, 1937.

40. Duncan, G. A.: Congenital coxa vara occurring in identical twins. Am. J. Surg., *37*:112, 1937.

41. Duncan, G. A.: Congenital and developmental coxa vara. Surgery, 3:741, 1938.

42. Dysek, M.: Coxa vara congenita. Acta Chir. Orthop. Traumatol. Ceh., *41*:350, 1974.

43. Elmslie, R. C.: Injury and deformity of the epiphysis of the head of the femur: Coxa vara. Lancet, *1*:410, 1907.

44. Elmslie, R. C.: Coxa Vara. London, Henry Frowde, 1913; Lancet, *1*:413, 1907; Jacksonian Prize Essay, 1905.

45. Etienne, E.: Traitement de la coxa-vara chez l'enfant et chez l'adolescent. Rev. Chir. Orthop., *41*:270, 1954.

46. Exner, G.: Vergleichende Untersuchungen über das verhalten des proximalen Femurendes bei angeborenen Femurdefect und Coxa vara congenita. Z. Orthop., *79*:624, 1950.

47. Fairbank, H. A. T.: Unusual case of congenital coxa vara. Proc. R. Soc. Med., *20*:237, 1926.

48. Fairbank, H. A. T.: Coxa vara due to congenital defect of the neck of the femur. J. Anat., *62*:232, 1928.

49. Fairbank, H. A. T.: Infantile or cervical coxa vara. In Robert Jones Birthday Volume. A Collection of Surgical Essays. London, Milford, 1928, p. 225.

50. Feiss, H. O.: Congenital coxa vara. J.A.M.A., *46*:565, 1906.

51. Fiorani, F.: Concerning a rare form of limping. Gazz. Osp., 2:717, 1881.

52. Finby, N., Jacobson, H. G., and Poppel, M. H.: Idiopathic coxa vara in childhood. Radiology, *67*:10, 1956.

53. Fisher, R. L., and Waskowitz, W. J.: Familial developmental coxa vara. Clin. Orthop. *86*:2, 1972.

54. Francke, K.: Zur Kasuistik der angeborenen Coxa vara. Z. Orthop., *15*:288, 1906.

55. Frost, H. M.: A simple method for achieving subtrochanteric valgus femoral osteotomy in infants and children. Clin. Orthop., *103*:18, 1974.

56. Goeminne, L., and Dujardin, L.: Congenital coxa vara, patella aplasia and tarsal synostosis: A new inherited syndrome. Acta Genet. Med. Gemellol. (Roma), *19*:534, 1970.

57. Goksan, M. A., Cilingiroğlu, K., and Sonmezler, H. A.: Trochanteric osteotomies in surgical treatment of coxa vara. Turk Tip Cem. Mec., *35*:452, 1969.

58. Golding, F. C.: Congenital coxa vara and the short femur. Proc. R. Soc. Med., *32*:641, 1938.

59. Golding, F. C.: Congenital coxa vara. J. Bone Joint Surg., *30-B*:160, 1948.

60. Greensfelder, L. A., and Blanchard, W.: Coxa vara. Trans. Chgo. Surg. Soc., Dec., 1905; Ann. Surg., *43*:630, 1906.

61. Greve, H.: Coxa vara congenita bei eineiigen Zwillingen. Arch. Orthop. Chir., *43*:309, 1944.

62. Guillemin, A.: Quelques observations de la coxa vara essentielle et d'ostéochondrite. Rev. Orthop., *11*:51, 1924.

63. Guilleminet, M.: Traitement chirurgical de la coxa-vara congénitale. Lyon Chir., *37*:350, 1941–1942.

64. Guilleminet, M., and Stagnara, P.: Valeur de l'ostéo-

tomie sous-trochantérienne dans le traitement de la coxa-vara congénitale à fissure verticale. Lyon Chir., 39:476, 1944.

65. Gutig, C., and Herzog, A.: Der berginn der sogenannten "coxa vara congenita" aseptische schenkelhalsnekrose. Beitr. Klin. Chir., 156:551, 1932.

66. Haas, S. L.: Lengthening of the femur with simultaneous correction of coxa vara. J. Bone Joint Surg., 15:219, 1933.

67. Hafezi, F. F.: Recurrent congenital coxa vara associated with primary hypoparathyroidism. A case report. Clin. Orthop., 79:127, 1971.

68. Hansen, F. W., Hansen-Leth, C., and Jensen, E. G.: Intertrochanteric osteotomy with A.O. technique in arthrosis of the hip. Acta Orthop. Scand., 44:219, 1973.

69. Hark, F. W.: Congenital coxa vara. Am. J. Surg., 80:305, 1950.

70. Hasue, M., Kimura, F., Funayama, M., and Ito, R.: An unusual form of coxa vara, characterized by varying degrees of metaphyseal changes and multiple slipped epiphyses. J. Bone Joint Surg., 50-A:373, 1968.

71. Helbing, C.: Die coxa vara. Z. Orthop. Chir., 15:502, 1906.

72. Henriksson, L.: Measurement of femoral neck anteversion and inclination. Acta Orthop. Scand., 186:1, 1980.

73. Hilgenreiner, H.: Zur Genese der Coxa vara. Med. Klin., 27:159, 1931.

74. Hofer, H.: Zur Atiologie und Therapie der Coxa vara congenita. Wien. Med. Wochensch., 122:413, 1972.

75. Hoffa, A.: Die angeborenen Coxa vara. Dtsche Med. Wochenschr., 31:1257, 1905.

76. Hofmeister, F.: Coxa vara, eine typische Form der Schenkelalsverbiegung. Beitr. Klin. Chir., 12:245, 1894.

77. Horwitz, T.: The treatment of congenital (or developmental) coxa vara. Surg. Gynecol. Obstet., 87:71, 1948.

78. Hoyt, W. A., Jr., and Greenberg, B. J.: Congenital coxa vara. In Tronzo, R. (ed.): Surgery of the Hip Joint. Philadelphia, Lea & Febiger, 1973.

79. Huc, G.: La coxa vara de l'enfance. Rev. Orthop., 17:445, 1930.

80. Ingelrans and Vendeuvre: Coxa-vara congénitale. Resultats du traitement dans cinq observations. Rev. Orthop., 32:368, 1956.

81. Iwamoto, M., Basmajian, J. V., and Strom, C. H.: A method for determining femoral neck-shaft and anteversion angles. Arch. Phys. Med. Rehabil., 53:253, 1972.

82. Jahss, M.: Congenital coxa vara (preliminary clinical follow-up). Bull. Hosp. Joint Dis., 13:342, 1952.

83. Janek, J.: Traitement opératoire de la coxa-vara de l'enfance. Zentralbl. Chir., 5:277, 1937.

84. Jerre, T.: Spontaneous recovery in coxa vara. Acta Orthop. Scand., 25:149, 1955.

85. Jerre, T., and Tilling, G.: Stable fixation in the intertrochanteric osteotomy. Acta Orthop. Scand., 40:466, 1969.

86. Johanning, K.: Coxa vara infantum. I. Clinical appearance and aetiological problems. Acta Orthop. Scand., 21:273, 1951.

87. Johanning, K.: Coxa vara infantum. II. Treatment and results of treatment. Acta Orthop. Scand., 22:100, 1952.

88. Jones, R., and Lovett, R. W.: Orthopaedic Surgery. London, Frowde, Hodder & Stoughton, 1923.

89. Jorrig, K., and Movin, R.: Experience with 79 subtrochanteric valgus osteotomies of the hip. Acta Orthop. Scand., 44:467, 1973.

90. Keetley, C. B.: Coxa vara. Lancet, 1:1115, 1900.

91. King, R. E., and Lovejoy, J. F., Jr.: Familial osteo-

92. Knowles, K. G.: Congenital coxa vara: Presentation of a case. R.I. Med. J., 46:594, 1963.

93. Konig, G.: Value and significance of various methods for x-ray determination of the real antetorsion and femoral neck-shaft angle. Z. Orthop., 111:663, 1973.

94. Konig, G.: Eine praktische Methode zur röntgenologischen Bestimmung des Antetorsions- und Kollodiaphysenwinkels. Z. Orthop., 110:76, 1972.

95. Kredel, L.: Coxa vara congenita. Zentralbl. Chir., 23:969, 1896.

96. Kreuz, L.: Kritische Betrachtungen zur Morphologie der angeborenen Coxa vara. Arch. Orthop. Unfallchir., 28:106, 1930.

97. Lahoenranta, V., and Pylkkanen, P.: Early and late results of Brackett's operation for pseudarthrosis of the neck of the femur in infantile coxa vara. A review of 30 operations. Acta Orthop. Scand., 48:74, 1977.

98. Lange, M.: Die Coxa-vara. Ihr klinisches Bild und ihre heutige Behandlung. Munch. Med. Wochenschr., 85:1637, 1938.

99. Langenskiöld, A., and Salenius, P.: Epiphyseodesis of the greater trochanter. Acta Orthop. Scand., 38:199, 1967.

100. Langenskiöld, F.: On pseudarthrosis of the femoral neck in congenital coxa vara. Acta Chir. Scand., 98:568, 1949.

101. Lasserre, C.: Subtrochanteric oblique osteotomy in coxa vara, with temporary external fixation of the fragments. J. Bone Joint Surg., 13:296, 1931.

102. Lasserre, M. J.: Ostéotomie en Y pour coxa-vara congénitale. Bordeaux Chir., 4:191, 1964.

103. Laurent, L. E.: Growth disturbances of the proximal end of the femur in the light of animal experiments. Acta Orthop. Scand., 28:255, 1959.

104. Le Mesurier, A. B.: Developmental coxa vara. J. Bone Joint Surg., 30-B:595, 1948.

105. Le Mesurier, A. B.: Developmental coxa vara (correspondence). J. Bone Joint Surg., 33-B:478, 1951.

106. Letts, R. M., and Shokeir, M. H. K.: Mirror-image coxa vara in identical twins. J. Bone Joint Surg., 57-A:117, 1975.

107. Lian, C.: Congenital coxa vara and Perthes' disease. Acta Orthop. Scand., 19:527, 1950.

108. Lindemann, K.: Das erbliche Vorkommen der angeborenen Coxa vara. Z. Orthop. Chir., 72:326, 1941.

109. Lindemann, K.: Zur Morphologie der Coxa vara congenita. Z. orthop., 78:47, 1949.

110. Lococo, S. J., Pusateri, W. M., and Newman, W. H.: Intramedullary fixation after subtrochanteric osteotomy for coxa vara and coxa valga deformities in children. South. Med. J., 66:1379, 1973.

111. MacEwen, G. D., and Shands, A. R.: Oblique trochanteric osteotomy. J. Bone Joint Surg., 49-A:345, 1967.

112. Magnusson, R.: Coxa vara infantum. Acta Orthop. Scand., 23:284, 1954.

113. Maquet, P.: Biomécanique de la gonarthrose. Acta Orthop. Belg., 38:33, 1972.

114. Martin, H.: Coxa vara congenita bei eineigen Zwillingen. Arch. Orthop. Chir., 42:230, 1943.

115. Masse, P.: Coxa-vara rachitiques et coxa-vara congénitales. Rev. Chir. Orthop., 42:362, 1956.

116. Mau, H.: Die Trochanterresektion als physiologische Behandlung der Coxa vara. Z. Orthop., 85:48, 1955.

117. Mayer, G.: Results of the transposition of the trochanter in symptomatic coxa vara. Beitr. Orthop. Traumatol., 23:79, 1976.

118. Merle D'Aubigne, R., and Descamps, L.: L'ostéotomie plane oblique dans la correction des déformations des membres. Mem. Acad. Chir., 78:271, 1952.

119. Merle D'Aubigne, R., and Vaillant, J. M.: Correction

simultanée des angles d'inclinaison et de torsion du col fémoral par l'ostéotomie plane oblique. Rev. Chir. Orthop., 47:94, 1961.

120. Michelsson, J. E., and Langenskiöld, A.: Coxa vara following immobilization of the knee in extension in young rabbits. Acta Orthop. Scand., 45:399, 1974.

121. Michelsson, J. E., and Langenskiöld, A.: Dislocation or subluxation of the hip; regular sequels of immobilization of the knee in extension in young rabbits. J. Bone Joint Surg., 54-A:1177, 1972.

122. Morandi, G.: L'osteotomia sotto trocanterica secondo Putti nel trattamento della coxa-vara congenita. Chir. Org. Mov., 35:141, 1957.

123. Morgan, J. D., and Somerville, E. W.: Normal and abnormal growth at the upper end of the femur. J. Bone Joint Surg., 42-B:264, 1960.

124. Muller, M. E.: Die huftnahen Femurosteotomien. Stuttgart, Thieme, 1971, p. 2.

125. Muller, M. E., Allgower, M., and Willenegger, H.: Manual of Internal Fixation. Techniques Recommended by the AO Group. 2nd Ed. New York, Springer Verlag, 1979.

126. Nagura, S.: Zur Ätiologie der Coxa vara, zugleich Beitrag zur Kenntnis der Transformation der Knochen. Arch. Klin. Chir., 199:533, 1940.

127. Nilsonne, H.: Beitrag zur Kenntnis der kongenitalen Form der Coxa vara. Acta Radiol., 3:153, 1924.

128. Nilsonne, H.: On congenital coxa vara. Acta Chir. Scand., 64:217, 1929.

129. Noble, T. P., and Hauser, E. D. W.: Coxa vara. Arch. Surg., 12:501, 1926.

130. Nove-Josserand and Pouzet: Coxa-vara traitée par l'ostéotomie sous-trochanterienne. Lyon Chir., 35:470, 1938.

131. Ollerenshaw, R.: The femoral neck in childhood. Proc. R. Soc. Med., 32:113, 1939.

132. Olszewski, W.: Surgical treatment of coxa vara. Chir. Narzadow Kuchu. Ortop. Pol., 42:563, 1977.

133. Omiadze, D. A., Marsagishvili, T. S. A., and Kacharova, N. N.: Method of treatment of coxa vara. Ortop. Travmatol. Protez, 6:74, 1977.

134. Papadopulos, J. S.: Ursachen absoluter Revalgisierung kindlicher Huftgelenke nach Varisierungs and Detorsions-Osteotomie. Arch. Orthop. Unfallchir., 70:189, 1971.

135. Papadopulos, J. S., and Hofmann, A.: Periosteal growth as the principal means of functional adaptations of the femoral neck–femoral shaft angle. Arch. Orthop. Unfallchir., 73:33, 1972.

136. Pauwels, F.: Zur Therapie der kindlichen Coxa vara. Z. Orthop., 64:372, 1936.

137. Pauwels, F.: Über die Coxa vara. (Deutschen orthopädischen Gesellschaft). Ver. Dtsch. Orthop. Ges., 24:8, 1930.

138. Pauwels, F.: Zur Therapie der klinischen Coxa vara. Verh. Dtsch. Orthop. Ges., 30:372, 1935.

139. Pauwels, F.: Uber die Bedentung einer Zuggurtung für die Beanspruchung eines Röhrenknochens und ihre Verwending zur Druckasteosynthes. Verh. Dtsch. Orthop. Ges., 52:231, 1966.

140. Pauwels, F.: Biomechanics of the Normal and Diseased Hip. New York, Springer, 1976.

141. Pavlansky, R., and Vondráček, L.: Experimental myodynamics of alterations in the coxa-femoral angle. Acta Chir. Orthop. Traumatol. Cech. (Prague), 37:67, 1970.

142. Peabody, C. W.: Subtrochanteric osteotomy in coxa vara. Arch. Surg., 46:743, 1943.

143. Peixinho, M., Cordeiro, E. N., and Kuroba, M. T.: Congenital coxa vara: Considerations on its surgical treatment. Rev. Paul. Med., 80:227, 1972.

144. Petersen, D.: Entstehung einer Coxa vara im Verlauf einer Huftgelenksluxations-behandlung. Arch. Orthop. Unfallchir., 56:208, 1964.

145. Picault, C.: Traitement de la coxa-vara congénitale. Rev. Chir. Orthop., 47:75, 1961.

146. Polivka, D., and Grigar, L.: Coxa vara congenita (operacni leceni v mcadsim detskem veku). Acta Chir. Orthop. Traumatol. Cech., 40:516, 1973.

147. Pompe Van Meerdervoort, H. F.: Congenital (infantile) coxa vara: A report of three cases and their treatment by interlocking high intertrochanteric osteotomy. S. Afr. J. Surg., 14:127, 1976.

148. Pouzet, F.: Evolution anatomique des aplasies du col fémoral. Coxa-vara à fissure verticale. Lyon Chir., 31:712, 1934.

149. Pouzet, F.: Le traitement de la coxa vara congénitale. Presse Méd., 46:1095, 1938.

150. Prat-Dalfo, J.: Berechnung der Langenanderung des Beines bei varisierender und valgisierender intertrochanterer Osteotomie. Z. Orthop., 102:163, 1966.

151. Pylkkänen, P. V.: Coxa vara infantum. Acta Orthop. Scand., Suppl. 48, 1960.

152. Ring, P. A.: Congenital abnormalities of the femur. Arch. Dis. Child., 36:410, 1961.

153. Roberts, W. M.: End results study of congenital coxa vara treated by the Haas trochanteric osteotomy. South. Med. J., 43:389, 1950.

154. Rocher, H. L., and Guérin, R.: Coxa-vara de l'enfance. Traitement par greffe osseuse. Journ. Orthop. Bordeaux, 7 et 8 juin, 1935; J. Med. Bordeaux, p. 678, 30 sept., 1935.

155. Ruszkowski, I., and Kovacic, S.: Biomechanische Analyse gestorter ossifikation bei coxa vara und ihre normalisierung nach korrektiven osteotomien. Arch. Orthop. Unfallchir., 74:338, 1973.

156. Sage, F. P.: Congenital coxa vara. In Crenshaw, A. H. (ed.): Campbell's Operative Orthopaedics: Congenital Anomalies. 6th Ed. St. Louis, Mosby, 1980, pp. 1899–1904.

157. Salenius, P., and Videman, T.: Growth disturbances of the proximal end of the femur—an animal experimental study with tetracycline. Acta Orthop. Scand., 41:199, 1970.

158. Savastano, A. A., and Bliss, T. F.: Contribution of the epiphyses of the greater trochanter to the growth of the femur. Int. Surg., 60:280, 1975.

159. Say, B., Taysi, K., Pirnar, T., Tokgozoglu, N., and Inan, E.: Dominant congenital coxa vara. J. Bone Joint Surg., 56-B:78, 1975.

160. Say, B., Tuncbilek, E., Pirnar, T., and Tokgozoglu, N.: Hereditary congenital coxa vara with dominant inheritance? Humangenetik, 11:266, 1971.

161. Schanz, A.: Zur Behandlung der Coxa vara. Munch. Med. Wochenschr., 70:1247, 1923.

162. Schanz, A.: Zur Behandlung der angeborenen Coxa vara. Z. Orthop., 44:261, 1924.

163. Scholder-Hegi, P.: Considérations sur l'ostéotomie intertrochantérienne oblique de dérotation-varisation. Rev. Chir. Orthop., 45:710, 1959.

164. Schulze, H., and Haike, H. J.: Die operative Behandlung der Coxa vara infantum. Z. Orthop., 98:477, 1964.

165. Schwarz, E.: Ueber die Coxa vara congenita. Beitr. Klin. Chir., 87:685, 1913.

166. Sebastiani, C.: Surgical correction of a severe case of congenital coxa vara. Arch. Putti Chir. Organi Mov., 27:231, 1976.

167. Simonetti, E., and Corradini, C.: La pseudoartrosis congenita di collo femore. Arch. Putti Chir. Organi Mov., 26:318, 1971.

168. Simons, B.: Die sogenannte Coxa vara congenita. Beitr. Klin. Chir., 161:205, 1935.

169. Skrzypczak, J.: Radiologic evaluation of the shape of

the upper femur end in congenital coxa vara. Chir. Narzadow Ruchu Ortop. Pol., *36*:497, 1971.

170. Steno, M., Vesely, I., and Majercik, D.: Coxa vara congenita. Acta Chir. Orthop. Traumatol. Cech., *45*:235, 1978.

171. Szarnagiel: Congenital infantile coxa vara. J. Bone Joint Surg., *34-B*:158, 1952.

172. Von Lanz, T., and Mayet, A.: Die Gelenkkorper des menschlichen Hüftgelenkes in der progredienten Phase ihrer umwegigen Ausformung. Z. Anat., *117*:317, 1953.

173. Von Lanz, T., and Wachsmuth, W.: Praktische Anatomie. Berlin, Springer, 1938, p. 138.

174. Walker, N.: Zur Coxa vara congenita. Verh. Dtsch Orthop. Ges., 59. Kongr. 1972, Berlin. Z. Orthop., *111*:612, 1973.

175. Walker, N.: Klinik und radiolog. Kriterien der sek. Coxa vara congenita. Z. Orthop., *111*:847, 1973.

176. Walker, N.: Proceedings: Primary and secondary congenital coxa vara—studies in differential diagnosis. Z. Orthop., *112*:589, 1974.

177. Walker, N., and Dietschi, C.: Die Behandlung der Coxa vara congenita. Z. Orthop., *111*:857, 1973.

178. Walter, H.: Sogenannte angeborene Coxa vara durch Umlagerung der Pseudarthrosenzone geheilt. Zentralbl. Chir., *60*:2359, 1933.

179. Weighill, F. J.: The treatment of developmental coxa vara by abduction subtrochanteric and intertrochanteric femoral osteotomy with special reference to the role of adductor tenotomy. Clin. Orthop., *116*:116, 1976.

180. Weinstein, J. N., Kuo, K. N., and Millar, E. A.: Congenital Coxa vara. A retrospective review. J. Pediatr. Orthop., *4*:70a, 1984.

181. White, J. W.: Cited by MacEwen, G. D., and Shands, A. R.: Oblique trochanteric osteotomy. J. Bone Joint Surg., *49-A*:345, 1967.

182. Zadek, I.: Congenital coxa vara. Arch. Surg., *30*:62, 1935.

183. Zimmerman, M.: Untersuchungen über Krankheitsbild und Aetiologie der "sogenannten Coxa vara congenita" oder "Coxa vara infantum." Z. Orthop., *68*:389, 1938.

CONGENITAL DISLOCATION AND SUBLUXATION OF THE KNEE

In this rare deformity, the tibia is displaced anteriorly in relation to the femur, and there may be varying degrees of rotatory and lateral subluxation.

Early descriptions of congenital dislocation of the knee date to Chanssier in 1812 (according to Rechmann) and to Chatelain in 1822 (as quoted by Shattock).[47, 48] During the past 50 years numerous reports have been given in the literature.[1–52]

Incidence

In Denmark, according to Jacobsen and Vopalecky, the incidence of congenital dislocation of the knee is 0.017 per thousand or approximately 1 per cent of the incidence of congenital dislocation of the hip.[22] Charif and Reichelder-

fer reported its incidence in the black community of Washington, D.C., to be 0.7 per thousand, but most of these cases were congenital hyperextension of the knee and not true congenital subluxation or dislocation.[9]

Involvement is more common in the female. In a review of 155 children in 17 Shriner's Hospitals, Katz and associates reported it in 99 girls and 56 boys.[25] Jacobsen and Vopalecky found a female to male ratio of 10 to 3.[22] In about a third of the cases, involvement is bilateral. Right and left sides are equally affected.

Etiology

It is possible that environmental factors are influential in causing this condition. Abnormal fetal position during pregnancy is one suggested by Shattock.[48] He proposed that, in utero, the feet may become locked beneath the mandible or in the axilla, causing hyperextension of the knee and eventual dislocation (Fig. 2–265). The incidence of congenital dislocation of the knee is higher among neonates born by breech presentation than in the general population.

The bony configuration of the early fetal knee differs from that of the adult. The femoral condyles are round, as compared with the elliptical adult condyles; the tibial plateau in the young fetus slopes posteriorly 35 degrees, whereas in the adult it slopes 10 degrees. By the twenty-eighth week the bony configuration of the knee joint in the fetus resembles that of the adult.

In the adult, anterior knee dislocation is prevented by the posterior joint capsule, the collateral ligaments, the cruciate ligaments, the hamstring tendons, and the heads of the gastrocnemius. In about 18 per cent of all pregnancies, the fetal knee is in hyperextended position, creating a force that tends to produce anterior dislocation of the knee. Absence or hypoplasia of the cruciate ligaments will allow the knee to become dislocated. Katz and associates surgically explored five congenitally dislocated knees and found the cruciate ligament to be absent or hypoplastic in all of them. They proposed the theory that the basic defect in the knee that causes dislocation is absence or hypoplasia of the cruciate ligaments, a trait that is either genetically inherited or induced in the developing embryo before nine weeks of age. On dissecting the knees of fetuses less than 28 weeks old, they found the cruciate ligaments to be the principal structures preventing anterior dislocation of the knee.[25]

Curtis and Fisher reported 15 congenitally hyperextended and anteriorly subluxated knees

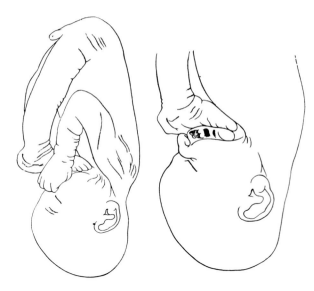

FIGURE 2–265. A stillborn infant with bilateral anterior dislocation of the knee and deformed mandible.

(From Shattock, S. G.: Genu recurvatum in a foetus at term. Trans. Pathol. Soc. London, *42*:280–292, London, Smith, Elder and Co., 1891; reproduced from Niebauer, J. J., and King, D.: J. Bone Joint Surg., *42-A*:207, 1960. Reprinted by permission.)

in 11 patients. Every case had associated congenital abnormalities of the hip, seven patients had clubfoot deformities, one had calcaneovalgus deformity of the foot at birth, and seven were believed to have arthrogryposis multiplex congenita. Fibrosis of the quadriceps mechanism, primarily its lateral portion, was found in all the knees they operated on. The patella was laterally placed in over half the cases. Curtis and Fisher did not observe absence or hypoplasia of any cruciate ligaments. They believed that the ligament abnormalities reported by Katz and associates were late adaptive changes.[11]

Injury to the knee during birth is an unlikely causative factor; it has been demonstrated that attempts to produce anterior dislocation of the knee in stillborn infants displace the distal femoral epiphysis before causing knee dislocation. Contracture of the quadriceps mechanism that holds the knee in hyperextension was suggested by Middleton as a cause of congenital dislocation.[40] Contracture of the quadriceps muscle and abnormalities of the distal femoral condyles are acquired, however, and are the result, rather than the cause, of the condition.

Heredity

Heredity appears to be a factor in some cases. A family was reported by McFarlane in which a mother and her three children by three different normal fathers had congenital dislocation of the knee.[36] Provenzano, in his review of 200 cases of congenital dislocation of the knee, found seven patients who had a positive family history of similar affection.[46]

The familial and hereditary cases cited in the literature probably represent Larsen's syndrome. Excluding the cases of Larsen's syndrome, it is doubtful whether the sporadic cases of congenital dislocation of the knee have a hereditary basis.

Associated Deformities

Congenital dislocation of the knee frequently is associated with other congenital abnormalities, the most commonly occurring one of the musculoskeletal system being congenital dislocation of the hip (present in 45 per cent of patients); next in frequency are congenital deformities of the feet (31 per cent); and then congenital dislocations of the elbow (10 per cent).[25] Associated anomalies of other systems include harelip, cleft palate, spina bifida, hydrocephalus, Down's syndrome, cryptorchidism, angiomata, facial paralysis, and imperforate anus.[17, 42] Camptodactyly of the little finger may accompany congenital dislocation of the knee. In arthrogryposis multiplex congenita the foot deformities are associated with congenital dislocation of the hip and of the knee. Larsen's syndrome is characterized by multiple congenital dislocations of the hips, knees, elbows, feet, and ankles—the distinctive facies with hypertelorism and prominent forehead completes and identifies the syndrome. Congenital dislocation of the hip is also encountered in syndromes related to ligamentous hyperlaxity, such as Ehlers-Danlos and Down's syndromes.

Pathologic Findings and Clinical Features

The displaced upper end of the tibia is anterior to the lower end of the femur. There may also be lateral subluxation and valgus deformity of the knee, in which case a contracture of the iliotibial band and the lateral intermuscular septum may be present. Rotatory subluxation may also occur. The tibia may be bowed anteriorly. The hamstrings, especially the medial semitendinosus and semimembranosus, may be displaced forward and actually function as extensors of the knee. The heads of the gastrocnemius may be located laterally. The anterior capsule of the knee is contracted. The patellar tendon and quadriceps muscle are shortened; the latter may be adhering to a mass of fibrous tissue that corresponds to the suprapatellar pouch. The patella may be underdeveloped and located more proximally than normal. The collateral ligaments are displaced anteriorly. The popliteal vessels and nerves are normal, indicating that the deformity is a slow developmental process.

The severity of deformity varies; it is classified in three grades (Fig. 2–266). In *Grade I* the subluxation is minimal; the knee is held in 15 to 20 degrees of hyperextension and can be passively manipulated into 45 to 90 degrees of flexion. This is the commonest form. In *Grade II* the displacement is moderate; the upper epiphysis of the tibia is displaced forward on the anterior aspect of the femoral condyles, but there is still some contact between the tibial and femoral articular surfaces. The long axes of the tibia and femur do not point at each other at the joint line. Clinically the knee is held in 25 to 45 degrees of hyperextension and can be flexed only to neutral position. In *Grade III* there is total displacement of the upper tibial

epiphysis in front of the femoral condyles; there is no contact between the articular surfaces of the two bones.

The clinical appearance at birth is striking: The knee is in severe hyperextension and the hip in hyperflexion with the toes touching the anterior chest wall or the mandible (Fig. 2–267). In the popliteal area, the femoral condyles are prominent and can be easily palpated. Transverse skin creases and folds are present on the anterior aspect of the knee joint.

Diagnosis

The appearance of the lower limb with the hyperextended knee is distinctive, and diagnosis can easily be made by inspection. On manipulation, knee flexion is limited and the knee springs back into hyperextension. The knee can readily be extended further from its already hyperextended posture.

Radiograms in the anterior and true lateral projections will demonstrate the partial or complete anterior displacement of the tibia over the femur. In frank dislocation there is total loss of all articular contact between the tibia and femur (Fig. 2–267 D). In the lateral view the tibial plateau is inclined posteriorly. The anteroposterior projection depicts lateral subluxation with valgus deformity of the knee and rotatory subluxation (Fig. 2–268). The ossification centers of the proximal tibia and distal femur are usually hypoplastic or occasionally absent. This picture is similar to that of delayed ossification of the capital femoral epiphysis in congenital dislocation of the hip. There may also be longitudinal

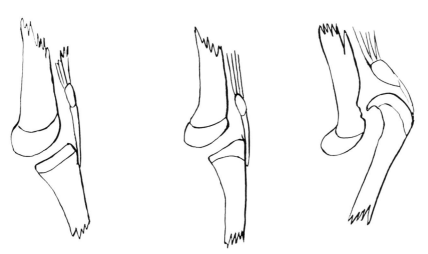

FIGURE 2–266. *Degrees of congenital subluxation and dislocation of the knee.*

(From Niebauer, J. J., and King, D. E.: Congenital dislocation of the knee. J. Bone Joint Surg., *42-A*:208, 1960. Reprinted by permission.)

deficiency and hypoplasia of the fibula. An air arthrogram may be obtained by gentle traction to determine the presence of a suprapatellar pouch; if unsuccessful, contrast arthrography is performed. Computed tomography and nuclear magnetic resonance studies are useful in delineating pathologic conditions in selected cases. Ultrasonography may depict the suprapatellar pouch.

Congenital dislocation of the knee may occur along with bone dysplasia or generalized congenital syndromes; in such instances, the associated findings are depicted on the radiogram.

Simple *genu recurvatum* should be distinguished from congenital dislocation of the knee. In genu recurvatum the knee is postured in hyperextension, but the tibia is *not* displaced anteriorly over the femur, whereas in congenital dislocation or subluxation there is hyperextension with actual anterior displacement of the tibia. Genu recurvatum may result from a variety of causes: namely, ligamentous hyperlaxity, fibrosis and contracture of the quadriceps mechanism, muscle imbalance between strong quadriceps and weak knee flexors, bony deformity of the distal femoral condyles or tibial plateau due to injury to the epiphysis, developmental affections, infection, or malunion of fractures.

Radiograms will rule out birth trauma such as fracture separation of the distal femoral or proximal tibial epiphyses. Ultrasonography may enable prenatal diagnosis of congenital dislocation of the knee.

Treatment

Treatment is begun as early as possible, preferably at birth. If subluxation is mild or moderate and is treated in the immediate neonatal period, reduction may be effected by manipulating the knee into flexion. The limb is then immobilized in a solid above-knee cast, with the knee in flexion in the reduced position. At two-week intervals, the solid casts are changed, and the knee is manipulated into more flexion. This regimen is continued until the knee becomes stable, ordinarily a period of six to eight weeks. Then the Pavlik harness is used at night and during part of the day to maintain the knee in flexion dynamically. The parents are instructed to exercise the knees into increasing flexion. The period of dynamic splinting of the knees in the Pavlik harness varies; usually it is two to three months.

The presence of rotatory lateral subluxation of the knees is a contraindication to splinting with the Pavlik harness. The proximal displace-

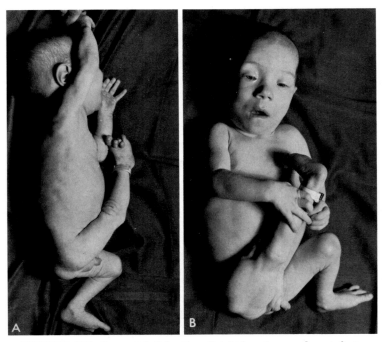

FIGURE 2–267. Congenital dislocation of right knee in a newborn infant.

A and **B.** Clinical appearance of patient's deformity. Note the prominence of the femoral condyles posteriorly in the popliteal area and the transverse skin folds and creases in the anterior aspect of the knee joint.

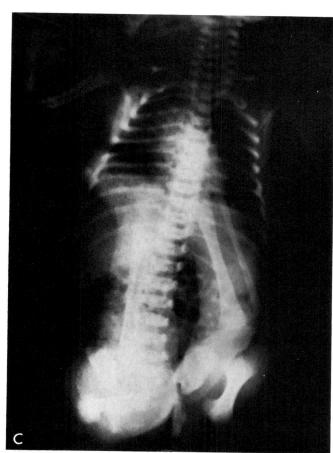

FIGURE 2–267 Continued Congenital dislocation of right knee in a newborn infant.

C and D. Radiograms of whole infant and of right knee showing the proximal end of the tibia displaced forward to the lower end of the femur.

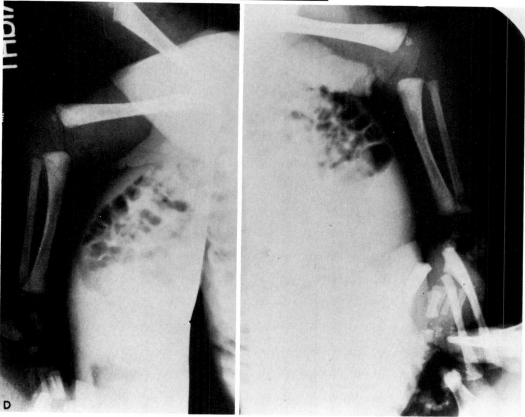

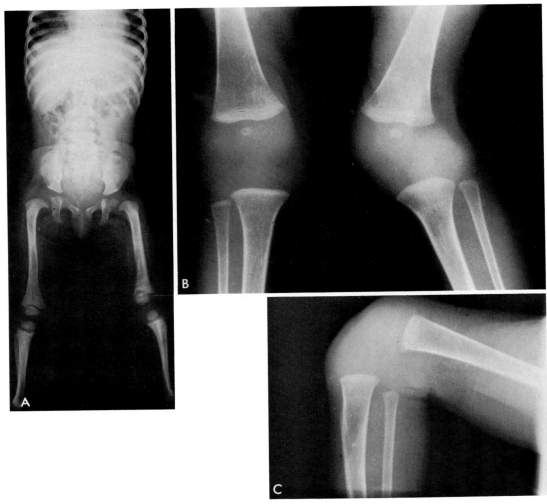

FIGURE 2–268. Congenital subluxation of left knee associated with bilateral congenital coxa vara.

A. Anteroposterior radiogram of lower limbs and torso. Note, on the left, genu valgum with lateral and external rotatory subluxation of the tibia over the femur. Bilateral coxa vara is evident. **B.** On passive manipulation and manual traction, the external rotation can be corrected but the lateral subluxation persists. **C.** Radiogram of left knee in flexion showing anterior displacement of the tibia over the lower end of the femur.

ment of the anterior stirrup will aggravate the lateral subluxation. It is safer to use removable plastic splints or bivalved casts to hold the knees in flexion at night and part-time during the day. When the knee is laterally subluxated, the period of partial immobilization of the knee in flexion is longer—depending on the degree and persistence of its lateral instability in extension—usually four to six months.

If the subluxation cannot be reduced immediately by manipulation, the affected limb is placed in skin traction with the infant in prone position. Traction forces are directed toward knee flexion. Knee flexion exercises are performed several times a day by a physical ther-

apist. Once the knee can be flexed to 45 to 60 degrees, the limb is immobilized in an above-knee solid cast. The cast is changed at weekly intervals and the knee manipulated into further flexion until 100 degrees is achieved. Then reduction is maintained in an above-knee plastic splint for 6 to 12 months, depending on the degree of knee instability.

The reduction of the dislocated knee usually requires skeletal traction with one threaded Kirschner wire in the distal femoral metaphysis and two threaded wires in the tibia, one through the proximal metaphysis and the other through the distal metaphysis. The pins are inserted under image intensifier radiographic control to avoid damage to the growth plate. If there are associated deformities of the foot, they are corrected by manipulation and application of a below-knee cast that incorporates the Kirschner wires. The cast will also assist in controlling rotatory subluxation of the knee. The weight on the distal femoral wire is directed anteriorly and proximally; the weights on the tibia are directed distally. The traction forces are initially in the line of deformity. Once the tibia is pulled distally to clear the lower end of the femur, the weights on the tibia are directed posteriorly to allow gradual knee flexion. Several times a day, the knees are gently manipulated in traction, bringing them into further flexion. Care should be taken to prevent iatrogenic fracture of the femur. The line of pull of traction forces is gradually changed to bring the knee into more flexion. Usually within a period of two to three weeks, the subluxation can be gently reduced. The limb is then immobilized in a solid cast for six to eight weeks, with subsequent management following the same principles as outlined for manipulative reduction.

Jacobsen and Vopalecky reported physeal fracture separation or tibial or femoral shaft fractures in 6 of 19 patients.[22]

An open reduction is indicated as soon as it is evident that closed methods are not successful. The timing of surgery is important; it should be performed before the infant begins to stand or bear weight on the dislocated knee. The procedure employed depends on the pathologic changes found in the affected knee. The possible operative procedures are outlined by Niebauer and King.[42] This author recommends the following technique:

An anteromedial approach is used to expose the knee joint. First, the pathologic anatomy is studied. The rectus femoris and vastus intermedius muscles with the adjoining quadriceps mechanism are usually found adhering to the femur by a mass of fibrous tissue, obliterating the suprapatellar pouch. The collateral ligaments and the hamstring tendons may be displaced anteriorly. The patellar ligament and the anterior joint capsule are contracted.

By medial and lateral parapatellar incisions, the quadriceps tendon, the patella, and the patellar ligament are dissected free from the underlying capsule. The muscle fibers of the vastus medialis should be preserved. The quadriceps tendon is lengthened by a Z-plasty or an inverted V-lengthening.[11] The iliotibial band and the lateral intermuscular septum, if contracted, are released. Ordinarily, this is not sufficient to effect reduction, and one has to

divide the anterior joint capsule transversely and free the quadriceps mechanism from the underlying bone. This allows the knee to go into flexion, reducing the anterior displacement of the tibia and bringing the hamstring tendons and collateral ligaments into their proper relationship to the joint. The cruciate ligaments are inspected next. If absent, they should be reconstructed to provide added stability to the joint. Katz and associates recommend using the retinaculum and the tendon medial to the patella in a modification of the Jones technique.[23, 25] This author prefers using the semitendinosus for reconstruction of the anterior cruciate ligament. If the anterior cruciate is present but elongated, its attachment may be transferred distally on the tibia to tauten it.[42] The capsule and quadriceps mechanism are sutured in their lengthened position, and a hip spica cast is applied for immobilization. Ordinarily, it is not necessary to fix the femur to the tibia to secure maintenance of reduction. Immobilization in the cast is continued for six weeks, following which a knee-ankle-foot arthosis is used with a stop to prevent hyperextension of the knee joint during walking. A night splint (a bivalved cast) is used to keep the knee in flexion during sleep. An illustrative case is shown in Figure 2–269.

In the adult patient with an untreated dislocated knee who has developed arthritis and marked disability, an arthrodesis may be indicated.

References

1. Alpsoy, C.: Congenital recurved knee and its surgery. Z. Orthop., 110:978, 1972.
2. Ahmadi, B., Shahriaree, H., and Silver, C. M.: Severe congenital genu recurvatum. J. Bone Joint Surg., 61-A:622, 1979.
3. Austwick, D. H., and Dandy, D. J.: Early operation for congenital subluxation of the knee. J. Pediatr. Orthop., 3:85, 1983.
4. Baldwin, C. H.: Congenital dislocation of the knee joint. J. Bone Joint Surg., 8:822, 1926.
5. Boorstein, S. W.: Congenital backward dislocation of the knee. Am. J. Dis. Child., 30:37, 1955.
6. Browne, D.: Congenital deformities of mechanical origin. Arch. Dis. Child, 30:107, 1929.
7. Carlson, D. H., and O'Connor, J.: Congenital dislocation of the knee. A.J.R., 127:465, 1976.
8. Carnera, G.: Contributo allo studio delle lussazioni congenite del ginocchio. Arch. Putti Chir. Organi Mov., 17:97, 1962.
9. Charif, P., and Reichelderfer, T. E.: Genu recurvatum congenitum in the newborn; its incidence, course, treatment, prognosis. Clin. Pediatr., 4:587, 1965.
10. Clayburgh, B. J., and Henderson, E. D.: Congenital dislocation of the knee. Proc. Mayo Clin., 30:396, 1955.
11. Curtis, B. H., and Fisher, R. L.: Congenital hyperextension with anterior subluxation of the knee. Surgical treatment and long-term observations. J. Bone Joint Surg., 51-A:255, 1969.
12. Curtis, B. H., and Fisher, R. L.: Heritable congenital

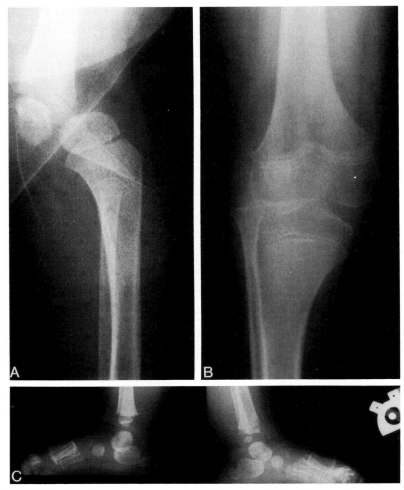

FIGURE 2–269. *Anterior dislocation of both knees in a child with Larsen's syndrome.*

A. Lateral projection of left knee. **B.** Anteroposterior view of both knees, showing the rotatory subluxation. **C.** Lateral projection of both feet, showing the accessory calcaneus, which is typical of Larsen's syndrome.

tibio-femoral subluxation. J. Bone Joint Surg., *52-A*:104, 1970.

13. Drehmann, G.: Die congenitalen Luxationen des Kniegelenkes. Z. Orthop. Chir., *7*:459, 1900.

14. Eikelaar, H. R.: Congenital luxation of the knee. Arch. Chir. Neerl., *23*:201, 1971.

15. Ferrone, J. D., Jr.: Congenital deformities about the knee. Orthop. Clin. North Am., *7*:323, 1976.

16. Finder, J. A.: Congenital hyperextension of the knee. J. Bone Joint Surg., *46-B*:783, 1964.

17. Forgon, M., and Szentpetery, J.: Über angeborene Kniegelenksverrenkung. Arch. Orthop. Unfallchir., *52*:599, 1961.

18. Giordani, C.: Dislocazioni congenite del ginocchio. Minerva Ortop., *9*:326, 1958.

19. Griswold, A. S.: Congenital dislocation of the knee joint. Case report. J. Bone Joint Surg., *9*:628, 1927.

20. Heyse, U.: Über die angeborene nichtfamiliäre Kniegelenksverrenkung. Kinderaerztl. Prax., *23*:354, 1955.

21. Ingelrans, P., and Saint-Aubert, P.: A propos de deux observations de luxations congénitales du genou traitées par l'opération de Leveuf. Soc. Belg. Orthop., *29*:601, 1963.

22. Jacobsen, K., and Vopalecky, F.: Congenital dislocation of the knee. Acta Orthop. Scand., *56*:1, 1985.

23. Jones, K. G.: Reconstruction of the anterior cruciate ligament. J. Bone Joint Surg., *45-A*:925, 1963.

24. Kaijser, R.: Über kongenitale Kniegelenksluxationen. Acta Orthop. Scand., *6*:1, 1935.

25. Katz, M. P., Grogono, B. J. S., and Soper, K. C.: The etiology and treatment of congenital dislocation of the knee. J. Bone Joint Surg., *49-B*:112, 1967.

26. Kennedy, J. C., Weinberg, H. W., and Wilson, A. S.: The anatomy and function of the anterior cruciate ligament as determined by clinical and morphological studies. J. Bone Joint Surg., *56-A*:223, 1974.

27. Klein, H.: Die erbliche, angeborene Kniegelenksluxation. Beitr. Orthop., *15*:101, 1968.

28. Knapp, R.: Ueber angeborene Kniegelenksverrenkung. Beitr. Orthop., *15*:572, 1968.

29. Kopits, E.: Beitrage zur Pathologie und Therapie der angeborenen Kniegelenkssubluxationen. Arch. Orthop. Unfallchir., *23*:593, 1925.

30. Lapeyrie, M., Pous, J. G., and Chaptal, P. A.: Subluxations congénitales du genou. Possibilités orthopédiques en periode néo-natale. Ann. Chir. Infant. (Paris), *6*:135, 1965.

31. Largot, F., Cohen-Solal, L., and Tordjeman, G.: Les dislocations congénitales du genou. A propos de trois cas. Pediatrie, *18*:102, 1963.

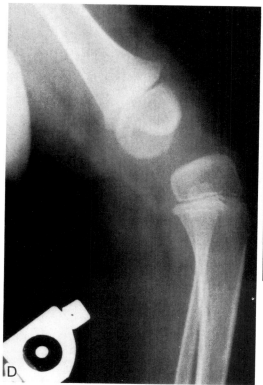
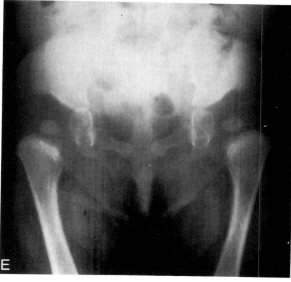

FIGURE 2–269 Continued *Anterior dislocation of both knees in child with Larsen's syndrome.*

D. Lateral view of left knee following open reduction. **E.** Anteroposterior view of both hips, showing the acetabular dysplasia.

32. Larsen, L. J., Schottstaedt, E. R., and Bost, F. C.: Multiple congenital dislocation associated with characteristic facial abnormality. J. Pediatr., *37*:574, 1950.

33. Laurence, M.: Genu recurvatum congenitum. J. Bone Joint Surg., *49-B*:121, 1967.

34. Leveuf, J., and Pais, C.: Les dislocations congénitales du genou. Rev. Orthop., *32*:313, 1946.

35. McFarland, B. L.: Congenital dislocation of the knee. J. Bone Joint Surg., *11*:281, 1929.

36. McFarlane, A. L.: A report on four cases of congenital genu recurvatum occurring in one family. Br. J. Surg., *34*:388, 1947.

37. Magnus, F.: Über totale congenitale Luxation der Kniegelenke bei drei Geschwistern. Dtsch. Z. Chir., *78*:555, 1905.

38. Marique, P.: Luxation congénitale héréditaire des genoux. Operation. Soc. Belg. Orthop., *29*:613, 1963.

39. Mayer, L.: Congenital anterior subluxation of the knee. Am. J. Orthop. Surg., *10*:411, 1913.

40. Middleton, D. S.: The pathology of congenital genu recurvatum. Br. J. Surg., *22*:696, 1935.

41. Murphy, D. P.: Familial finger contracture and associated familial knee joint subluxation. J.A.M.A., *86*:395, 1926.

42. Niebauer, J. J., and King, D. E.: Congenital dislocation of the knee. J. Bone Joint Surg., *47-A*:207, 1960.

43. Nogi, J., and MacEwen, G. D.: Congenital dislocation of the knee. J. Pediatr. Orthop., *2*:509, 1983.

44. Perricone, G.: Dislocazioni congenite del ginocchio. Chir. Organi. Mov., *37*:247, 1952.

45. Porter, D. D.: Congenital dislocation of the knee. Case report. St. Joseph Hosp. Med. Surg., *7*:28, 1972.

46. Provenzano, K. W.: Congenital dislocation of the knee. Report of a case. N. Engl. J. Med., *236*:360, 1947.

47. Rechmann, L.: Beitrag zur Therapie der kongenitalen Luxation des Kniegelenkes. Arch. Orthop. Unfallchir., *13*:227, 1914.

48. Shattock, S. G.: Genu recurvatum on a foetus at term. Trans. Pathol. Soc., London, *42*:280, 1891.

49. Silvermann, F. N.: Larsen's syndrome: Congenital dislocation of knees and other joints, distinctive facies and, frequently, cleft palate. Ann. Radiol., *15*:297, 1972.

50. Uher, M.: Die angeborene Kniegelenksverrenkung. Arch. Orthop. Unfallchir., *61*:327, 1967.

51. Weiss, S. M., and Brooks, D. B.: A simplified method of splinting for congenital dislocation of the knee. Clin. Orthop., *123*:40, 1977.

52. Zwierzchowska, D., Olejniczak, A., and Faflik, J.: Results of treatment of congenital dislocation of the knee. Chir. Narzadow Ruchu Ortop. Pol., *36*:735, 1971.

GENU RECURVATUM

The knees of normal babies up to the age of three to four months have a flexion deformity of 10 to 20 degrees. In a baby born by breech delivery, the knees may be hyperextended up to 20 degrees. Also, in perinatal dislocation of the hip the knees are hyperextendable. In familial ligamentous hyperlaxity, hyperextension of the knees is common. It should be noted, however, that in these conditions, the anterior part of the upper articular surface of the tibia has contact with the lower articular surface of the femur. Genu recurvatum should be distinguished from congenital subluxation of the knee, in which there is loss of contact between the lower end of the femur and the upper end of the tibia. No treatment is indicated for congenital hyperextension deformities of the knee. As the child gets older, ligamentous tissue will tauten, and the knees will become stable.

CONGENITAL DISLOCATION OF THE PATELLA

Congenital dislocation of the patella is a very rare abnormality in which there is lateral malrotation of the quadriceps mechanism due to failure of medial rotation of the myotome that contains the quadriceps. The patella is dislocated on the lateral side of the lateral femoral condyle, and the displacement is fixed and cannot be reduced even when the knee is extended passively. The patella is hypoplastic and has no ridges. The lateral femoral condyle is flattened anteriorly, and the tibia is rotated and subluxated laterally with genu valgum of varying degrees. The quadriceps functions as a flexor and lateral rotator of the tibia. The condition may be unilateral or bilateral, and there is a familial tendency.[7, 9]

Dislocation is present at birth but is rarely diagnosed in infancy. It should be suspected when an infant presents with fixed flexion deformity of the knee with excessive lateral rotation of the tibia. On palpation of the knee, one can easily feel the femoral condyle, but not the patella, which is displaced posteriorly immediately above the fibular head. The function of the quadriceps muscle is weakened, with a loss of active, complete extension of the knee. As the child gets older and begins walking, the flexion deformity of the knee and lateral displacement of the patella increase. The patella does not ossify until the age of three years and, therefore, is not visualized in the infant, but the normal quadriceps soft-tissue shadow in the lateral projection is not seen anteriorly. In the anteroposterior projection the quadriceps shadow is found to be on the lateral side of the lateral femoral condyle. Lateral rotation of the tibia at the knee is evident. When the patella ossifies at the age of three to four years, the diagnosis is readily made.[14, 15]

Treatment

Closed manipulation to reduce the dislocation is not feasible, and treatment consists of open surgical realignment of the quadriceps mecha-

nism and reduction of the lateral dislocation of the patella (Fig. 2–270). The operative technique is as follows:

An anterolateral incision is made beginning 7 cm. above the lateral condyle of the femur and extending distally to the joint line, and then curved medially and distally for a distance of 5 cm. The subcutaneous tissue is divided in line with the skin incision, the fascia lata is incised laterally, and the vastus lateralis is fully mobilized from the lateral intermuscular septum. The vastus medialis is transferred distally and laterally.

By blunt and sharp extraperiosteal dissection, the quadriceps muscle is elevated from the anterolateral aspect of the femur and displaced medially. The thick patellar retinaculum on the lateral aspect of the patella is divided, and the fibrotic bands of the iliotibial tract are sectioned from the patella. The patella is displaced medially to its normal position in the intercondylar groove. This author recommends the Galleazi-Dewar operation, i.e., the semitendinosis tendon is detached at its musculotendinous junction, and its distal segment is tenodesed to the patellar tendon. Frequently the patellar tendon is split and the lateral portion transferred under the medial half and sutured as far medially as possible. Often one may have to detach the patellar tendon at its insertion, taking care not to damage the proximal tibial tubercle, and transfer the whole tendon distally and medially and suture it through a hole in the medial metaphysis of the tibia. If the flexor muscles are very taut, one may have to perform a fractional lengthening of the hamstring muscles. This is especially important in the older child with fixed knee flexion deformity. The wound is closed, and an above-knee cylinder cast is applied for six weeks. Then the knee is gradually mobilized, and active exercises to develop motor strength are performed. These children must wear a night orthosis with a lateral buttress to hold the patella medially with pads; the Engen principle is utilized to force the knee into complete extension. This night brace may have to be worn for 6 to 12 months. During the day, a patellar immobilizer is worn for four to eight weeks.

References

1. Alarcon, P. O., and Costiorena, R.: Luxacion congenita de la rotula—concioderaciones acerca del tratamiento en los adultos. Rev. Ortop. Traumatol., 8:176, 1938.
2. Boitchev, B.: Follow-up on the surgery for congenital dislocation of the patella. Ortop. Traum. Protez. (U.S.S.R.), 20:34, 1959.
3. Bourgeau, D.: Luxation congénitale de la rotule. Un cas suivi dupuis la naissance. Rev. Chir. Orthop., 56:697, 1970.

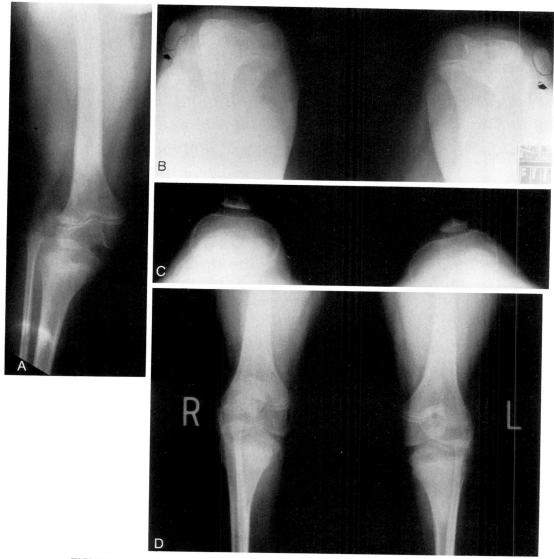

FIGURE 2–270. Bilateral congenital dislocation of the patellae in an eight-year-old girl.

A and **B.** Preoperative radiograms showing the complete lateral dislocation *(arrows)*. **C** and **D.** Postoperative radiograms showing reduction.

4. Conn, H. R.: A new method of operative reduction for congenital luxation of the patella. J. Bone Joint Surg., 7:370, 1925.

5. Fruend, R.: Ein Beitrag zur habituellen und angeborenen Luxation der Patella. Z. Mensch. Vererb. Konstitutionslehre, 83:253, 1953.

6. Goldthwait, J. E.: Permanent dislocation of the patella. Ann. Surg., 29:62, 1899.

7. Green, J. P., and Waugh, W.: Congenital lateral dislocation of the patella. J. Bone Joint Surg., 50-B:285, 1968.

8. Jones, R. D. S., Fischer, R. L., and Curtis, B. H.: Congenital dislocation of the patella. Clin. Orthop., 119:177, 1976.

9. Lanny, L.: Le traitement de la luxation congénitale de la rotule. Bull. Soc. Chir. (Paris), 27:419, 1936.

10. Mumford, E. B.: Congenital dislocation of the patella. J. Bone Joint Surg., 29:1083, 1947.

11. Nefedeva, N. N.: Congenital dislocation of the patella and its surgical treatment. Ortop. Traum. Protez (U.S.S.R.), 26:35, 1965.

12. Rooney, J. R., Baker, C. W., and Harmony, K. J.: Congenital lateral luxation of the patella in the horse. Cornell Vet., 61:670, 1971.

13. Singer, R.: Ein Fall von angeborener volstaendiger Verrenkung der beiden Kniescheiben nach aussen, bei guten Gebrauch der Gleidmassen. Aerzte Wien., 12:295, 1956.

14. Stanisavljevic, S., Zemenick, G., and Miller, D.: Congenital, irreducible, permanent lateral dislocation of the patella. Clin. Orthop., 116:190, 1976.

15. Stern, M.: Persistent congenital dislocation of the patella. Int. Coll. Surg. J., 41:654, 1964.

16. Tesoriere, A.: Lussazione congenita della rotula. Settim. Med., 17:137, 1939.

17. Vinditti, D., and Forcella, G.: Un nuovo intervento

per il trattamento della lussazione congenita della rotula: La doppia osteotomia di torsione della diafisi femorale. Chir. Organi Mov., 45:502, 1958.

CONGENITAL ABSENCE OF THE PATELLA

Congenital absence of the patella is very rare, often bilateral, and often associated with other malformations such as talipes equinovarus, congenital dislocation of the hip, and the nail-patella syndrome. Occasionally it presents as an isolated lesion.[1]

On clinical examination, the anterior aspect of the knee is flattened, which is more evident when the knee is flexed. Disability is minimal if the quadriceps mechanism is intact. If the absence of the patella is associated with a defective quadriceps mechanism, however, the patient will have weakness of knee extension and will develop progressive flexion deformity of the knee. Because the ossification center of the patella appears around the third year of life, it is difficult to detect the absence of the patella on the radiogram (Fig. 2–271). Treatment consists of exercises to develop quadriceps motor strength, but if the quadriceps motor function is trace or poor, the medial and lateral hamstrings are transferred laterally to provide active knee extension.

References

1. Bernhang, A. M., and Levine, S. A.: Familial absence of the patella. J. Bone Join Surg., 55-A:1088, 1973.
2. Carbonara, P., and Alpert, M.: Hereditary osteo-ony-cho-dysplasia (HOOD). Am. J. Med. Sci., 248:139, 1964.
3. Duncan, J. G., and Souter, W. A.: Hereditary onycho-osteodysplasia. The nail-patella syndrome. J. Bone Joint Surg., 45-B:242, 1963.
4. Kutz, E. R.: Congenital absence of the patellae. J. Pediatr., 34:760, 1949.

CONGENITAL BIPARTITE OR TRIPARTITE PATELLA

The patella, instead of arising from one center of ossification, may arise from two or more centers in one of seven cases. The separate center of ossification may not fuse with the main body but persist as a separate fragment and attach to the main body of the patella by fibrocartilaginous tissue. The condition is usually bilateral. In about 75 per cent of cases, the accessory patella is located on the superolateral pole; in 20 per cent, on the lateral margin; and in 5 per cent, on the inferior pole.

Trauma may separate the accessory fragment from the main part of the patella. There is local tenderness on pressure. In the radiograms, the bipartite patella is characterized by a regular, smooth, half moon–shaped defect between the fragment and the patella. Often, the defect is bilateral. It is important to make radiograms of both knees. The painful bipartite patella is treated by immobilization in an above-knee cylinder cast for two to three weeks. Excision of the accessory patella is rarely indicated.

CONGENITAL LONGITUDINAL DEFICIENCY OF THE FIBULA (PARAXIAL FIBULAR HEMIMELIA)

Congenital deficiency of the fibula is not an isolated malformation but rather a part of a spectrum of dysplasia of the entire lower limb. The fibular deficiency ranges from partial absence to complete absence. Associated congenital anomalies of the femur are present in three fourths of the patients. The tibia is almost always shortened and, in complete aplasia of the fibula, often bowed anteromedially. In addition there are other associated malformations such as ball-and-socket ankle joint, tarsal coalition, equinovalgus deformity of the hindfoot, and absence of the lateral rays of the foot.

The fibula is more commonly absent than any other long bone, next in order of frequency being the radius, femur, tibia, ulna, and humerus.[18] The exact incidence of paraxial fibular hemimelia is unknown; it is a relatively uncommon anomaly. The right side is more often involved than the left. Occasionally, involvement is bilateral. It is more prevalent in boys than in girls.

Etiology

Its pathogenesis is obscure. Heredity does not appear to be an etiologic factor. Whatever the primary cause, the aberration of this musculoskeletal organogenesis must occur prior to the eighth fetal week, as the anlage of the limbs is formed by the sixth or seventh week of embryonic life.[10] Mechanical and metabolic disturbances affecting the embryo before limb bud formation can cause such defects. Experimentally, teratogenic insults such as irradiation, injection of insulin, and dietary deficiency have produced congenital absence of the fibula as well as other anomalies.[8] Middleton, in 1934, postulated a theory that absence of the fibula is a defect secondary to a primary lesion of the muscles, which failed to mature and grow in length.[48] The shortening of the peroneal and triceps surae muscles places undue stress on

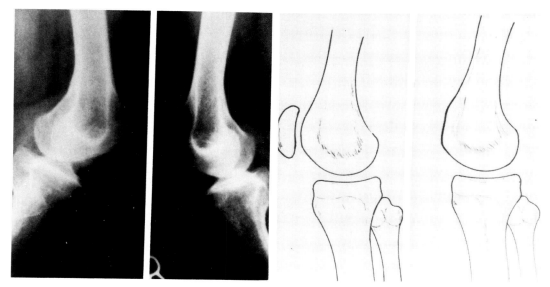

FIGURE 2–271. Congenital absence of the patella.

the tibia and foot, causing bowing of the leg and equinovalgus deformity of the foot.[67]

Classification

Achterman and Kalamchi devised an anatomic classification to distinguish minimal hypoplasia of the fibula from complete aplasia. In Type I there is partial or incomplete absence of the fibula. Type I is further subdivided into two forms: in Type IA the entire fibula is present, but it is shortened and small, with the proximal fibular epiphysis distal to the upper physis of the tibia and the distal fibular physis proximal to the ankle joint line (Fig. 2–272 A). In Type IB, the more severe form, there is partial

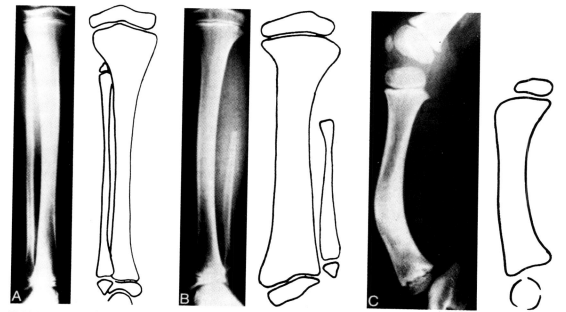

FIGURE 2–272. Classification of congenital longitudinal deficiency of the fibula according to Achterman and Kalamchi.

A. In Type IA the fibula is hypoplastic. Note the proximal epiphysis of the fibula is distal to the upper tibial physis and the distal fibular physis is above the dome of the talus. **B.** Type IB. There is partial absence of the upper third of the fibula. The lower end of the fibula is present but elevated and does not support the ankle. **C.** Type II. The entire fibula is absent. (From Achterman, C., and Kalamchi, A.: Congenital deficiency of the fibula. J. Bone Joint Surg., *61-B*:133, 1979. Reprinted by permission.)

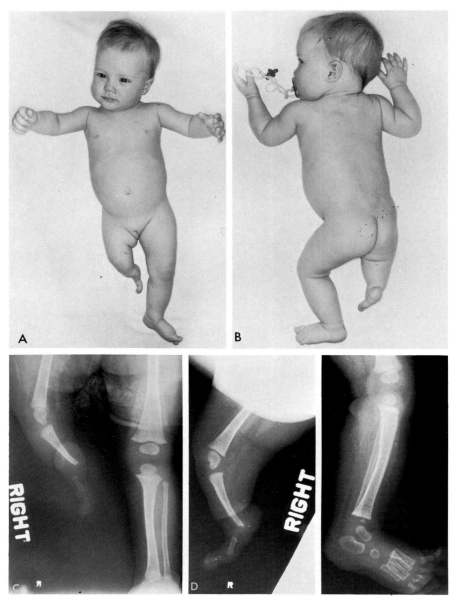

FIGURE 2–273. *Congenital absence of the fibula with absence of the lateral four rays of the foot and marked hypoplasia of the tibia.*

Note that the foot is nonfunctional and the limb length inequality is very severe. In such an instance the foot is retained as a means of lengthening the below-knee component in a prosthesis.

absence of the upper fibula (30 to 50 per cent of its length), and distally the lower fibular epiphysis is present but elevated and not supporting the ankle (Fig. 2–272 B). In Type II the entire fibula is absent, or only a distal vestigial fibrocartilaginous or fibrous fragment is present (Fig. 2–272 C).[2]

Coventry and Johnson subdivided congenital deficiency of the fibula into three main types based on the progressive severity of deformity and prognosis. In *Type I* only one limb is affected, and the degree of deficiency ranges from a shortened fibula to partial absence of its upper part. Shortening of the tibia and limb length inequality are usually minimal, and there are no associated anomalies of the foot. The prognosis is good. In *Type II*, again, the involvement is unilateral, but deficiency of the fibula is complete, with absence of the entire bone, or sometimes a vestigial anlage is present distally. There is severe dysplasia of the entire lower limb. The shortening of the limb is marked, usually 5 to 7 cm. in childhood and 12 to 15 cm. in adult life. The tibia is bowed or angulated anteromedially, and the foot is malformed. The prognosis is rather poor, cosmetically and functionally (Fig. 2–273). *Type III* is the most severe malformation, and the prognosis the poorest. Involvement may be bilateral, or the deformity may occur in association with other major congenital malformations such as partial or complete absence of the upper limb, proximal focal femoral deficiency, and partial or complete absence of the contralateral tibia and foot.[18]

Diagnosis

The affected limb is abnormally short and diminished in girth in varying degrees, depending on the type and severity of the deficiency of the fibula. Both the tibial and femoral segments are shortened, with the greatest reduction in length in the tibia. Generally the tibial shortening increases as the fibular deficiency becomes more marked.

The tibia is bowed or angulated anteromedially. There is usually a dimpling of the skin at the apex of the curve over the anterior aspect of the tibia. These features are characteristically present in Type II deficiency (Achterman and Kalamchi, Coventry and Johnson). Occasionally, however, they may be found in Type I limbs.[2, 18] In complete absence of the fibula, a fibrocartilaginous or fibrous anlage of the bone extends from the upper end of the tibia to the calcaneus. This taut band exerts a tethering force, deforming the tibia and pulling the hindfoot into equinovalgus posture.

At the ankle, in Type II, the lateral malleolus cannot be palpated, whereas in Type I the distal tip of the fibula is high, extending to the ankle but not providing adequate lateral support to the joint. The distal tibial epiphysis may be dysplastic laterally. The tibiotalar joint is usually stable in Type I. In Type II, however, varying degrees of instability and lateral subluxation of the tibiotarsal joints are usually present. The deltoid ligament may be interposed between the articular surfaces of the medial malleolus and the talus, preventing anatomic repositioning of the talus under the tibia.[58]

The foot, especially in Type II, is commonly in equinovalgus position owing to contracture of the triceps surae, the peroneals, and the fibrous anlage of the fibula; however, in Type I, occasionally the foot may be in equinovarus, calcaneovalgus, or simple equinus position.

Rigidity or restriction of range of motion of the hindfoot is commonly due to coalition of the tarsal bones. The most frequent pattern is fusion of the talus to the calcaneus, and next in order is coalition of the talus to the navicular and calcaneus. Calcaneocuboid and calcaneonavicular coalitions may be occasionally encountered.

The lateral rays of the foot (usually the fourth and fifth) are frequently absent (Fig. 2–274).

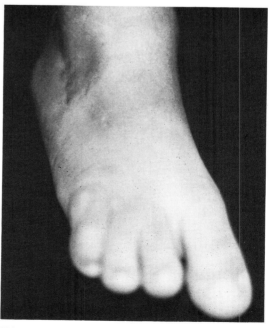

FIGURE 2–274. Congenital absence of the fibula Type IA.

Note the absence of the lateral two rays of the foot and coalition of the talus and the calcaneus.

Occasionally the cuboid bone may be aplastic. Ossification of the tarsal bones is delayed.

The knee is in varying degrees of valgus angulation; this is due to hypoplasia of the lateral condyle, lack of lateral support at the knee owing to absence or hypoplasia of the fibula, and contracture of lateral soft tissues.[65] Anteroposterior instability of the knee is common because of absence of either anterior or posterior cruciate ligaments or both. The patella is small and high-riding; occasionally it may be absent. Recurrent lateral patellofemoral subluxation may occur.

Congenital shortening of the femur is a common associated anomaly (about three fifths of the cases in the series reported by Achterman and Kalamchi). Additional findings may be coxa vara and proximal femoral focal deficiency.

Other associated anomalies include defects in the upper limb, such as absence of the ulnar rays, syndactyly, and absence of part of or an entire upper limb (Fig. 2–275). Anomalies of the viscera, e.g., cardiac or renal, can occur but are very rare.

In the differential diagnosis congenital absence of the tibia may cause a problem, as in both conditions the affected leg is short and atrophied. There are, however, certain definite differences in gross appearance. In congenital absence of the tibia the medial malleolus is absent, the entire foot is displaced medially and is in varus position, whereas in congenital absence of the fibula the foot and ankle are in valgus position and the lateral malleolus cannot be palpated. Dislocation of the knee with a laterally riding fibular head and the absence of the anterior bowing of the leg are other features indicating paraxial tibial hemimelia. In radiograms, the lack of tibial articulation with the femur will establish the diagnosis of congenital absence of the tibia.

Congenital pseudarthrosis of the tibia, shortening of the lower limb without absence of the fibula, and congenital posteromedial angulation of the tibia are other entities to be considered in the differential diagnosis.

Treatment

The objectives of treatment are to equalize the lengths of the lower limbs and to provide a functional foot for weight-bearing. Therefore, the form of treatment depends on the extent of lower limb length discrepancy at maturity and the severity of malformation of the foot and ankle.

It is vital to predict the likely shortening at skeletal maturity. The relative difference in length between the lower limbs remains constant throughout growth; this was demonstrated for congenitally short femora by Ring, and for congenitally short tibiae by Hootnick and associates, Moseley, and Westin and associates.[34, 49, 54, 65] Both the tibia and femur are often short in congenital deficiency of the fibula; therefore, it is essential to include the femur in the calculation. The final discrepancy is calculated as follows: first, measure the lengths of the normal and abnormal tibia and femur in the radiograms. Second, determine the percentage differences between the normal and abnormal femora and tibiae. Third, from the tables of Anderson, Green, and Messner, predict the lengths of the normal femur and tibia at skeletal maturity. Fourth, deduct the initial percentage of deficiency from the normal femoral and tibial lengths to predict the lengths of the short femur and tibia. Fifth, calculate the total shortening at maturity by deducting the projected length of the short abnormal limb from that of the long normal limb. The following case is given to illustrate the method of prediction of eventual shortening at skeletal maturity. The patient is a three-year-old boy with Type II complete congenital deficiency of the left fibula. In the orthoroentgenograms the right femur measures 21 cm., and the left femur, 19 cm. The length of the short femur as a percentage of normal is 90 per cent. The right tibia measures 17 cm., and the left tibia, 14 cm. The length of the short tibia as a percentage of normal is 82 per cent. The lengths of the normal femur and tibia were mean average. At skeletal maturity the length of the normal right femur is predicted to be 47 cm., and that of the normal right tibia 37 cm. By deducting the initial percentage deficiency from the normal femoral and tibial lengths one can predict the length of the short femur at skeletal maturity to be 40.3 cm., and that of the short tibia, 30.3 cm. The calculated shortening at skeletal maturity is, therefore, 6.7 cm. in the femur ($47 - 40.3 = 6.7$ cm.) and 6.7 cm. in the tibia ($37.0 - 30.3 = 6.7$ cm.) or a total shortening of 13.4 cm.

In general the degree of tibial shortening increases as the fibular deficiency becomes more severe, and is directly related to the state of preservation of the foot—the greater the number of missing lateral rays, the greater the tibial shortening. In addition, anterior tibial bowing or angulation (kyphosis) indicates a poor prognosis for tibial length. Although shortening of the femur is frequently associated with tibial

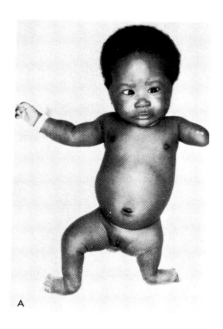
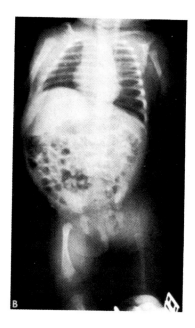
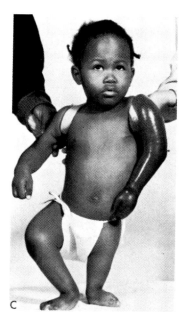

FIGURE 2–275. *Congenital absence of the fibula on the left associated with major congenital malformations.*

Note the absence of the forearm and distal half of the arm on the left and the proximal femoral focal deficiency on the left.

shortening in congenital deficiency of the fibula, there is no apparent correlation between the two segments.

Deformity and malalignment of the foot and ankle are the next factors determining the plan of treatment. Can one provide a stable and functional weight-bearing foot? The ankle tends to subluxate into valgus posture because of the absence of the lateral malleolus and the lack of lateral ligamentous support. The foot is usually in equinovalgus position because of the deforming forces of the contracted peroneals, triceps surae, and fibrous anlage of the fibula. In some cases the associated ball-and-socket ankle joint may limit plantar flexion of the foot. The absence of the lateral rays and the coalition or absence of some of the tarsal bones make provision of a plantigrade functional foot more difficult. The muscle strength and motor control of the foot and ankle should be carefully assessed.

An additional factor to consider is the psychologic effect and the social aspects of multiple surgical procedures and repeated hospitalizations. Also, some parents may not consent to ablation of the foot at an early age.

Treatment of hypoplasia or partial absence of the fibula (Type I) is relatively simple. Conservatism is appropriate. If the lower limb length discrepancy is greater than 2 cm. and the spine is decompensated, an elevated shoe is worn on the affected side. Discrepancy of the growth of the lower limbs is followed, and at an appropriate age, an epiphyseodesis is performed on the contralateral longer limb to equalize leg lengths. Alignment of the foot and ankle is maintained by passive stretching exercises and splinting at night, if necessary. In congenitally short fibula with progressive ankle valgus deformity, diaphyseal lengthening of the fibula by the Wagner technique (described in the section on leg lengthening) may be indicated. Supramalleolar varus osteotomy of the tibia to correct the valgus deformity of the ankle is a simpler method with fewer problems than fibular lengthening.

Complete absence of the fibula (Type II of Achterman and Kalamchi) presents difficult problems in management: namely, the instability of the ankle, the deformed foot, and the marked limb length inequality.

Syme's amputation is indicated as the treatment of choice if the deformity of the foot is so severe that operative procedures to provide a plantigrade and functional foot, satisfactorily reduced under the tibia, and to maintain it so, would most probably be unsuccessful. Another indication is marked limb length inequality (Fig. 2–276). Opinion varies as to how much that is. Westin and associates recommend amputation when limb length discrepancy is 7.5 cm. or more, actual or predicted, by the time skeletal maturity is attained.[65] Hootnick, Boyd, Fixsen, and Lloyd-Roberts advise Syme amputation when the overall limb length inequality is between 3.7 and 5 cm. at one year of age because the ultimate shortening at skeletal maturity will be within the range of 10 to 12.5 cm.[34] They believe discrepancy of this magnitude is beyond redemption by shortening of the normal side within acceptable limits. In their experience tibial lengthening has proved to be a particularly difficult undertaking, with delayed union, need for repeated bone grafting, and varying degrees of loss of function.

With lengthening of the short limb and shortening of the long limb, a final discrepancy of 5 cm. may be achieved, but often the foot is deformed and rigid, requiring a specially made and often ugly raised shoe. In conclusion, Hootnick, Boyd, Fixsen, and Lloyd-Roberts recommend that if the predicted shortening is (1) less than 8.7 cm., conservative treatment seems appropriate; (2) between 8.7 and 15 cm., amputation is indicated; and (3) beyond 15 cm., the foot should be retained because it has some advantage as a means of lengthening the below-knee component, provided it can be placed in full equinus position without valgus deformity. If the valgus angulation cannot be corrected surgically, amputation is preferable, for the prosthesis becomes difficult to fit and cumbersome.[34]

Pappas, Hanawalt, and Anderson recommend early Syme amputation if the limb length discrepancy is 4 cm. or over at one year of age and the foot is so deformed that it cannot be relocated with casts or soft-tissue surgery to bring it under the tibia in satisfactory alignment. If the discrepancy is 4 cm. or less at one year of age, however, and provision of a plantigrade foot and ankle by operative procedures seems probable, early constructive surgery is carried out.[51] This author believes that the present methods of femoral and tibial lengthening have opened new vistas. If the predicted limb length inequality at skeletal maturity is less than 12.5 cm., and if the foot is functional and plantigrade or such a foot can be provided by appropriate surgical measures, the foot is retained, and the femur and tibia are lengthened by the Ilizarov, DeBastiani, or Wagner technique (described in the section on limb length inequality). In other words, the indica-

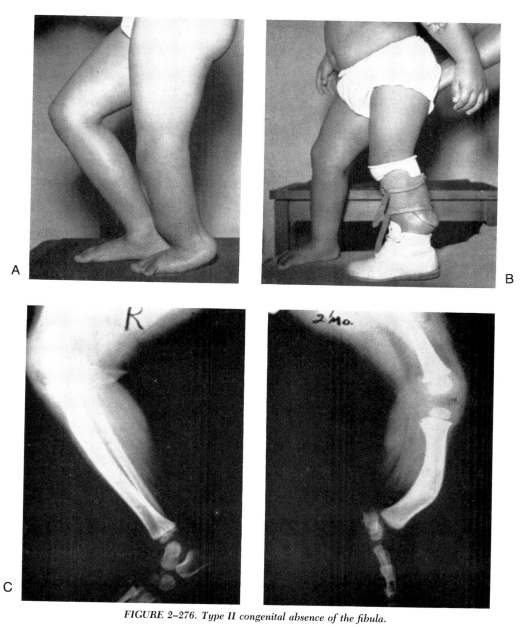

FIGURE 2–276. *Type II congenital absence of the fibula.*

Note the severe shortening and anterior bowing of the tibia.

Illustration continued on following page

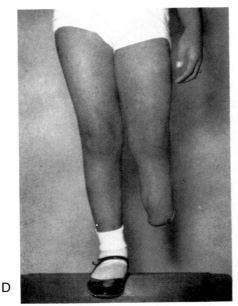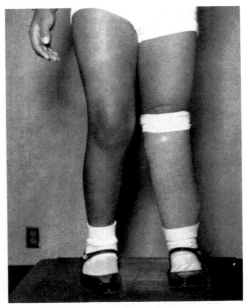

D E

FIGURE 2–276 Continued Type II congenital absence of the fibula.

tions for a Syme amputation are a rigid, severely deformed foot and a limb length inequality greater than 12.5 cm.

If primary amputation is chosen as the definitive procedure it should be performed prior to the child's entering school, preferably when he begins to stand and walk independently. The earlier the better for the child and the family. The technique of the Syme amputation is described and illustrated in Plate 32. The operation should be performed carefully. Migration of the heel pad usually is not a problem in children; often normal skin will hypertrophy and allow weight-bearing without difficulty. Anterior angulation of the tibia, however, tends to displace the heel flap posteriorly away from the weight-bearing area. If the tibial kyphosis is moderate it is best to secure the heel flap to the tibia by a Kirschner wire. In severe tibial kyphosis, correction of anterior angulation of the tibia by osteotomy may be indicated; this is carried out at the time of amputation, the heel flap and tibial osteotomy being secured with the same Kirschner wire. Excision of the cartilaginous apophysis of the calcaneus should be complete. Leaving behind a sliver of cartilagi-

nous apophysis and securing it to the distal tibia to prevent migration of the heel pad is not recommended. The cartilaginous fragment will ossify and form a painful ossicle, requiring excision.

Syme amputation gives an end-bearing stump that can be walked on with or without a prosthesis.[31, 32, 42, 43, 51, 65] It provides better proprioception in gait. Revision of a Syme amputation is rarely required in children. Preservation of the normal heel tissue beneath the distal tibia provides an excellent cushion for fitting the prosthesis and a biologic feedback mechanism that allows the heel skin and stump to grow with the intact distal tibial physis. When the Syme amputation is performed at an early age, no large bulk forms at the end of the stump; it appears the distal tibial epiphysis is not stimulated to enlarge in the absence of the ankle joint.[23, 51, 65]

When the foot is to be preserved, it should be anatomically aligned under the distal end of the tibia. It is commonly in equinovalgus posture with varying degrees of lateral subluxation of the ankle. In the neonate and young infant the contracted soft tissues are elongated by

Text continued on page 634

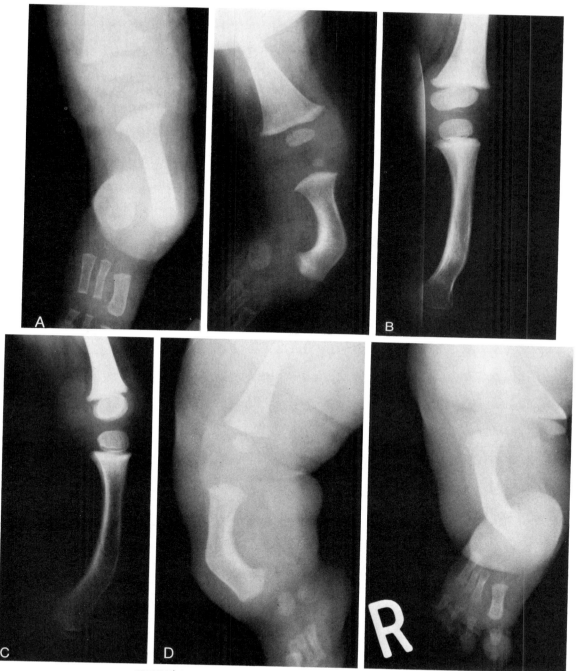

FIGURE 2–277. Congenital absence of the fibula on the left.

A to E. Preoperative radiograms.

Syme's Amputation

The objective of Syme's amputation is to provide a good end-bearing stump. Skin incisions are very vital. A single posterior heel flap is utilized. The heel pad resists pressure of the static force of body weight because of its specialized elastic adipose tissue consisting of dense septa of elastic fibrous tissue enclosing spaces filled with fat. Each loculus containing fat is separated and isolated from the adjacent loculi. This specialized subcutaneous tissue of the heel should be preserved when making incisions for Syme's amputation.

OPERATIVE TECHNIQUE

A. *Skin Incisions.* A *dorsal incision* is made to open into the ankle joint; it extends from the inferior tip of the fibular malleolus, passes across the anterior aspect of the ankle joint at the level of the distal end of the tibia, and terminates 1.5 cm. distal to the tip of the medial malleolus. The *plantar incision* is carried vertically downward perpendicular to the sole of the foot and passing across the plantar aspect of the foot to join the medial and lateral dorsal starting joints.

B and **C.** The subcutaneous tissue on the front and sides of the ankle is divided in line with the skin incision. Subcutaneous veins are clamped and coagulated, and sensory nerves are divided with a sharp scalpel. The anterior tibial, long toe extensor, peroneal, and posterior tibial tendons are pulled down and sectioned to retract proximally. The anterior tibial vessels are isolated, ligated, and divided. The capsule of the ankle joint is divided anteriorly, medially, and laterally.

D. The foot is manipulated into marked plantar flexion, and the posterior part of the deltoid ligament is divided. A bone hook is placed on the posterior part of the dome of the talus, and the hindfoot is pulled into extreme equinus position. With a long knife the posterior capsule of the ankle joint is sectioned.

Plate 32. Syme's Amputation

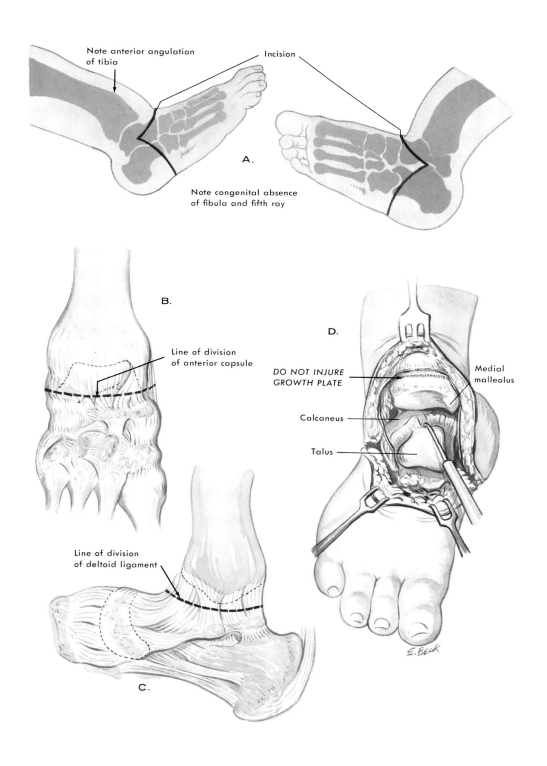

A.

Note anterior angulation of tibia

Incision

Note congenital absence of fibula and fifth ray

B.

Line of division of anterior capsule

C.

Line of division of deltoid ligament

D.

DO NOT INJURE GROWTH PLATE

Medial malleolus

Calcaneus

Talus

E. BECK

Syme's Amputation (Continued)

E. The Achilles tendon is identified and sectioned at its insertion in the posterior part of the calcaneus.

F. Next, the bone hook is placed on the back of the calcaneus, and the heel is pulled into plantar flexion. With a periosteal elevator, the calcaneus is dissected subperiosteally and the entire tarsus is removed, leaving the heel flap behind. Excision of the cartilaginous apophysis of the calcaneus should be complete. Do not leave behind any slivers of cartilage because as they ossify they will form painful ossicles that require excision.

G. The distal end of the tibia is exposed by retracting the heel flap posteriorly. The growth plate of the distal tibia is identified. Caution! It should not be injured. Then, the articular end of the tibia is sectioned perpendicular to the weight-bearing line. The resected surface of the tibia should be parallel to the floor when the patient is standing. The medial and lateral plantar nerves are sharply divided. The posterior tibial vessels are isolated, ligated, and divided.

H. The heel flap is cleaned of all muscle. The tourniquet is released, and after complete hemostasis the wound is closed in the usual fashion over two catheters for Hemovac suction. A compression dressing is applied.

POSTOPERATIVE CARE

Complications in the immediate postoperative period are hematoma in the stump and ecchymosis in the skin flap. Hemostasis and closed suction should make it possible to avoid these problems. Slough may develop occasionally in the plantar flap, requiring skin grafting.

A definitive prosthesis is fitted within six to eight weeks. The prosthesis is end-bearing and has a flexible inner wall for suspension of a patellar tendon–bearing type of socket. A new prosthesis is usually required every one and one half to two years by the growing child.

Plate 32. Syme's Amputation

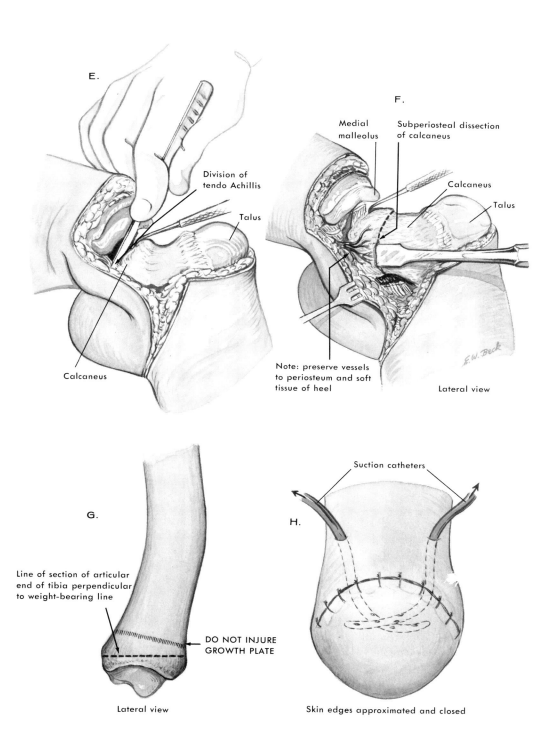

E.

Division of tendo Achillis

Talus

Calcaneus

F.

Medial malleolus

Subperiosteal dissection of calcaneus

Calcaneus

Talus

Note: preserve vessels to periosteum and soft tissue of heel

Lateral view

E.W. Beck

G.

Line of section of articular end of tibia perpendicular to weight-bearing line

DO NOT INJURE GROWTH PLATE

Lateral view

H.

Suction catheters

Skin edges approximated and closed

repeated passive manipulative stretching and retention in an above-knee cast. When satisfactory alignment of the foot and ankle is achieved it is maintained at night in a splint. When the child is 6 to 12 months of age, the fibrous or cartilaginous anlage of the fibula is thoroughly excised. This taut band extending to the calcaneus exerts a tethering force, pulling the hindfoot into eversion; it should be removed. The lateral ligament of the ankle is lengthened by Z-lengthening. The peroneus longus and brevis muscles are lengthened fractionally at their musculotendinous junctions. Equinus deformity is corrected by sliding or Z-lengthening of the tendo Achillis and capsulotomies of the tibiotalar and talocalcaneal joints (if the talocalcaneal joint is not fused). The lateral intermuscular septum and deep fascia encasing the muscles are completely excised. If tibial lengthening is contemplated in the future, all contracted soft tissues proximally tethering the peroneal nerve are released and excised. This soft-tissue release should be very meticulous to prevent development of peroneal nerve compression and palsy.

Occasionally the deltoid ligament is entrapped between the articular surfaces of the medial malleolus and the talus, preventing anatomic repositioning of the talus under the tibia. In such an instance a separate medial incision is made to dislodge the deltoid ligament.[51, 59]

After reduction of the foot and confirmation by radiograms, a Steinmann pin is inserted in the os calcis and drilled proximally into the talus, across the ankle joint, and into the tibia. It is essential to maintain anatomic reductions of the ankle joint by internal fixation. Relocation of the foot is maintained in an above-knee solid cast for a period of 4 to 6 weeks. Later, splints are used at night to keep the foot in neutral position. Active exercises are performed to strengthen muscles, and passive exercises will maintain range of motion of the ankle joint. The objective is to provide a plantigrade and functional foot.

Serafin, according to the suggestions of Gruca, developed a reconstructive operation to maintain the foot in line with the longitudinal axis of the tibia.[28, 57] The objectives of the procedure are to create a lateral malleolus containing a viable growth plate that can grow along with the lower tibial physis, to stabilize the tibiotalar joint and prevent lateral subluxation and valgus deformity of the foot by reconstructing a forklike shape for the tibio-

talar joint, and to preserve motion of the ankle joint.

The operative technique is as follows: a longitudinal incision is made beginning from a point 7 cm. superior to the ankle joint and extending to the neck of the talus. The subcutaneous tissue and deep fascia are divided in line with the skin incision. The tendons of the extensor digitorum longus and extensor hallucis longus are retracted medially along with the corresponding neurovascular bundle. A vertical incision is made in the periosteum and capsule of the ankle joint between the lateral third and medial two thirds of the tibia. The periosteum on the lateral and posterolateral surface of the tibia should not be disturbed. Periosteal stripping should be kept to a minimum. Next, with an oscillating electric saw, the tibia is sectioned obliquely in the vertical plane, beginning at a point between the lateral and middle thirds of the lower articular surface of the distal tibial epiphysis and extending obliquely cephalad and medially for a distance of about 7 cm. (Fig. 2–278 A). The medial tibial fragment is mobilized and displaced upward and medially for a distance of about 1.5 cm. The gap between the fragments above the physis is packed with cancellous and cortical bone taken from the upper tibial metaphysis or ilium (Fig. 2–278 B). This author fills the space at the site of the growth plate with adipose tissue taken from the buttocks following the Langenskiöld technique. The tibial fragments are transfixed by two positional screws (Fig. 2–278 C). The wound is closed, and an above-knee cast is applied. The cast is bivalved, and range-of-motion exercises are performed. Weight-bearing is not allowed until there is complete healing of the osteotomy, which usually takes place within eight weeks. The sharp linear section of the lower tibial physis does not disturb growth; fat interposition prevents formation of a bony bridge across the physis. By preserving attachments of soft tissues one can avoid impairing the blood supply and viability of the two tibial fragments. The hindfoot is shifted medially in relation to the longitudinal axis of the tibia, correcting valgus deformity of the heel.

Serafin reported the results in three children aged four, eight, and eight years who were treated by this bifurcation operation of Gruca (Fig. 2–279). The follow-up was for 17 and 27 months. In his experience, the Gruca operation did produce a new lateral malleolus with an epiphysis that grew at the same rate as the remainder of the epiphysis of the tibia, did not

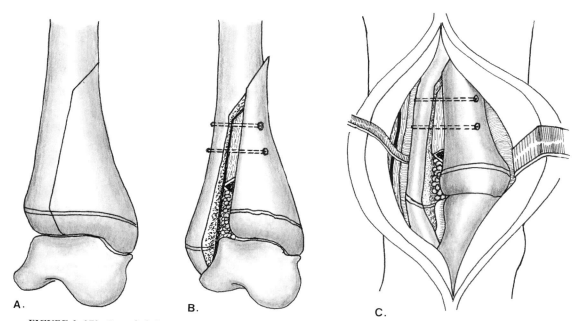

A.   B.   C.

FIGURE 2–278. Gruca's bifurcation operation on the lower end of the tibia in congenital absence of the fibula.

A. Line of osteotomy. **B.** Medial fragment is mobilized and displaced upward and medially for about 1.5 cm. Note the cancellous and cortical bone graft between the two fragments above the physis and the interposition of fat at the physis. **C.** The two fragments are transfixed securely with two positional screws.

FIGURE 2–279. Gruca's bifurcation operation for congenital absence of the fibula.

A. Preoperative radiogram in child eight years of age. **B.** Postoperative radiogram one year later. Note the satisfactory position of the talus and foot and the preservation of the physis. (From Serafin, J.: A new operation for congenital absence of the fibula. J. Bone Joint Surg., *49-B*:59, 1967. Reprinted by permission.)

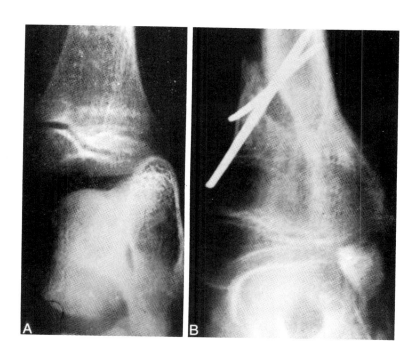

A   B

affect the rate of growth of the tibial physis, prevented recurrence of deformity, and preserved mobility of the tibiotalar joint. He recommended that the operation be performed in children two to seven years of age in order to give the limb the best chance to develop normally. Serafin believed that the operation may be done at the same time as soft-tissue release and reduction of ankle joint subluxation.[57] Mr. Peter Williams of Melbourne, Australia, has performed Gruca's operation and has found it to have very satisfactory results.[66]

References

1. Acker, R. B.: Congenital absence of the femur and fibula. Report of two cases. Clin. Orthop., *15*:203, 1959.
2. Achterman, C., and Kalamchi, A.: Congenital absence of the fibula. J. Bone Joint Surg., *61-B*:132, 1979.
3. Aitken, G. T.: Amputation as a treatment for certain lower-extremity congenital abnormalities. J. Bone Joint Surg., *41-A*:1267, 1959.
4. Aitken, G. T.: Congenital short femur with fibular hemimelia. J. Bone Joint Surg., *56-A*:1306, 1974.
5. Amstutz, H. C.: Natural history and treatment of congenital absence of the fibula. J. Bone Joint Surg., *54-A*:1349, 1972.
6. Arnold, W. D.: Congenital absence of the fibula. Clin. Orthop., *14*:20, 1959.
7. Badgley, C. E., O'Connor, S. J., and Kudner, D. F.: Congenital kyphoscoliotic tibia. J. Bone Joint Surg., *34-A*:349, 1952.
8. Bagg, H. J.: Disturbances in mammalian development produced by radium emanation. Am. J. Anat., *30*:133, 1922.
9. Bannister, P.: Congenital malformations: Preliminary report of an investigation of reduction of deformities of the limbs, triggered by a pilot surveillance system. Can. Med. Assoc. J., *103*:466, 1970.
10. Bardeen, C. R., and Lewis, W. H.: Development of the limbs, body-wall, and back in man. Am. J. Anat., *1*:1, 1901.
11. Bensahel, H., and Baum, C.: Aplasie congénitale du perone. Ann. Chir. Infant., *15*:103, 1974.
12. Blockey, N. J.: Observations on the fate of fibular transplants for congenital absence of the radius. J. Bone Joint Surg., *49-B*:762, 1967.
13. Bohne, W. H. O., and Root, L.: Hypoplasia of the fibula. Clin. Orthop., *125*:107, 1975.
14. Bose, K.: Congenital diastasis of the inferior tibiofibular joint. Report of a case. J. Bone Joint Surg., *58-A*:886, 1976.
15. Boyd, H. B.: Amputation of the foot with calcaneotibial arthrodesis. J. Bone Joint Surg., *21*:997, 1939.
16. Clark, M. W.: Autosomal dominant inheritance of tibial meromelia. Report of a kindred. J. Bone Joint Surg., *57-A*:262, 1975.
17. Corner, E. M.: The clinical picture of congenital absence of the fibula. Br. J. Surg., *1*:203, 1913.
18. Coventry, M. B., and Johnson, E. W., Jr.: Congenital absence of the fibula. J. Bone Joint Surg., *34-A*:941, 1952.
19. Davidson, W., and Bohne, W. H. O.: The Syme amputation in children. J. Bone Joint Surg., *57-A*:905, 1975.
20. Dieulafe, R., and Chahuzac, M.: Un cas d'absence partielle congénitale du péroné avec dissection. Bordeaux Chir., *6*:196, 1935.
21. Dubost-Perret, T.: Le Traitement des Absences Congénitales du Pérone et ses Résultats. Lyon, Imprimerie des Beaux-Arts, 1950.
22. Duraiswami, P. K.: Experimental causation of congenital skeletal defects and its significance in orthopedic surgery. J. Bone Joint Surg., *34-B*:646, 1952.
23. Eilert, R. E., and Jayakumar, S. S.: Boyd and Syme ankle amputations in children. J. Bone Joint Surg., *58-A*:1138, 1976.
24. Emami-Ahari, Z., and Mahloudji, M.: Bilateral absence of the tibias in three sibs. Birth Defects, *10*:197, 1974.
25. Farmer, A. W., and Lauren, C. A.: Congenital absence of the fibula. J. Bone Joint Surg., *42-A*:1, 1960.
26. Fitch, N.: Letter: Congenital absence of the fibula. J. Pediatr., *87*:839, 1975.
27. Frantz, C. H., and O'Rahilly, R.: Congenital skeletal limb deficiencies. J. Bone Joint Surg., *43-A*:1202, 1961.
28. Gruca, A.: Chirurgia Ortopedyczna, PZWL, 329, 1959.
29. Haim, E.: Über angeborenen Mangel der Fibula. Arch. Orthop. Unfallchir., *1*:31, 1903.
30. Harmon, P. H., and Fahey, J. J.: The syndrome of congenital absence of the fibula. Report of three cases with special reference to pathogenesis and treatment. Surg. Gynecol. Obstet., *64*:876, 1937.
31. Harris, R. I.: Syme's amputation. The technical details essential for success. J. Bone Joint Surg., *38-B*:614, 1956.
32. Harris, R. I.: The history and development of Syme's amputation. Artif. Limbs, *6*:4, 1961.
33. Hechard, P., and Carlioz, H.: Practical method of prediction of leg length inequality. Rev. Chir. Orthop., *64*:81, 1978.
34. Hootnick, D., Boyd, N. A., Fixsen, J. A., and Lloyd-Roberts, G. C.: The natural history and management of congenital short tibia with dysplasia or absence of the fibula. J. Bone Joint Surg., *59-B*:267, 1977.
35. Jansen, K., and Andersen, K. S.: Congenital absence of the fibula. Acta Orthop. Scand., *45*:446, 1974.
36. Karimova, L. F.: Surgical treatment of children with congenital defects in the development of the fibula. Vestn. Khir., *108*:82, 1972.
37. Kruger, L. M.: Fibular hemimelia. *In* Aitken, G. T. (ed.): Selected Lower-Limb Anomalies. Washington, D. C., National Academy of Science, 1971, pp. 49–71.
38. Kruger, L. M., and Talbott, R. D.: Amputations and prosthesis as definitive treatment in congenital absence of the fibula. J. Bone Joint Surg., *43-A*:625, 1961.
39. LaPasset, and Cahuzac, M.: Absence congénitale du pérone. Rev. Orthop., *22*:110, 1935.
40. Lefort, J., Carlioz, H., and Pere, C.: Fibular aplasia and associated malformations. 62 cases. Rev. Chir. Orthop., *62*:621, 1976.
41. Lowry, R. B.: Congenital absence of the fibula and craniosynostosis in sibs. J. Med. Genet., *9*:227, 1972.
42. McCullough, N. C., Matthews, J. G., Traut, A., and Cowell, J.: Early opinions concerning the importance of bony fixation of the heel pad to the tibia in the juvenile amputee. N.Y.U. Inter-Clin. Inf. Bull., *3*:1–16, Aug., 1964.
43. McKenzie, D. S.: The prosthetic management of congenital deformities of the extremities. J. Bone Joint Surg., *39-B*:233, 1957.
44. Martin du Pan, C. H.: Absence congénitale du pérone sans déformation du tibia. Rev. Orthop., *11*:227, 1924.
45. Matthews, W. E., Mubarak, S. J., and Carroll, N. C.: Diastasis of the tibiofibular mortise, hypoplasia of the tibia, and clubfoot in a neonate with cleft hand and cardiac anomalies. A case report. Clin. Orthop., *126*:216, 1977.
46. Mattner, H. R.: Treatment of congenital defect of fibula. Beitr. Orthop. Traumatol., *15*:586, 1968.
47. Mazet, R., Jr.: Syme's amputation. A follow-up study of fifty-one adults and thirty-two children. J. Bone Joint Surg., *50-A*:1549, 1968.

48. Middleton, D. S.: Studies of prenatal lesions of striated muscle as a cause of congenital deformity. I. Congenital tibial kyphosis. II. Congenital high shoulder. III. Myelodysplasia foetalis deformans. Edinburgh Med. J., *41*:401, 1934.

49. Moseley, C. F.: A straight-line graph for leg length discrepancies. J. Bone Joint Surg., *59-A*:174, 1977.

50. O'Rahilly, R.: Morphological patterns in limb deficiencies and duplications. Am. J. Anat., 89:135, 1951.

51. Pappas, A. M., Hanawalt, B. J., and Anderson, M.: Congenital defects of the fibula. Orthop. Clin. North Am., 3:187, 1972.

52. Pratt, A. D., Jr.: Apparent congenital absence of the tibia with lethal congenital cardiac disease. Am. J. Dis. Child., *122*:452, 1971.

53. Putti, V.: Cura del'assenza congenita della tibia del perone. Chir. Organi Mov., 13:513, 1929.

54. Ring, P. A.: Congenital short femur. J. Bone Joint Surg., *41-B*:73, 1959.

55. Schoneberg, H., and Forster, H. P.: Bilateral aplasia of the proximal part of the fibula. Klin. Paediatr., *188*:186, 1976.

56. Scranton, P. E., McMaster, J. H., and Kelly, E.: Dynamic fibular function. A new concept. Clin. Orthop., *118*:76, 1976.

57. Serafin, J.: A new operation for congenital absence of the fibula. J. Bone Joint Surg., *49-B*:59, 1967.

58. Syme, J.: Amputation at the ankle joint. London and Edinburgh Month. J. Med. Sci., 3:93, 1843.

59. Thompson, T. C., Straub, L. R., and Arnold, W. D.: Congenital absence of the fibula. J. Bone Joint Surg., *39-A*:1229, 1957.

60. Tsukimura, T., Tomita, S., and Okouchi, R.: Case of congenital absence of the fibula. Orthop. Surg. (Tokyo), 17:910, 1966.

61. Tuli, S. M., and Varma, B. P.: Congenital diastasis of tibio-fibular mortise. J. Bone Joint Surg., *54-B*:346, 1972.

62. Warkany, J., Nelson, R. C., and Schraffenberger, E.: Congenital malformations induced in rats by maternal nutritional deficiency. III. The malformations of the extremities. J. Bone Joint Surg., 25:261, 1943.

63. Weiner, D. S., Greenberg, B., and Shamp, N.: Congenital reduplication of the femur associated with paraxial fibular hemimelia. Report of a case. J. Bone Joint Surg., *60-A*:554, 1978.

64. Weinert, C. R., McMaster, J. H., Scranton, P. E., and Ferguson, R. J.: Human fibular dynamics. *In* Bateman, J. E. (ed.): Foot Science. Philadelphia, Saunders, 1976, pp. 1–6.

65. Westin, G. W., Sakai, D. N., and Wood, W. L.: Congenital longitudinal deficiency of the fibula. J. Bone Joint Surg., *58-A*:492, 1976.

66. Williams, P.: Personal communication, 1980.

67. Wood, W. L., Zlotsky, N., and Westin, G. W.: Congenital absence of the fibula: treatment by Syme amputation. Indications and technique. J. Bone Joint Surg., *47-A*:1159, 1963.

CONGENITAL LONGITUDINAL DEFICIENCY OF THE TIBIA

This is an extremely rare anomaly with an incidence of about one per million live births.[6] The first report was given by Otto in the German literature in 1841 (as quoted by Myers).[29] It is frequently associated with other malformations in the same limb, such as proximal femoral focal deficiency, absence of one or more rays of the foot, duplication of the femur, and synostosis of the tarsal bones.

According to Kalamchi and Dawe, two thirds of the affected children in their series had associated anomalies.[21] Reported elsewhere in the literature are anomalies of the hand (lobster claw hand, syndactyly, polydactyly, and absence of thumbs or bifid thumbs), equinovarus deformity of the feet, hypoplasia of the femur, bifid femur, hernia, cryptorchidism, varicocele, congenital heart disease, scoliosis, absence of the radius, duplication of the ulna and fibula, and diastasis of the distal tibiofibular syndesmosis. This author has had three patients with duplication of the femur (Fig. 2–280).

Classification

Based on clinical and radiographic findings, three types of congenital longitudinal deficiency of the tibia can be delineated. According to Kalamchi and Dawe, in Type I, there is total absence of the tibia, the foot is in marked inversion and adduction, and occasionally the medial rays are absent. The knee has marked flexion contracture with proximal displacement of the fibular head, and the distal femur is markedly hypoplastic with delayed ossification of its distal epiphysis and reduction in the width of the lower metaphysis. Quadriceps motor strength is very weak or absent (Fig. 2–281).[21]

In Type II, the distal half of the tibia is absent, but the proximal part is present to a varying degree. The femorotibial articulation is well preserved, but the proximal fibula has migrated superiorly. The flexion contracture of the knee is less marked, being about 25 to 30 degrees.

In the radiograms, sometimes the proximal tibia is not visible because it is cartilaginous, but its presence is indicated by the normal development of the distal femur with normal width of the distal femoral metaphysis and ossification of the epiphysis (Fig. 2–282).

In Type III, the distal tibia is dysplastic, with diastasis of the distal tibiofibular syndesmosis of varying degree. The foot is tilted into varus position, the fibular malleolus is prominent, and the distal tibia is hypoplastic and shortened (Fig. 2–283).

Treatment

The type of treatment varies according to the severity of the deficiency and whether involvement is unilateral or bilateral.

In Type I deficiency with only one limb involved, the function of the quadriceps muscle

Text continued on page 643

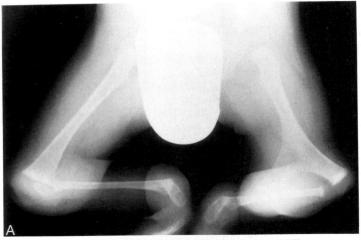

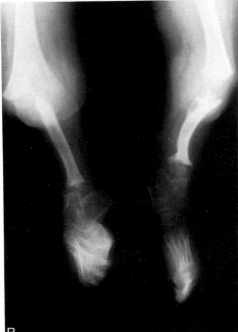

FIGURE 2–280. Bilateral congenital longitudinal deficiency of the tibia with duplication of the left femur.

A. Preoperative radiogram of both lower limbs and hips. **B** and **C.** Anteroposterior and lateral views following excision of the accessory femur and centralization of the fibula under the lower end of the femur.

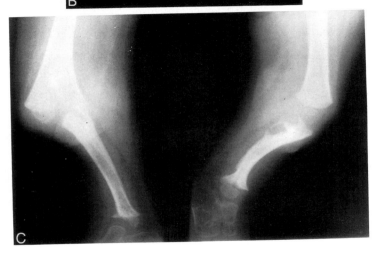

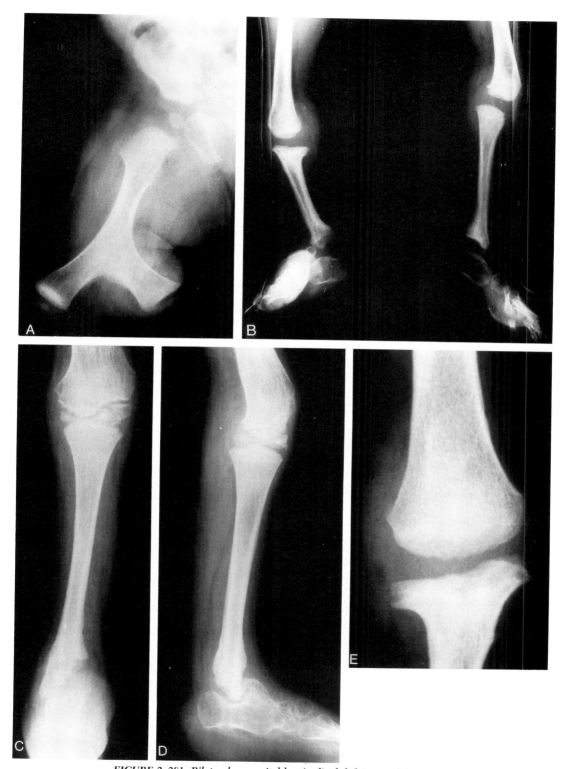

FIGURE 2–281. Bilateral congenital longitudinal deficiency of the tibia.

A. Preoperative radiogram showing duplication of the femur. **B.** Following centralization of the fibula under the lower end of the femur. **C** and **D.** Following centralization of the distal fibula into the fused talocalcaneal bones. **E.** Anteroposterior radiogram of the knee, showing the formation of a joint.

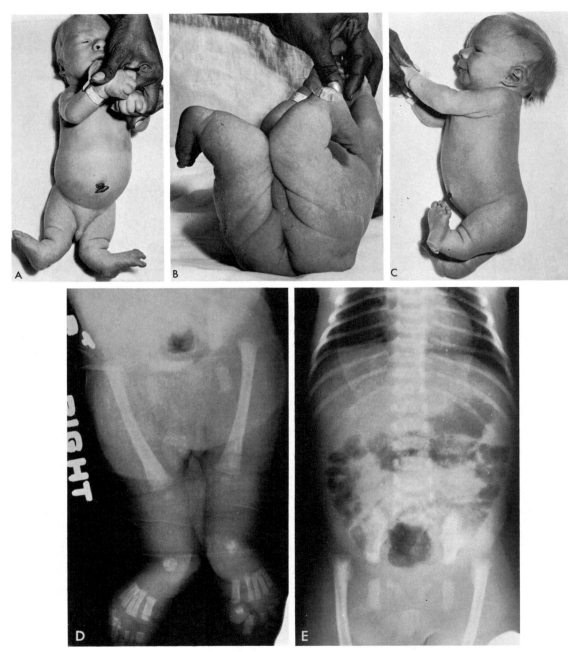

FIGURE 2–282. Bilateral partial absence of the tibia and fibula.

A to **C.** Clinical appearance of the patient at two months of age. Note the markedly short legs, severe genu recurvatum, and calcaneal valgus deformity of the feet. **D** and **E.** Anteroposterior radiograms of both lower limbs and spine, showing absence of ossification of the tibiae and teratologic dislocation of the hips.

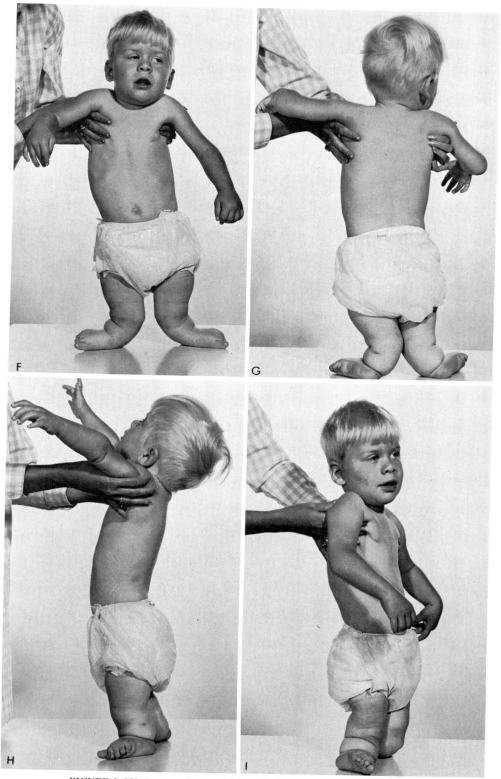

FIGURE 2–282 *Continued Bilateral partial absence of the tibia and fibula.*

F to I. Clinical appearance of patient at three years of age.

Illustration continued on following page

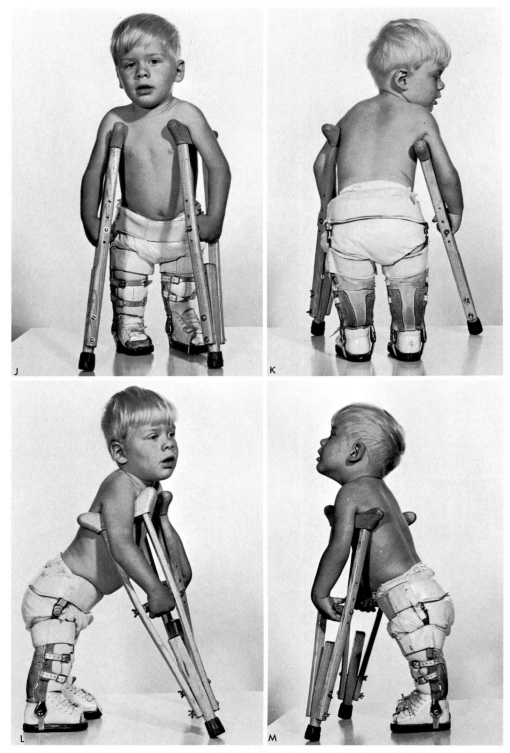

FIGURE 2–282 Continued Bilateral partial absence of the tibia and fibula.

J to **M.** Patient is fitted with braces with a pelvic band and can walk with crutches and a four-point gait.

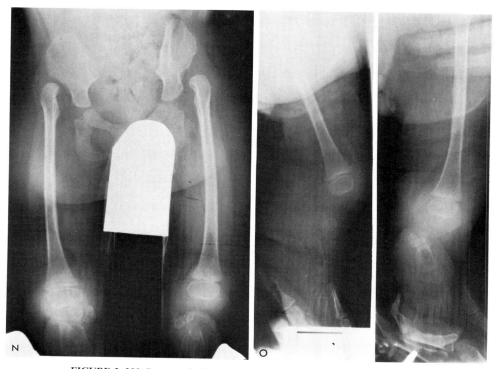

FIGURE 2–282 *Continued Bilateral partial absence of the tibia and fibula.*

N and O. Anteroposterior and lateral radiograms of both lower limbs. There is suggestion of ossification of the distal third of the tibial diaphysis. The hips are still dislocated.

is an important consideration and whether there is associated hypoplasia of the femur is another. If quadriceps muscle function is poor, knee reconstruction by fibulofemoral arthroplasty should not be performed, because results are poor. Persistent knee flexion contracture with very little knee joint motion makes prosthetic fitting difficult, cumbersome, and esthetically poor. If the projected length of the femur at skeletal maturity is normal, it is best to perform knee disarticulation at two to three years of age and fit a conventional above-knee amputation prosthesis. Early in life when the child begins to stand, he can be fitted with an extension orthosis.

If the ipsilateral femur is short, provision of maximal length of the affected limb is important. The proximal end of the fibula is fused into the intercondylar notch of the femur, and a Syme amputation is performed. With weight-bearing stresses, the fibula will hypertrophy. Lengthening of the thigh segment by femoro-fibular fusion improves the lever arm of the limb.

An above-knee amputation should not be performed, because bony overgrowth of the stump causes skin problems, and a short thigh segment does not provide adequate control of rotation of the prosthesis.

If there is adequate motor strength of the quadriceps muscle in unilateral cases, one may attempt reconstruction of the knee by Brown's fibulofemoral arthroplasty (Plate 33).[5, 6] This procedure is controversial; long-term results indicate that the reconstructed knee may develop arthritis.

Historically the credit for the construction of a functional fibulofemoral arthroplasty should be given to Myers.[29, 30] Brown reintroduced and popularized the procedure in 1965, and his modification of fibular transfer by shortening the fibula has made the operation relatively simple.[5, 6] Results of the operation in unilateral cases are illustrated in Figure 2–284.

In bilateral cases, this author has attempted to salvage the lower limbs by Brown's femoro-fibular arthroplasty. If the foot is functional it is salvaged by implanting the distal end of the fibula into the talus (or the calcaneus if the talus is absent). The reconstruction of the ankle joint

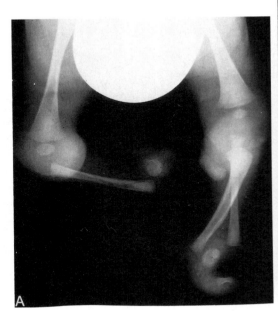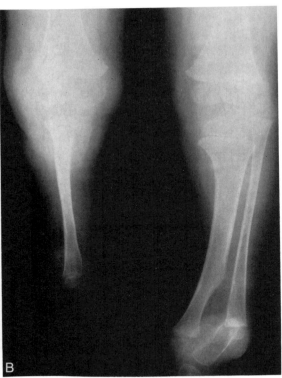

FIGURE 2–283. *Longitudinal deficiency of the tibia: Type III on the left and Type I on the right.*

A. At birth. **B.** At age two years. On the right side, with complete absence of the tibia, the fibula has been centralized under the lower end of the femur and a Syme amputation has been performed. On the left side, note the diastasis of the distal tibiofibular syndesmosis.

is staged separately, not performed simultaneously with femorofibular arthroplasty. The distal third and end of the fibula is exposed through an anterolateral approach. A medial and lateral soft-tissue release is carried out to mobilize the fibula. An appropriate segment (usually 1 to 1.5 cm. long) of the lower fibular shaft is excised. Distal fibular shortening will facilitate anatomic alignment of the fibula over the superior surface of the talus. The tip of the fibular epiphysis is squared by partial excision without disturbing the distal fibular physis. A niche is made in the dome of the talus, and by retrograde insertion of a smooth Steinmann pin, the fibula is fixed into it. The limb is immobilized in a single spica cast.

An illustrative case is shown in Figure 2–285. This technique differs from the second-stage Putti operation—in which the distal fibula is implanted in the talus and the foot is fixed in marked equinus posture so that the weight is borne on the metatarsal head—the purpose being to increase length of the lower limb.[37]

In Type II deficiency (Kalamchi and Dawe) the objective of treatment is to provide a stable knee joint; this is best achieved by proximal tibiofibular side-to-side fusion. In unilateral cases, lower limb length disparity is very marked, and an extension prosthesis will be required to equalize limb lengths. An end-bearing stump is provided by implanting the distal end of the fibula into the body of the talus and partially ablating the foot (a modified Boyd amputation). It is vital to preserve the distal physis of the fibula to provide maximal stump length. A below-knee amputation should not be performed because of problems with stump overgrowth and skin ulceration.

In bilateral Type II tibial deficiency the feet are preserved by reconstructive surgery; this will allow independent function without prostheses.

In Type III deficiency (Kalamchi and Dawe) the hindfoot is stabilized and foot function improved by calcaneofibular fusion. If the degree of tibial shortening and ankle diastesis is marked and the talus is displaced proximally, talectomy, synostosis of the distal tibia and fibula, and modified Boyd amputation are recommended.

In the very rare case of aplasia of the proximal

Text continued on page 651

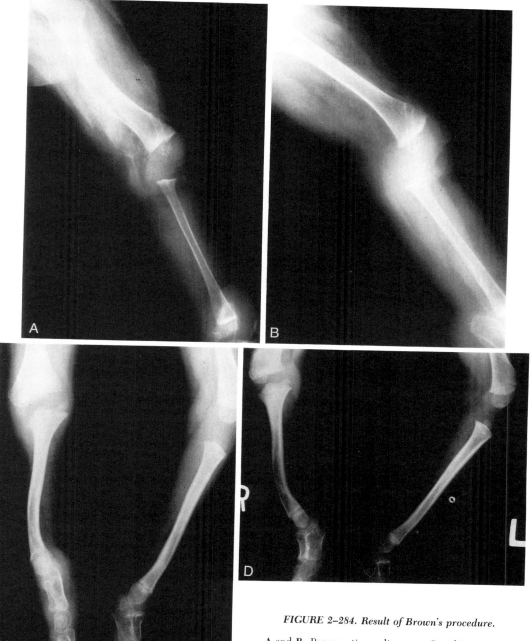

FIGURE 2–284. Result of Brown's procedure.

A and B. Preoperative radiograms. C and D. Postoperative radiograms.

Brown's Femorofibular Arthroplasty With Shortening of the Upper Fibular Shaft

OPERATIVE TECHNIQUE

A. A lazy S–shaped incision is made. It begins laterally and distally at the junction of the upper one fourth and lower three fourths of the fibula and extends proximally to the knee joint level, where it curves medially and then upward to the lower fourth of the thigh. Subcutaneous tissue is divided in line with the skin incision. The skin flaps are developed and retracted. (Note: In Brown's original description, a U-shaped incision was made on the anterior aspect of the knee joint; this makes exposure of the upper part of the fibula and fibular shortening very difficult.)

B. Next, the patella and patellar tendon are identified, and a longitudinal incision is made through the capsular structures lateral to the patella.

C. The patellar tendon is traced as far distally as possible, sectioned at its lowest point, and reflected proximally. The knee joint capsule is incised, and the lower end of the femur exposed.

D. By blunt and sharp dissection, the upper fibular shaft is exposed. Stay anterior to avoid injury to the common peroneal nerve. About 0.5 to 1 cm. of the tip of the epiphysis is resected to create a flat surface at the upper end of the fibula.

Plate 33. Brown's Femorofibular Arthroplasty With Shortening of the Upper Fibular Shaft

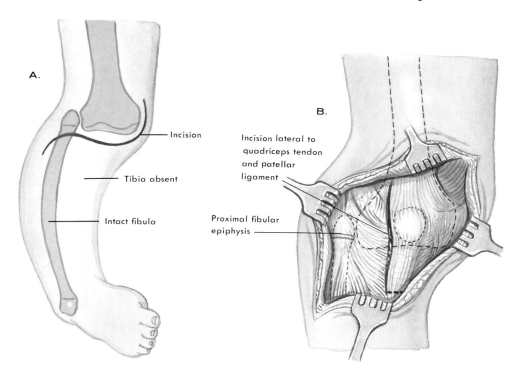

A.

Incision

Tibia absent

Intact fibula

B.

Incision lateral to quadriceps tendon and patellar ligament

Proximal fibular epiphysis

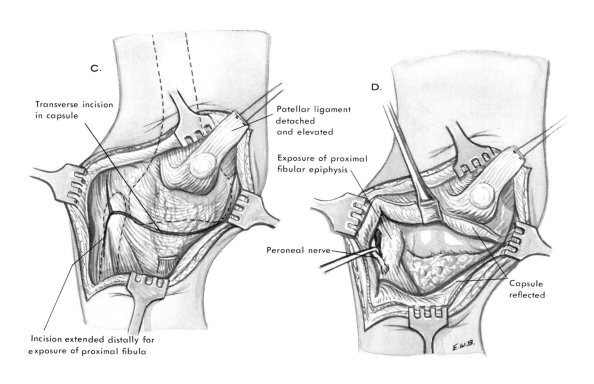

C.

Transverse incision in capsule

Patellar ligament detached and elevated

Exposure of proximal fibular epiphysis

Incision extended distally for exposure of proximal fibula

D.

Peroneal nerve

Capsule reflected

E.W.B.

Brown's Femorofibular Arthroplasty With Shortening of the Upper Fibular Shaft (Continued)

E. One to two centimeters of the upper diaphysis of the fibula is resected at its metaphyseal junction, and all soft-tissue attachments between the upper end of the fibula and the distal femur are released. The upper segment of the fibula is placed in weight-bearing alignment below the femoral condyles.

F. An intramedullary Steinmann pin is inserted into the fibular segments and driven into the femoral condyle in the intercondylar notch.

G and **H.** The patellar tendon is reattached, and the quadriceps mechanism repaired. The wound is closed in the usual manner, and a hip spica cast is applied for immobilization.

POSTOPERATIVE CARE

In about four to six weeks the intramedullary pin is removed, and an above-knee cast is applied for an additional two to four weeks until the fibular osteotomy is healed. After removal of the cast, passive and active exercises are gradually instituted to restore range of motion of the knee and to develop motor strength of the quadriceps muscle.

Initially the limb is supported in an above-knee orthosis with a drop lock knee and a plastic ankle-foot component to maintain alignment of the foot and knee. Splinting at night is continued for a prolonged period; this will prevent development of flexion contracture of the knee and varus deviation of the foot and ankle.

Plate 33. Brown's Femorofibular Arthroplasty With Shortening of the Upper Fibular Shaft

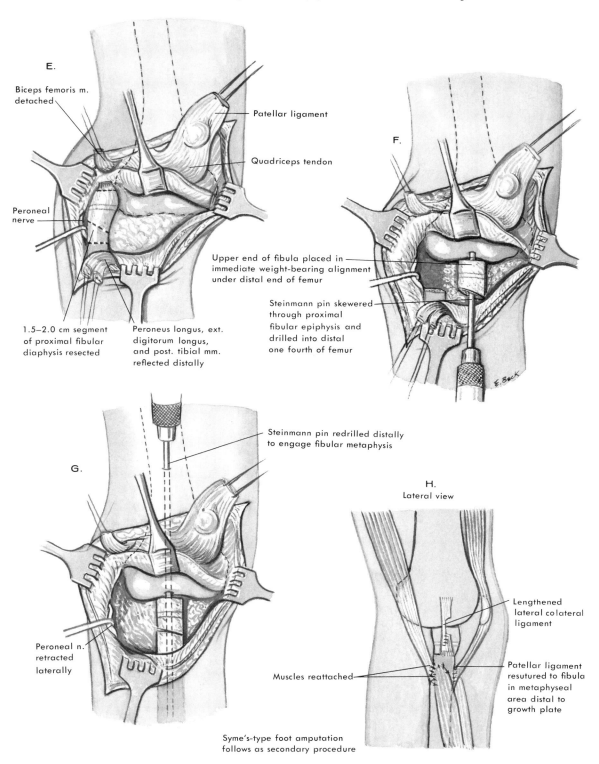

E.

Biceps femoris m. detached

Patellar ligament

Quadriceps tendon

Peroneal nerve

Upper end of fibula placed in immediate weight-bearing alignment under distal end of femur

Steinmann pin skewered through proximal fibular epiphysis and drilled into distal one fourth of femur

1.5–2.0 cm segment of proximal fibular diaphysis resected

Peroneus longus, ext. digitorum longus, and post. tibial mm. reflected distally

F.

E. Beck

Steinmann pin redrilled distally to engage fibular metaphysis

G.

H.
Lateral view

Peroneal n. retracted laterally

Lengthened lateral colateral ligament

Muscles reattached

Patellar ligament resutured to fibula in metaphyseal area distal to growth plate

Syme's-type foot amputation follows as secondary procedure

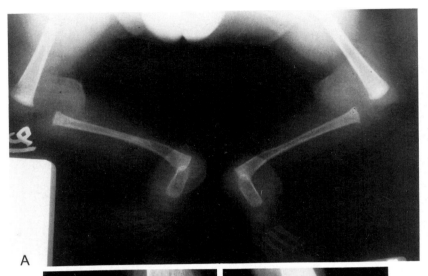

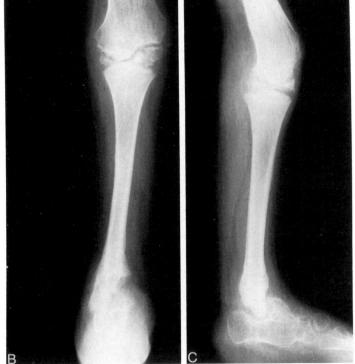

FIGURE 2–285. *McFarland bypass procedure.*

A. Preoperative anteroposterior and lateral radiogram. **B** and **C.** Postoperative anteroposterior and lateral radiograms.

tibia, Brown's femorofibular arthroplasty is performed with synostosis of the distal tibia and fibula.

References

1. Aitken, G. T.: Tibial hemimelia. *In* Aitken, G. T. (ed.): Selected Lower Limb Anomalies. Washington, D.C., National Academy of Science, 1971, p. 2.
2. Allenbach, E.: Absence du tibia congénitale et familiale. Rev. Fr. Pediatr., 5:368, 1929.
3. Bertola, V. -J.: Transplante del perone pro tibia. Prensa Med. Argent., 43:2074, 1939.
4. Bose, K.: Congenital diastasis of the inferior tibiofibular joint. J. Bone Joint Surg., 58-A:886, 1976.
5. Brown, F. W.: Construction of a knee joint in congenital total absence of the tibia. A preliminary report. J. Bone Joint Surg., 47-A:695, 1965.
6. Brown, F. W.: The Brown operation for total hemimelia tibia. *In* Aitken, G. T. (ed.): Selected Lower Limb Anomalies. Washington, D.C., National Academy of Science, 1971, pp. 20–28.
7. Brown, F. W., and Pohnert, W. H.: Construction of a knee joint in meromelia tibia (congenital absence of the tibia). A 15 year follow-up study. J. Bone Joint Surg., 54-A:1333, 1972.
8. Canki, N.: Syndactylia, polydactylia and absence of thumbs associated with tibial hypoplasia and a nose abnormality in 2 generations: A new syndrome. Rev. Med. Liege, 35:464, 1980.
9. Clark, M. W.: Autosomal dominant inheritance of tibial meromelia. J. Bone Joint Surg., 57-A:262, 1975.
10. Congdon, R.-T.: Congenital absence of both tibiae, treated by bone transplants. Northwest Med., 21:214, 1922.
11. Dankmeijer, J.: Congenital absence of the tibia. Anat. Rec., 62:179, 1935.
12. Dennison, W. M.: Delayed ossification of the tibia in apparent congenital absence. Br. J. Surg., 28:101, 1940.
13. Elmslie, R. C.: Congenital absence of the tibiae. Proc. R. Soc. Med., 13:224, 1920.
14. Emami-Ahari, E., and Mahloudji, M.: Bilateral absence of the tibias in three sibs. *In* Bergsma, D. (ed.): Limb Malformations. Case Report. New York, Stratton, 1976, pp. 197–200.
15. Evans, E. L., and Smith, N. R.: Congenital absence of the tibia. Arch. Dis. Child., 1:194, 1926.
16. Gaenslen, F. J.: Congenital defects of the tibia and fibula. Am. J. Orthop. Surg., 12:453, 1915.
17. Gray, J. E.: Congenital absence of the tibia. Anat. Rec., 101:265, 1948.
18. Gurkan, K. J.: Aplasie totale du tibia. Rev. Orthop. Chir., 35:389, 1949.
19. Hootnick, D., Boyd, N. A., Fixsen, J. A., and Lloyd-Roberts, G. C.: The natural history and management of congenital short tibia with dysplasia or absence of the fibula. J. Bone Joint Surg., 59-B:267, 1977.
20. Jones, D., Barnes, J., and Lloyd-Roberts, G. C.: Congenital aplasia and dysplasia of the tibia with intact fibula. J. Bone Joint Surg., 60-B:31, 1978.
21. Kalamchi, A., and Dawe, R. V.: Congenital deficiency of the tibia. J. Bone Joint Surg., 67-B:581, 1985.
22. Karchinov, K.: Congenital diplopodia with hypoplasia or aplasia of the tibia. J. Bone Joint Surg., 55-B:604, 1973.
23. Koebke, J., and Brade, A.: Anatomical investigations on the lower leg and foot in cases of hypoplasia and aplasia of the tibia. Anat. Anz., 148:350, 1980.
24. Laurin, C. A., Favreau, J. C., and Labelle, P.: Bilateral absence of the radius and tibia with bilateral reduplication of the ulna and fibula. J. Bone Joint Surg., 46-A:137, 1964.
25. Loder, R. T., and Herring, J. A.: Fibular transfer for

26. Matthews, W. E., Mubarak, S. J., and Carroll, N. C.: Diastasis of the tibiofibular mortise, hypoplasia of the tibia and clubfoot, in a neonate with cleft hand and cardiac anomalies. A case report. Clin. Orthop., 126:216, 1977.
27. McKenzie, D. S.: The prosthetic management of congenital deformities of the extremities. J. Bone Joint Surg., 39-B:232, 1957.
28. Michel, C. R., and Guilleminet, M.: Le traitement de l'absence congénitale du tibia et ses résultats éloignés. Rev. Chir. Orthop., 44:125, 1958.
29. Myers, T. H.: Congenital absence of tibia: Transplantation of head of the fibula: Arthrodesis at the ankle-joint. Am. J. Orthop. Surg., 3:72, 1905.
30. Myers, T. H.: Further report on a case of congenital absence of the tibia. Am. J. Orthop. Surg., 8:398, 1910.
31. Narang, I. C., Mysorekar, V. R., and Mathur, B. P.: Diplopodia with double fibula and agenesis of tibia. A case report. J. Bone Joint Surg., 64:206, 1982.
32. Nutt, J. J., and Smith, E. E.: Total congenital absence of the tibia. A.J.R., 46:841, 1941.
33. Ollerenshaw, R.: Congenital defects of the long bones of the lower limb. J. Bone Joint Surg., 7:528, 1925.
34. Pashayan, H., Fraser, F. C., McIntyre, J. M., and Dunbar, J. S.: Bilateral aplasia of the tibia, polydactyly and absent thumb in father and daughter. J. Bone Joint Surg., 53-B:495, 1971.
35. Pfeiffer, R. A., and Roeskau, M.: Agensie der Tibia, Fibulaverdoppelung und spiegelbildliche Polydaktylie (Diplopodie) bei Mutter und Kind. Z. Kinderheilk., 111:38, 1971.
36. Pratt, A. D., Jr.: Apparent congenital absence of the tibia with lethal congenital cardiac disease. Am. J. Dis. Child., 122:452, 1971.
37. Putti, V.: The treatment of congenital absence of the tibia or fibula. Chir. Organi Mov., 7:513, 1929.
38. Reber, M.: Un syndrome osseux peu commun associant une heptadactylie et une aplasie des tibias. J. Genet. Hum., 16:15, 1967–68.
39. Williams, L., Weintroub, S., Getty, C. J., Pincott, J. R., Gordon, I., and Fixsen, J. A.: Tibial dysplasia. A study of the anatomy. J. Bone Joint Surg., 65-B:157, 1983.
40. Rocher, H.-L., and Baranger, J.: Deux observations d'absence congénitale du tibia. Considérations cliniques et thérapeutiques. Mem. Acad. Chir., 79:171, 1953.
41. Sulamaa, M., and Ryoppy, S.: Congenital absence of the tibia. Acta Orthop. Scand., 34:337, 1964.
42. Tuli, S. M., and Varma, B. P.: Congenital diastasis of the tibio-fibular mortise. J. Bone Joint Surg., 54-B:346, 1972.

CONGENITAL POSTEROMEDIAL ANGULATION OF THE TIBIA AND FIBULA

In this deformation the tibia and fibula are bowed posteromedially at the junction of the middle and distal thirds of their shafts. The etiology is unknown. It most probably is the result of a developmental failure of the lower tibia and fibula occurring in the embryonic period, rather than an intrauterine fracture, constriction from taut structures, or intrauterine malposture because of fetal packing.[5, 7, 9, 16, 17] The degree of angulation varies from 25 to 65

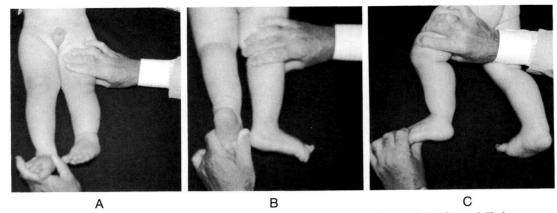

A   B   C

FIGURE 2–286. Clinical appearance of congenital posteromedial angulation of the tibia and fibula.

A to C. Photographs of the patient. Anterior, posterior, and lateral views. Note the short leg, the posteromedial angulation, and the dimple at the apex of the angulation.

degrees, with the angle of bowing in the medial and posterior directions being of almost the same degree. The foot is hyperdorsiflexed on the concave anterior surface of the leg in marked calcaneovalgus posture (Fig. 2–286). The anterior crural muscles are shortened, limiting plantar flexion of the foot (usually to neutral position); there is no bony deformity of the foot or ankle. The subtalar and midtarsal joints have normal flexibility.

The calf of the affected leg is atrophied, and there is a varying degree of weakness of the triceps surae. On clinical mensuration, the calf of the involved side averages 1 cm. less in circumference than that of the contralateral normal side. Often there is a posteromedial dimple at the apex of the angulation (Fig. 2–287). An extra crease in the soft tissues may be present at the level of the dimple; this should not be mistaken for the annular band of the congenital constriction band syndrome.

Involvement is unilateral. The affected tibia

and fibula are shortened to a varying degree, the fibula a little more than the tibia. The average difference between the normal and angulated tibiae averages 12 to 13 per cent (range 5 to 27 per cent) at all ages. There appears to be a direct relationship between the amount of tibial shortening and the degree of angulation; the greater the bowing, the more severe is the lower limb length discrepancy.[13] The proportionate difference in length between the normal tibia and the angulated one remains stable throughout growth. The shortening is progressive, the absolute discrepancy increasing steadily with age (Fig. 2–288). The average tibial length difference is 1.2 cm. in the first two months of life, 2.4 cm. at five years of age, 3.3 cm. at ten years of age, and 4.1 cm. (with a range of 3.3 to 6.9 cm.) at maturity.[17] After one year of age, when the secondary epiphyses have ossified and the acute bowing has decreased, one can quite accurately determine the lower limb length disparity at skeletal maturity. First, the predicted mature length of the normal tibia as judged by its present length relative to the norm on the Anderson-Green growth charts is determined. Second, the probable length of the bowed tibia at maturity is assessed by the percentage of shortening of the involved side. The ultimate disparity in tibial length at completion of growth is then calculated.

The progressive shortening appears to be caused by the inhibition of growth and tardy development of the secondary ossification center of the distal tibial epiphysis. The proximal tibial and fibular physeal growth is normal.

On the radiograms the intramedullary osseous structure appears normal. The cortices on the concave side of the bow (lateral and anterior)

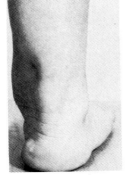

FIGURE 2–287. Posteromedial skin dimple at the apex of the angulation.

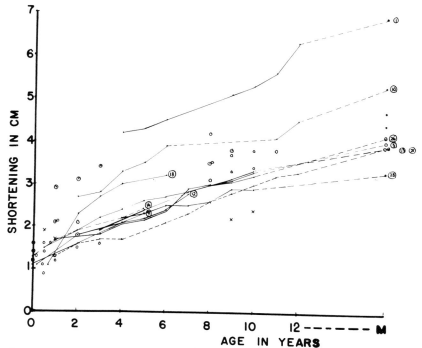

FIGURE 2–288. *Progressive increase of tibial length discrepancy with age in congenital posteromedial angulation of the tibia and fibula.*

Lengths of tibiae are measured on teleo- or orthoroentgenograms of 28 patients. Discrepancy in tibial lengths between the involved and normal legs is plotted against age. M, maturity. (From Pappas, A. M.: Congenital posteromedial bowing of the tibia and fibula. J. Pediatr. Orthop. 4:525, 1984. Reprinted by permission.)

are thickened, a response to stress (Fig. 2–289). There is no increased susceptibility to fracture; none of the patients develop pathologic fractures or pseudarthrosis. The distal parts of the affected tibial and fibular shafts are broader than the contralateral normal ones.

With growth and development the posteromedial bowing of the tibia and fibula decreases. During the first six months of life the correction of bowing is strikingly rapid; by the age of two years about 50 per cent of the angulation corrects itself, but after three years of age, diminution of bowing proceeds at a much slower rate. The posterior component of the angulation straightens more rapidly than the medial component, and the angle of fibular bowing persists longer. This is to be expected because the tibia is subjected to greater weight-bearing stress than the fibula.

The calcaneovalgus deformity of the foot gradually improves within the first nine months of life; however, some degree of pes planovalgus persists into adolescence. The calcaneovalgus posture of the foot is secondary to the posterior bowing of the tibia and weakness of the triceps surae.

Treatment

Treatment should be commenced soon after birth. In the neonatal period and early infancy passive stretching exercises are performed several times a day to elongate shortened muscles on the anterolateral aspect of the leg; in severe cases an anterior plastic splint or an above-knee cast may be applied to hold the foot in maximal plantar flexion and inversion. Within three to six weeks, ordinarily, fixed calcaneovalgus deformity of the foot can be fully corrected. Once the foot is brought into normal alignment, passive and active exercises are performed to maintain the correction. In severe cases night splints are worn to hold the foot in plantar flexion and inversion. After the age of two to three years, UCBL foot orthoses may be worn to support the severe planovalgus foot.

Initially Heyman and Herndon recommended the use of an orthosis to diminish the deforming force of the backward thrust at the apex of the curve. They also believed it might correct the deformity because of the pliability of growing bone.[11] In their later report, however, they thought the use of an orthosis unnecessary.[12]

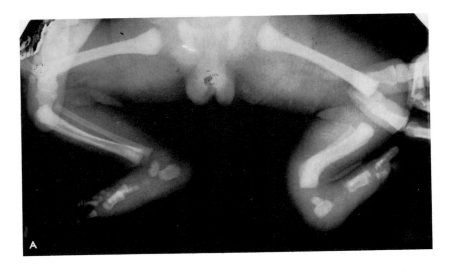

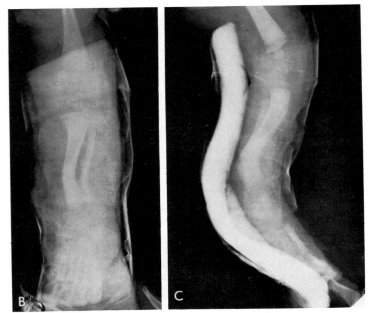

FIGURE 2–289. Congenital posteromedial angulation of the leg with talipes calcaneovalgus in a four-week-old girl.

A. Lateral radiogram of both lower limbs. Note the calcaneovalgus deformity of left foot. **B** and **C.** Anteroposterior and lateral radiograms of left leg showing the leg cast correcting the calcaneovalgus deformity.

Osteotomy to correct posteromedial bowing of the tibia is not ordinarily indicated. If after the age of three to four years, severe medial bowing of the leg persists, corrective osteotomy may be considered. Bone healing is not a problem in congenital posteromedial angulation of the tibia and fibula. In all the cases reported in the literature, healing has taken place without any delayed union or the necessity of bone grafting. Whether osteotomy at an early age has any beneficial effect in decreasing the eventual tibial shortening is not known at present; further longitudinal data are required to determine its usefulness. All the patients who have had corrective osteotomy have also required later limb length equalization.

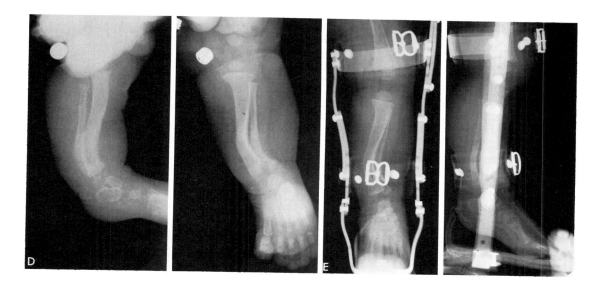

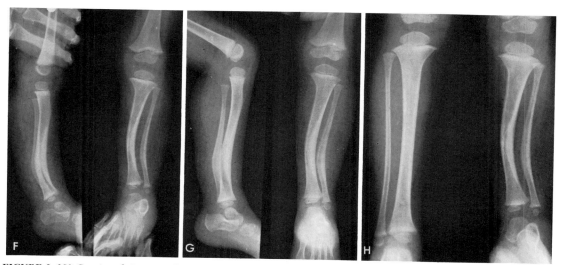

FIGURE 2–289 Continued *Congenital posteromedial angulation of the leg with talipes calcaneovalgus in a four-week-old girl.*

D. At three months of age. The foot rests in neutral position. The posteromedial bowing of the tibia is obvious. A night splint was used to hold the foot in plantar flexion, and passive stretching exercises of the shortened muscles on the anterior aspect of the leg were performed to maintain the correction. **E.** Anteroposterior and lateral radiograms of the leg in the orthosis that was given when the child began to walk. Use of the orthosis is optional. It was thought beneficial in lessening the deforming force of the backward thrust at the apex of the curve. **F.** Radiograms at two years and, **G,** at three years of age. Note the decrease in the degree of deformity. **H.** Anteroposterior radiograms of both tibiae at six years of age show the shortening of the left.

The lower limb length discrepancy is observed and the rate of growth of the short tibia versus the long normal leg is determined by serial scanograms. A contralateral proximal tibial and fibular epiphysiodesis will often be required to equalize limb lengths (30 of the 33 in the series of Pappas).[17] This author has lengthened the short tibia in two cases in which the projected disparity of limb length was greater than 5 cm. at skeletal maturity and the patients were of short stature. A preliminary staged soft-tissue release is crucial to prevent neurovascular complications.

References

1. Andersen, K. S., Bohr, H., and Sneppen, O.: Congenital angulation of the lower leg. Acta Orthop. Scand., 39:387, 1968.
2. Angle, C. R.: Congenital bowing and angulation of long bones. Pediatrics, 13:257, 1954.
3. Badgley, C. E., O'Connor, S. J., and Kudner, D. F.: Congenital kyphoscoliotic tibia. J. Bone Joint Surg., 34-A:349, 1952.
4. Beals, R. K., and Fraser, W.: Familial congenital bowing of the tibia with pseudarthrosis and pectus excavatum. J. Bone Joint Surg., 58:545, 1976.
5. Caffey, J.: Prenatal bowing and thickening of tubular bones, with multiple cutaneous dimples in arms and legs. Am. J. Dis. Child., 74:543, 1947.
6. Carvell, J. E.: The relationship of the periosteum to angular deformities of long bones. Experimental operations in rabbits. Clin. Orthop., 173:262, 1983.
7. Dawson, G. R.: Intrauterine fractures of the tibia and fibula. J. Bone Joint Surg., 31-A:406, 1949.
8. Dooley, B. J., Menelaus, M. B., and Paterson, D. C.: Congenital pseudarthrosis and bowing of the tibia. J. Bone Joint Surg., 56-B:739, 1974.
9. Freund, E.: Congenital defect of femur, fibula, and tibia. Arch. Surg., 33:349, 1936.
10. Hardinge, K.: Congenital anterior bowing of the tibia. Ann. R. Coll. Surg. Eng., 51:17, 1972.
11. Heyman, C. H., and Herndon, C. H.: Congenital posterior angulation of the tibia. J. Bone Joint Surg., 31-A:571, 1949.
12. Heyman, C. H., Herndon, C. H., and Heiple, K. G.: Congenital posterior angulation of the tibia with talipes calcaneus. A long-term report of eleven patients. J. Bone Joint Surg., 41-A:476, 1959.
13. Hofmann, A., and Wenger, D. R.: Posteromedial bowing of the tibia. Progression of discrepancy in leg lengths. J. Bone Joint Surg., 63-A:384, 1981.
14. Kling, T. F., and Hensinger, R. N.: Angular and torsional deformities of the lower limbs on children. Clin. Orthop., 176:136, 1983.
15. Krida, A.: Congenital posterior angulation of the tibia: A clinical entity not related to pseudarthrosis. Am. J. Surg., 82:98, 1951.
16. Miller, B. F.: Congenital posterior bowing of the tibia with talipes calcaneo-valgus. J. Bone Joint Surg., 33:50, 1951.
17. Pappas, A. M.: Congenital posteromedial bowing of the tibia and fibula. J. Pediatr. Orthop., 4:525, 1984.
18. Rabinowitz, M. S.: Congenital curvature of the tibia. Bull. Hosp. Joint Dis., 12:63, 1951.
19. Rathgeb, J. M., Ramsey, P. L., and Cowell, H. R.: Congenital kyphoscoliosis of the tibia. Clin. Orthop., 103:178, 1974.
20. Sadiq, S. A., and Varshney, G. K.: Congenital posterior angulation of the tibia. Int. Surg., 62:48, 1977.
21. Yadav, S. S., and Thomas, S.: Congenital posteromedial bowing of the tibia. Acta Orthop., 51:311, 1980.

"CONGENITAL" PSEUDARTHROSIS OF THE TIBIA

Congenital pseudarthrosis of the tibia is a complex affection in which there are dysplasia of bone with failure of normal bone formation in its distal half and consequent segmental weakening of the bone, anterolateral angulation of the tibia, and pathologic fracture. Hamartomatous tissue forms at the fracture site, and pseudarthrosis results because normal callus does not form. Congenital pseudarthrosis of the tibia was first described by Hatzoecher in 1708.[81]

It is only in the minority that the fracture and pseudarthrosis are present at birth; therefore the pseudarthrosis is not truly congenital, and the term *congenital pseudarthrosis of the tibia* is not correct. Some authors have proposed *infantile* instead of *congenital*; because of its general use in the literature, however, it is best to continue to call it congenital; perhaps the word should be used in quotes—"congenital."

Incidence

The condition is very rare. Andersen has estimated the incidence to be one per 190,000 live births.[8] Pais reported only 50 cases in 50 years at the Institute Rizzoli, Bologna.[134] Sofield found congenital pseudarthrosis of the tibia in fewer than 0.1 per cent of patients treated in the Shriners' Hospitals in the United States.[165] McFarland did not find a single case among 48,000 newborns.[114] The left side is affected slightly more often than the right. Bilateral involvement is very rare.

Etiology

The exact cause of congenital pseudarthrosis of the tibia is unknown. In the past many theories have been proposed, such as intrauterine trauma, "birth posture," metabolic disturbance, and vascular malformations, but all have since been discarded.

The disorder is not a single separate entity but rather a manifestation of several different pathologic conditions. It is vital to understand the composite nature of this complex abnormality.

Congenital pseudarthrosis of the tibia and neurofibromatosis seem to be related. The relationship was first noted by Ducroquet, who reported that of 11 patients with congenital pseudarthrosis 9 had café-au-lait spots and, of those, 2 had actual skin nodules of neurofibromatosis.[49] In the American literature, Barber in 1939 first described five patients with congenital pseudarthrosis and pigmental spots, in whose immediate families there was evidence of neurofibromatosis, thus emphasizing the relationship of congenital pseudarthrosis of the tibia with von Recklinghausen's disease.[12] Intraosseous neurofibroma at the site of congenital pseudarthrosis was first reported by Green and Rudo.[70] A less well-substantiated case is that of Jacobs and associates, whose patient might exemplify Albright's disease.[88] A relation between fibrous dysplasia, congenital pseudarthrosis, and neurofibromatosis was suggested by Aegerter, who believed that the fibroblastic masses encountered in all three conditions were due to alterations in the nerve pathways to those areas that produce abnormal growth and maturation of the tissues supplied.[1]

Sofield found evidence of neurofibromatosis in 42 of 106 cases (40 per cent), Hardinge found it in 55 per cent of the patients, and Andersen found it in 80 per cent of the cases.[6, 79, 165] Andersen considered the diagnosis of neurofibromatosis to be positive when the patient showed typical café-au-lait spots and had a positive family history of neurofibromatosis; when the family history was negative, the diagnosis of neurofibromatosis was considered positive only when the child had more than five typical café-au-lait spots, each more than 0.5 cm. in diameter.[7] Lloyd-Roberts and Shaw noted that café-au-lait spots and, especially, neurofibromatous nodules are often absent at birth; these stigmata of neurofibromatosis appear later on in life; their absence in infancy should not be accepted as evidence against the diagnosis. This difficulty in making the diagnosis of neurofibromatosis in infants and young children accounts for the considerable variation in its reported incidence in congenital pseudarthrosis of the tibia.[107]

Neurofibromatosis is of autosomal dominant inheritance. Information relating to the transmission of congenital pseudarthrosis of the tibia is not available. Most cases occur sporadically.

Beals and Fraser described a syndrome of congenital bowing of the tibia, fibular hypoplasia, and pectus excavatum transmitted as an autosomal dominant trait. In the reported family all grades of severity were found, from anteriorly bowed tibiae with no fracture to frank pseudarthrosis and tibiae with cystic changes. In one patient there was an apparently healed congenital pseudarthrosis of the ulna. It appears that in some cases congenital pseudarthrosis of the tibia is hereditary and congenital.[18]

The site of pseudarthrosis is usually surrounded by a thickened periosteum and a heavy cuff of fibrous tissue. This was initially observed by McElvenny and has been consistently noted since.[112] He believed the presence of this hamartomatous proliferated soft tissue interfered with bone production and normal callus formation. It was proposed that the tautly adherent thickened band of fibrous tissue constricts the bone, decreases its blood supply, and causes osseous atrophy due to pressure.

Kullmann and Wouters implanted a cellophane strip around the tibial diaphysis in young rats and experimentally produced pseudarthrosis of the tibia, which on radiographic and histologic examination appeared to be similar to congenital pseudarthrosis of the tibia in man. This experimental work suggests that an intraosseous mechanical factor may be pathogenic in the development of congenital pseudarthrosis.[98] A possible relationship between congenital pseudarthrosis to the congenital ring syndrome and congenital amputation of limbs was suggested by McElvenny.[112] Zych and Ballard reported a case of a congenital band causing pseudarthrosis of the tibia and impending gangrene of the leg.[189]

Briner and Yunis studied the ultrastructure of tissue from congenital pseudarthrosis of the tibia from three patients with the stigmata of neurofibromatosis. The vast majority of the cells lacked a basement membrane and were thought to be fibroblasts in the stationary phase; Schwann's cells, perineural cells, and axons were absent. No basement membrane could be demonstrated around them. Electron microscopy of neurofibromas and in neurofibromatosis has demonstrated that these tumors consist of Schwann's cells, fibroblasts, and occasional unmyelinated axons. The interosseous tissue from the site of congenital pseudarthrosis of the tibia shows a dense fibrillar structure with cellular areas that is indistinguishable from tissue found in pseudarthrosis due to other causes. It is, however, different from that of neurofibromas and neurolemmomas.[31]

Brown and associates studied the ultrastructure of bone in 17 patients with pseudarthrosis, 16 of the tibia and 1 of the radius; 8 had neurofibromatosis clinically, 3 had fibrous dysplasia, and 6 had no evidence of either neurofibromatosis or fibrous dysplasia. Electron microscopy failed to distinguish between neurofibromatous pseudarthrosis and pseudarthrosis without either neurofibromatosis or fibrous dysplasia. Electron microscopy did not shed any light on the origin of congenital pseudarthrosis of the tibia, nor did it support the concept of a neural or vascular derivation.[32]

A primary defect in the cartilaginous anlage of the tibia has been proposed as the cause in some cases of congenital pseudarthrosis of the tibia not associated with neurofibromatosis.[11, 128] This premise is supported by the observation of Badgley and associates that the site of the maximal angulation of the tibia and of the narrowest point of the medullary canal was the primary ossification center of the bone.[11] Is there a cartilage anomaly with failure of ossification?

Congenital pseudarthrosis is a complex disorder with perhaps several pathogenic factors in its causation.

Classification

There are three principal types of "congenital" pseudarthrosis of the tibia—dysplastic, cystic, and late. The *dysplastic type* is characterized by narrowing of the diameter of the tibia and sometimes the fibula as well, with sclerosis and partial or complete obliteration of the medullary cavity (Fig. 2–290). The hourglass constriction of the long bones is characteristic. The tibia is bowed anteriorly or anterolaterally. Fracture may be present at birth; more often spontaneous fracture and subsequent pseudarthrosis of the tibia develop when the infant begins to stand and walk at an average age of 12 months. Following fracture, the bone ends taper, the periosteum thickens, and there is hamartomatous proliferation of fibrous tissue at the fracture site, filling the defect. The pseudarthrosis is well established at 18 months of age. The fibula may also be bowed, thinned, and have pseudarthrosis. Bilateral involvement is very rare. The dysplastic type is notoriously prone to nonunion and refracture. According to Andersen, neurofibromatosis is always present in the dysplastic type.[7] In the series reported by Morrissy and associates, 19 of the 40 pseudarthroses of the tibia were classified as dysplastic; 11 patients had neurofibromatosis and 8 did not.[126]

In the *cystic type* there is no significant narrowing of the diameter of the tibia or fibula. In the lower third of the tibia (and sometimes of the fibula) there are cystlike rarefactions, the contents of which resemble fibrous dysplasia tissue (Fig. 2–291). At birth the leg is not angulated, but in the first few months of life, slight but definite anterior angulation of the tibia gradually develops. The fracture occurs at an average age of eight months. According to Andersen, neurofibromatosis is not associated with the cystic type; however, of the ten cystic cases reported by Morrissy and associates, three of the patients had neurofibromatosis and seven did not.[7, 126]

In the *late type* the leg appears to be normal early in life. There may be slight lower limb length discrepancy, the affected leg being shorter. After minimal trauma a stress fracture–like break occurs with consequent development of pseudarthrosis (Figs. 2–292 and 2–293). The pseudarthrosis should be classified as *late* when it occurs in a child five years old or older. The late type is not associated with neurofibromatosis. None of the patients with late pseudarthrosis or their families had any evidence of neurofibromatosis.

Andersen has described a clubfoot-type congenital pseudarthrosis in which the fracture is present at birth in a leg with marked anterior angulation. The involved or the contralateral lower limb has other associated congenital abnormalities such as constriction band or clubfoot.[5] This clubfoot type should *not* be considered a *true* congenital pseudarthrosis.

Pseudarthrosis may develop after a corrective osteotomy in a tibia that is angulated anteriorly in a child in whom neurofibromatosis has been diagnosed. In the roentgenogram there are no signs of bone dysplasia. This author must stress the importance of exercising restraint in treating a bowed tibia in these patients. Andersen refers to this deformity as *angulated pseudarthrosis*; it should not, however, be regarded as true congenital pseudarthrosis.[4] Congenital pseudarthrosis of the fibula is a separate entity and is described later.

Treatment

Management of congenital pseudarthrosis is one of the most challenging problems in orthopedics. In spite of improvements in bone grafting techniques and internal fixation, more sophisticated microvascular live fibular transplanting, electric bone stimulators, and the recent Ilizarov technique of distraction-compression osteogenesis, pessimism as to the outcome prevails; the future of the leg is uncertain. The problems of obtaining and maintaining union are not yet solved. Often multiple oper-

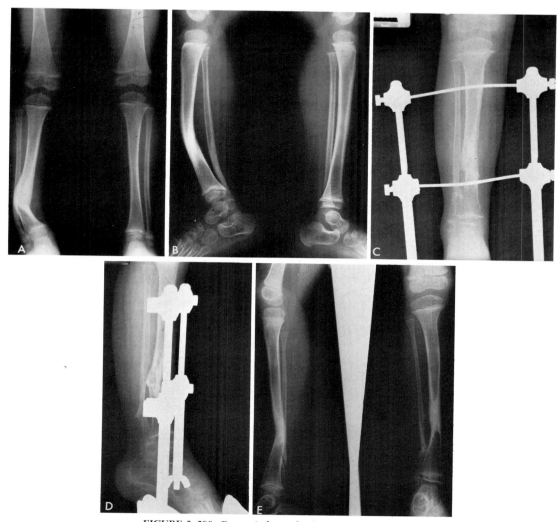

FIGURE 2–290. Congenital pseudarthrosis of right tibia.

A and **B.** Anteroposterior and lateral radiograms of both tibiae. Note the anterior and lateral angulation of the right tibia with sclerosis and almost complete obliteration of the medullary canal. **C** and **D.** Postoperative radiograms following excision of hamartomatous fibrous tissue, excision of sclerotic bone ends, and dual bone grafting. Note the Steinmann pins and Charnley clamp compressing the bone ends. The anterior angulation at the site of pseudarthrosis has been converted to a posterior one. **E.** One-year-postoperative radiogram. The fracture has healed, but the sclerosis of the medullary canal persists. The lower limb is protected in a long leg brace with a leather corset on the leg.

Illustration continued on following page

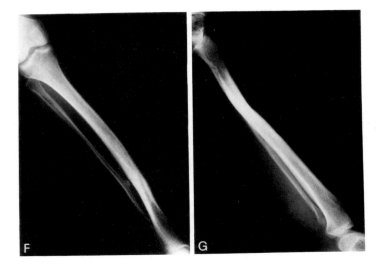

FIGURE 2–290 Continued Congenital
pseudarthrosis of right tibia.

F and **G.** Fifteen-year follow-up radiograms.

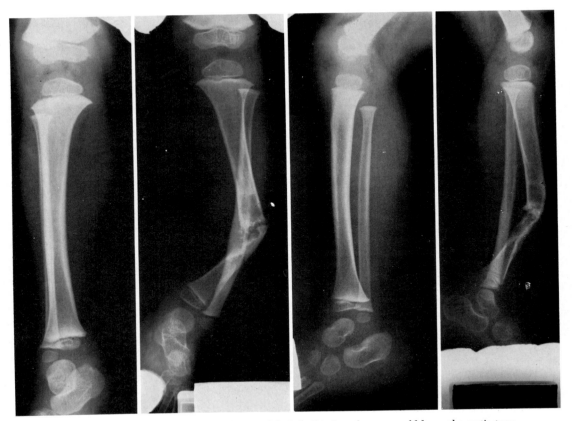

FIGURE 2–291. Congenital pseudarthrosis of the left tibia in a three-year-old boy—the cystic type.

Anteroposterior and lateral radiograms show the anterolateral angulation of the fracture and the nonunion. This patient had no clinical evidence of neurofibromatosis.

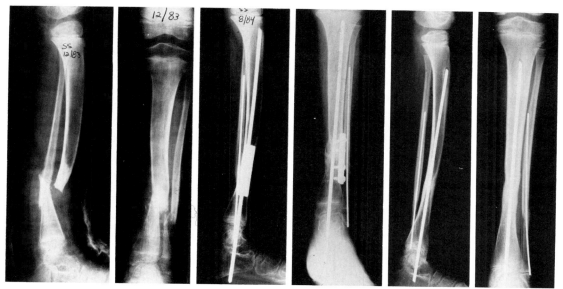

FIGURE 2–292. Congenital pseudarthrosis of the tibia—late type.

ations are necessary. The result may be a markedly short, dystrophic, and unstable leg. These problems and the fact that the eventual outcome may be amputation should be clearly explained to the parents at the outset to prevent misunderstanding.

The etiology and treatment of congenital pseudarthrosis of the tibia remain enigmas. Enigmas in medicine stimulate surgeons to propose numerous methods for treatment, which indicates there is no one best method. Boyd and Sage reported 23 variations of operations in 167 procedures in 91 patients, ranging from conservative measures such as cast fixation to

such radical means as amputation. They cited the advantages and disadvantages of the various operative procedures advocated in the literature.[29]

The dual onlay graft is technically complex, and secure fixation of the grafts to the distal fragment is difficult; to find cortical bone of adequate substance is an additional problem.[26, 72, 74, 75, 117, 155] Purvis and Holder modified Boyd's technique of dual grafting by performing the operation in two stages and by using an intramedullary Steinmann pin in the fibula for internal fixation. Like Boyd, they excised the hamartomatous tissue, resected sclerotic bone

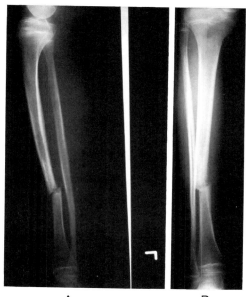

FIGURE 2–293. Anteroposterior and lateral radiograms of congenital pseudarthrosis of the tibia.

A and **B.** Note the narrowing of the medullary canal of the fibula in the distal third and also of that of the tibia at the fracture site.

A   B

ends, opened the medullary canal in both directions with a drill, and used twin onlay cortical grafts and cancellous bone. They reported solid union in six patients so treated.[143]

The composite pedicle graft procedure used by Farmer has the potential for infecting the uninvolved tibia and is technically difficult.[56] Two-stage fibular transplantation has its complexities and requires two operations.[86, 185] The use of the fibula, from either the opposite leg or the same side, as an onlay graft has proved to be unsuitable. The delayed autogenous bone graft advocated by Moore requires two operations on the normal leg and depends on hypertrophy of a small graft or upon numerous regrafting procedures of the area to obtain a tibia solid enough not to refracture.[123, 124] In the use of multiple chip grafts alone or in wide resection of the periosteum, security of fixation of the fragments depends on cast immobilization, which is not adequate.[78, 112] Because of the constant threat of refracture, Charnley and Van Nes have employed intramedullary tarsotibial pinning to maintain continuous internal fixation, thus reducing the possibility of refracture.[38, 179] The ankle joint and the distal tibial epiphyseal growth plate may, however, be injured. Another problem is spontaneous extrusion of the nail through the sole of the foot.

Sofield and Millar reported solid union in three patients with congenital pseudarthrosis of the tibia treated by fragmentation of the shaft and intramedullary fixation.[166] The technique is illustrated in Figure 2–294. The entire shaft of the tibia is exposed through a longitudinal incision. Both the proximal and distal metaphyseal areas are osteotomized, and the diaphysis is removed from the limb in two pieces (Fig. 2–294 A). Care should be taken not to injure the growth plate. If the distal fragment is short and atrophied, it is discarded and a substantial bone graft is used instead. The sclerotic and tapered ends of the fragments are resected, and their medullary cavities opened by drilling. The fragments are reversed so that the base of the proximal fragment is against the distal tibial metaphysis and the distal fragment or the bone graft is against the metaphyseal area just below the knee (Fig. 2–294 B). The fragments are threaded on a medullary nail, which is then securely fixed into the distal and proximal metaphyseal areas (Fig. 2–294 C). The periosteum is sutured as much as possible, and the wound is closed in the routine manner. The limb is immobilized in an above-knee plaster cast until solid union takes place.

In the past this author used the Sofield-Millar

technique when the distal fragment was too small and tapered. The area was reinforced with posteriorly and laterally placed onlay grafts; and a well-molded, snug, single hip spica cast was applied, allowing the patient to bear weight on the leg in three weeks to stimulate osteogenesis. Unfortunately, the failure rate was so high that he abandoned this technique.

Baw, in 1975, described a technique of transarticular graft in which a pointed graft (preferably autogenous) is driven into the medullary cavity of the distal tibia and across the ankle joint and the body of the talus before fixation to the proximal tibia.[17] Newer techniques are the vascularized fibular graft, which has the advantages of removing the diseased tibia and replacing it with a live fibular graft, and of making leg lengthening and correction of deformity feasible at the same time as grafting; and electric stimulation of bone healing by either direct current or pulsing electromagnetic fields. Recently, the Ilizarov technique of distraction osteogenesis opened new vistas in the management of congenital pseudarthrosis of the tibia and fibula.[86a]

The treatment modality employed will depend on the type of congenital pseudarthrosis of the tibia and whether the "pseudarthrosis" is in its incipient stage or the fracture has occurred and the pseudarthrosis developed.

THE PRE-PSEUDARTHROSIS OR INCIPIENT PHASE

The anteriorly or anterolaterally bowed tibia with partial sclerosis and narrowing of its medullary cavity is vulnerable to fracture and development of pseudarthrosis. In the young infant these precarious tibiae with impending fractures are supported in above-knee orthoses to prevent stress fracture. Between the ages of six and nine months, i.e., before the infant pulls himself up to standing and takes steps to walk and fall, this author strongly recommends a modification of McFarland's posterior bypass autogenous bone graft operation with the objective of reducing the risk of fracture.[114] The graft is placed posteriorly, spanning the pseudarthrosis in the normal biomechanical longitudinal axis of weight-bearing and protecting the anteriorly bowed weak tibial segment. No attempt is made to mobilize the impending "pseudarthrosis" and correct anterior angulation of the tibia; the deformity of a shortened and anteriorly angulated tibia is accepted. This author recommends using a delayed autogenous graft from the opposite tibia, as described by Moore and endorsed by Green and by Eyre-Brook and

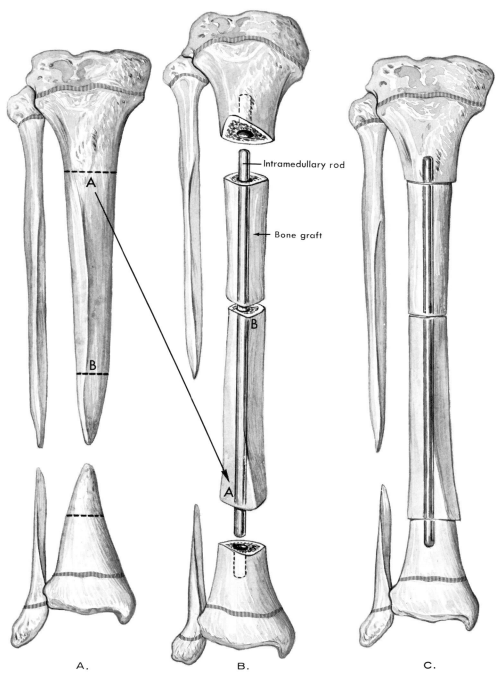

Intramedullary rod

Bone graft

A. B. C.

FIGURE 2–294. Treatment of congenital pseudarthrosis of the tibia.

Technique of Sofield and Millar (see text for explanation). (Drawing modified from Sofield, H. A., and Millar, E. A.: J. Bone Joint Surg., *41-A*:1384, 1959.)

associates.[55, 69, 123] With an oscillating saw a longitudinal graft with the periosteum intact is elevated from the anteromedial surface of the normal tibia; the graft is then replaced in its bed. Injury to the proximal and distal physes of the tibia should be avoided; use radiographic control if in doubt. An interval of four to six weeks should elapse before the graft is again lifted and inserted as a bypass graft into the affected posterior surface of the tibia. The delayed autogenous graft has enhanced osteogenic properties and is stouter and stronger than a graft taken immediately.

During the bypass operation it is vital to handle the leg with caution and gentleness. The operative procedure is performed under tourniquet ischemia. The posterior surface of the tibia is exposed through a sinuous posteromedial longitudinal incision. Avoid injury to the saphenous vein. An advantage of the procedure is that, because the tibia is exposed extraperiosteally, there is no devitalizing effect on the bone ends from extensive stripping of periosteum. The flexor digitorum longus, soleus, and posterior tibial muscles are extraperiosteally elevated and retracted posteriorly. The heavy cuff of proliferated fibrous ("hamartomatous") tissue surrounding the bone "ends" at the impending "pseudarthrosis site" is meticulously dissected and completely excised. The thickened periosteum on the posterior concave surface of the tibia at the potential "pseudarthrosis" site is also resected. It is important to release thoroughly any tethering soft-tissue contracture posteriorly on the concave posterior surface of the anteriorly angulated tibia. Heel cord lengthening is performed when there is equinus deformity of the ankle. Under radiographic control, the distal tibial metaphysis is identified, and a unicortical slot of appropriate size is made in the center of its posterior surface into which the graft is inserted. Proximally the bone graft is placed in a slot and secured, preferably with a unicortical cancellous screw. The graft should be on the posterior surface of the tibia, lying vertically, with its upper end as far above the apex of the curve as possible. For added security one may prefer to make holes with a small drill at each end of the graft, insert Mersiline sutures into them, and pass the sutures through power equipment–drilled holes in the proximal and distal tibial segments. This ensures secure anchorage of the graft in the desired position. It is vital that the graft be stable, lying vertically, under compression between the knee and ankle, and that its ends be embedded in healthy cancellous bone proximally and distally, well away from the lesion. The space between the longitudinal strut graft and the impending pseudarthrosis site is packed with long graft slivers and cancellous bone chips. It is also best to place some cancellous bone grafts at each end of the bypass graft to ensure and enhance its rate of incorporation. The tourniquet is released and, after complete hemostasis and insertion of a Hemovac drainage tube, the wound is closed in the usual fashion. Both lower limbs are immobilized in above-knee casts with the knees flexed 45 degrees.

In four to six weeks the normal leg from which the graft was harvested can be out of the cast, but the leg with the incipient "pseudarthrosis" is immobilized in a non–weight-bearing above-knee cast for four weeks. Then the patient is allowed to bear weight in an above-knee cast for an additional four weeks. Usually by then the graft is incorporated. The cast is removed and the limb protected in a knee-ankle-foot polypropylene orthosis with an anterior shell and drop-lock knee. As the child gets older and more stable in gait, and the graft incorporation becomes more solid, the orthosis can be for the ankle and foot only. For the initial 6 to 12 months the leg is protected in a night orthosis, but later on it may be free at night.

In the *cystic type* of incipient "pseudarthrosis" this author recommends gently curetting the cyst in the tibia and grafting cancellous autogenous bone in the cystic cavities. Do not break the tibia! The posterior bypass bone graft is performed as described for the dysplastic pre-pseudarthrosis type.

In the literature there is some controversy as to the value and effectiveness of the McFarland posterior bypass operation. McFarland reports success in 9 of 11 cases.[114] Morrissy and associates reported the results of prophylactic grafting in seven cases (four dysplastic, one cystic, and two of unknown type). The results were good in one and poor in two, and four came to amputation. The average age of preventive grafting was 13.4 months (range 5 to 24 months). The interval between prophylactic graft and fracture averaged 14 months, ranging from 4 to 55 months; and the average age at which fracture occurred was 27.4 months.[126]

This author has had success in five cases; an illustrative one is shown in Figure 2–295. All cases were treated before fracture had occurred. Modifications of the technique of McFarland and prolonged protection of the limb are probable factors in the successful prevention of fracture. As Lloyd-Roberts states, if grafting

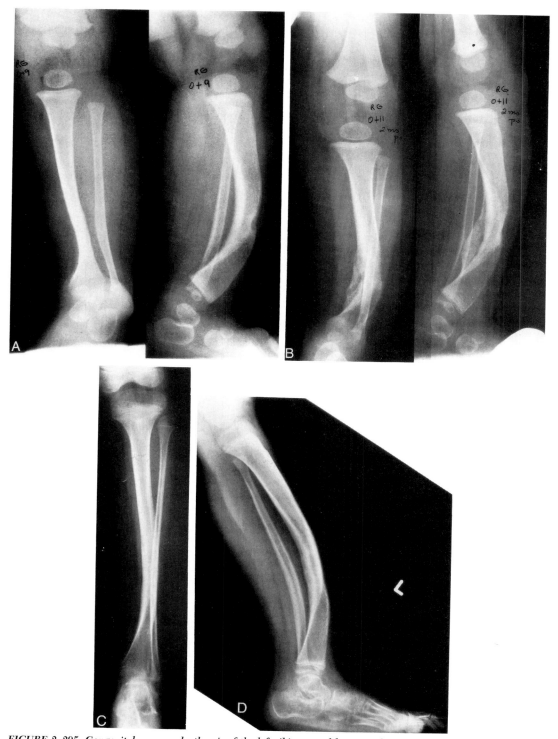

FIGURE 2–295. Congenital pre-pseudarthrosis of the left tibia treated by McFarland's posterior bypass operation.

A. Anteroposterior and lateral radiograms showing the anterior angulation with a cystic area at the apex. **B.** Two-months-postoperative radiograms showing the bone graft posteriorly and medially. **C** and **D.** Eight years postoperatively, radiograms showing incorporation of the graft. There is a medullary cavity. The patient had no fracture.

does no more than delay the age of fracture, it is an advantage because the delay puts the child at a more favorable age for successful grafting. Of five patients in whom Lloyd-Roberts and Shaw performed grafts, one ended with amputation, one with pseudarthrosis, and one with union, but with a very short period of follow-up (only nine months); two cases were regarded as successes because the patients had unbroken tibiae at ages seven and nine years.[107] In the series of four consecutive cases reported by

Eyre-Brook and associates, the bypass graft was performed after the fracture; one patient ended with amputation; one healed with fibrous dysplasia, which carries a good prognosis; one fracture united, but the period of follow-up was short; and another patient, whose case is illustrated in Figure 2–296, had follow-up to skeletal maturity (age 19 years) with an excellent result.[55]

The value of electric stimulation without surgical grafting as a prophylactic measure in treat-

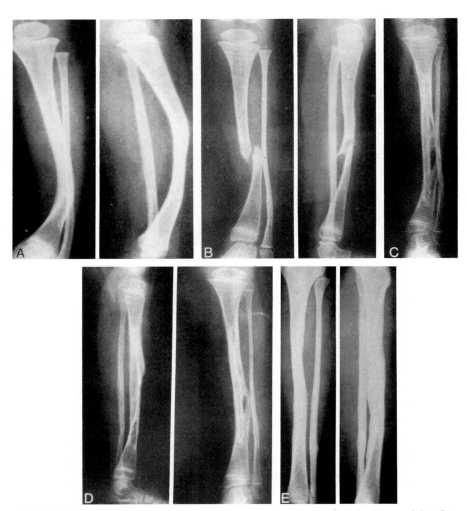

FIGURE 2–296. *Result of McFarland bypass operation for congenital pseudarthrosis of the tibia.*

A. Congenital pseudarthrosis of the tibia with typical sclerosis and bowing anteriorly and laterally in a nine-month-old child. **B.** At the age of three years and nine months there is nonunion of the fracture that had occurred a year earlier. **C.** Seven months after a delayed bypass graft, there is good incorporation at each end. The child is now five years old. **D.** Radiogram a year and a half later. The bypass graft has consolidated, and the pseudarthrosis has united. **E.** Fifteen years after grafting, the leg is strong and straight, and there is no shortening. The patient is 19 years old. (From Eyre-Brook, A. L., Baily, R. A. J., and Price, C. H. G.: Infantile pseudarthrosis of the tibia; three cases treated successfully by delayed autogenous by-pass graft, with some comments on the causative lesion. J. Bone Joint Surg., *51-B*:604, 1969. Reprinted by permission.)

ment of pre-pseudarthrosis is uncertain. It has been used by Crawford with a certain degree of success.[45] This author, however, has been disappointed with the results and at present does not recommend its use.

ESTABLISHED PSEUDARTHROSIS

If a pseudarthrosis has already developed, surgery is the only means of obtaining union. In the past, there has been some variance of opinion as to the best age for operation. Because the older the patient, the better the chances of union, it has been advised that surgical correction be delayed until five or six years of age, the affected leg being protected in the meantime with a knee-ankle-foot orthosis with an anterior shell to prevent injury and increased bowing deformity. The end result, however, will be much better if union is obtained as early as possible, because deformity and shortening of the leg associated with congenital pseudarthrosis increases as the child grows. Early use of the leg and weight-bearing minimize growth retardation and stimulate development of normal bone. At present the procedure of choice is the fixation of the tibial segments by Ilizarov wires and circular apparatus and utilization of compression distraction osteogenesis to stimulate healing. Experience with this procedure in North America is very limited; it appears to be biologically and biomechanically sound. Time will tell. Long-term results are not available, and it is not established as to the best age for surgery. Ilizarov recommends waiting until two to four years of age; however, this author feels that physically and biologically it is best to promote healing in the first year of life before the patient starts standing and walking. If there is no marked shortening, the tibia should not be elongated proximally, as the pseudarthrosis site is compressed distally. In the older patient with marked shortening, the tibia can be elongated at the proximal diaphyseal region and the distal pseudarthrosis can be compressed. Early experience of this author has shown that this is an excellent way to handle an established pseudarthrosis of the tibia in children. Refracture is still a problem; the leg should be protected postoperatively.

The operative procedure with which this author has had adequate success during the past 25 years is thorough excision of all hamartomatous and fibrous tissue at the pseudarthrosis site, removal of all sclerotic bone, conversion of anterior angulation of the tibia to slight posterior angulation, intramedullary fixation, and autogenous bone grafting. The fibula, if involved, is managed similarly to tibial pseudarthrosis. Progressive ankle valgus should be prevented by distal metaphyseal tibiofibular bone grafting (Langenskiöld procedure). If the fibula is normal and long, it is shortened proximally, in order to allow compression of tibial segments. The operative technique is described and illustrated in Plate 34. In the author's experience this technique has been the most suitable to achieve and maintain union (Fig. 2–297). At present this author favors the use of Ilizarov wires and circular apparatus for fixation, especially if the distal tibial segment is short. Leg length discrepancy should be followed in the growing child and an epiphysiodesis performed at the appropriate age to equalize limb lengths.

Problems and Complications Following Obtaining Union

Refracture. The achievement of union is the initial problem; maintaining union and preventing refractures is the greater challenge. At the beginning of treatment the grave problems of maintenance of union and refracture should be explained to both the parents and the patient. Following consolidation of the pseudarthrosis, the affected limb is protected with a knee-ankle-foot orthosis with an anterior shell on the leg and a rigid ankle and drop-lock knee; later on, for the older child with more mature union, an ankle-foot orthosis with an anterior shell on the leg is prescribed. The importance of the anterior shell, padded with Plastizolte and snugly fitted to the anterior convexity of the tibia, cannot be overemphasized. This orthotic device is worn until there is normal canalization of the medullary cavity of the tibia and preferably until the patient reaches skeletal maturity. In the hyperactive and uncontrollable child the leg is supported at night also. The child may refracture the bone when getting out of bed to go to the bathroom or while playing in bed or falling out of bed. Refractures have occurred in adult life when the brace is discontinued.

The intramedullary rod acts as an internal splint; it is kept in the tibia as long as possible.

If the follow-up radiograms show recurrence of sclerosis and narrowing of the medullary cavity and progressive tapering and hourglass constriction at the healed old pseudarthrosis site, one should not hesitate to reoperate before a fracture is sustained. At surgery all hamartomatous soft-tissue scarring is excised, and the sclerotic bone is repeatedly drilled with a very small drill point and regrafted.

Text continued on page 675

Treatment of Congenital Pseudarthrosis of the Tibia by Dual Graft

OPERATIVE TECHNIQUE

A. Over the anteromedial aspect of the tibia a gently arched incision is made, starting just distal to the proximal tibial tubercle; then it curves posteriorly and extends distally parallel with the posteromedial margin of the tibia. At the distal end of the tibia the incision swings forward to end at the anterior border of the tibia.

B. The subcutaneous tissue and the fascia are incised in line with the skin incision. The wound flaps are mobilized and retracted to their respective sides. The saphenous vein and nerve are identified and protected from injury. The veins that cross the field are clamped, divided, and coagulated. The site of pseudarthrosis is exposed.

C. The heavy cuff of proliferated fibrous tissue and thickened periosteum surrounding the bone at the pseudarthrosis site is meticulously dissected. This should be very thorough posteriorly. To expose the posterior surface of the tibia, the periosteum is dissected longitudinally and immediately in front of the anterior margin of the flexor digitorum longus and soleus muscles, which are extraperiosteally elevated and retracted posteriorly. The thickened periosteum and dense fibrous tissue are completely excised down to healthy muscle and bone.

Plate 34. Treatment of Congenital Pseudarthrosis of the Tibia by Dual Graft

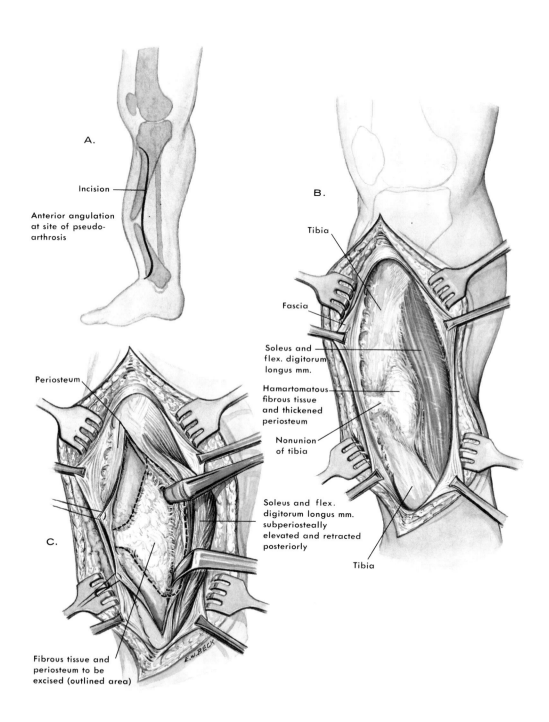

A.

Incision

Anterior angulation at site of pseudo-arthrosis

B.

Tibia

Fascia

Soleus and flex. digitorum longus mm.

Hamartomatous fibrous tissue and thickened periosteum

Nonunion of tibia

Soleus and flex. digitorum longus mm. subperiosteally elevated and retracted posteriorly

Tibia

Periosteum

C.

Fibrous tissue and periosteum to be excised (outlined area)

E.W.BECK

Treatment of Congenital Pseudarthrosis of the Tibia by Dual Graft (Continued)

D. The sclerotic bone from the ends of the proximal and distal fragments is resected with a rongeur, preserving as much length of the bone as possible.

E. Next, the medullary canal of the ends of each fragment is drilled in both directions with progressively larger sizes of diamond-head hand drills.

F. Then, by manipulation, the anterior bowing of the tibia is corrected completely, and the viable ends of the bone fragments are impacted and telescoped together. At times, the Achilles tendon may have to be lengthened through a separate incision to correct the anterior bowing. If the fibula is intact and is holding the tibial bone fragments apart, it is essential to resect an adequate segment through a lateral incision.

G. An intramedullary Steinmann pin of appropriate size is used to impact and hold the fibular fragments firmly together. It is best to insert the Steinmann pin retrograde, i.e., first from the proximal end of the distal fragment of the fibula, drilling out through the lateral malleolus, and then holding the fibular fragments together and drilling the pin into the proximal fragment. The Steinmann pin through the fibula also provides better fixation and more secure alignment of the tibial fragments.

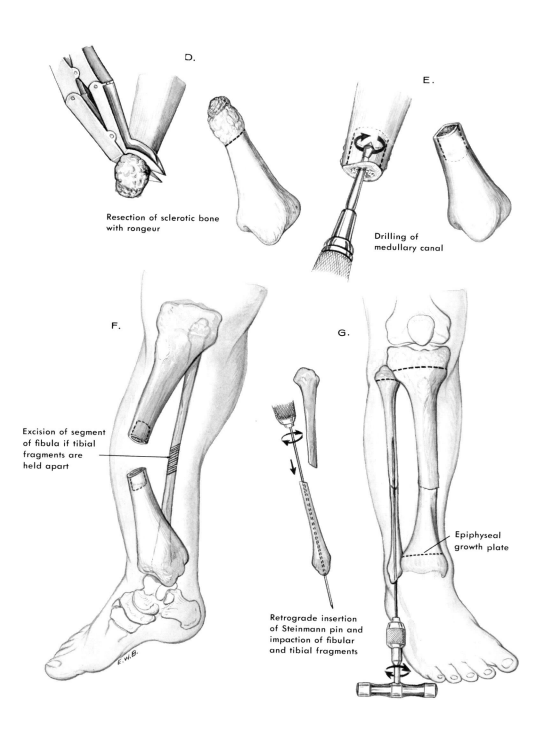

D.

Resection of sclerotic bone with rongeur

E.

Drilling of medullary canal

F.

Excision of segment of fibula if tibial fragments are held apart

G.

Retrograde insertion of Steinmann pin and impaction of fibular and tibial fragments

Epiphyseal growth plate

671

Treatment of Congenital Pseudarthrosis of the Tibia by Dual Graft (Continued)

H. During the manipulative reduction it is best to convert the anterior bowing of the tibia to 15 to 20 degrees of posterior angulation.

I and **J.** Next, the beds for the grafts on the lateral and posterior surfaces of the tibia are prepared by removing a shaving of bone with an osteotome or gauge. The bone grafts should extend at least 2 to 3 inches on the proximal fragment and as far distally as possible on the distal fragment, but without injuring the distal tibial epiphyseal plate.

An osteoperiosteal bone graft is removed from the patient's normal tibia and is divided transversely in half. At each end of the grafts a hole is made with a sharp towel clip or drill, and 0 or 00 Tycron sutures are inserted through the holes. One half of the graft is placed on the posterior surface and the second half on the lateral surface of the tibia, and they are sutured to the proximal and distal tibial fragments. The space between the grafts and the site of pseudarthrosis is packed with long bone graft slivers and cancellous bone chips.

K. Next, an external fixator is applied. In this drawing, a Wagner lengthening apparatus with two Schanz screws proximally and two Schanz screws distally is illustrated. At present this author recommends the use of the Ilizarov wires and apparatus—fixation is more secure and allows compression-distraction osteogenesis.

With a few interrupted sutures, the flexor digitorum longus, gastrocnemius soleus, and anterior tibial muscles are reattached to the tibia. Skin and subcutaneous tissue are closed in the usual manner. Abundant sterile sheath wadding is applied.

L and **M.** When the distal fragment is short, instead of using the Wagner, De Bastiani Orthofix, or Ilizarov lengthening apparatus, the tibial fragments are fixed with a large intramedullary Steinmann pin. The Steinmann pin is drilled distally from the proximal end of the distal fragment across the center of the distal tibial epiphysis, across the ankle and subtalar joints, and out of the skin through the plantar aspect of the heel. Then the tibial fragments are aligned and held together and the Steinmann pin is drilled into the proximal tibial fragment. The pin is directed in such a way that its proximal end will engage the posterior cortex of the tibia 1 to 2 inches distal to the proximal tibial epiphyseal plate. The distal end of the pin is cut just under the skin, and the heel is well padded while the cast is applied.

POSTOPERATIVE MANAGEMENT

Cast immobilization is continued until there is radiologic evidence of definite bony union. This may take as long as six months or more. The cast is changed every six to eight weeks, as necessary. The Wagner lengthening apparatus and Steinmann pins are removed in two to three months. If an intramedullary tarsotibial nail is used, it is taken out when cast immobilization is discontinued.

Following removal of the cast, the child should use an above-knee orthosis with an anterior shell on the leg, and ankle and knee joints that are free to allow normal weight-bearing stresses for stimulation of bone formation. The brace protection is continued until skeletal maturity or until the medullary canal of the tibia has normal diameter and there are no areas of sclerosis.

If the hamartomatous fibrous tissue regenerates, it should be excised before bony changes are produced.

Plate 34. Treatment of Congenital Pseudarthrosis of the Tibia by Dual Graft

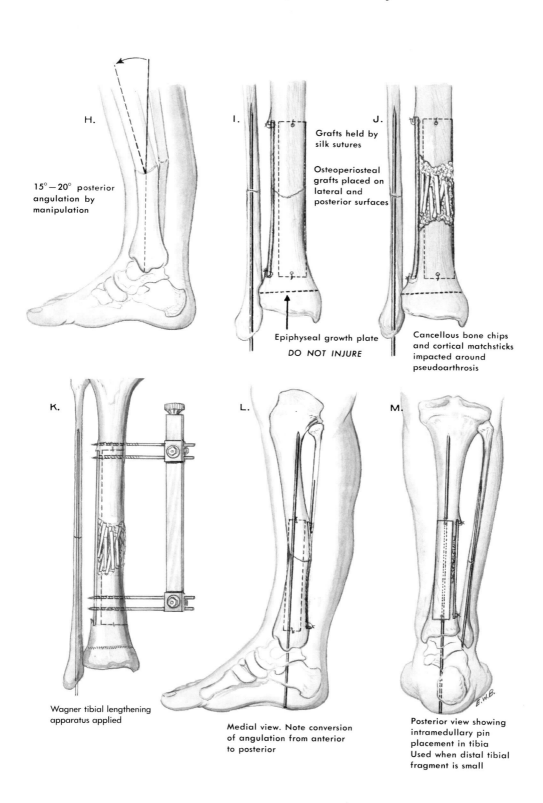

H.

15°—20° posterior angulation by manipulation

I.

Epiphyseal growth plate
DO NOT INJURE

J.

Grafts held by silk sutures

Osteoperiosteal grafts placed on lateral and posterior surfaces

Cancellous bone chips and cortical matchsticks impacted around pseudoarthrosis

K.

Wagner tibial lengthening apparatus applied

L.

Medial view. Note conversion of angulation from anterior to posterior

M.

Posterior view showing intramedullary pin placement in tibia
Used when distal tibial fragment is small

E.W.B.

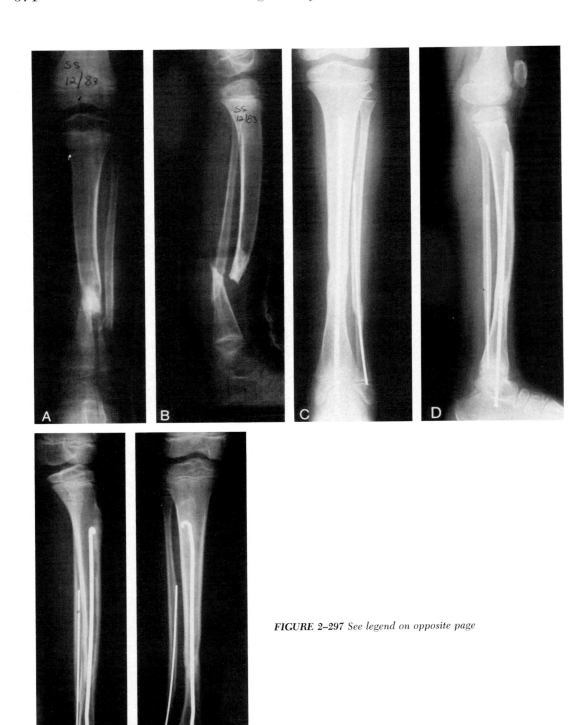

FIGURE 2-297 See legend on opposite page

Stiffness of the Ankle and Subtalar Joint.
This is caused by prolonged immobilization of the joints in the cast and by transfixation of the joints by the intramedullary rod. It is a calculated risk and a drawback that is often unavoidable; it should be explained to the parents at the outset. After skeletal growth, when the intramedullary rod has migrated upward into the distal tibial epiphysis, attempts are made to mobilize the ankle joint by continuous passive motion at night; in the experience of this author some functional degree of range of ankle motion is often restored.

Shortening of the Limb. This is common; in the detailed study of 67 patients by McBryde and Stelling the average shortening was 5 cm.[109] It is in part due to growth retardation of the distal tibial physis. The appearance of the ossification center of the distal tibia is often delayed. Bone imaging with ^{99m}technetium-polyphosphatase shows uptake to be decreased in the distal tibial physis as compared with the contralateral normal side. Follow-up radiograms show apparent distal migration of the pseudarthrosis; this is caused by normal growth of the proximal tibial physis and growth retardation of the distal tibial physis. Lack of the stimulus of weight-bearing and muscular atrophy are other factors in the pathogenesis of lower limb length discrepancy. At surgery the sclerotic bone ends of the tibia are resected until "raw" bleeding live bone is exposed—this shortens the leg to a varying degree. The presence of the intramedullary rod across the distal physis is another potential pathogenic factor; the rod is smooth, and despite all efforts at central placement, it may retard the growth of the distal tibial physis. The shortening of the affected lower leg is often progressive; the greater the severity of pseudarthrosis and the number of failed surgical attempts to obtain union, the greater the amount of shortening.

Treatment of lower limb length discrepancy depends on the degree of shortening and the age of the patient. Epiphysiodesis of the contralateral proximal tibia and, in some cases, of the distal femur, will be adequate to equalize limb length if the discrepancy is 5 cm. or less and the procedure is performed at the appropriate skeletal age. One should not forget to calculate the inhibition factor due to the growth retardation of the affected distal tibial physis. It is important to carry out serial limb length determinations by either orthoroentgenography or computed tomography.

Limb lengthening is a high-risk procedure with potential for grave complications. It can be tried if the alternative choice is amputation; parents and patient should accept it as a possible antecedent to limb ablation. In the literature there is a case report by McKellar, who lengthened the tibia successfully with corrective osteotomy seven years after the pseudarthrosis had healed.[115] Coleman has also successfully lengthened the tibia after healing of the pseudarthrosis.[43] Recently, lengthening at the proximal metaphyseal-diaphyseal level by either the Ilizarov technique or the DeBastiana callotasis technique has been successful in the experience of this author. It is recommended that it be tried.

Amputation and prosthetic fitting is the simplest and most pragmatic method of managing severe lower limb length discrepancy in congenital pseudarthrosis of the tibia.

Valgus Ankle. This is often caused by asymmetrical growth of the distal tibial physis, which is thinner laterally; there is more growth medially than laterally. The distal tibial epiphysis is wedged laterally. Another cause of valgus ankle is the high-riding fibular malleolus resulting from pseudarthrosis of the fibula. The distal fibula is attenuated, providing no lateral stability to the ankle joint.

Ankle valgus deviation can be prevented by synostosis of the distal metaphysis of the fibula to that of the tibia (Langenskiöld procedure). When there is pseudarthrosis of both the tibia and the fibula, intramedullary rod fixation and excision of the fibrous nonunion and bone grafting should be performed simultaneously on both.

When the pseudarthrosis of the tibia has healed, a medial displacement varus osteotomy of the distal tibia, through normal bone in the metaphyseal region, can be performed. This author prefers the Wiltse technique.[186]

Occasionally the tibiotalar joint is subluxated laterally and is very rigid and painful; the severe valgus deformity of the ankle makes the lower leg biomechanically weak, the skin over the prominent medial malleolus breaks down from shoe pressure, shoe wear is abnormal, and

---

FIGURE 2–297.
Congenital pseudarthrosis of the tibia and fibula.

A. and **B.** Preoperative radiograms. **C.** and **D.** Postoperative anteroposterior and lateral radiograms showing intramedullary pinning of the tibia. The hamartomatous soft tissue was excised and the pseudarthrosis site grafted with autogenous bone. **E.** and **F.** Four years later showing healing of the pseudarthrosis. The intramedullary pins have been changed. Note that the distal tibial and fibular physes are intact and that the ankle and knee mortise is well aligned.

adequate shoes are very difficult to find. In such cases ankle fusion may be the only solution to the problem.

Progressive Anterior Angulation of the Tibia. Ordinarily this occurs at the old site of pseudarthrosis. Soft-tissue contracture posteriorly may be an aggravating factor. The deformity is corrected several years after union by osteotomy—anterior closing wedge—through the distal tibia through normal metaphyseal bone below the affected area. It is best to graft simultaneously with cancellous bone and utilize secure internal fixation. An above-knee cast should be applied for immobilization.

Infection. Repeated operations, soft-tissue scarring, bone grafting, and internal fixation with metal increase the risk of osteomyelitis. This is a disastrous complication that may require amputation through the pseudarthrosis site.

Amputation. Amputation is not recommended as primary treatment; esthetically and anatomically, it is neither ideal nor acceptable to the parents and the patient. It is, however, a fact that some cases will end in amputation. In a series of 106 patients reported by Sofield, 25 underwent amputation; six of the amputations were done for resistant infection.[165] Andersen reported that 18 of 46 patients (39 per cent) had amputation of the limbs—the indication for ablation was shortening or nonunion in 15 and chronic osteomyelitis in 3.[6] Morrissy and associates reported amputations in 14 of 40 patients (35 per cent).[126] Therefore, it is best that early in the course of treatment the surgeon explain and prepare the parents and the patient for such an eventuality. It is difficult to set forth absolute criteria for ablation. Tapering and sclerosis with narrowing of the intramedullary canal at the pseudarthrosis indicate a poor prognosis for healing. Rapid resorption of the bone graft and spreading destruction at the site of pseudarthrosis are ominous. As a general rule amputation is indicated when two or three attempts to obtain union by conventional methods of treatment have resulted in failure: after intramedullary rodding and autogenous bone grafting, the grafts have been absorbed, and the pseudarthrosis has persisted; a subsequent attempt at microvascular live fibular transplant from the opposite leg has been performed, and it also has failed; and the result is a lower limb that is unstable, weak, deformed, with acute angulation at the pseudarthrosis site causing marked restriction of ankle and subtalar motion, functionally useless, markedly atrophic, and so shortened that leg length equalization would produce an extremely short-statured, corpo-

really deformed person. In such a patient there should be no question that amputation is the treatment of choice. The Ilizarov has also been tried and has been unsuccessful.

The psychological response of some patients may be absolutely against amputation, despite the fact that they are totally dissatisfied with the appearance and function of their affected limbs. Such emotional attachment to the affected limb is due to the enormous amount of energy invested by them in the multitude of operations, the years in cast, and the thought of social stigma.

Another factor to consider in patients with neurofibromatosis is their ultimate prognosis for life. Statistically, 25 per cent of patients with neurofibromatosis associated with congenital pseudarthrosis of the tibia will develop a glioma of the central nervous system in early adult life. The patients with glioma will either die because of the malignancy of the neoplasm or end up in extreme paralysis. The quality of living in the shortened span of life is an important consideration. This high incidence of glioma in patients with neurofibromatosis should temper the surgeon's enthusiasm.

Level of Amputation. In the literature, both Aitken and Murray and Lovell recommended below-knee amputation either through or above the pseudarthrosis site.[2, 127] This author believes the only indication for below-knee amputation is chronic osteomyelitis at the site of pseudarthrosis; otherwise a Syme or Boyd amputation is recommended. The disadvantages of the below-knee amputation are that the stump is short, which causes difficulties with prosthetic fitting, and the scarred skin flaps on the stump are subject to frequent skin ulceration, wound breakdown, and stump overgrowth that will require repeated revision. The advantages of the Syme or Boyd amputation are that it preserves limb length and growth from the distal tibial physis, which provides a better gait, and stump overgrowth is not a problem.[53] A Syme amputation implies the advantage of a weight-bearing heel pad.

Jacobsen and associates reported a follow-up study of eight patients with congenital pseudarthrosis of the tibia who had Syme amputations. The average age at amputation was 8.2 years. At an average follow-up of 5.9 years, none of the pseudarthroses had healed, and independent nonprosthetic weight-bearing was not achieved. Only three of the eight patients underwent bone grafting of the pseudarthrosis in conjunction with the amputation. Despite the fact that healing ordinarily will not take place in a patient with congenital pseudarthrosis of the tibia after a Syme amputation, Jacobsen and associates recommend the use of the Syme procedure instead of below-knee ablation.[89]

The operative technique of Syme amputation is described and illustrated in Plate 32.

Healing of the pseudarthrosis in one patient was reported by Edvardsen, who excised the fibrous nonunion of the tibia, resected part of the fibular shaft to allow impaction of the tibial segments, and followed with a Boyd amputation. Early weight-bearing allowed exertion of direct compressive forces across the vertically aligned tibial fragments.[52] This author shares Edvardsen's experience in a case and recommends performing this procedure simultaneously with the Boyd or Syme amputation. The cancellous bone from the ablated tarsus and the matchsticks of bone from the metatarsals are used for autogenous bone graft. The importance of fibular resection to allow impaction, thorough excision of the pseudarthrosis site in the tibia, conversion of the anterior angulation of the tibia to slight posterior angulation, and adequate intramedullary fixation cannot be overemphasized. Before amputation, a final effort should be made for independent nonprosthetic weight-bearing.

Free Vascularized Fibular Transplant. The use of a free vascularized fibular graft in the treatment of congenital pseudarthrosis of the tibia has been advocated by Gilbert, Chen and associates, Pho and associates, and Weiland and Daniel.[39, 65, 141, 183] In the past, the free vascularized fibular graft has been successfully used in bridging a bony defect of the tibia, reconstruction of bone defects after tumor excision, traumatic nonunions, and congenital nonunion.[3, 140, 141, 174, 183]

The operation is very sophisticated, technically demanding, of long duration (up to eight hours), and a multidisciplinary procedure, requiring the expertise of a microvascular surgeon and an orthopedic surgeon. It should be performed only in a few specialized centers. The operative technique is as follows:

Two to three weeks before the definitive operation, the vascular anatomy of the donor and recipient lower limb is determined. The operative procedure is long, requiring insertion of a Foley catheter in the bladder to monitor urinary output and appropriate measures to control and maintain body temperature. Team effort, i.e., the microvascular surgeon harvesting the fibular graft and the orthopedic surgeon preparing the bed for the graft, will curtail the operative time. The operation is divided into five stages: harvesting of the vascularized fibula with the peroneal vascular pedicle, excision of the pseudarthrosis, fixation of the vascularized fibula in situ, anastomosis of the vessels, and skin closure.

First, the fibula is taken from the contralateral normal limb through a posteromedial incision. The length of fibula that is required is measured and exposed extraperiosteally. With an osteotome or an oscillating electric saw, the distal and proximal fibular cuts are made. Superiorly, great care should be exercised not to injure the anterior vessels and nerves, which traverse in close proximity to the periosteum of the fibula. The fibula is gently elevated from its bed; bone hooks will facilitate its delivery. Anteriorly, the extensor muscles and the interosseous membrane are carefully dissected from the branches of the deep peroneal nerve. Proximally the dissection is subperiosteal to ensure avoiding injury to the anterior tibial vessels. Posteriorly, the posterior tibial neurovascular bundle is identified and dissected free in the plane between the gastrocnemius and soleus muscles. The musculoperiosteal vessels are preserved by sectioning a 0.5 cm. fringe of the soleus muscle with the fibula. About 2.5 cm. below the bifurcation of the popliteal artery, the posterior tibial vessels branch off and run distally parallel to the fibula. Next, with great attention to detail, the fibula together with its peroneal vascular pedicle and the musculoperiosteal vessels is dissected free from the surrounding muscles. The vascular pedicles are then sectioned, completing the harvest of the fibula.

Next, the pseudarthrosis site is explored through a longitudinal anteromedial incision. All abnormal soft tissue and sclerotic bone are excised. It is vital that the entire sclerotic portion of the medullary canal of the tibia be removed.

The harvested fibular graft is then slotted into grooves in the osteotomized ends of the involved recipient tibia, first into the proximal tibial fragment and then into the distal tibial fragment. If there is shortening, one may have to use substantial traction to restore length, or sometimes to apply a Wagner limb lengthening device to restore the desired length of the involved leg. Once the graft is in position, it is fixed with screws. Utilization of transverse screws checks telescoping of the transplanted fibula into the medullary canal of the recipient tibia. Telescoping is a more common problem with the distal tibial fragment because of its enlarged medullary cavity and porosis. An additional fixation safeguard is to use a transepiphyseal Kirschner wire, which will give axial stability (Fig. 2–298).

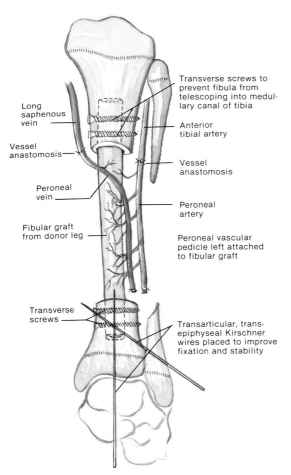

Transverse screws to prevent fibula from telescoping into medullary canal of tibia

Long saphenous vein

Anterior tibial artery

Vessel anastomosis

Vessel anastomosis

Peroneal vein

Peroneal artery

Fibular graft from donor leg

Peroneal vascular pedicle left attached to fibular graft

Transverse screws

Transarticular, transepiphyseal Kirschner wires placed to improve fixation and stability

FIGURE 2–298. *The free vascularized fibular transplant.*

(After Pho, R. W. H., Levack, B., Satku, K., and Patradul, A.: Free vascularized fibula graft in the treatment of congenital pseudarthrosis of the tibia. J. Bone Joint Surg., 67-B:64, 1985.)

The next step is anastomosis of the vessels between the donor peroneal artery and the recipient anterior tibial artery, and between the venae comitantes of the peroneal artery and the long saphenous vein or the venae comitantes of the recipient anterior tibial artery. It is important to anastomose normal vessel to normal vessel. There should be no tension or external compression. The wound is closed in the usual fashion.

Postoperatively the limb is immobilized in an above-knee plaster of Paris cast, and the cast is changed as necessary until bony union has taken place, when weight-bearing is begun.

The advantages of a free vascularized fibular transplant in the treatment of congenital pseudarthrosis of the tibia are that it allows radical excision of all diseased tissue and should effectively prevent recurrence; that it allows primary lengthening of the shortened tibia; and that the angular deformity of the tibia is corrected simultaneously at one operation. An illustrative case is shown in Figure 2–299.

The procedure appears to be very promising, achieving satisfactory bony union. In five cases of congenital pseudarthrosis of the tibia, successful healing was reported by Pho and associates. The follow-up period has been short, with a mean of 17.5 months and a range from 5 to 34 months. The operation has its problems. *Fixation* of the transplanted fibula to the recipient tibia is difficult, because the tibia is small and porotic and has a very short distal segment. Bone fixation should not impair vascular supply to the graft. Pho recommends the use of intramedullary fixation, as it allows maximal contact between the vascularized fibular graft and the recipient tibia. Telescoping of the fibula into the tibial medullary canal is prevented by using transverse screws, which also improve stability of fixation. Axial stability at the short, porotic distal tibial segment is provided by a transarticular, transepiphyseal Kirschner wire.

Delay in Bony Union. Theoretically the normal vascularized fibular transplant should unite in the time a normal fracture takes to heal. The problem is that the "fractures" at the ends of the fibular transplant are biologically segmental in nature, inadequately fixed, and open. In the series of five cases reported by Pho and associates, eight of the ten "fractures" occurred a mean of 4.5 months (range of 3 to 7 months) after operation.[141] Distal union is a greater problem. Non-union here is treated by autogenous cancellous bone grafting from the ilium. One may also use rigid fixation with small plates.

Stress Fracture. An annoying problem, stress fracture may occur when the patient commences weight-bearing in a plaster of Paris cast or, at times, when all external support is discarded. The fracture site is *not painful*, because the vascularized fibular graft is denervated. The stress fracture presents as a painless lump with some local erythema.

Valgus Deformity of the Ankle. This is difficult to correct at the time of fibular transplant, and with growth of the tibia the valgus ankle is exacerbated. It is best to treat the pseudarthrosis of the distal fibula simultaneously with that of the tibia, by synostosis of the distal fibular metaphysis to that of the tibia (Langenskiöld procedure). When the ankle valgus deformity is rigid and severe, osteotomy of the distal tibia through normal metaphyseal bone may be performed years after complete healing.

Progressive Valgus Deviation of the Donor Leg. A troublesome problem, especially in children under five years of age, it is prevented by

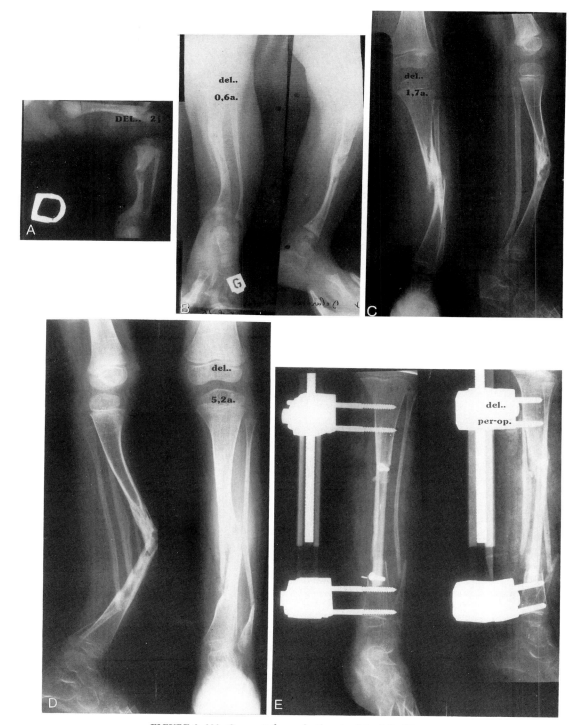

FIGURE 2–299. *Congenital pseudarthrosis of the left tibia.*

A. Radiogram of the left tibia in a two-day-old boy showing congenital pseudarthrosis of the tibia with neurofibromatosis. **B.** It was treated by surgical currettage and bone grafting at four months of age. A radiogram at six months of age shows healing. **C.** At 17 months of age the child sustained a fracture. This was treated by cast immobilization but failed to unite. **D.** A McFarland bypass operation was performed, which failed. **E.** Immediate postoperative radiogram following lengthening and free 11-cm. fibular vascularized bone graft transfer with Wagner external fixation.

Illustration continued on following page

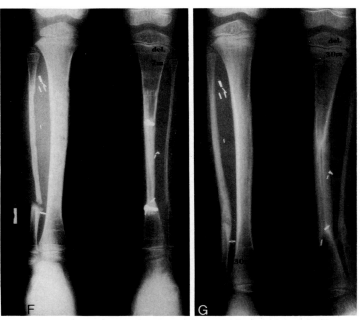

FIGURE 2–299 Continued Congenital pseudarthrosis of the left tibia.

F. Seven months postoperatively the lesion had healed. The screws were removed at eight months. **G.** Thirty-months-postoperative radiogram showing healing. The complication is valgus deviation of the ankle.

synostosis of the distal fibula to the tibia. The potential for deformity of the donor leg should be explained beforehand to the parents and patient.

Electric Stimulation of Bone Healing. Stress-generated electric potential in bone originates from the organic components of osseous tissue and is not dependent on cellular viability; the potentials arising in mechanically stressed bone are electropositive in areas of tension and electronegative in areas of compression.[14, 158] Bioelectric potential in bone is dependent on cellular activity and not on mechanical stress; it is electronegative in areas of active growth and repair, and electropositive in less active areas.[62] Investigations on the effect of electric current in bone have demonstrated stimulation of osteogenesis at the site of the cathode, or negative pole.[15, 131]

Promising results of research to determine the effect of electric stimulation in an animal model of delayed union of the tibia led to clinical trial in humans.[138, 139] It is evident that electricity stimulates osteogenesis. Types of electricity available are constant direct current, pulsed direct current, and magnetically induced current. At present it has not been determined which form of electric energy is the most efficient stimulator of osteogenesis. The various techniques available for applying current to bone are totally invasive, totally noninvasive, and semi-invasive

The *totally invasive* method employs electrodes and a power pack implanted in the limb. An open operation is required to implant a considerable amount of foreign material, and the risk of infection is increased. The implant must then be removed at a second operation. This technique was developed by Sir Dennis Paterson and co-workers.[136, 137] Its advantages are the free mobility and nonconfinement of the patient and the continuous administration of the therapy. The disadvantages are that two open operations are required and the considerable amount of implanted foreign material with its consequent risk of infection. A totally *noninvasive* method employs a pair of magnetic coils placed external to the limb. The electric current is provided by a pulse generator that produces a uniform time-varying electromagnetic field. The technique was developed by Bassett and associates.[14] The advantages of the noninvasive technique are that the potential complication of infection due to surgical implantation is avoided and a second operation is not required to remove the power pack and coils. Its disadvantages are that during the treatment period the patient must remain stationary and in a confined area, and compliance at home may be a problem. A *semi-invasive* method employs one or more electrodes inserted percutaneously into the area of nonunion; the power pack, which supplies direct continuous current, is external to the skin. This method was developed by Brighton and associates.[30] Its advantages are that no incision is required, the risk of infection is minimized, and the patient can be up and around.

"Successful" treatment of congenital pseudarthrosis of the tibia by electric stimulation of osteogenesis is reported by Lavine and associates, Paterson and associates, Basset and associates, and Sutcliffe and Goldberg.[14, 101, 137, 171] The rate of success varies. So far, the follow-up period has been short, and as the patients are followed for longer periods, the failure rate increases. With the present state of knowledge, this author does not recommend electric bone stimulation as the sole method of treatment of congenital pseudarthrosis of the tibia. The primary treatment is surgical. Electric bone stimulation may be used as an adjunct to augment osteogenesis. Because it is utilized concomitantly with open surgery, this author utilizes the totally invasive technique. Delivery of electric current is continuous, there is no interference with the child's mobility, and compliance is not a problem. The direct source of electric stimulation, the power pack, is placed proximally in the upper medial part of the leg, away from the site of repair of the pseudarthrosis, and lasts for a year. One can easily check whether the electricity is being generated.

Simonis and Paterson reported the results of treatment of 27 congenital pseudarthroses of the tibiae in 25 patients by full correction of the tibial deformity, stabilization with an intramedullary rod, and augmentation of bone formation by cancellous bone grafting and an implanted bone growth stimulator. The lower limb was protected in plaster until there was sound clinical and radiographic healing. Successful union was obtained in 20 pseudarthroses within an average time of 7.2 months (range 3 to 18 months). The average age of the child at the time of union was 7.4 years, with union occurring in one child at two years of age, and in three other children under four years of age. The causes of failure were lack of correction of anterior bowing of the tibia, inadequate internal fixation, and premature removal of the intramedullary rod before skeletal maturity, which resulted in refracture.[160]

References

1. Aegerter, E. E.: The possible relationship of neurofibromatosis, congenital pseudarthrosis and fibrous dysplasia. J. Bone Joint Surg., 32-A:618, 1950.
2. Aitken, G. T.: Amputation as a treatment for certain lower-extremity congenital anomalies. J. Bone Joint Surg., 41-A:1267, 1959.
3. Allieu, Y., Gomis, R., Yoshimura, M., Dimeglio, A., and Bonnel, F.: Congenital pseudarthrosis of the forearm: Two cases treated by free vascularized fibular graft. Hand Surg., 6:475, 1981.
4. Andersen, K. S.: Congenital angulation of the lower leg and congenital pseudarthrosis of the tibia in Denmark. Acta Orthop. Scand., 43:539, 1972.
5. Andersen, K. S.: Radiological classification of congenital pseudarthrosis of the tibia. Acta Orthop. Scand., 44:719, 1973.
6. Andersen, K. S.: Congenital pseudarthrosis of the leg. Late results. J. Bone Joint Surg., 58-A:657, 1976.
7. Andersen, K. S.: Congenital pseudarthrosis of the tibia and neurofibromatosis. Acta Orthop. Scand., 47:108, 1976.
8. Andersen, K. S.: Congenital pseudarthrosis of the tibia. Thesis, Copenhagen, 1978.
9. Andersen, K. S., Bohr, II., and Sheppen, O.: Congenital angulation of the lower leg. Acta Orthop. Scand., 39:387, 1968.
10. Apoil, A.: Les pseudarthroses congénitales de jambe. Rev. Chir. Orthop., 56:120, 1970.
11. Badgley, C. E., O'Connor, S. J., and Kudner, D. G.: Congenital kyphoscoliotic tibia. J. Bone Joint Surg., 34:349, 1952.
12. Barber, C. G.: Congenital bowing and pseudarthrosis of the lower leg. Manifestations of von Recklinghausen's neurofibromatosis. Surg. Gynecol. Obstet., 69:618, 1939.
13. Bassett, C. A.: Biophysical principles affecting bone structure in the biochemistry and physiology of bone. In Development and Growth. 2nd Ed. New York, Academic, 1971. Vol. 3, pp. 1–76.
14. Bassett, C. A., Caulo, N., and Kort, J.: Congenital "pseudarthrosis" of the tibia: Treatment with pulsing electromagnetic fields. Clin. Orthop., 154:136, 1981.
15. Bassett, C. A., Pawluk, R. J., and Pilla, A. A.: Augmentation of bone repair by inductively coupled electromagnet fields. Science, 198:575, 1974.
16. Bassett, C. A., Pilla, A. A., and Pawluk, R. J.: A nonoperative salvage of surgically resistant pseudarthrosis and non-unions by pulsating electromagnetic fields. A preliminary report. Clin. Orthop., 124:128, 1977.
17. Baw, S.: The transarticular graft for infantile pseudarthrosis of the tibia. A new technique. J. Bone Joint Surg., 57-B:63, 1975.
18. Beals, R. K., and Fraser, W.: Familial congenital bowing of the tibia with pseudarthrosis and pectus excavatum: Report of a kindred. J. Bone Joint Surg., 58-A:545, 1976.
19. Bergami, P. L., and De Iure, T.: La nostra esperienze nel trattamento delle pseudoartrosi di gamba con gravi perdite della tibia. Chir. Organi Mov., 57:34, 1968.
20. Berk, L., and Mankin, H. J.: Spontaneous pseudarthrosis of the tibia occurring in a patient with neurofibromatosis. J. Bone Joint Surg., 46-A:619, 1964.
21. Berkshire, S. B., Jr., Maxwell, E. N., and Sams, B. F.: Bilateral symmetrical pseudarthrosis in a newborn. Radiology, 97:389, 1970.
22. Birkett, A. N.: Note on pseudarthrosis of the tibia in childhood. J. Bone Joint Surg., 33-B:47, 1951.
23. Bischofberger, C.: Erfahrungen in der operativen Behandlung der kongenitalen Unterschenkelpseudarthrose. Z. Orthop., 78:423, 1949.
24. Boron, Z., Zagalski, J., Wrzask, J., and Kucowicz, P.: Die angeborene Pseudoarthrose der Tibia. Fortschr. Roentgenstr., 1065:579, 1967.
25. Bosch, J.: Beitrag zur Behandlung der kongenitalen Unterschenkelpseudarthrosen. Arch. Orthop. Unfallchir., 49:333, 1957.
26. Boyd, H. B.: Congenital pseudarthrosis. Treatment by dual bone grafts. J. Bone Joint Surg., 23:497, 1941.
27. Boyd, H. B.: Pathology and natural history of congenital pseudarthrosis of the tibia. Clin. Orthop., 166:5, 1982.
28. Boyd, H. B., and Fox, K. W.: Congenital pseudar-

throsis. Follow-up study after massive bone-grafting. J. Bone Joint Surg., *30-A*:274, 1948.

29. Boyd, H. B., and Sage, F. P.: Congenital pseudarthrosis of the tibia. J. Bone Joint Surg., *40-A*:1245, 1958.

30. Brighton, C. T., Freidenberg, Z. A., Zemsky, L. M., and Pollis, P. R.: Direct current stimulation of non-union and congenital pseudarthrosis. J. Bone Joint Surg., *57-A*:368, 1975.

31. Briner, J., and Yunis, E.: Ultrastructure of congenital pseudarthrosis of the tibia. Arch. Pathol., *95*:97, 1973.

32. Brown, G. A., Osebold, W. R., and Ponseti, I. V.: Congenital pseudarthrosis of long bones: A clinical, radiographic, histologic and ultrastructural study. Clin. Orthop., *128*:228, 1977.

33. Buttner, A., and Eysholdt, K.-G.: Die angeborenen Verbiegungen und Pseudarthrosen des Unterschenkels, Ergb. Chir. Orthop., *36*:165, 1953.

34. Campanacci, M.: Displasia osteofibrosa delle ossa lunghe. Una nuova entita anatomoclinica. Ital. J. Orthop. Traumatol., *2*:221, 1976.

35. Campanacci, M., Nicoll, E. A., and Pagella, P.: The differential diagnosis of congenital pseudarthrosis of the tibia. Int. Orthop., *4*:283, 1981.

36. Campanacci, M., Giunti, A., Leonessa, C., Pagani, P., and Trental, C.: Pseudarthrose infantile della tibia. Ital. J. Orthop. Traumatol., Suppl. 25, 1973.

37. Camurati, M.: Le pseudartrosi congenite della tibia. Chir. Organi Mov., *15*:1, 1930.

38. Charnley, J.: Congenital pseudarthrosis of the tibia treated by the intramedullary nail. J. Bone Joint Surg., *38-A*:283, 1956.

39. Chen, C. W., Yu, Z. J., and Wang, Y.: A new method of treatment of congenital tibial pseudarthrosis using free vascularised fibular graft: A preliminary report. Ann. Acad. Med. Singapore, *8*:465, 1979.

40. Cheng, Z. W.: A new treatment for congenital tibial pseudarthrosis—free fibula graft with microvascular anastomosis: A preliminary report of 12 cases. (Author's transl.) Chung Hua Wai Ko Tsa Chih., *17*:147, 1979.

41. Chino, F., and Tsuruhara, T.: Electron microscopic study on von Recklinghausen's disease. Jpn. J. Med. Sci. Biol., *21*:249, 1968.

42. Codivilla, A.: On the care of congenital pseudarthrosis of the tibia by means of periosteal transplantation. Am. J. Orthop. Surg., *4*:163, 1906.

43. Coleman, S.: Personal communication, 1985.

44. Compere, E. L.: Localized osteitis fibrosa in the newborn and congenital pseudarthrosis. J. Bone Joint Surg., *18*:513, 1936.

45. Crawford, A.: Personal communication, 1984.

46. Delcourt, P.: Considérations sur le traitement de la pseudarthrose congénitale du tibia. Acta Chir. Belg., *52*:801, 1953.

47. Dillehunt, R. B., and LeCocq, J. F.: Pseudarthrosis of the tibia in young children. J.A.M.A., *90*:1615, 1928.

48. Dooley, B. J., Menelaus, M. B., and Paterson, D. C.: Congenital pseudarthrosis and bowing of the fibula. J. Bone Joint Surg., *56-B*:739, 1974.

49. Ducroquet, R.: A propos des pseudarthroses et inflexions congénitales du tibia. Mem. Acad. Chir., *63*:863, 1937.

50. Ducroquet, R., and Cottard,: Pseudarthrose congénitale de jambe. Deformation osseuse de la neurofibromatose. J. Chir., *53*:483, 1939.

51. Duhaime, M., Simoneau, R., Daziond, L., Favreau, J. C., Gauthier, B., and Labelle, P.: Les pseudarthroses congénitales du tibia. Union Med. Can., *101*:1832, 1972.

52. Edvardsen, P.: Resection osteosynthesis and Boyd amputation for congenital pseudarthrosis of the tibia. J. Bone Joint Surg., *55-B*:179, 1973.

53. Eilert, R. E., and Jayakumar, S. S.: Boyd and Syme ankle amputations in children. J. Bone Joint Surg., *58-A*:1138, 1976.

54. Exner, G.: Zur klinik und Pathogenese der angeborenen Verbiegungen und Pseudarthrose des Unterschenkels. Z. Orthop., *82*:50, 1952.

55. Eyre-Brook, A. L., Baily, R. A. J., and Price, C. H. G.: Infantile pseudarthrosis of the tibia; three cases treated successfully by delayed autogenous by-pass graft, with some comments on the causative lesion. J. Bone Joint Surg., *51-B*:604, 1969.

56. Farmer, A. W.: The use of a composite pedicle graft for pseudarthrosis of the tibia. J. Bone Joint Surg., *34-A*:591, 1952.

57. Fevre, M.: Les pseudarthroses de jambes du nouveau-né secondaires aux dystrophies kystiques congénitales. Rev. Chir. Orthop. (Paris), *40*:305, 1954.

58. Fienman, N. L., and Yakovac, W. C.: Neurofibromatosis in childhood. J. Pediatr., *76*:339, 1970.

59. Folschveiller, J., and Jenny, G.: Le traitement de la pseudarthrose infectée grave du tibia par la solidarisation tibiopéronière supérieure et inférieure. Rev. Chir. Orthop., *50*:490, 1964.

60. Fontana, G., and Gallinotto, G.: Considerations on the remote results of the fibular pro-tibia operation in pseudoarthrosis of the tibia. Minerva Med., *58*:4001, 1967.

61. Fraser, W.: Congenital pseudarthrosis of the tibia. J. Bone Joint Surg., *46-B*:167, 1964.

62. Freidenberg, Z. B., and Brighton, C. T.: Bioelectric potentials in bone. J. Bone Joint Surg., *48-A*:915, 1966.

63. Froelich, L.: Kongenitale Verbiegungen und Pseudarthrosen des Unterschenkels. Wert der Periosttransplantationen. Verh. Dtsch. Ges. Orthop. Chir., *9*:270, 1910.

64. Gaenslen, F. J.: Congenital defects of the tibia and fibula. Am. J. Orthop. Surg., *12*:453, 1915.

65. Gilbert, A.: Personal communication, 1985.

66. Gordon, E. J.: Solitary interosseous neurolemmoma of the tibia. Clin. Orthop., *117*:271, 1976.

67. Gossett, J.: La greffe enéclisse (inlay de Chant) dans les pseudarthroses basses du tibia. Mem. Acad. Chir. Paris. *81*:584, 1955.

68. Grassi, E., Rossi, E., and Boidi-Trotti, M.: La pseudoartrosi congenita della tibia (studio clinico-radiologico). Minerva Nipiol., *15*:284, 1965.

69. Green, W. T.: Personal communication, 1960.

70. Green, W. T., and Rudo, N.: Pseudarthrosis and neurofibromatosis. Arch. Surg., *46*:639, 1943.

71. Gui, A.: Studio anatomico in due casi di pseudartrosi congenita della tibia. Arch. Ortop., *57*:393, 1942.

72. Guilleminet, M.: Pseudarthrose congénitale du tibia. Rev. Chir. Orthop., *39*:690, 1953.

73. Guilleminet, M., and Cabanac, J.: Valeur de l'enclouage médullaire dans les formes graves de pseudarthroses congénitales du tibia. Lyon Chir., *54*:373, 1958.

74. Guilleminet, M., and Ricard, R.: Sur le traitement de la pseudarthrose congénitale du tibia. Valeur de la double greffe vissée. Rev. Chir. Orthop., *39*:3, 1953.

75. Guilleminet, M., and Ricard, R.: Pseudarthrose congénitale du tibia et son traitement. Paris, Masson, 1958.

76. Guilleminet, M., Stagnara, P., and Faysse, R.: Résultats du traitement des pseudarthroses congénitales du tibia. Lyon Chir., *46*:848, 1951.

77. Hagen, K. F., and Buncke, H. J.: Treatment of congenital pseudarthrosis of the tibia with free vascularized bone graft. Clin. Orthop., *166*:34, 1982.

78. Hallock, H.: The use of multiple small bone transplants in the treatment of pseudarthrosis of the tibia of congenital origin or following osteotomy for the correction of congenital deformity. J. Bone Joint Surg., *20*:648, 1938.

79. Hardinge, K.: Congenital anterior bowing of the tibia.

The significance of the different types in relation to pseudarthrosis. Ann. R. Coll. Surg., *51*:17, 1972.

80. Hasselmann, W.: Heilung einer angeborenen Tibiapseudarthrose mittels Marknagel und Tibiaspan. Z. Orthop., *80*:93, 1950.

81. Hatzoecher: cited by Camurati; in turn cited by Henderson and Clegg, Proc. Mayo Clin., *16*:769, 1941.

82. Henderson, M. S.: Congenital pseudarthrosis of the tibia. J. Bone Joint Surg., *10*:483, 1928.

83. Henderson, M. S., and Clegg, R. S.: Pseudarthrosis of the tibia: Report of a case. Proc. Mayo Clin., *16*:769, 1941.

84. Herbst, E., and von Satzger, G.: Electrical pulsed current stimulation in five cases of congenital pseudarthrosis of the tibia. *In* Brighton, C. T., Black, J., and Pollack, S. R. (eds.): Electrical Properties of Bone and Cartilage. New York, Grune & Stratton, 1975, p. 639.

85. Hsu, L. C., O'Brien, J. P., Yau, A. C., and Hodgson, A. R.: Valgus deformity of the ankle in children with fibular pseudarthrosis. J. Bone Joint Surg., *56-A*:503, 1974.

86. Huntington, T. W.: Case of bone transference; use of a segment of fibula to supply a defect in the tibia. Ann. Surg., *41*:249, 1905.

86a. Ilizarov, G.: Paper presented at Pediatric Orthopedic International Seminar, San Francisco, 1988.

87. Inglis, K.: The pathology of congenital pseudarthrosis of the tibia. J. Coll. Surg. Austr., *1*:194, 1928.

88. Jacobs, J. E., Kimmelstiel, P., and Thompson, K. R., Jr.: Neurofibromatosis and pseudarthrosis; report of a case. Arch. Surg., *59*:232, 1949.

89. Jacobsen, S. T., Crawford, A. H., Millar, E. A., and Steel, H. H.: The Syme amputation in patients with congenital pseudarthrosis of the tibia. J. Bone Joint Surg., *65*:533, 1983.

90. Johnson, L. C.: Congenital pseudarthrosis, adamantinoma of long bone and intracortical fibrous dysplasia of the tibia. *In* Proc. A.A.O.S., Washington, D.C., Feb., 1972. Abstract in J. Bone Joint Surg., *54-A*:1355, 1972.

91. Jonasch, E.: Die angeborenen Verbiegungen und Pseudarthrosen des Unterschenkels. Arch. Orthop. Unfallchir., *56*:56, 1964.

92. Joveneau, G.: Pseudarthrose de la diaphyse fémorale chez un enfant de quatre ans. Acta Orthop. Belg., *27*:247, 1961.

93. Judet, J., Judet, R., Rigault, P., and Roy-Camille, R.: Traitement des pseudarthroses congénitales de la jambe par décortication, fixateur externe et greffe secondaire de renforcement. Rev. Chir., *54*:503, 1968.

94. King, K. F.: Periosteal pedicle grafting in dogs. J. Bone Joint Surg., *58-B*:117, 1976.

95. Kite, J. H.: Congenital pseudarthrosis of the tibia and fibula. Report of fifteen cases. South. Med. J., *34*:1021, 1941.

96. Knofler, E. W.: Behandlung und Ergebnisse bei angeborenen Unterschenkelpseudarthrosen. Beitr. Orthop. Traumatol., *16*:629, 1969.

97. Kort, J. S., Schink, M. M., Mitchell, S. N., and Bassett, C. A.: Congenital pseudarthrosis of the tibia: Treatment with pulsing electromagnetic fields. Clin. Orthop., *165*:124, 1982.

98. Kullmann, L., and Wouters, H. W.: Modellexperiment der kongenitalen Unterschenkelpseudarthrose. Arch. Orthop. Unfallchir., *73*:55, 1972.

99. Langenskiöld, A.: Pseudarthrosis of the fibula and progressive valgus deformity of the ankle in children: Treatment by fusion of the distal tibial and fibular metaphyses. J. Bone Joint Surg., *49-A*:463, 1967.

100. Langenskiöld, A.: Hahn's operation for pseudarthrosis after osteomyelitis of the tibia in children. A report of three cases. Acta Orthop. Scand., *54*:714, 1983.

101. Lavine, L. S., Lustrin, I., and Shamos, M. H.:

Treatment of congenital pseudarthrosis of the tibia with direct current. Clin. Orthop., *124*:69, 1977.

102. Lawsing, J. F., III, Puglisi, A., Fielding, J. W., and Liebler, W. A.: Congenital pseudarthrosis of the tibia: Successful one stage transposition of the fibula into the distal tibia. Clin. Orthop., *110*:101, 1975.

103. Leung, P. C.: Congenital pseudarthrosis of the tibia. Three cases treated by free vascularized iliac crest graft. Clin. Orthop., *175*:45, 1983.

104. Lindemann, K.: Die Pathogenese der angeborenen Unterschenkelpseudarthrose. Z. Orthop., *74*:256, 1943.

105. Lindemann, K.: L'évaluation de l'implantation de la greffe à la pseudarthrose congénitale du tibia. Rev. Chir. Orthop., *39*:708, 1953.

106. Lindemann, K.: Die angeborenen Deformitäten des Unterschenkels. *In* Hohmann, G. (ed.): Handbuch der Orthopädie. Stuttgart, Thieme, 1961, Vol. IV, Part II, pp. 741–780.

107. Lloyd Roberts, G. C., and Shaw, N. E.: The prevention of pseudarthrosis in congenital kyphosis of the tibia. J. Bone Joint Surg., *51-B*:100, 1969.

108. Lombard, P.: Notes sur la pathogénie des courbures et pseudarthroses congénitales de jambe. Rev. Chir. Orthop., *40*:314, 1954.

109. McBryde, A. M., Jr., and Stelling, F. H.: Infantile pseudarthrosis of the tibia. J. Bone Joint Surg., *54-A*:1354, 1972.

110. McCarthy, R. E.: Amputation for congenital pseudarthrosis of the tibia. Indication and techniques. Clin. Orthop., *166*:21, 1982.

111. McElhannon, F. M., Jr.: Congenital pseudarthrosis of the tibia. South. Med. J., *68*:824, 1975.

112. McElvenny, R. T.: Congenital pseudo-arthrosis of the tibia. Findings in one case and a suggestion as to possible etiology and treatment. Q. Bull. Northwest. Univ. Med. Sch., *23*:413, 1949.

113. McFarland, B.: "Birth fracture" of the tibia. Br. J. Surg., *27*:706, 1939.

114. McFarland, B.: Pseudarthrosis of the tibia in childhood. J. Bone Joint Surg., *33-B*:36, 1951.

115. McKellar, C. C.: Congenital pseudarthrosis of the tibia—treatment by tibial lengthening and corrective osteotomy seven years after successful bone graft. A case report. J. Bone Joint Surg., *55-A*:193, 1973.

116. Madsen, E. T.: Congenital angulations and fractures of the extremities. Acta Orthop. Scand., *25*:242, 1956.

117. Makin, A. S.: Congenital pseudarthrosis of tibia treated by twin grafts. Proc. R. Soc. Med., *38*:71, 1944.

118. Masserman, R. L., Peterson, H. A., and Bianco, A. J., Jr.: Congenital pseudarthrosis of the tibia. A review of the literature and 52 cases from the Mayo Clinic. Clin. Orthop., *99*:140, 1974.

119. Merle d'Aubigne, R., Meary, R., Postel, M. F., Thomine, J.-M.: L'homogreffe en manchon dans le traitement des pseudarthroses congénitales de jambe. Rev. Chir. Orthop., *56*:77, 1970.

120. Milgram, J. E.: Impaling (telescoping) operation for pseudarthrosis of long bones in childhood. Bull. Hosp. Joint Dis., *17*:152, 1956.

121. Moore, B. H.: Some orthopaedic relationships of neurofibromatosis. J. Bone Joint Surg., *23*:109, 1941.

122. Moore, B. H.: Peripheral-nerve changes associated with congenital deformities. J. Bone Joint Surg., *26*:282, 1944.

123. Moore, J. R.: Delayed autogenous bone graft in the treatment of congenital pseudarthrosis. J. Bone Joint Surg., *31-A*:23, 1949.

124. Moore, J. R.: Congenital pseudarthrosis of tibia. A.A.O.S. Instruct. Course Lect., *14*:222, 1957.

125. Morrissy, R. T.: Congenital pseudarthrosis of the tibia. Factors that affect results. Clin. Orthop., *166*:21, 1982.

126. Morrissy, R. T., Riseborough, E. J., and Hall, J. E.:

Congenital pseudarthrosis of the tibia. J. Bone Joint Surg., 63-B:367, 1981.

127. Murray, H. H., and Lovell, W. W.: Congenital pseudarthrosis of the tibia. A long-term follow-up study. Clin. Orthop., 166:14, 1982.

128. Newell, R. L., and Durbin, F. C.: The aetiology of congenital angulation of tubular bones with constriction of the medullary canal and its relationship to congenital pseudarthrosis. J. Bone Joint Surg., 58-B:444, 1976.

129. Nicolato, A., and Zanolla, V.: A case of congenital pseudarthrosis of tubular bones with constriction of the medullary canal, and its relationship to congenital pseudarthrosi. J. Bone Joint Surg., 58-B:444, 1976.

130. Nicoll, E. A.: Editorials and annotations. Infantile pseudarthrosis of the tibia. J. Bone Joint Surg., 51-B:589, 1969.

131. Noguchi, K.: Study on dynamic callus and electric callus. J. Jpn. Orthop. Surg. Soc., 31:641, 1957.

132. Ondrouch, A.: Beitrag zur Behandlung der angeborenen Pseudarthrose des Unterschenkels. Arch. Orthop. Unfallchir., 60:138, 1966.

133. Pagella, P.: La pseudartrosi congenita della tibia. Ital. J. Orthop. Traumatol., 4:47, 1978.

134. Pais, C.: La pseudarthrose congénitale du tibia. Rev. Chir. Orthop., 39:701, 1953.

135. Paterson, D. C., and Simonis, R. B.: Electrical stimulation in the treatment of congenital pseudarthrosis of the tibia. J. Bone Joint Surg., 67-B:454, 1985.

136. Paterson, D. C., Lewis, G. N., and Cass, C. A.: Treatment of delayed union and nonunion with an implanted direct current stimulator. Clin. Orthop., 148:117, 1980.

137. Paterson, D. C., Lewis, G. N., and Cass, C. A.: Treatment of congenital pseudarthrosis of the tibia with direct current stimulation. Clin. Orthop., 148:129, 1980.

138. Paterson, D. C., Hillier, T. M., Carter, R. F., Ludbrook, J., Maxwell, G. M., and Savage, J. P.: Electrical bone-growth stimulation in an experimental model of delayed union. Lancet, 1:278, 1977.

139. Paterson, D. C., Hillier, T. M., Carter, R. F., Ludbrook, J., Maxwell, G. M., and Savage, J. P.: Experimental delayed union of the dog tibia and its use in assessing the effect of an electrical bone growth stimulator. Clin. Orthop., 128:340, 1977.

140. Pho, R. W. H.: Free vascularised fibular transplant for replacement of the lower radius. J. Bone Joint Surg., 61-B:362, 1979.

141. Pho, R. W. H., Levack, B., Satku, K., and Patradul, A.: Free vascularised fibular graft in the treatment of congenital pseudarthrosis of the tibia. J. Bone Joint Surg., 67-B:64, 1985.

142. Pierer, H.: Ein beitrag zur Hahnschen operstion. Monatsschr. Unfallheilkd., 56:202, 1953.

143. Purvis, G. D., and Holder, J. E.: Dual bone graft for congenital pseudarthrosis of the tibia: Variations of technic. South. Med. J., 53:926, 1960.

144. Rajgopal, C., Dhariwal, H. S., Nauth-Misir, T.: Congenital pseudarthrosis of tibia and fibula. Br. J. Clin. Pract., 33:332, 1979.

145. Rathgeb, J. M., Ramsey, P. L., and Cowell, H. R.: Congenital kyphoscoliosis of the tibia. Clin. Orthop., 103:178, 1976.

146. Riseborough, E. J., Morrissy, R. T., Hall, J. E., Bernal, J., and Trott, A. W.: Congenital pseudarthrosis of the tibia: Results in forty patients. J. Bone Joint Surg., 56-A:1312, 1974.

147. Romano, B.: La cura chirurgica della pseudoartrosi congenita della gamba. Bull. Sci. Mediche, 139:332, 1967.

148. Rose, G. K.: Restraint in the treatment of bowed tibia associated with neurofibromatosis. Acta Orthop. Scand., 46:704, 1975.

149. Ruszkowski, Y.: Traitement chirurgical des Pertes de substance du tibia par implantation du péroné. Rev. Chir. Orthop., 51:719, 1965.

150. Sabatini, R., de Peretti, and Gola: Un cas de pseudarthrose congénitale du tibia (neurofibromatose). Pediatrie, 48:523, 1961.

151. Sage, F. P.: Congenital anomalies. In Crenshaw, A.

152. Sane, S., Yunis, E., and Greer, R.: Subperiosteal or cortical cyst and intramedullary neurofibromatosis—uncommon manifestations of neurofibromatosis. A case report. J. Bone Joint Surg., 53-A:1194, 1971.

153. Schier, H.: Zur kongenitalen Tibiapseudarthrose. Z. Orthop., 102:469, 1967.

154. Schmickel, R. D., Heidelberger, K. P., and Poznanski, A. K.: The Campomelique syndrome. J. Pediatr., 82:299, 1973.

155. Scott, C. R.: Congenital pseudarthrosis of the tibia. A.J.R., 42:104, 1939.

156. Seewald, K.: Zur Lokalisation und Behandlung der angeborenen Schienbeinpseudarthrose. Z. Orthop., 96:42, 1962.

157. Semian, D. W., Willis, J. B., and Bowe, K. E.: Congenital fibrous defect of the tibia mimicking fibrous dysplasia. J. Bone Joint Surg., 57-A:854, 1975.

158. Shamos, M. H., Lavine, L. S., and Shamos, M. I.: Piezoelectric effect in bone. Nature, 197:81, 1963.

159. Sharrard, W.: Pediatric Orthopedics and Fractures. 2nd Ed. Oxford, Blackwell, 1979, pp. 466–483.

160. Simonis, R. B., and Paterson, D.: Electric stimulation in the treatment of congenital pseudarthrosis of the tibia. J. Bone Joint Surg., 66-B:283, 1984.

161. Simons, G.: Personal communication, 1985.

162. Skrede, D.: Congenital pseudoarthrosis of the lower leg. J. Oslo City Hosp., 24:177, 1976.

163. Soeur, R.: La pseudarthrose du tibia. Ses causes, son traitement chirurgical. Acta Orthop. Belg., 12:48, 1946.

164. Soeur, R.: Une nouvelle conception du traitement de la pseudarthrose congénitale du tibia. Rev. Orthop., 32:15, 1946.

165. Sofield, H. A.: Congenital pseudarthrosis of the tibia. Clin. Orthop., 76:33, 1971.

166. Sofield, H. A., and Millar, E. A.: Fragmentation, realignment, and intramedullary rod fixation of deformities of the long bones in children. A ten-year appraisal. J. Bone Joint Surg., 41-A:1371, 1959.

167. Sofield, H. A., Page, M. A., and Mead, N. C.: Multiple osteotomies and metal rod fixation for osteogenesis imperfecta. Paper presented at the American Academy of Orthopedic Surgeons, January 1952.

168. Solomon, J. D.: Infantile pseudarthrosis of the tibia. J. Bone Joint Surg., 54-B:203, 1972.

169. Soustelle, J.: A propos des pseudarthroses diaphysaires des membres. Marseille Chir., 5:320, 1953.

170. Sulamaa, M., and Vikki, P.: Congenital pseudarthrosis of the tibia. Acta Orthop. Scand., 33:312, 1963.

171. Sutcliffe, M. L., and Goldberg, A. A.: The treatment of congenital pseudarthrosis of the tibia with pulsating electromagnetic fields. A survey of 52 cases. Clin. Orthop., 166:45, 1982.

172. Syme, J.: Amputation at the ankle joint. London and Edinburgh Month. J. Med. Sci., 3:93, 1843.

173. Taylor, G. I., Buncke, H. J., Jr., Watson, M., and Murray, W.: Vascularised osseous transplantation for reconstruction of the tibia. In Serafin, D., and Buncke, H. J., Jr. (eds.): Microsurgical Composite Tissue Transplantation. St. Louis, Mosby, 1978.

174. Taylor, G. I., Miller, G. D. H., and Ham, F. J.: The free vascularized bone graft: Clinical extension of microvascular techniques. Plast. Reconstr. Surg., 55:533, 1975.

175. Timmermans, G.: La pseudarthrose congénitale de la jambe. Acta Orthop. Belg., 31:865, 1965.

176. Tooms, R. E.: Amputations. In Crenshaw, A. H. (ed.): Campbell's Operative Orthopedics. 5th Ed. St. Louis, Mosby, 1971, p. 852.

177. Tschokanow, K.: Behandlung der angeborenen Tibiapseudarthrose mit der ersten Etappe nach Putti. Beitr. Orthop. Traumatol., *15*:583, 1968.

178. Umber, J. S., Moss, S. W., and Coleman, S. S.: Surgical treatment of congenital pseudarthrosis of the tibia. Clin. Orthop., *166*:28, 1982.

179. Van Nes, C. P.: Congenital pseudarthrosis of the leg. J. Bone Joint Surg., *48-A*:1467, 1966.

180. Vilkki, P.: Preventive treatment of congenital pseudarthrosis of tibia. J. Pediatr. Surg., *12*:91, 1977.

181. Von Satzger, G., and Herbst, E.: Surgical and electrical mode in the treatment of congenital and post-traumatic pseudarthrosis of the tibia. Clin. Orthop., *161*:82, 1981.

182. Wellwood, J. M., Bulmer, J. H., and Graff, D. J. C.: Congenital defects of the tibia in siblings with neurofibromatosis. J. Bone Joint Surg., *53-B*:314, 1971.

183. Weiland, A. J., and Daniel, R. K.: Congenital pseudarthrosis of the tibia: Treatment with vascularized autogenous fibular grafts. A preliminary report. Johns Hopkins Med. J., *147*:89, 1980.

184. Williams, E. R.: Two congenital deformities of the tibia: Congenital angulation and congenital pseudarthrosis. Br. J. Radiol., *16*:371, 1943.

185. Wilson, P. D.: A simple method of two-stage transplantation of the tibia for use in cases of complicated and congenital pseudarthrosis of the tibia. J. Bone Joint Surg., *23*:639, 1941.

186. Wiltse, L. L.: Valgus deformity of the ankle as a sequel to acquired or congenital anomalies of the fibula. J. Bone Joint Surg., *54-A*:595, 1972.

187. Witt, A. N., and Refior, H. J.: Weitere Erfahrungen in der Behandlung des Crus curvatum congenitum und der kongenitalen Unterschenkelpseudarthrose. Arch. Orthop. Unfallchir., *68*:230, 1970.

188. Zippel, H., and Gummel, J.: Zur operativen Behandlung des Crus varum congenitum und der kongenitalen Unterschenkelpseudarthrose. Beitr. Orthop. Traumatol., *20*:193, 1973.

189. Zych, G. A., and Ballard, A.: Congenital band causing pseudarthrosis and impending gangrene of the leg. J. Bone Joint Surg., *65-A*:410, 1983.

CONGENITAL PSEUDARTHROSIS OF THE FIBULA

Congenital pseudarthrosis of the fibula may present in varying grades of severity: (1) as fibular bowing without fibular pseudarthrosis, (2) as fibular pseudarthrosis without ankle deformity, (3) as fibular pseudarthrosis with valgus deformity of the ankle but without late development of tibial pseudarthrosis, or (4) as fibular pseudarthrosis with the late development of pseudarthrosis of the tibia.[4]

Isolated congenital pseudarthrosis of the fibula is very rare; the disorder is often associated with pseudarthrosis of the tibia. When it apparently does occur, it behooves the orthopedic surgeon to scrutinize the tibia carefully to rule out sclerosis of its medullary cavity and incipient pseudarthrosis.

Clinically the condition may remain undetected until valgus deformity of the ankle develops. Radiograms will disclose the narrowed or obliterated medullary cavity, the fracture, and the tapered and sclerotic bone ends of the fibula shaft. The site of pseudarthrosis is almost always in the lowest fourth of the diaphysis.

Treatment

Treatment varies according to the severity of the condition. Bowing of the fibula without pseudarthrosis does not require treatment. Pseudarthrosis of the fibula without valgus deformity of the ankle may be treated either by excision of the pseudarthrosis, bone grafting, and intramedullary fixation, or by fusion of the distal tibial and fibular metaphyses (Langenskiöld procedure).[7, 8] This author recommends fibular-tibial synostosis because the procedure is simple, and the fusion heals rapidly and controls the development of valgus ankle. The operative technique is as follows:

The distal part of the fibular shaft is exposed through a longitudinal incision. The site of pseudarthrosis is exposed, and under image intensifier radiographic control, the level of the distal fibular physis is determined. Next, with an electric burr or small sharp osteotomes, a hole is made on the lateral aspect of the tibia at the site of the attachment of the interosseous membrane. The size of the tibial hole should correspond to the diameter of the fibula, it should be at a level parallel with the upper cut surface of the fibular metaphysis, and in depth it should extend well into cancellous bone of the tibia. Next, a 1- to 2-cm. square of the periosteum above the hole in the tibia is excised. Autogenous bone is then taken from the ilium for the graft; it should be long enough to extend from the lateral surface of the fibula into the cancellous bone of the tibial metaphysis, and its width should correspond to the diameter of the cut surface of the fibula. The iliac bone graft is inserted into the hole in the tibia perpendicular to the long axis of the tibia and extending laterally in close approximation to the upper cut surface of the fibula (Fig. 2–300). The space between the lateral surface of the tibia and the graft is packed with strips of cancellous bone from the ilium. A below-knee cast is applied for a period of three to four months. Full weight-bearing is not permitted for the first two months.

If the valgus deformity of the ankle is severe, supramalleolar osteotomy of the tibia is required to correct it. If the tibia is involved, however, one should not osteotomize it because the consequent development of pseudarthrosis will become a serious problem.

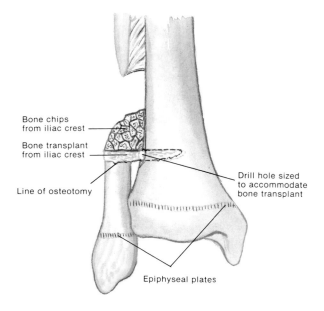

Bone chips
from iliac crest

Bone transplant
from iliac crest

Line of osteotomy

Drill hole sized
to accommodate
bone transplant

Epiphyseal plates

FIGURE 2–300. Diagram illustrating the Langenskiöld technique for treating congenital pseudarthrosis of the fibula by fusion of the distal tibial and fibular metaphyses by iliac bone graft.

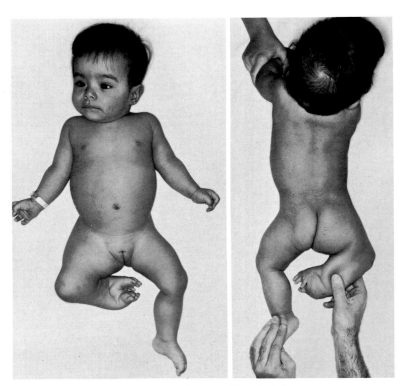

FIGURE 2–301. Duplication of long limb bone.

A one-year-old infant with duplication of the foot and tibia. (Courtesy of Dr. C. Pease.)

References

1. Andersen, K. S.: Congenital pseudarthrosis of the leg: Late results. J. Bone Joint Surg., *58-A*:657, 1976.
2. Boyd, H. B.: Congenital pseudarthrosis: Treatment by dual bone grafts. J. Bone Joint Surg., *23*:497, 1941.
3. Boyd, H. B., and Sage, F. P.: Congenital pseudarthrosis of the tibia. J. Bone Joint Surg., *40-A*:1245, 1958.
4. Dooley, B. J., Menelaus, M. B., and Paterson, D. C.: Congenital pseudarthrosis and bowing of the fibula. J. Bone Joint Surg., *56-B*:739, 1974.
5. Hsu, L. C. S., O'Brien, J. P., Yau, A. C. M. C., and Hodgson, A. R.: Valgus deformity of the ankle in children with fibular pseudarthrosis: Results of treatment by bone-grafting of the fibula. J. Bone Joint Surg., *56-A*:503, 1974.
6. Lambert, K. L.: The weight-bearing function of the fibula: A strain gauge study. J. Bone Joint Surg., *53-A*:507, 1971.
7. Langenskiöld, A.: Pseudarthrosis of the fibula and progressive valgus deformity of the ankle in children: Treatment by fusion of the distal tibial and fibular metaphyses; a review of three cases. J. Bone Joint Surg., *49-A*:463, 1967.
8. Merkel, K. D., and Peterson, H. A.: Isolated congenital pseudarthrosis of the fibula: Report of a case and review of the literature. J. Pediatr. Orthop., *4*:100, 1984.

DUPLICATION OF LONG BONES

Duplication of long bones in the lower limb is rare. An illustrative case is shown in Figure 2–301. The deformities are grotesque, requiring major reconstructive surgery. The accessory parts are excised, and muscle tendon transfers are performed to restore function.

References

1. British Medical Journal: Posterior dichotomy: A three-legged boy. Br. Med. J., *1*:1528, 1898.
2. Carlson, B. M.: Morphogenetic interactions between rotated skin cuffs and underlying stump tissues in regenerating axolotl forelimbs. Dev. Biol., *39*:263, 1974.
3. Cornah, M. S., and Dangerfield, P. H.: Reduplication of the femur. Report of a case. J. Bone Joint Surg., *56-B*:744, 1974.
4. Davis, R. G., and Farmer, A. W.: Mirror hand anomaly. A case presentation. Plast. Reconstr. Surg., *21*:80, 1958.
5. Deboo, S. N.: A three legged person. Med. Bull. Bombay, *11*:339, 1943.
6. Gruneberg, H.: The Pathology of Development. A Study of Inherited Skeletal Disorders in Animals. New York, Wiley & Sons, 1963.
7. Kino, Y.: Morphogenesis of congenital limb defects. Clin. Orthop. Surg. (Japan), *6*:664, 1971.
8. Kusswetter, W., Matzen, K. A., and Baumann, D.: Bifurcation of the distal femur. Acta Orthop. Scand., *47*:648, 1976.
9. Laurin, C. A., and Farmer, A. W.: Congenital absence of ulna. Can. J. Surg., *2*:204, 1959.
10. Norman, W. H.: A child with three lower extremities. J. Bone Joint Surg., *46-A*:1755, 1964.
11. Ogden, J. A.: Ipsilateral femoral bifurcation and tibial hemimelia. A case report. J. Bone Joint Surg., *58-A*:713, 1976.
12. O'Rahilly, R.: Morphological patterns in limb deficiencies and duplications. Am. J. Anat., *89*:135, 1951.
13. Sanguinetti, C., and Unger, F.: La dimelia peroneale. Arch. Putti Chir. Organi Mov., *24*:361, 1969.
14. Smillie, I. S., and Murdoch, J. H.: Man with three legs. J. Bone Joint Surg., *34-B*:630, 1952.
15. Srivastava, K. K., and Garg, L. D.: Reduplication of bones of lower extremity. J. Bone Joint Surg., *53-A*:1445, 1971.
16. Taniguchi, K., Aoki, Y., Kurimoto, H., and Okamura, T.: Baby with a third leg. J. Pediatr. Surg., *10*:143, 1975.
17. Tschumi, P. A.: The growth of the hindlimb bud of Xenopus laevis and its dependence upon the epidermis. J. Anat., *91*:149, 1957.
18. Warkany, J.: Congenital malformations: Notes and comments. Chicago, Year Book, 1971.
19. Weiner, D. S., Greenberg, B., and Shamp, N.: Congenital reduplication of the femur associated with paraxial fibular hemimelia. J. Bone Joint Surg., *60-A*:554, 1978.
20. Zwilling, E., and Hansborough, L. A.: Interaction between limb bud ectoderm and mesoderm in the chick embryo. III. Experiments with polydactylous limbs. J. Exp. Zool., *132*:219, 1956.

Index

Index

Note: Page numbers in *italics* refer to illustrations; page numbers in boldface refer to surgical plates. Page numbers followed by the letter t refer to tables.

Brachymesophalangy, 283
Brachymetacarpalia, 283
Brachymetatarsia, 2633, *2634–2636*, 2637
Brachytelephalangy, 283
Brain, in myelomeningocele, 1778
Brand thumb opposition restoration, 2057, **2068–2069**
Braumann's angle, 3066, *3066*
Breech posture, development of, 2422, *2423*
Breech presentation, in congenital dysplasia of hip, 302–303, *303*
Brevicollis, 128–136. See also *Klippel-Feil syndrome.*
Brown's fibulofemoral arthroplasty, in congenital longitudinal deficiency of tibia, 643, *645*, **646–649**
Brucellar osteomyelitis, 1123–1124
Bryant's traction, in congenital dysplasia of hip, 343, *344*
    in femoral shaft fracture, *3256–3259*, 3256–3261
    modified, in femoral shaft fracture, *3261*, 3261–3262
Buck-Gramcko technique, **262–267**
Buckminister Brown brace, in congenital torticollis, *119*
Bunion, *2626–2628*, 2626–2629
    dorsal, in poliomyelitis, *1945*, *1946–1948*, *1950–1951*
Bursitis, 2181–2182
    infectious or suppurative, 2182
    traumatic, 2181–2182

C

Cadence, 6
Café-au-lait spots, in fibrous dysplasia, 1229
    in neurofibromatosis, 1290, *1290*
Caffey's disease, 817–824. See also *Cortical hyperostosis, infantile.*
Caffey's sign, in Legg-Calvé-Perthes disease, 949
Caisson disease, 689
Calcaneal lateral wedge resection, of Dwyer, in pes cavus, 2700–2701, **2702–2703**
Calcaneal osteotomy, Baker's horizontal, 1703, *1704*
    Dwyer's, 1702–1703
        in talipes equinovarus, 2517, **2518–2519**, 2520–2521
Calcaneocuboid synostosis, 2579
Calcaneofibular tenodesis, in myelomeningocele, 1805, **1806–1807**
Calcaneonavicular coalition, 2601, **2602–2607**, 2608
Calcaneus, fracture of, 3341
    in talipes equinovarus, 2435
    unicameral bone cyst of, 2780, *2786*
Calcification, of intervertebral disc, 2391–2393, *2392*
Calcinosis, of foot, 2780, *2780*
Calcium, vitamin D metabolism and, 897–898
Callotasis, for lengthening of femur, 2896
    for lengthening of tibia, 2896, **2960–2971**
Campanacci syndrome, 1242–1246, *1243–1245*
Campylodactyly, 284–285
    diagnosis of, 284–285, *285*
    disorders associated with, 284t
    etiology of, 284
    treatment of, 285, *286*
Camurati-Engelmann disease, 804–807, *805*
    clinical features of, 804
    differential diagnosis of, 806
    etiology and heredity in, 804
    infantile cortical hyperostosis vs., 806
    pathology in, 804, *805*
    radiography and scintigraphy in, 806
    treatment of, 806–807

Carbenicillin, in septic arthritis, 1424t
Cardiovascular system, in Klippel-Feil syndrome, 131
    in Marfan's syndrome, 832
Carpenter's syndrome, 856
Carpus, centralization over distal ulna of, 199–205, **200–203**
    stabilization of, in Madelung's deformity, 221
Cartilage, articular, nutrition of, 1411
    destruction of, in septic arthritis, 1417–1419
Cartilaginous exostosis, multiple, 1172–1190. See also *Exostosis, multiple.*
Caster cart, in myelomeningocele, 1855, *1855*
Cat-scratch fever, 1133
Cavovarus deformity, in arthrogryposis multiplex congenita, 2099
Cavovarus test, 2681, *2682–2683*
Cavus deformity, in myelomeningocele, *1816*, 1816–1817
Cefotaxime, in septic arthritis, 1424t
Ceftriaxone, in septic arthritis, 1424t
Cefuroxime, in septic arthritis, 1424t
Cellulitis, pyogenic osteomyelitis vs., 1092–1093
    septic arthritis vs., 1422
Cephalothin, in septic arthritis, 1424t
Cerebellar ataxia, dentate, 1980t
    gait in, 26, 1613
    hereditary, 1980t
Cerebellar disorders, differentiation of, 1602t-1603t, 1604
Cerebellar tumor, 1980t
Cerebral cortex, developmental changes in, 42
Cerebral palsy, 1605–1757
    anesthesia in, 70
    arm in, 1717, 1722–1747
        abduction contracture of shoulder in, 1747, *1747*, *1754*
        cosmetic appearance of, 1717, 1722, *1722*
        finger deformities in, 1738–1744
            flexion, 1738–1739, **1740–1743**
            swan-neck, 1739, 1744
                Swanson sublimis tenodesis of proximal interphalangeal joints in, 1739, 1744
        flexion deformity of elbow in, 1746–1747
        flexion deformity of wrist in, *1744–1745*, 1744–1746, **1748–1753**
        function of, 1717
        Green's flexor carpi ulnaris transfer in, 1746, **1748–1753**
        preoperative assessment of, 1717
        pronation contracture of forearm in, 1746
        thumb-in-palm deformity of, 1722–1738
            adductor myotomy of thumb in, 1730, **1732–1733**
            adductor pollicis release in, **1726–1729**, 1730
            bivalved long arm cast in, 1730, *1730*
            brachioradialis transfer in, **1734–1737**
            extensor pollicis longus rerouting in, 1731
            metacarpophalangeal capsulorrhaphy in, 1731, 1738
            opponens splint in, 1724, *1725*
            tendon transfers for thumb motor function in, 1730–1731
            treatment of, 1724–1738
            types of, 1722–1724, *1724*
    classification of, 1605t-1608t, 1605–1608
        American, 1605, 1605t
        Crothers and Paine's, 1606, 1608t
        Ingram and Balf's, 1606, 1608t
        Minear's, 1606, 1607t
        Perlstein's, 1606, 1606t
    clinical features of, 1614–1620
        epilepsy in, 1616